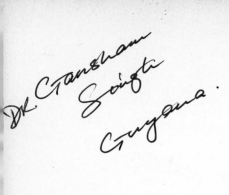

EMERGENCY PEDIATRICS

A Guide to Ambulatory Care

6

EMERGENCY PEDIATRICS
A Guide to Ambulatory Care

Editor

ROGER M. BARKIN, M.D., M.P.H., F.A.A.P., F.A.C.E.P.

Associate Professor of Pediatrics and Surgery,
University of Colorado Health Sciences Center;
Director, Pediatric Emergency Services, Rose Medical Center;
Associate Attending Physician, Department of Emergency Medicine,
Denver General Hospital, Denver, Colorado

Associate Editor

PETER ROSEN, M.D.

Professor of Surgery, University of Colorado
Health Sciences Center; Director, Emergency Medical Services,
Denver Department of Health and Hospitals; Program Director,
Emergency Medicine Residency Combined Program,
Denver General Hospital, St. Anthony Hospital Systems, and
St. Joseph Hospital, Denver, Colorado

SECOND EDITION

With 56 illustrations

The C. V. Mosby Company

ST. LOUIS • WASHINGTON, D.C. • TORONTO   1987

MOSBY

A TRADITION OF PUBLISHING EXCELLENCE

Assistant editor: Ellen Baker Geisel
Project editor: Sylvia B. Kluth
Manuscript editor: Sheila Walker
Book design: Gail Morey Hudson
Production: Florence Fansher

SECOND EDITION

The C.V. Mosby Company
11830 Westline Industrial Drive, St. Louis, Missouri 63146

Library of Congress Cataloging-in-Publication Data

Emergency pediatrics.

    Includes bibliographies and index.
    1. Pediatric emergencies. I. Barkin, Roger M.
II. Rosen, Peter, 1935-   . [DNLM: 1. Emergencies—
in infancy & childhood. 2. Pediatrics.
WS 200 E53]
RJ370.E44 1986   618.92′0025   86-5431
ISBN 0-8016-0479-6

GW/VH/VH 9 8 7 6 5 4 3   0/2B/272

Contributors

GARY K. BELANGER, D.D.S.

Assistant Professor and Chairman, Pediatric Dentistry, Department of Growth and Development, University of Colorado School of Dentistry, Denver, Colorado

PAMELA W. BOURG, R.N., M.S., C.E.N.

Assistant Clinical Professor, University of Colorado Health Sciences Center; Assistant Director of Nursing, Emergency Medical Services and Outpatient Department, Denver General Hospital, Denver, Colorado

STEPHEN V. CANTRILL, M.D.

Attending Staff Physician, Department of Emergency Medicine, Denver General Hospital, Denver, Colorado; Assistant Clinical Professor, Department of Emergency Medicine, Oregon Health Science University, Portland, Oregon

PAUL S. CASAMASSIMO, D.D.S., M.S.

Associate Professor and Chairman, Department of Growth and Development, School of Dentistry, University of Colorado Health Sciences Center; Attending Physician, Dental Medicine, University Hospital, Denver, Colorado

ROGER H. GILLER, M.D.

Assistant Professor of Pediatrics, Department of Pediatrics, University of Iowa College of Medicine, Iowa City, Iowa

WILLIAM V. GOOD, M.D.

Resident, Department of Ophthalmology, University of California at San Francisco, San Francisco, California; Former Assistant Professor of Psychiatry,

University of Colorado Health Sciences Center, Denver, Colorado

BENJAMIN HONIGMAN, M.D.

Assistant Professor of Emergency Medicine, Department of Surgery, University of Colorado Health Sciences Center; Director, Emergency Department, University Hospital, Denver, Colorado

ROBERT C. JORDEN, M.D.

Director, Division of Emergency Services, Department of Medicine, University of Mississippi Hospital, Jackson, Mississippi

KENNETH W. KULIG, M.D.

Assistant Professor of Pediatrics, University of Colorado Health Sciences Center; Director, Clinical Toxicology Training Program, Rocky Mountain Poison Center, Denver General Hospital, Denver, Colorado

RONALD D. LINDZON, M.D.

Lecturer, Department of Medicine, Coordinator, Postgraduate Emergency Medicine Resident Program, University of Toronto; Staff Emergency Physician Toronto General Hospital, Toronto, Ontario, Canada

VINCE J. MARKOVCHICK, M.D.

Assistant Professor of Emergency Medicine, Department of Surgery, University of Colorado Health Sciences Center; Assistant Director, Emergency Medical Services, Department of Emergency Medicine, Denver General Hospital, Denver, Colorado

JOHN A. MARX, M.D.

Associate Professor of Emergency Medicine, Oregon Health Sciences University, Portland, Oregon; Attending Staff Physician, Department of Emergency Services, Denver General Hospital, Denver, Colorado

DOUGLAS V. MAYEDA, M.D.

Associate Staff, Department of Emergency Medicine, Denver General Hospital, Denver, Colorado; Associate Staff, Emergency Department, Penrose Hospital, Colorado Springs, Colorado

JAMES C. MITCHINER, M.D.

Staff Physician, Department of Emergency Medicine, Elmhurst Memorial Hospital, Elmhurst, Illinois

ANTHONY F. PHILLIPS, M.D.

Associate Professor of Pediatrics, Assistant Professor of Obstetrics and Gynecology, The University of Connecticut Health Center, Farmington, Connecticut

PETER T. PONS, M.D.

Assistant Professor of Surgery, Department of Surgery, University of Colorado Health Sciences Center; Associate Director, Emergency Department, University Hospital, Denver, Colorado

BARRY H. RUMACK, M.D.

Professor of Pediatrics, University of Colorado School of Medicine; Director, Rocky Mountain Poison and Drug Center, Denver General Hospital, Denver, Colorado

AILEEN B. SEDMAN, M.D.

Assistant Professor, Department of Pediatrics and Communicable Diseases, University of Michigan Medical Center, Ann Arbor, Michigan

JAMES SPRAGUE, M.D.

Clinical Associate Professor, Department of Ophthalmology, Georgetown University, Washington, D.C.; Staff Physician, Fairfax Hospital, Fairfax, Virginia

REGINALD L. WASHINGTON, M.D.

Assistant Professor of Pediatric Cardiology, Department of Pediatrics, University of Colorado School of Medicine; Director of Pediatric Cardiology, Non-Invasive Laboratories, Department of Pediatric Cardiology, The Children's Hospital, Denver, Colorado

ROCHELLE A. YANOFSKY, M.D.

Assistant Professor, Department of Pediatrics, Division of Hematology and Oncology, University of Alberta Hospital; Pediatric Hematologist-Oncologist, Cross Cancer Institute, Edmonton, Alberta, Canada

GREGORY W. ZOLLER, M.D.

Associate Attending Physician, Department of Emergency Medicine, Denver General Hospital; Director, Emergency Medical Staff, Porter Memorial Hospital, Denver, Colorado

To C. Henry Kempe
a master clinician, teacher, and scientist; a man of vision,
insight, and sensitivity; and a model for those who have cared for
children in the past and will treat them in the future

To Suzanne
who provided support, encouragement, and understanding

To Adam and Michael
who have taught me much of what I know about pediatrics, and

To children
who have been our partners in learning and whose needs will,
I hope, be better served through the use of this book

R. M. B.

Foreword

DR. GANSHAM SINGH GUYANA.

Over the past 36 years, a great number of medical students and some residents have told me something like the following: "I am afraid I cannot handle medicine as a career. Last night I worked in the emergency department, and a desperately ill accident victim was brought in for treatment. My only thought was to flee out the back door, and I was in a panic." I have always replied that I was so pleased to hear that because only people devoid of conscience will run toward such acute disasters with joy; to be scared is to be honest as well as intelligent.

The unprepared student soon acquires experience by working alongside senior role models, nurses, paramedics, and other physicians—learning that team care is essential. All emergencies require more than one set of hands. Practitioners must be well trained and intellectually as well as emotionally prepared to deal with anything that comes through the door. I always urge practicing physicians, residents, and students to "play" at situations where a mother rushes her child to the office or to the emergency department or where an urgent call comes from a ward and the immediate needs for survival must be practiced: an airway established, breathing ensured, and the vascular bed brought back to a capacity to carry oxygen to all organs. The entire team must maintain its competency to maximize each patient's chances. The ability to tell a four-star from a one-star emergency is learned with time.

Often the patient's history is obtained while urgent care for life support is given. It isn't easy to do both at the same time, yet both are required. This is no moment for textbooks or lengthy dissertations; ready access to a broad range of diagnostic and therapeutic information is needed. The basics are crucial and must be learned by heart. Where are vital medications? Where is a working laryngoscope? Who will assist the primary members of the team? What are the most important drug dosages, fluids, and electrolytes? Practice, expertise, organization, and cooperation make the components flow smoothly.

Emergency care is always a bit scary, and it should be! It needs the best kind of quick and broadly based diagnostic thought and action. Yet, regardless of where the emergency is treated—even in the best equipped and trained units—some patients will die. This is always a very bad time for all who have worked so hard to pull a youngster through. Recriminations between parents and relatives abound.

Among the members of the health care team, there are similar frustrations, anger, and sorrow, and the temptation to scapegoat somebody must be avoided at all costs. It is best to lock the door, pick up, clean the dead child, and have the last provisional rites of baptism administered to a Catholic child.* Important too is taking a few minutes to calm down before talking to the parents in a quiet place and with plenty of time.

---

*Note that any person of any faith can administer provisional last rites: "I baptize you in the name of the Father, the Son, and the Holy Spirit. Amen."

The response to "I am sorry we lost your baby" is often disbelief. Properly run emergency departments will already have seen that a supportive relative or a minister is in the waiting room. Relatives usually want to see the child, and they will remember these next moments forever.

Then follows the time of questioning. It is simply bad medicine to blame anyone, tempting though it may be. It is useless to tell a mother that she should have brought in the child 2 hours earlier or that the child's regular doctor should have diagnosed the problem better and sooner, even though that may be true. A devastated family needs compassion and support, wherever it can be found. In my experience, when families have been treated with respect and kindness, permission for diagnostic autopsies is routinely given.

The field of emergency care is continuing to expand rapidly and well. Recent technical advances have made for better survival rates, and greater understanding of physiology has led to new and better medications. Thus emergency medicine has become a new and highly sophisticated specialty. Yet all physicians are expected to perform basic life-support procedures in any setting and, sometimes, without any help or tools.

This book addresses the field of pediatric emergencies in a comprehensive and readily accessible format, focusing on information that is immediately required. It contains these priority items, as well as those many conditions that permit more thought and time. It prepares the conscientious physician, resident, student, and other members of the team to overcome and thus lessen the anxiety that signifies a good conscience while capably performing all that is needed in an outwardly calm manner. In this field, experience allows rapid growth in building the confidence that management will be proficient.

I shall always trust and admire the competent, yet honestly frightened, practitioner.

The late **C. Henry Kempe, M.D.** (1922-1984)

Former Professor of Pediatrics and Microbiology, University of Colorado Health Sciences Center, Denver, Colorado

Preface

The emergently ill child presents the clinician with a necessity for immediate action. Access to a broad range of diagnostic and therapeutic data is needed before making clinical judgments. This book deals with that need and has evolved over many years of practicing pediatrics and emergency medicine. Representing the combined efforts of pediatricians and emergency medicine physicians, it is designed to bring together in an accessible outline format that which is immediately required for the care of the acutely ill child by the health care provider, whether that individual be pediatrician, emergency physician, family practitioner, nurse practitioner, or student of medicine. *Emergency Pediatrics* is a resource for the clinician to consult, analyze, alter, and add to as experience dictates but certainly not to leave on the bookshelf for leisure reading.

Although the basic organization of the book remains unchanged, this second edition incorporates many of the suggestions of readers and reflects the rapid expansion of available pharmacologic agents. Furthermore, the scope of treatment has expanded as emergency departments increasingly become community clinics for children in many settings; the new material accounts for these factors. In updating this book and expanding its coverage, we hope to be even more responsive to those in the "front lines."

The initial sections emphasize both nontraumatic and traumatic conditions that are life threatening, presenting strategies and diagnostic considerations crucial to stabilization. Resuscitation of the newborn and the young child are prominently covered.

To provide a consistent approach to the patient, information throughout this book is structured into diagnostic categories. Alphabetic order is maintained when appropriate. Differentials are encompassed within the mnemonic categories of *i*nfection/*i*nflammation, *n*eoplasms, *d*egenerative/*d*eficiency, *i*ntoxication, *c*ongenital, *a*utoimmune/*a*llergy, *t*rauma, *i*ntrapsychic, *v*ascular, and *e*ndocrine (INDICATIVE). Extensive use of tables throughout the book facilitates access to material. In these tables, commonly encountered conditions are set in boldface type for ease of identification.

The latter part of the book, which focuses on diagnostic entities, is organized as a systems approach to provide a comprehensive resource for diagnostic and management data on the vast majority of children's problems seen at any ambulatory facility. Specific attention is given to parental education to encourage appropriate follow-up, counseling, and preventive medicine. Whenever possible, instructions should be given to the individual responsible for providing ongoing care and observation. For easy access, parental instruction sheets are included both as an Appendix and in the relevant sections of the text. Other Appendixes consist of procedures, reference standards, and a formulary. All are intended to expedite patient care and provide a data base for the "competent, yet honestly frightened, practitioner."

Children present a unique challenge and a rare opportunity to the health care professional. Medical and traumatic illnesses tend to progress rapidly in the pediatric patient, but the vast majority are treatable with appropriate and timely health care and may be expected to leave the child without sequelae and with a full life ahead.

The child is often frightened, and the history may be obtainable only from parents. Further, the history rarely provides specific data on which to focus a diagnostic and therapeutic plan. Frustrations often are encountered in gaining cooperation during the course of a physical examination or necessary tests and procedures.

The clinician's anxiety is often greater if experience with children is limited, and the threat to life is often viewed as more significant. The purpose of this book is to assist the clinician in synthesizing the many data sources and reaching a good clinical judgment. Perhaps more than in any other area of medicine, when the data base conflicts with the clinical assessment, the clinician must go with judgment and gestalt. For those who lack confidence, it is easy to endow laboratory numbers with infallibility and ignore pertinent clinical findings.

Children's dependency on their familial environment compels the practitioner to be particularly sensitive to the concerns, fears, anxieties, and grief of families whose youngsters are experiencing major illness. Children are constantly looking for support from parents, who simultaneously are seeking small reassurances from a child, such as an infrequent smile or nod. This dependency is exaggerated during illness and must be recognized. It requires careful nurturing and support in moments of stress because, on occasion, these relationships break down.

Emergency Pediatrics is designed to help clinicians who care for children combine experience, reason, and an appropriate data base in making better clinical judgments. This synthesis must form the basis for our care for children.

Roger M. Barkin
Peter Rosen

Acknowledgments

A book such as this is the product of the medical, nursing, and administrative staffs of the many great institutions in which we have had the pleasure to serve in the last two decades. It must necessarily be the synthesis of many individuals' knowledge, experience, concerns, and sensitivities toward patient care in general and the child in particular.

We are grateful to the members of the Departments of Pediatrics and Surgery at the University of Colorado Health Sciences Center and the Department of Emergency Medical Services of the Denver Department of Health and Hospitals for their ongoing support during the development of this book. Beyond the numerous authors who have generously contributed chapters, special thanks go to Drs. Allen Adenoff, John Brooks, Henry Cooper, Alden Harken, Ronald Gotlin, Arnold Silverman, and William Weston. Marjorie Leggitt did the superb illustrations.

Karen Berger, Ellen Baker Geisel, and Sylvia Kluth's unending support and frequent reminders and hints made our effort a pleasure throughout the process of conception to completion.

We would like also to thank our readers, who we hope will take this book with them to the front lines and use it with expertise and confidence in the care of the pediatric patients to whom all our efforts are dedicated.

NOTE: The indications for and dosages of medications recommended conform to practices at the present time. References to specific products are incorporated to serve only as guidelines; they are not meant to exclude a practitioner's choice of other, comparable drugs. Many oral medications may be given with more scheduling flexibility than implied by the specific time intervals noted. Individual drug sensitivity and allergies must be considered in drug selection. Adult doses are provided as a gauge of the maximum dose commonly used.

Every attempt has been made to ensure accuracy and appropriateness. New investigations and broader experience may alter present dosage schedules, and it is recommended that the package insert for each drug be consulted before administration. Often there is limited experience with established drugs for neonates and young children. Furthermore, new drugs may be introduced, and indications for use may change. This rapid evolution is particularly noticeable in the use of antibiotics and cardiopulmonary resuscitation. The clinician is encouraged to maintain expertise concerning appropriate medications for specific conditions.

Contents

INITIAL ASSESSMENT

1 Triage

The expansion of emergency services is a response to a growing demand for accessible, efficient, and superior health care facilities,* and the variety of patients treated on an emergency basis reflects this growth. Fewer than 2% of pediatric patients require admission, emphasizing the noncritical nature of most encounters. Many parents with private health care resources have been frustrated in their attempts to schedule an appointment, and they demand immediate attention to relieve their children's discomfort. Others prefer the anonymity of the emergency facility and use it as their primary source of health care, whereas a significant number of patients have been directed to the emergency facility by health care professionals.

Increased knowledge of the spectrum of illness has intensified the necessity of developing mechanisms to rapidly identify children with life-threatening conditions, while providing expeditious care to less seriously ill patients to meet their immediate needs and provide ongoing care.

---

*Hereafter referred to as the emergency department (ED).

Many approaches to triage have been used. Both nursing and nonprofessional systems have been developed, and they must be modified and restructured for individual patient care settings. Tables 1-1 and 1-2 provide a foundation for triage and effective screening that may serve as a basis for formalization of pediatric triage protocols.

REFERENCES

Fifield, G.C., Magnuson, C., Carr, W.P., and Deinard, A.S.: Pediatric emergency care in a metropolitan area, J. Emerg. Med. 1:495, 1984.

Halperin, R., Meyers, A.R., and Alpert, J.J.: Utilization of pediatric emergency services: a critical review, Pediatr. Clin. North Am. 26:747, 1979.

Hilker, T.L.: Nonemergency visits to a pediatric emergency department, J.A.C.E.P. 7:3, 1978.

Russo, R.M., Gururaj, V.J., Bunye, A.S., et al. Triage abilities of nurse practitioner versus pediatrician, Am. J. Dis. Child. 129:673, 1975.

Sacchetti, A., Carraccio, C., Warden, T., and Gazak, S.: Community hospital management of pediatric emergencies: implications for pediatric emergency medical services, Am. J. Emerg. Med. 4:10, 1986.

Wilson, F.P., Wilson, L.O., Butler, A.B., et al.: Algorithm-directed triage of pediatric patients, JAMA 243:1528, 1980.

CHAPTER 1

TABLE 1-1. Major pediatric triage categories

Emergent				Urgent*
Abnormal vital signs				**Abuse, child**
Age	BP (sys)	Pulse	Resp	**Abuse, sexual**
0-2 yr	<60	<80	<10 or >40	**Acute symptoms in child <2-3 mo**
2-5 yr	<70	<60	<10 or >30	**Behavioral alteration**
>5 yr	<90	<50	<5 or >25	**Bite, poisonous snake**
Respirations				**Bleeding, moderate**
Irregular				**Dehydration**
Apneic				**Drowning (near)**
Labored				**Eye: alkali, acid, or chemical burn**
Pulse				**Fever ≥40° C**
Irregular				**GI hemorrhage**
Dysrhythmic				**Headache: acute and severe**
Coma				**Hypertension**
Cyanosis				**Hyperthermia**
Status epilepticus				**Hypothermia**
Multiple or major trauma				**Neck pain or stiffness**
Head				**Pain: acute and severe**
Loss of consciousness				**Poisoning**
Altered mental status				**Rash** (isolate patient)
Changing neurologic or asymmetric neurologic findings				**SIDS** (near)
CSF leak				
Depressed fracture				
Neck or spinal injury				
Chest				
Abdomen				
Orthopedic				
Two or more long bone fractures				
Pelvic fracture				
Potential neurovascular compromise				
Amputation				
Major burn				
Bleeding: acute and significant				

If none of these emergent or urgent conditions are present, the patient should be appropriately screened and treated according to normal facility flow patterns unless there is a complicating condition. Repeat visits or very anxious parents may require that the visit be categorized as urgent.

*May be emergent, depending on patient's condition.

TABLE 1-2. Initial nursing assessment: pediatric patients

Condition	Temp	Resp	Pulse	BP	CBC	UA	Other	Parent instruction sheet	Comments
Abdominal pain	+		±	±0	±	+	±Gravindex		
Anemia					+				Do reticulocyte count, assess diet
Asthma	+	+	+	+				Yes	Assess medications
Burn	+	+	+	+	±	+	±Electrolytes	Yes	Notify MD if >5%
Child abuse				+			Growth parameters		Reassure, observe
Communicable disease	+	+	+						Isolate patient
Cough	+	+						Yes	
Croup	+	+						Yes	Notify MD
Diabetic ketoacidosis	+	+	+	+0		+	Glucose,* acetone		±IV
Diarrhea	+	+	+	±0	±	+	±Electrolytes	Yes	Assess hydration
Dysuria (painful urination)	+			+		+ and urine culture		Yes	
Earache	+							Yes	
Eye infection	+	+						Yes	
Eye injury									Screen vision
Fever <3 mo old	+	+	+			+		Yes	Notify MD
>3 mo old	+	+	+			+		Yes	±Antipyretics
Head injury		+	+	+				Yes	Do brief neuro
Headache	+			+					Do brief neuro, ±vision screen
Ingestion		+	+	+			Toxicology screen		Obtain history, do neuro, ±ipecac, prevention talk
Laceration			+	±0				Yes	Clean
Nosebleed			+	±0	±			Yes	Apply pressure
Rash	+								±Isolate patient
Seizure	+	+	+	+			Glucose*		Give O₂, maintain airway, ±IV, ±antipyretics, do neuro
Sore throat	+	+					±Throat culture	Yes	
Sprain/fracture			±	±0			±x-ray	Yes	
Vaginal bleeding		+	+	+0	+		Gravindex		
Vomiting	+	+	+	±0	±	+	±Electrolytes	Yes	Assess hydration

+, Perform procedure; ±, perform if indicated by patient's condition; 0, obtain orthostatic BP if appropriate.
*May be performed initially by bedside techniques (Dextrostix or Chemstrip).

INITIAL NURSING ASSESSMENT: PEDIATRIC PATIENTS

Determine on all patients:

1. Age
2. Chief complaint
3. Previous medical history
4. Weight
5. Medications
6. Allergies
7. Immunizations: Identify any deficiencies, and encourage parent to make health maintenance appointment at usual health care facility.
8. Source of routine care

NOTE:

a. Vital signs and laboratory tests must be individualized for each patient.
b. If abnormalities in pulse, respiration, or blood pressure are recorded, notify MD.
c. Antipyretics should be initiated in children with temperatures above 39° C if none have been given in last 4-6 hr (e.g., acetaminophen 10-15 mg/kg/dose PO).
d. Any patient seen at a health care facility earlier in the day and brought back in a few hours is a source of concern. Notify MD.
e. Document concerns about parenting and home environment.

---

2 The nurse's role

PAMELA W. BOURG

In many institutions where emergently ill children are treated, the nurse is the first professional to encounter the sick or injured child. The responsibility of sorting out or "triaging" the sick child from the well child falls initially on the nurse, unless an effective prehospitalization system has initiated this process. The nurse must act on observations and assessments and thus plays a pivotal role in this initial stage.

The ED nurse must look beyond just taking vital signs. The "typical" pediatric patient often arrives with nonspecific and vague complaints, and the nurse must develop the skills to identify children with life-threatening and high-risk problems. Rapid deterioration is common, and early intervention is crucial.

The professional nurse is the hub of the wheel that provides continuity and consistency. The physician relies on the nurse to screen valid information and to initiate therapy in emergencies. There must be a close relationship between nurses and physicians, with both functioning independently and interdependently.

The nurse brings to the health care team a broad psychosocial base, often facilitating the interaction with children and families. Unique sensitivities are important. The child is responding to separation anxiety and fear of pain. The parents may experience a sense of guilt, which may decrease their coping skills and require both the parents and child to be treated as patients. Furthermore, the nurse may assist the family in understanding emergency medical services, emphasizing appropriate use patterns, and preparing the child and family for procedures.

The emergency pediatric patient constitutes a small percentage of ED visits. Protocols facilitate patient management in defining these emergent problems, outlining screening criteria for common complaints, and serving as guidelines for staff. These ensure that each patient's needs are met and that communication among staff members in the various services is maximized.

Staff expertise is of course essential. The responsibility for achieving high-quality care is the dual responsibility of the nursing leader and individual staff nurse. Knowledge and skill must be maintained through chart reviews, direct observation, peer review, continuing education, and the availability of readily accessible management information.

Communication is vital in facilitating the efforts of all members of the health care team. It provides the basis for team functioning and interactions. If problems develop, direct empathic confrontation is appropriate. Emergency care is stressful enough without the additional stress of ongoing interpersonal conflicts.

A coordinated team effort is paramount to an effective, efficient, and responsive health care delivery system. The emergency nurse facilitates this process, and within an environment of sharing, communication, and trust, patient care can be optimally delivered.

CHAPTER 2

REFERENCES

Anderson, D., and Cosgrift, J.: The practice of emergency nursing, Philadelphia, 1975, J.B. Lippincott Co.

Hansen, B., and Evans, M.: Preparing a child for procedures, Matern. Child. Nurs. J. **6:**392, 1981.

Hawley, D.D.: Postoperative pain in children: misconceptions, descriptions, and interventions, Pediatr. Nurs. **10:**20, 1984.

McCaffery, M.: Nursing management of the patient with pain, Philadelphia, 1972, J.B. Lippincott Co.

3 Transport of the pediatric patient

ALERT: Do not decrease the intensity of resuscitation and stabilization efforts once transport has been arranged. Aggressive medical management can be lifesaving throughout this period and should not be postponed until arrival at the receiving facility.

A parent often brings a child to an institution that can provide adequate stabilization but that may lack personnel and equipment to deal with the acute or long-term medical problems of the child beyond immediate stabilization. Transfer becomes a necessity.

Before transport can be considered, resuscitation must be initiated and immediate therapy instituted. The airway requires stabilization, and adequate ventilation must be ensured, often through administration of oxygen and active airway management. An intravenous line (or lines) should be started to permit fluid resuscitation and administration of life-saving medications.

An urgent evaluation is appropriate. The physical examination should be completed, baseline laboratory values obtained, and x-ray tests performed as indicated by the presenting medical or traumatic condition. Early pharmacologic therapy, including antibiotics, anticonvulsants, beta-adrenergic agents, and bronchodilators, should be initiated as necessary. Traumatic injuries may require surgical, neurosurgical, or orthopedic intervention before transport.

Once rapid stabilization has been achieved, the physician must carefully analyze facilities that can adequately care for the child from the perspective of personnel, equipment, and distance. Special needs such as dialysis, intensive care, or cardiac catheterization programs should be considered. The institution selected should be contacted and transport discussed and arranged. It is imperative that communication at this time be adequate between physician and nursing staffs of the two hospitals to ensure a smooth transfer.

The mechanism of transfer should be a joint decision of the referring and receiving institutions, focusing on equipment, speed, distance, and on the level of expertise of medical personnel required to care for the child. The concept of "pick up and run" is usually not appropriate with the current sophistication of air and ground transport systems. Once the decision is made to transport, arrangements should be expedited to permit a rapid transfer of the patient and parents to the receiving institution.

Charts, x-ray films, laboratory results, and past records should be duplicated and readied for transport with the patient.

Parents and patients should be involved throughout the resuscitation and stabilization processes to assist them to feel comfortable with the transfer and understand its benefits.

II ADVANCED CARDIAC LIFE SUPPORT

4 Cardiopulmonary arrest

ALERT: Cardiopulmonary arrest in children is commonly respiratory in origin, emphasizing the importance of stabilization of the airway, breathing, and then circulation (the ABCs). The coordinated effort of a team of professionals is required for optimal care.

The outcome of cardiopulmonary arrests in hospitalized pediatric patients, when contrasted with older patients, is reassuring. In one center with a cardiac arrest team, 78% of patients had a return of cardiac function. Of those surviving the initial episode, 87% were alive at 24 hr and 68% after 5 days; 47% left the intensive care unit, and 88% of those who were followed had no sequelae. Out-of-hospital cardiac arrests in patients under 18 yr are most commonly a result of sudden infant death syndrome (SIDS), drowning, and respiratory arrest, and they occur most commonly in children under 1 yr of age. Only 7%-29% of patients with prehospital or ED cardiac arrests were discharged alive.

ETIOLOGY

Cardiopulmonary arrest in the pediatric age-group is primarily respiratory in origin, stemming from obstruction and hypoxia, secondarily leading to cardiac arrest. Hypoxia may be acute or chronic, resulting from either an acquired or underlying disease. Respiratory arrest and hypoxia almost always precede cardiac standstill. The precipitating causes are often preventable and identifiable before such catastrophic events:

1. Respiratory disease (Chapters 20 and 84)
   a. Upper airway obstruction: croup, epiglottitis, foreign body, suffocation, strangulation, and trauma
   b. Lower airway disease: pneumonia, asthma, bronchiolitis, foreign body aspiration, near-drowning, smoke inhalation, and pulmonary edema
2. Infection: sepsis and meningitis
3. Intoxication: narcotic depressants, sedatives, and antidysrhythmics (Chapter 54)
4. Cardiac disorders: congenital heart disease, myocarditis, pericarditis, and dysrhythmias, often associated with congestive heart failure (CHF) and pulmonary edema
5. Shock: cardiogenic, hypovolemic, or distributive (Chapter 5)
6. CNS: meningitis, encephalitis, head trauma, anoxia, and other causes of hypoventilation (Chapter 81)
7. Trauma/environment: multiple organ failure, child abuse, hypothermia or hyperthermia, and near-drowning
8. Metabolic: hypoglycemia, hypocalcemia, and hyperkalemia
9. Near–sudden infant death syndrome (SIDS) (Chapter 22)

TEAM APPROACH

The management of cardiorespiratory arrest in children requires the combined efforts of a team of professionals. The team captain must be immediately identifiable and provide direction, expertise, and coordination in a precise way. This individual must be responsible for ensuring that everything gets done through delegating responsibility rather than singlehandedly assuming all duties. Beyond dealing with the immediate logistics of procedures and medication and monitoring their effects, the leader must also be able to delineate issues that are crucial to the outcome and that may alter management.

1. Etiology
   a. What caused the arrest?
   b. Why is the patient in shock (hypovolemic, distributive, or cardiogenic)?
   c. Why are we not making progress (e.g., cardiac tamponade, pneumothorax, electromechanical dissociation, electrolyte or acid-base disturbance, inadequate ventilation, or coagulopathy)?
2. Time
   a. How long have we been treating the patient?
   b. How much time (including time before arrival in the ED) has elapsed since initiating cardiopulmonary resuscitation (CPR), and how long was the patient in arrest before CPR was begun?
3. End point. When do we stop, and what criteria do we have for stopping?
4. Evaluation
   a. Can we learn about our performance from this resuscitation?
   b. How can we improve techniques, equipment, personnel training, and team functioning?

ADVANCED LIFE SUPPORT (Fig. 4-1)

The principles of basic life support for the child parallel those evolved for adults. The importance of (A) stabilizing the airway and (B) establishing adequate breathing and (C) circulation cannot be overemphasized. Basic cardiopulmonary resuscitation, employing the ABC's, should be interrupted only for defibrillation or intubation. However, the logistics vary.

1. Establish unresponsiveness or respiratory difficulty. Gently shake patient who, if conscious, should display motor activity. Check carotid or femoral pulse.
2. Call for help.
3. Position the patient for basic life support without subjecting to further injury.

Airway

Patency should be established by one of several techniques, once it is determined that the patient is unconscious or having respiratory difficulty. Options are restricted if there is a question of neck trauma.

1. Lift the occiput slightly off the bed or flat surface by placing a towel roll or hand under the occiput (sniffing position).
2. Tilt head and lift chin. With one hand under the neck and the other on the forehead, lift the neck slightly and push the head back with gentle pressure on the forehead. Maintain extension of the head by pressure on the forehead while using the tips of the fingers of the hand that had been under the neck to lift the bony part of the jaw near the chin forward.

The following adjuncts to airway management may be used:

1. Oxygen: administered by hood, mask, or cannula: 3-6 L/min by mask or cannula produces a forced inspiratory oxygen (FIo_2) of 40%-50%. To get higher oxygen (O_2) concentrations, a mask with reservoir is required (100% or nonrebreathing bag).
2. Oropharyngeal airway: a semicircular-shaped apparatus of plastic curved to fit over the back of the tongue and inserted into the lower posterior pharynx. It is introduced into the mouth backward and rotated as it approaches the posterior wall of the pharynx near the back of the tongue (poorly tolerated in conscious patients).

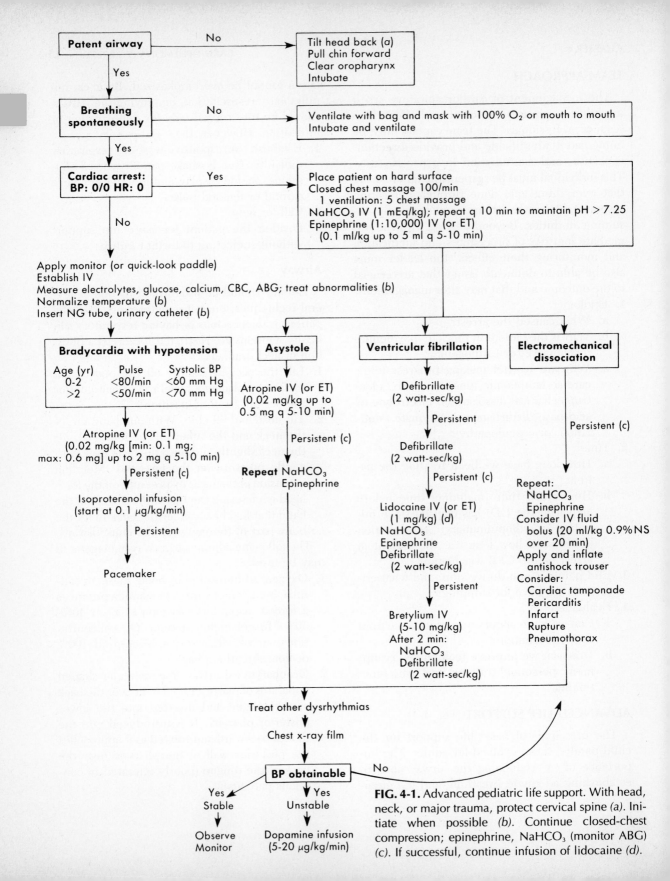

FIG. 4-1. Advanced pediatric life support. With head, neck, or major trauma, protect cervical spine *(a)*. Initiate when possible *(b)*. Continue closed-chest compression; epinephrine, NaHCO₃ (monitor ABG) *(c)*. If successful, continue infusion of lidocaine *(d)*.

3. Nasopharyngeal airway: a soft rubber or plastic tube inserted into the nose close to the midline along the floor of the nostril and into the posterior pharynx behind the tongue (tolerated fairly well in conscious patients).
4. Endotracheal (ET) intubation: provides and protects a stable airway for more efficient ventilation. The size of the ET tube varies with the age and size of the child but may be estimated by selecting a tube that approximates the diameter of the patient's little finger. An estimate also may be made by adding 16 to the child's age (up to 16 yr) and dividing this total by 4. Below the age of 7 or 8 yr, uncuffed tubes are used; cuffed tubes are used in older children. Cuffed tubes must be treated as if they were 0.5 mm larger in size (e.g., 6.0 cuffed = 6.5 mm uncuffed tube). Cole tubes with the tapered end should be avoided. Although patient-to-patient variability exists, the following guidelines may be useful in estimating the correct tube size (Appendix C-2):

Newborn	2.5-3.5 mm	4-5 yr	5.0-6.0 mm
1 mo	3.5 mm	6-8 yr	6.0-6.5 mm
12 mo	4.0 mm	10-12 yr	7.0 mm
2-3 yr	4.5 mm	14 yr	7.5-8.5 mm

   a. Prepare by checking the laryngoscope to ensure adequate functioning and light source. Be certain that suction is available. In the newborn, a DeLee trap suction may be helpful. If a stylet is used, it should not protrude beyond the tip of the ET tube. Lighted stylets are available.
   b. Oxygenate patient and attach heart monitor. Position patient into sniffing position.
   c. Visualize the esophagus, epiglottis, and cords. Laryngeal pressure may be helpful.
   d. Whether orally or nasotracheally intubating the patient, watch the tube pass through the cords, and pass it 1-2 cm beyond.
   e. If the patient becomes bradycardic or cyanotic, abort the procedure, administer oxygen, and ventilate. Start again once signs have stabilized.
   f. Check the position of the tube by listening on both sides of upper chest and stomach. Make sure the tube is not in the right stem bronchus or esophagus. Confirm by x-ray film. The tip should be at T2-T3 vertebral level or at the level of the lower edge of the medial aspect of the clavicle.
   g. Stabilize the tube with adhesive tape or other device. The skin to which adhesive tape is to be affixed should be cleansed and dried, followed by an application of tincture of benzoin.
5. Cricothyroidotomy is indicated as a temporizing measure in children over 3 yr when acute upper airway obstruction cannot otherwise be relieved. It is, however, rarely needed.
6. If unable to ventilate on an emergent basis with intubation, bag and mask, or cricothyroidotomy, a 14-gauge catheter over the needle may be inserted into the cricothyroid membrane. The adapter from a 3 mm nasotracheal or ET tube may be inserted into the Luer adapter of the catheter for application of oxygen and positive pressure for a limited period of time.
7. Patients with pure respiratory arrests unassociated with trauma often respond rapidly to bag and mask or mouth to mouth (mouth to mouth and nose) ventilation. However, if there is no response within 60 sec, intubation should be considered. Respiratory arrests that are complicated by such findings as cyanosis and hypotension usually require intubation.
8. Prophylactic intubation of nontraumatized patients in the ED setting is rarely indicated because of concern about depression of respirations, secondary to pharmacologic management of such diseases as seizures with diazepam (Valium) or phenobarbital and agitation (sedatives).
9. Although, ultimately, judgment becomes the

prime determinant of a patient's need for intubation, each situation must be individualized to consider the patient's condition, progression of disease, potential therapeutic maneuvers, personnel, and equipment availability.

Breathing

Breathing is demonstrated by movement of the chest and abdomen with ventilation, by feeling air moving through the mouth, or by hearing noise during expiration.

1. If the patient is a nonbreathing infant, cover both the mouth and the nose (mouth to nose and mouth), and establish a seal. If the child is too large, cover the mouth (mouth to mouth) of the child while pinching the nose.
2. Initially, give two quick breaths to check for airway obstruction. If air enters freely and the chest rises, proceed to check the pulse while maintaining ventilation. If there is no movement, an obstruction may be present.

   NOTE: Airway obstruction can be caused by a foreign body or an infection such as croup or epiglottitis. If a foreign body is suspected, relieve by a series of manual thrusts without the use of a finger sweep (p. 600).

3. Limit ventilation to the amount of air needed to cause the chest to rise (excessive volumes exacerbate gastric distention and increase the risk of pneumothorax).
4. Use a self-inflating resuscitation bag whenever possible, optimally with a pop-off valve or in-line manometer. A gas reservoir increases the concentration of oxygen delivered (nonrebreathing bag). The volume of a bag for a newborn should be no larger than 300 ml. Bags are available, with appropriate masks, in infant, child, and adult sizes.

Circulation

Circulation must be assessed by checking brachial, femoral, or carotid pulses. All patients should be monitored if possible.

1. External chest compression should be initiated if there is no effective pulse. Compression of the sternum should be maintained for 50% of each cycle. Interposed abdominal compression combined with closed chest compression may improve efficacy but has not been adequately studied. Pulse and blood pressure should be monitored during compression. Children over 1 yr of age require a hard surface. The following is recommended:

	Age-group		
	< 1 yr	1-8 yr	> 8 yr
Compression			
Site	Midsternum*	Lower third	Lower third
Mechanism	Two hands or two fingers encircle chest	Heel of hand	Two hands
Depth (in)	½-1	1-1½	1½-2
Rate/min	100	80-100	80-100
Cardiac: ventilatory ratio	5:1	5:1	5:1

*Draw an imaginary line between the nipples and compress below.

2. Intravenous cannulation is achieved by a variety of peripheral modalities; most common are the butterfly or scalp vein–type needle or the catheter over the needle. Although any vein may be used, those that should be remembered in the acute situation include the saphenous, femoral, and external jugular veins. The size and type of catheter depend on the clinician's level of comfort and the availability of sites. If access if difficult, a cutdown should be done early in the resuscitation (p. 628).

3. Atropine, epinephrine, lidocaine, and naloxone also may be administered by ET tube. A higher than standard dose of medication may be required.

4. Recently, in extraordinary circumstances, intraosseous infusion of crystalloid has been used successfully. An 18-gauge spinal or bone marrow needle is inserted into the anterior tibia (midline flat surface of the tibia) 2-3 cm below the tibial tuberosity. With aseptic technique the needle is inserted perpendicular to the skin or 60 degrees inferior to it. The needle is in marrow when the following conditions occur: a lack of resistance on passing through the cortex, the needle stands straight up without support, bone marrow can be aspirated with a syringe, and infusion flows smoothly (p. 629). The safety of infusion of hypertonic or strongly alkaline solutions has not been established.

5. Central venous catheters, preferably inserted into the internal jugular, may be used by the experienced practitioner. The middle approach is preferred but still carries a risk of pneumothorax. Often a small guide needle is used to locate the internal jugular before insertion of the larger catheter. The external jugular with a guide-wire technique also may be used (p. 630).

6. If there is any question of hypovolemia, a rapid infusion of normal saline or lactated Ringer's solution at 20 ml/kg over 20-30 min should be given. If there is no response and patient is not hypovolemic, dopamine 5-20 μg/kg/min IV should be initiated and a rapid evaluation for shock begun (Chapter 5).

Essential medications and measures

First-line drugs are given to virtually all patients who suffer a cardiopulmonary arrest and who do not respond to relief of airway obstruction and ventilatory assistance:

1. Oxygen
2. Epinephrine: (1 : 10,000) : 0.1 ml/kg/dose (maximum: 5 ml) q 2-3 min IV, ET
3. Bicarbonate: 1 mEq/kg/dose q 10 min IV, as indicated by arterial blood gases

These are outlined in Fig. 4-1 and Table 4-1.

Monitoring of blood pressure, pulse, and rhythm must be constant throughout the resuscitation to ensure that therapeutic intervention is appropriate. Additional steps include treatment of:

1. Electromechanical dissociation (EMD). The role of calcium blockers in cerebral resuscitation is under investigation. Calcium salts may not be beneficial in EMD.
2. Dysrhythmias (Chapter 6)
3. Seizure (Chapter 21)
4. Malignant hypertension (Chapter 18)
5. Increased intracranial pressure (Chapter 57)
6. Congestive heart failure (Chapter 16)

Ancillary data

Laboratory tests beyond those required for evaluation of the patient's underlying disease must be obtained:

1. CBC with hematocrit done in ED
2. Chemistries: electrolytes, blood urea nitrogen (BUN), creatinine, sugar, calcium, phosphorus
3. Arterial blood gases (ABG)
4. X-ray film: chest x-ray study for underlying disease, placement of ET and nasogastric

TABLE 4-1. Commonly used measures in cardiopulmonary resuscitation

Drug availability	Dose/route	Indications	Adverse reactions	Comments
Atropine (0.1, 0.4, 1.0 mg/ml)	0.01-0.03 mg/kg/dose (minimum: 0.1 mg/dose) (adult: 0.6-1.0 mg/dose; maximum 2 mg) q 5 min prn IV, ET	Bradycardia, asystole, ↑ vagal tone Heart block (temporary)	Tachycardia, dysrhythmias, anticholinergic	Parasympatholytic (Table 6-3)
Bicarbonate, sodium (NaHCO$_3$) (8.4%-50 mEq/50 ml) (7.5%-44.5 mEq/50 ml)	1 mEq/kg/dose q 10 min prn IV	Metabolic acidosis Hyperkalemia	Metabolic alkalosis, hyperosmolarity, hypernatremia	Dilute 1:1 with D5W or sterile water; incompatible with calcium, catecholamine infusion; monitor ABG
Bretylium (50 mg/ml)	5 mg/kg/dose IV followed prn by 10 mg/kg/dose q 15 min IV up to 30 mg/kg	Ventricular dysrhythmias refractory to lidocaine	Hypotension (orthostatic), bradyrhythmias	Blocks adrenergic nerve endings; do not give ET (Table 6-3)
Calcium chloride (10%-100 mg/ml) (1.36 mEq Ca/ml)	20-30 mg (0.2-0.3 ml)/kg/dose (maximum: 500 mg/dose) q 10 min prn IV slowly	Hyperkalemia Clacium channel blocker OD	Rapid infusion causes bradycardia, hypotension Extravasation—necrosis	Inotropic; monitor; use caution with digitalized patient; preferred in shock because no need to metabolize anion substrate; probably no benefit in asystole or electromechanical dissociation
Calcium gluconate (10%-100 mg/ml) (0.45 mEq Ca/ml)	100 mg (1.0 ml)/kg/dose (maximum: 1,000 mg/dose) q 10 min prn IV slowly	Hyperkalemia Calcium channel blocker OD	Rapid infusion causes bradycardia, hypotension Extravasation—necrosis	Inotropic; monitor; use caution in digitalized patient; probably no benefit in asystole or electromechanical dissociation
Crystalloid 0.9%NS, LR, D5W.9%NS, D5WLR	20 ml/kg over 20-30 min IV	Hypovolemia		Monitor volume status
Defibrillation	2 watt-sec/kg (adult: 200 watt-sec)	Ventricular fibrillation		Use correct paddle size and paste; cardioversion (1-2 watt-sec/kg)
Dexamethasone (Decadron) (4,24 mg/ml)	0.25 mg/kg/dose IM, IV	Cerebral edema, croup, asthma		Delayed onset
Diazepam (Valium) (5 mg/ml)	0.2-0.3 mg/kg/dose (maximum: 10 mg/dose) IV	Status epilepticus	Respiratory depression	Also begin maintenance medication (Table 81-6)
Diazoxide (Hyperstat) (15 mg/ml)	1-3 mg/kg q 4-24 hr IV	Hypertension	Hypotension, hyperglycemia	Monitor (very prompt onset) (Table 18-2)
Digoxin (0.1, 0.25 mg/ml)	Premie: 0.01-0.02 mg/kg/TDD IV	Congestive heart failure	Dysrhythmia, heart block, vomiting	Monitor ECG; may also load PO in nonarrest situ-

Drug (concentration)	Dose	Indication	Side effects/toxicity	Comments
	2 wk-2 yr: 0.03-0.05 mg/kg/TDD IV Newborn and >2 yr: 0.04 mg/kg/TDD IV ½ TDD initially, then ¼ q 4-8 hr IV × 2	Supraventricular tachycardia		ation; if mild CHF, may give PO without loading (Table 16-2)
Dopamine (200 mg/5 ml)	Low: 2-5 µg/kg/min IV Mod: 5-20 µg/kg/min IV High: >20 µg/kg/min IV	Cardiogenic shock (mod dose) Maintain renal perfusion	Tachycardia, bradycardia, vasoconstriction (increase with higher doses)	Beta adrenergic; avoid in hypovolemic shock; may use in combination with isoproterenol or levarterenol (norepinephrine) (Table 5-2)
Dobutamine (Dobutrex) (vial: 250 mg)	1-15 µg/kg/min IV	Cardiogenic shock	Tachycardia	Beta adrenergic; positive inotropic; maybe synergistic with dopamine or isoproterenol
Epinephrine (1:10,000)	0.1 ml/kg/dose (maximum: 5 ml/dose) q 3-5 min prn IV, ET	Ventricular standstill Ventricular fibrillation (fine)	Tachycardia, dysrhythmia, hypertension, decreased renal and splanchnic blood flow	Alpha and beta—adrenergic; inotropic; not effective if acidotic
Furosemide (Lasix) (10 mg/ml)	1 mg/kg/dose q 6-12 hr IV up to 6 mg/kg/dose; may repeat q 2 hr prn	Fluid overload, pulmonary edema, cerebral edema	Hypokalemia, hyponatremia, prerenal azotemia	Reduce dosage in newborn to q 12 hr if no response in urine output in 30 min, repeat; do not use if hypovolemic (Table 16-3)
Glucagon 1 mg (1 unit)/ml	0.03-0.1 mg/kg/dose q 20 min prn IV, SC, IM	Beta-blocker overdose Hypoglycemia		Not adequate as only glucose support in neonate Inotropic
Glucose (D50W-0.5 g/ml)	0.5-1.0 g (2-4 ml D25W or 1-2 ml D50W)/kg/dose IV	Hypoglycemia, with coma or seizure		Draw glucose; if possible use D25W
Hydralazine (Apresoline) (20 mg/ml)	0.1-0.2 mg/kg/dose q 4-6 hr IV/IM	Hypertension	Tachycardia, tachyphylaxis	Prompt onset (Table 18-2)
Hydrocortisone (Solu-Cortef) (100, 250, 500 mg)	Shock: 50 mg/kg/dose (maximum: 500 mg/dose) IV	Septic shock (controversial)		Lower dose for status asthmaticus (4-5 mg/kg/dose) (Table 74-2)
Isoproterenol (1 mg/5 ml)	0.05-1.5 µg/kg/min Begin at 0.1 µg/kg/min and increase q 5-10 min prn	Bradycardia or heart block (S/P atropine)	Tachyrhythmias	Beta adrenergic; avoid in hypovolemic shock; do not use with digoxin (Table 5-2)
Lidocaine (1%-10 mg/ml)	1 mg/kg/dose 5-10 min IV, ET up to 5 mg/kg, then 20-50 µg/kg/min	Ventricular dysrhythmias Cardiac arrest caused by ventricular fibrillation	Hypotension, bradycardia with block, seizures	↓ automaticity (Table 6-3)

TDD, Total digitalizing dose.

Continued.

TABLE 4-1. Commonly used measures in cardiopulmonary resuscitation—cont'd

Drug availability	Dose/route	Indications	Adverse reactions	Comments
Methylprednisolone (Solu-Medrol) (40, 125, 500, 1,000 mg)	Shock: 30-50 mg/kg/dose (maximum: 500 mg/dose) IV	Septic shock (controversial)		Lower dose for status asthmaticus (1-2 mg/kg/dose q 6 hr IV) (Table 74-2)
Morphine (8, 10, 15 mg/ml)	0.1-0.2 mg/kg/dose (maximum: 15 mg/dose) q 2-4 hr IV	Pulmonary edema Tetralogy spell Reduce preload and afterload Analgesic	Hypotension, respiratory depression	Antidote: naloxone (Narcan)
Naloxone (Narcan) (0.4 mg/ml) (1 mg/ml)	0.1 mg/kg/dose (maximum: 0.8 mg) IV, ET; if no response in 10 min give 2 mg (5 vials) IV	Narcotic overdose, ? septic shock		Give empirically in suspected opiate overdose; may be given ET
Nitroprusside (50 mg/vial)	0.5-10 µg (average: 3 µg)/kg/min IV	Hypertensive emergency Afterload reduction	Hypotension, cyanide poisoning	Monitor closely; light sensitive (Table 18-2)
Oxygen	100% mask, ET	Hypoxia Major injury	Toxicity not a problem with acute short-term use	Use high flow (3-6 L/min); monitor ABG
Pancuronium (Pavulon) (1, 2 mg/ml)	0.04-0.1 mg/kg/dose IV; may repeat 0.01-0.02 mg/kg/dose q 20-40 min IV prn	Muscle relaxation	Tachycardia	Rapid onset; support respirations; lower dose in newborn
Phenobarbital (65 mg/ml)	15 mg/kg load IV/IM (adult: 100 mg/dose q 20 min prn × 3), then 5 mg/kg/24 hr PO, IV, IM	Seizures	Sedation	If not controlled after load, repeat 10 mg/kg/dose IV; administer <50 mg/min (Table 81-6)
Phenytoin (Dilantin) (50 mg/ml)	15 mg/kg load IV slowly, then 5-10 mg/kg/24 hr PO, IV q 12-24 hr	Seizures	Hypotension, bradycardia when given too fast; cerebral disturbance	Do not give faster than 40 mg/min; dilute in normal saline (Table 81-6)
	5 mg/kg/dose IV q 5-20 min × 2 prn	Dysrhythmia	Dysrhythmia	
Succinylcholine (20 mg/ml)	1 mg/kg/dose IV	Muscle relaxation	Dysrhythmia Hypotension	Must be able to control ventilation

(NG) tubes, and monitoring of potential complications

5. ECG and ongoing cardiac monitoring

Termination

Efforts should be terminated if there is obvious brain death, remembering that the brain of the infant and child is relatively resistant to hypoxic damage. Clinical evidence that is useful includes the oculocephalic reflex (doll's eyes reflex), oculovestibular reflex (calorics), absent corneal reflex, and fixed, dilated pupils. Resuscitation should be continued if there is evidence of drug depression or hypothermia. Underlying disease may modify the aggressiveness of resuscitation.

Psychologic support

Support of the entire family and child is essential throughout the resuscitation period. The child is separated from the parents and is in a strange environment, surrounded by unfamiliar doctors and nurses. If the resuscitation is successful and vital signs and consciousness restored, time should be taken to calm and reassure the child.

1. A member of the health care team should be assigned to provide the family with information, explanations, and emotional support. The decision regarding whether to allow parents to stay with the child must be personalized, based on the child's medical condition and state of consciousness and the emotional status of the family. Family members should be allowed privacy in order to express their feelings and emotions. Often there are specific individuals such as relatives or clergy who can be supportive and should be called.

2. If the child dies, support and compassion are needed, while attempting to relieve the family of feelings of guilt and facilitating the normal grieving process. Most parents will want to touch and hold the child after the youngster has been made as presentable as possible (see Foreword). Arrangements should be made for follow-up support during the ensuing days and weeks to ensure that appropriate resources have been mobilized to assist the family.

NOTE: Advanced pediatric life support recommendations are currently under review.

REFERENCES

American Heart Association: Standards and guidelines for cardiopulmonary resuscitation (CPR) and emergency cardiac care (ECC), JAMA **255:**2905, 1986.

American Heart Association: Textbook of advanced cardiac life support, Dallas, 1981, The Association.

Crane, R.D., and Shapiro, E.A.: Mechanical ventilatory support, JAMA **254:**87, 1985.

Cummins, R.O., and Eisenberg, M.S.: Prehospital cardiopulmonary resuscitation, JAMA **253:**2408, 1985.

Ehrlich, R., Emmett, S.M., and Rodriques-Torres, R.: Pediatric cardiac resuscitation team: a 6 year study, J. Pediatr. **84:**152, 1974.

Eisenberg, M., Bergner, L., and Hallstrom, A.: Epidemiology of cardiac arrest and resuscitation in children, Ann. Emerg. Med. **12:**672, 1983.

Goldenheim, P.D., Kazemi, H.: Cardiopulmonary monitoring of critically ill patients, N. Engl. J. Med. **311:**717,776, 1984.

Levin, D.L., Morriss, F.C., and Moore, G.C.: A practical guide to pediatric intensive care, St. Louis, 1984, The C.V. Mosby Co.

Ludwig, S., Kettrick, R.G., and Parker, M.: Pediatric cardiopulmonary resuscitation: review of 130 cases, Clin. Pediatr. **23:**71, 1984.

Mayer, T.A.: Emergency pediatric vascular access: old solutions to an old problem, Am. J. Emerg. Med. **4:**98, 1986.

Orlowski, J.P.: Cardiopulmonary resuscitation in children, Pediatr. Clin. North Am. **27:**495, 1982.

Sanders, A.B., Meislin, H.W., and Eng, G.A.: The physiology of cardiopulmonary resuscitation: an update, JAMA **252:**3283, 1984.

5 Shock

ALERT: After stabilization of the airway and ventilation, it is essential, in approaching the cardiovascular system, to determine the type and stage of shock. Fluids and pharmacologic agents are usually required.

Shock occurs when acute circulatory dysfunction is marked by progressive impairment of blood flow to the skin, muscles, kidneys, mesentery, lungs, heart, and brain. Patients in shock have diminished perfusion manifested by decreased blood pressure, tachycardia, poor capillary refill, decreased skin temperature, altered mental status, diminished urinary output, and multiple system failure. In children hypovolemia is the most common cause. Compensatory mechanisms initially prevent functional deterioration, but with progression, there are cellular metabolic changes marked by anaerobic metabolism, leading to further injury and eventually cell death and release of proteolytic enzymes and cellular by-products.

Blood pressure is dependent on cardiac output (rate and volume) and peripheral resistance. Although normal blood pressure and pulse values are summarized in Appendix C-2, it is useful to remember that the maximum effective heart rate in infants is 200 beats/min; in preschool children, 150 beats/min; and in older individuals, 120 beats/min. Normal systolic blood pressures in individuals 1-20 yr of age can be estimated by adding twice the age in years to 80. Diastolic blood pressure is usually two thirds of systolic. Normal blood volume is 80 ml/kg.

STAGES OF SHOCK AND DIAGNOSTIC FINDINGS
Compensated shock

Vital organ functions are maintained by intrinsic compensatory mechanisms that stabilize vital signs. As fluid loss progresses, venous capacitance may decrease by 10%-25%, fluid shifts from the interstitial to intravascular compartments, and arteriolar constriction increases. With compensation the central venous pressure (CVP) is decreased, as is stroke volume and urine output; heart rate and systemic vascular resistance increase. Perfusion to the periphery (skin and muscles) and to the kidneys and intestine may be compromised, even in the absence of major alterations in blood pressure. Ultimately, the efficacy of compensatory mechanisms is dependent on the patient's preexisting cardiac and pulmonary status and the rate and volume of blood loss.

Diagnostic findings

Orthostatic changes (systolic blood pressure decreases ≥ 15 mm Hg or pulse increases ≥ 20 beats/min from supine to seated or erect position) reflect primarily intravascular volume but are difficult to delineate in the child under 5 yr of age.

1. An acute volume deficit of 10% may be

marked by an increase in pulse rate of 20 beats/min, and a 20% deficit has an associated heart rate increase of 30 beats/min, with a variable decrease in blood pressure. Larger volume deficits will have a consistent blood pressure decrease ($\geq$15 mm Hg) and pulse increase ($\geq$30 beats/min).

2. A 10%-15% gradual volume loss produces minimal physiologic change. On the other hand, a 20%-30% gradual volume deficit is marked by compensation, but there is no related hypotension. Progressive hypotension is noted with 30%-50% gradual volume loss.

In acute blood loss, *supine* blood pressure may remain normal with a 20% or greater deficit. Orthostatic changes *must* be measured. Acidosis, which may be the most sensitive indicator of inadequate perfusion, must also be monitored closely.

Uncompensated shock

Cardiovascular dysfunction and impairment of microvascular perfusion lead to lowered perfusion pressures, increased precapillary arteriolar resistance, and further contraction of venous capacitance; with progressive blood stagnation, anaerobic metabolism and release of proteolytic enzymes and vasoactive substances occur. This exacerbates myocardial depression. Platelet aggregation and release of tissue thromboplastin produce hypercoagulability and disseminated intravascular coagulation (DIC).

Diagnostic findings

Hypotension, tachycardia, decreased cardiac output, and variable central venous pressures are observed. Multiple organ system failure occurs with adult respiratory distress syndrome (ARDS), liver and pancreatic failure, coagulopathies with DIC, oliguria and renal failure, gastrointestinal bleeding, impaired mental status, acidosis, abnormal calcium and phosphorus homeostasis, and ongoing cellular damage. Although variability does exist, the following observation may be useful:

Type of shock	Appearance of skin	Neck veins
Hypovolemic	Cold, clammy, pale	Flat
Cardiogenic	Cold, clammy, pale	Bulging
Distributive	Warm, dry, flushed; then cold, clammy	Variable

Terminal shock

Irreversible damage to the heart and brain as a result of altered perfusion and metabolism ultimately leads to death.

ETIOLOGY AND DIAGNOSTIC FINDINGS
(box on p. 22)

The clinical presentation and progression of findings partially reflect the underlying condition and the stage and classification of shock. Patients evidence altered vital signs associated with tachycardia, poor capillary refill (abnormal if over 2 sec), cool, mottled, and pale skin, and altered mental status, and they may have evidence of impaired cardiac function. Blood pressure changes may develop, often preceded by earlier orthostatic changes. Respiratory alkalosis and metabolic acidosis are common. Specific focus must be directed toward defining the underlying disease and its specific sequelae and complications and understanding the pathophysiology of the disease process.

Hypovolemic shock

Reduction in circulating blood volume produces progressive dysfunction:

1. Decreased preload through capillary pooling and leakage accompanied by extrinsic and intrinsic loss of intravascular volume and decreased cardiac output
2. Increased afterload secondary to arteriolar constriction
3. Myocardial ischemia resulting from impairment of subendocardial blood flow and decreased supply of oxygen to myocardium. Concurrently, an increased myocardial oxygen requirement is associated with tachycardia, increased afterload, and cardiac distension

ETIOLOGIC CLASSIFICATION OF SHOCK

HYPOVOLEMIC

1. Hemorrhage
   a. External: laceration
   b. Internal: ruptured spleen or liver, vascular injury, fracture (neonate: intracerebral/intraventricular hemorrhage)
   c. Gastrointestinal: bleeding ulcer, ruptured viscus, mesenteric hemorrhage
2. Plasma loss
   a. Burn
   b. Inflammation or sepsis: leaky capillary syndrome
   c. Nephrotic syndrome
   d. Third spacing: intestinal obstruction, pancreatitis, peritonitis
3. Fluid and electrolyte loss
   a. Acute gastroenteritis
   b. Excessive sweating (cystic fibrosis)
   c. Renal pathology
4. Endocrine
   a. Adrenal insufficiency, adrenal-genital syndrome
   b. Diabetes mellitus
   c. Diabetes insipidus
   d. Hypothyroidism (myxedema coma)

CARDIOGENIC

1. Myocardial insufficiency
   a. Dysrhythmia: bradycardia, atrioventricular (AV) block, ventricular tachycardia, supraventricular tachycardia
   b. Cardiomyopathy: myocarditis, ischemia, hypoxia, hypoglycemia, acidosis
   c. Drug intoxication
   d. Hypothermia
   e. Myocardial depressant effects of shock
   f. Status post cardiac surgery
2. Filling or outflow obstruction
   a. Pericardial tamponade
   b. Pneumopericardium
   c. Tension pneumothorax
   d. Pulmonary embolism
   e. Congenital heart disease, including patent ductus arteriosus (PDA)–dependent lesion such as coarctation of the aorta or critical pulmonary stenosis

DISTRIBUTIVE (VASOGENIC)

1. High or normal resistance (increased venous capacitance)
   a. Septic shock
   b. Anaphylaxis
   c. Barbiturate intoxication
2. Low resistance, vasodilation: CNS injury (i.e., spinal cord transection)

4. Excessive aldosterone secretion with sodium and water retention, leading to pulmonary edema and further hypoxia

Initial compensatory homeostasis is achieved at the expense of regional blood flow initially to the skin and muscles and then to the kidneys, mesentery, lungs, heart, and brain. Since children have highly reactive vascular beds, an adequate blood pressure can be maintained, even in the presence of significant intravascular volume depletion; when hypotension does develop, it is profound and rapid.

Cardiogenic shock

Dysfunction of the heart with depressed cardiac output may result from myocardial insufficiency or mechanical obstruction to flow of blood into and out of the heart. Inadequate preload, with accompanying hypovolemia, capillary injury, vascular instability, decreased cardiac output, and tissue perfusion, produces a rapid downhill spiral of microcirculatory failure. Children rarely go through a compensated phase.

Hemodynamically, patients have decreased cardiac output, elevated central venous pressure

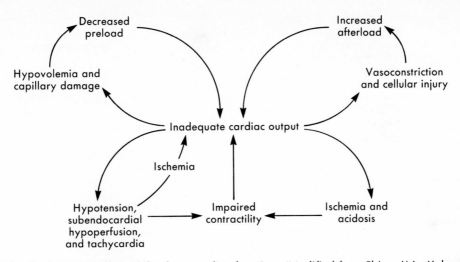

FIG. 5-1. Pathophysiology of effect of shock on cardiac function. (Modified from Shine, K.I., Kuhn, M., Young, L.S., and Tillisch, J.H.: Ann. Intern. Med. **93:**723, 1980.)

and pulmonary wedge pressure, and systemic vascular resistance. These may be the terminal events associated with primary shock of other etiology (Fig. 5-1).

Distributive or vasogenic shock (Table 5-1)

Distributive or vasogenic shock is associated with an abnormality in the distribution of blood flow, initially resulting from acute arteriolar dilation and increased venous capacitance accompanied by decreased intravascular volume secondary to leaky capillaries. This early hyperdynamic phase is associated with decreased afterload; it is less common in children than adults. The early phase is followed by rapid decompensation with decreased cardiac output and increased systemic vascular resistance secondary to hypoxemia and acidosis and increased venous capacitance. Clinically, warm, dry, flushed skin may be noted initially. This occurrence is followed by rapid progression to a vasoconstrictive phase.

In septic shock the endotoxin inhibits platelet

function while injuring the endothelium and activating intrinsic clotting factors with subsequent DIC.

Although the initial hyperdynamic phase is rare in children, when present it may respond to volume therapy. With progression, volume administration must be rapidly combined with agents that decrease peripheral resistance (alpha effect), whereas cardiac function is improved with positive inotropic agents (beta$_1$).

Complications

Complications are common, reflecting the stage of shock, rapidity of response, underlying disease process, and problems secondary to therapy.
1. Adult respiratory distress syndrome (ARDS) (p. 25)
2. Acute tubular necrosis (ATN) with renal failure (p. 615)
3. Myocardial dysfunction with failure (p. 98)
4. Stress ulcers, gastrointestinal (GI) bleeding, ileus

TABLE 5-1. Stages of distributive or septic shock

Early: hyperdynamic	Late: cardiogenic
BEDSIDE OBSERVATIONS	
Tachycardia	Tachycardia
Tachypnea	Respiratory depression
Fever	Hypothermia
Warm extremities	Cool, pale extremities
Bounding pulses	Decreased pulses
Normal capillary refill	Prolonged capillary refill
Normal or elevated systemic systolic blood pressure	Hypotension
Wide pulse pressure	Narrow pulse pressure
Elevated cardiac index	Depressed cardiac index
Decreased systemic vascular resistance	Increased systemic vascular resistance
Adequate urine output or polyuria	Oliguria
Mild mental confusion, occasional hallucinations	Lethargy or coma
LABORATORY MEASUREMENTS	
Hypoxemia	Hypoxemia
Respiratory alkalosis	Respiratory acidosis
Metabolic acidosis (not always present in early phase)	Metabolic acidosis
Marked pulmonary shunt	Minimal pulmonary shunt
Narrow arteriovenous oxygen saturation difference	Wide arteriovenous O_2 saturation difference
Hyperglycemia	Hypoglycemia
Mild coagulation abnormalities	Marked coagulopathy
Normal or mild elevation of blood lactate	Markedly elevated blood lactate

From Perkin, R.M., and Levin, D.L.: J. Pediatr. **101:**163, 1982.

Ancillary data

1. Chest x-ray studies on all patients to evaluate for cardiac size, pneumothorax, pneumonia, and pulmonary edema
2. ABG to monitor progression of diffusion and ventilation problems associated with respiratory distress syndrome
3. ECG and echocardiography to evaluate cardiac function, exclude dysrhythmias, monitor preload, and exclude effusion
4. Chemistries: electrolytes, BUN, creatinine, glucose, liver functions, calcium, phosphorus, cardiac enzymes, as indicated
5. Hematology: complete blood count (CBC), platelets, coagulation (prothrombin time [PT], partial thromboplastin time [PTT]), and DIC (fibrinogen, fibrin split products) screening (p. 522). Hemoglobin (Hb) and hematocrit (Hct) may be artifically normal in the face

of markedly decreased intravascular volume and must be measured on a continuing basis.
6. Type and cross-match because of the potential of hemorrhage, DIC, or intravascular hemolysis, which are common
7. Urinalysis to exclude hematuria, proteinuria, and infection. Output must be continuously monitored.
8. Cultures of blood and urine. Spinal fluid as indicated. Counterimmunoelectrophoresis (CIE) may be useful with negative cultures.

MANAGEMENT

Initial resuscitation must be followed by a systematic approach to fluid therapy, pharmacologic support, and diagnostic evaluation. It is imperative to constantly monitor perfusion through hemodynamic parameters, including blood pressure, heart rate and capillary refill, urine output, acid-base status, and mental alertness. If one approach is not effective, adjusting the fluid and pharmacologic approach must be tried on an empiric basis.

Following stabilization of the airway and ventilation and initiation of resuscitation of the cardiovascular system, the underlying disease process requires urgent attention.

Airway and ventilation

1. Administer oxygen at 3-6 L/min via cannula, mask, etc.
2. Determine need for intubation and mechanical ventilation. The indications for intubation include:
   a. Arterial oxygen tension (PaO_2) <50 mm Hg (sea level) when oxygen is administered with FIO_2 of 50%
   b. Arterial carbon dioxide tension ($PaCO_2$) >50 mm Hg (unless caused by compensation from prolonged condition such as bronchopulmonary dysplasia, cystic fibrosis)
   c. Decreasing vital capacity, increasing respiratory rate, or rapidly progressive disease
   d. Severe metabolic acidosis
   e. Inability to protect airway
   f. Severe pulmonary edema or marked respiratory distress following drowning or similar pathology requiring positive end expiratory pressure (PEEP)

Adult respiratory distress syndrome (ARDS) may develop with increased extravascular pulmonary water, thereby increasing both the work of breathing and the permeability secondary to damage of the alveolar epithelium and the pulmonary capillary endothelium. Because of this cellular injury, the pulmonary capillaries become permeable, and proteinaceous fluid leaks into the interstitial space and alveoli. This is characterized clinically by progressive hypoxemia, hypercapnia, respiratory alkalosis, increased shunting, and decreased compliance.

Ventilation with early introduction of positive-end expiratory pressure (PEEP) is essential if PaO_2 does not respond to only PEEP or if other indications for intubation are present. Initially start with a PEEP of 3-6 cm H_2O, and titrate upward using an adequate PaO_2 as the end point, without decreasing cardiac output. Chest x-ray films and arterial blood gases should be monitored.

NOTE: PEEP may increase intrapulmonary shunting, with a potential decrease in cardiac output and decreased delivery of oxygen to the tissues. This usually does not occur until PEEP reaches >15 cm H_2O.

Intravenous fluids

Fluids should be initiated following insertion of one or two large-bore intravenous (IV) lines. In administering IV fluids, it is essential to remember the relationship between preload and stroke volume described by the Frank-Starling curve; excessive fluid administration actually may impair cardiac function, emphasizing the importance of monitoring the central venous pressure or pulmonary capillary wedge pressure (PCWP).

Hypovolemic shock (Fig. 5-2)
1. Administer 0.9%NS at a rate of 20 ml/kg over 20 min. Use D5W.9%NS if the cause is gastroenteritis. Monitor urine output, pulse, perfusion, and blood pressure.
2. If no response, repeat the infusion once with ongoing evaluation of ventilatory status, temperature, electrolytes, glucose, ABG, and ECG.
3. Place a CVP line if no response after two infusions. Observe CVP or PCWP for 10 min after fluid challenge.
   a. If elevated (>10 mm Hg CVP* or >12 mm Hg PCWP), consider other etiologies, including tension pneumothorax, pericardial tamponade, myocardial insufficiency, congestive heart failure, PDA–dependent lesion with closing of PDA (coarctation of aorta in newborn), or myocarditis.

---

*0.75 mm Hg = 1 cm H_2O.

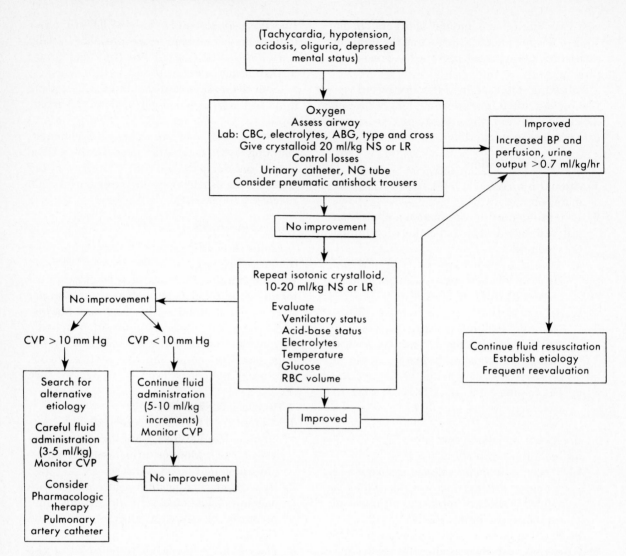

FIG. 5-2. Management of hypovolemic shock. (Modified from Perkin, R.M., and Levin, D.L.: J. Pediatr. **101:**319, 1982.)

b. If decreased (≤10 mm Hg CVP or ≤12 mm Hg PCWP), administer crystalloid (0.9%NS) in increments of 5-10 ml/kg over 20-30 min while monitoring CVP response. Observe response for at least 10 min after infusion. If CVP returns to within 3 mm Hg of the preinfusion value, continue infusion and repeat until either hemodynamic parameters are corrected or the CVP persistently exceeds the initial value by 3 mm Hg.

c. CVP may not reflect left ventricular function. PCWP may be needed, particularly if positive pressure ventilation is used, if pulmonary disease or mitral stenosis is present, or if there is evidence of failure of either the left or right side of the heart.

4. If hemorrhage is the cause of the hypovole-

mia, type specific or cross-matched *blood* should be administered following an initial crystalloid resuscitation. Once 40-50 ml/kg of crystalloid has been infused during the infusion, it is increasingly important to administer blood. Whole blood is particularly useful for massive ongoing acute bleeding; however, packed red blood cells may be appropriate following the infusion of large amounts of crystalloid in an acute situation or in a more chronic process.

a. If completely cross-matched blood is not available, administer type-specific blood. It is usually available within 10-15 min after delivery of a clot to the blood bank. O-negative blood should be reserved for those patients in profound shock secondary to hypovolemia who have no response to crystalloid or who are in cardiac arrest following trauma.

b. Fresh frozen plasma and platelets are often indicated to rapidly correct coagulation defects. Coagulation status should be monitored.

c. Massive blood transfusions (equivalent to one blood volume of 80 ml/kg) require the use of blood warmers and micropore filters.

5. If hypovolemia exists concurrently with hypoproteinemia or cardiac, respiratory, or renal failure, use 5% *albumin* in 0.9%NS (Plasmanate) or fresh frozen plasma at 5-10 ml/kg over 30 min with careful monitoring. This infusion may be repeated until the patient is hemodynamically stable or the CVP increases.

6. The role of *colloid* in severe shock or capillary leak syndromes is controversial. There may be a role for 5% albumin or products like 6% hetastarch combined with crystalloid to improve intravascular blood flow, but this has not been consistently demonstrated to be superior to crystalloid. Colloid is not used for initial burn therapy.

Cardiogenic shock

1. A fluid push may improve cardiac output by increasing filling pressure in accordance with the Frank-Starling curve, particularly if the CVP is ≤15 mm Hg. The PCWP is a more reliable measure of the response to fluid challenge in cardiogenic shock and should be measured if possible, but insertion of a Swan-Ganz catheter should not delay aggressive stabilization. 0.9%NS at 5 ml/kg over 30 min may be administered with careful monitoring of response.

2. Pressor agents (Table 5-2) are usually necessary with an inadequate response to IV fluid challenge. Ultimately, inotropic and vasodilating drugs may be needed to normalize blood pressure.

3. Evaluation of the adequacy of preload by CVP or PCWP measurements and afterload is essential in monitoring the efficacy of therapy. Monitoring by echocardiography in consultation with a cardiologist is extremely important.

Distributive shock

1. Septic shock. Intravenous fluids do not usually improve vital signs because cardiac output actually decreases when preload is increased. Pressor agents commonly are required after adequate preload has been established and documented. Filling pressure should be kept at the lowest level consistent with adequate tissue perfusion.

2. Anaphylaxis (Chapter 12)

3. Head and spinal cord trauma (Chapters 57 and 61). Pressor agents are usually required after adequate preload has been established and documented.

Cardiac function

1. Treatment of **dysrhythmias** (Chapter 6). Bradycardia, AV block, and tachyrhythmias are particularly detrimental to cardiac output. Predisposing conditions include electrolyte abnormalities, acidosis, alkalosis, drugs, fever, and pericardial disease, as well as ischemic or hypoxic damage.

2. **Inotropic agents** (Table 5-2). Although an evaluation of the adequacy of preload by ech-

TABLE 5-2. Commonly used drugs for shock*

Drug	Mechanism			Dose (IV)	Comments
	Alpha	Beta₁	Beta₂		
Isoproterenol (Isuprel)	±	+++	+++	0.05-1.5 µg/kg/min	Positive inotropic and chronotropic effect; peripheral vasodilation; increases cardiac oxygen requirement; relatively large increase in heart rate for given increase in cardiac output; decreases coronary blood flow Use: decreased cardiac contractility; bradycardia and third-degree AV block
Dopamine (Intropin)	At high dose	++ to +++	±	Low: 2-5 µg/kg/min Mod: 5-20 µg/kg/min High: >20 µg/kg/min	Low: increased renal and mesenteric blood flow, little effect on heart (dopaminergic effect) Mod: increased renal blood flow, heart rate, cardiac contractility, and cardiac output High: systemic vasoconstriction May be used synergistically with isoproterenol or dobutamine
Dobutamine (Dobutrex)	±	++ to +++	±	1-15 µg/kg/min (usually 10-15 µg/kg/min)	Positive inotropic effect with minimal chronotropic; minimal beta₂; useful in cardiogenic shock; may use with low dose dopamine
Norepinephrine (Levophed)	+++	+++	±	0.1-1.0 µg/kg/min	Positive inotropic; intense alpha vasoconstrictor, with compromised peripheral tissue and organ perfusion Useful in cardiogenic shock caused by myocardial insufficiency; seldom used without an alpha blocker

Drug				Dose	Comments
Epinephrine (Adrenalin)	+++	+++	+++	0.05-0.5 μg/kg/min	Use only when isoproterenol and dopamine are ineffective; positive inotropic and chronotropic effects; renal and mesenteric ischemia; tachyarrhythmia; increased cardiac oxygen requirements; intense alpha effect if >0.3 μg/kg/min. Use in asystole: 0.1 ml (1:10,000)/kg/dose (max: 5 ml/dose) q 3-5 min IV, ET prn
Sodium nitroprusside (Nipride)				0.5-10 μg/kg/min (average: 3 μg/kg/min)	Arterial and venous dilator; afterload reduction; rapid response, short duration
Phentolamine (Regitine)	Antagonist			0.05-0.1 mg/kg/dose q 1-4 hr IV prn	Counteracts vasoconstriction; useful in face of high CVP or in combination with vasoconstrictive drug; rapid onset, short activity; may also be given by continuous infusion
Hydrocortisone (Solu-Cortef)				50 mg/kg/dose	Use in septic shock; increases cardiac output; decreases peripheral resistance
Naloxone (Narcan)				0.1 mg/kg/dose (0.8-2.0 mg/dose) IV q 3-5 min × 2 prn	May be useful in septic shock; endorphin antagonist; alternative regimen: bolus of 0.03 mg/kg, then 0.03 mg/kg/hr IV infusion
Calcium chloride				0.2-0.3 ml/kg/dose q 10 min prn IV slowly (20-30 mg/kg/dose) (maximum: 0.5 g)	Positive inotropic and chronotropic; may cause bradycardia; controversial role

+, ++, +++, relative degree present; ±, variable.

*Inotropic agents are not useful in hypovolemic shock; volume replacement is required.

ocardiography, CVP, or PCWP optimally should be done before initiating pharmacologic support, it must not delay aggressive stabilization. The efficacy of the agent can then be measured. Inotropic agents have no role in hypovolemic shock, but they are fundamental components of therapy for cardiogenic and distributive shock.

a. Classification

	Mechanism/effect		
Effector Organ	Alpha	Beta$_1$	Beta$_2$
Heart			
Rate		Increase	Increase
Contractility		Increase	
Conduction velocity		Increase	
Arterioles	Constrict		Dilate
Veins	Constrict		Dilate
Lung-bronchiolar smooth muscles	Constrict		Dilate

b. If local infiltration of an agent with significant alpha effects (vasoconstriction) occurs during infusion, there is a significant risk of skin necrosis and ulceration. To minimize this when infiltration occurs, phentolamine (alpha antagonist) 1-5 mg diluted in 1-5 ml of 0.9%NS, depending on the size of the child, is infiltrated locally.

c. Often a combination of pressor agents is required to maximize the clinical effect. A typical combination includes dopamine in low doses (0.5-3 µg/kg/min) as one drug to maintain renal perfusion by dilating the splanchnic and renal vascular beds and a second drug such as dobutamine (5-15 µg/kg/min). Continuous infusions of isoproterenol and epinephrine may be used in severe, unresponsive situations.

3. Vasodilators

a. An evaluation of the adequacy of preload and cardiac function by echocardiography and CVP or PCWP measurement should be done before pharmacologic therapy is initiated, carefully monitoring improvement of function with intervention.

b. In cardiogenic shock, vasodilators such as nitroprusside (0.5-10 mg/kg/min IV) (p. 123) may be helpful for pulmonary congestion. Vasodilators are useful when there is peripheral hypoperfusion and when the patient is hypervolemic or a major outflow obstruction secondary to arteriolar vasoconstriction exists. Vasodilators are usually employed in combination with an inotropic drug. These agents may simultaneously reduce the preload, and therefore volume repletion may be required.

Hypovolemic shock

Inotropic agents are not indicated for hypovolemic shock.

Cardiogenic shock

1. Inotropic agents (e.g., dopamine, dobutamine) should be initiated if there is poor peripheral perfusion after an initial infusion of fluids to improve cardiac function. Periodically during inotropic therapy a fluid challenge should be administered to reassess intravascular volume status.

2. If pulmonary congestion exists or there is peripheral hypoperfusion in hypervolemic patients, vasodilators (e.g., nitroprusside) may be useful adjunctive therapy.

Distributive shock

Primary therapy is to initiate positive inotropic agents while maintaining intravascular volume. In the early hyperdynamic phase (rare in children) there is a decreased afterload requiring volume administration. Later, with the decreased cardiac output and increased systemic vascular resistance secondary to hypoxemia and acidosis, isoproterenol (0.1-1.0 µg/kg/min) is particularly useful because it decreases peripheral resistance and has a positive inotropic effect.

Ancillary procedures

These procedures require appropriate priority in the initial evaluation and stabilization.

1. Elevate legs unless respiratory distress or pulmonary edema is present.

2. If available, inflate pneumatic military an-

tishock trousers (MAST) to the extent necessary if the patient has hypovolemia that is not controlled by the initial intravenous fluids and if there is no evidence of pulmonary edema or cardiogenic shock. The trousers provide an autotransfusion into the upper circulation by compression of the venous beds in the legs and abdomen. Complications include acidosis, ventilatory and renal compromise, and reduced visibility of the patient. Mast rarely have been used on children.

3. Insert nasogastric tube to initiate decompression and provide information of GI bleeding.
4. Place urinary catheter to monitor renal output and evaluate renal injury.
5. Normalize temperature (Chapters 50 and 51).
6. Consider and perform peritoneal lavage to exclude peritoneal blood loss (Chapter 13) or peritonitis after trauma or, if appropriate, in the patient with ascites.
7. Insert CVP catheter. This is particularly important in hypovolemic shock if positive pressure ventilation is not required and there is no significant pulmonary or cardiac disease. A Swan-Ganz catheter permits measurement of the PCWP, which is particularly useful in cardiogenic or distributive shock.
8. Perform pericardiocentesis (Appendix A-5) to exclude pericardial tamponade, or do thoracentesis (Appendix A-9) to treat tension pneumothorax if specific indications are present.

Other considerations

1. *Electrolyte* and *acid-base* abnormalities must be corrected since they impair ventilation, depress the myocardium, predispose to dysrhythmias, and alter response to catecholamines. All corrections require frequent monitoring of response.
   a. *Acidosis* is a consistent finding, which must be at least partially corrected if the pH is less than 7.15. Early treatment of a pattern of deteriorating acid-base status may prevent complications. If acidosis is a result of hypoventilation, consider ac-

tive airway management. If the cause is metabolic, give 1-2 mEq/kg sodium bicarbonate ($NaHCO_3$) over 5 min IV. Repeat according to ABG. Correct only to 7.25-7.30, but monitor closely. Calculation: deficit mEq HCO_3^- = weight (kg) $\times$ base excess $\times$ 0.3.
   b. *Hypocalcemia* develops with decreased serum ionized calcium; it is associated with impaired tissue perfusion. Hypocalcemia depresses myocardial function as does hypophosphatemia. Give $CaCl_2$ 10% 10-20 mg/kg (0.1-0.2 ml/kg) IV slowly, optimally through a central venous line while monitoring vital signs. Simultaneously check phosphorus, a deficit being treated with KPO_4 5-10 mg/kg slowly if K^+ is normal. If phosphorus is high, care must be exercised in administering calcium.
2. *Urine output* is optimally maintained at 1-2 ml/kg/hr. Pharmacologic agents may be required to supplement volume repletion in maintaining urine flow. The choice of regimen must be individualized, reflecting the experience of the clinician and the response to one or more of the agents. Oliguria is a common finding secondary to prerenal failure and acute tubular necrosis (p. 615). It is essential to know the intravascular volume before initiating pharmacologic therapy. Treatment options in addition to fluid therapy include:
   a. Furosemide (Lasix) 1 mg/kg/dose up to 6 mg/kg/dose q 2-6 hr IV as needed
   b. Mannitol 0.25-1.0 g/kg/dose q 4-6 hr IV
   c. Low dose dopamine (0.5-3 μg/kg/min IV continuous infusion)
   d. Monitoring input and output meticulously and replacing urine output milliliter by milliliter.
   e. Dialysis, which is required in the face of unresponsive hyperkalemia, acidosis, or hypervolemia
3. *Corticosteroids* are controversial and without proved efficacy in the treatment of septic

shock, and there is at least preliminary data that they are detrimental. However, many clinicians do use them early in the course of disease because of the lack of definitive data.
   a. Methylprednisolone (Solu-Medrol) 30-50 mg/kg/dose IV; **or**
   b. Hydrocortisone (Solu-Cortef) 50 mg/kg/dose IV
4. *Antibiotics* are appropriate because of the nonspecific nature of the clinical presentation. The critically ill child with shock from unknown cause is thus treated empirically. Ideally, antibiotics are initiated after obtaining at least one blood culture and optimally all other relevant cultures. Broad-spectrum antibiotics should be used initially to cover all potential pathogens and then modified to reflect the results of culture and sensitivity data.
   a. Ampicillin 200-300 mg/kg/24 hr q 4 hr IV **and** chloramphenicol 100 mg/kg/24 hr q 6 hr IV; **or**
   b. Cefotaxime 50-100 mg/kg/24 hr q 4-6 hr IV (or ceftriaxone 50-75 mg/kg/24 hr q 12 hr IV; **or** cefuroxime 100 mg/kg/24 hr q 6-8 hr IV). In the newborn, ampicillin should be added and the dose altered.
These antibiotics should be modified if there are specific clinical indications such as a perforated abdominal organ or toxic shock syndrome.
5. *Coagulopathy* may occur after shock of any etiology. Disseminated intravascular coagulation (DIC) is common (p. 522). With many coagulopathies associated with shock, fresh frozen plasma is a rapid approach to correcting abnormalities and additionally provides volume expansion.
6. Naloxone (Narcan) use is controversial; it serves as an endorphin antagonist and has some questionable efficacy in the treatment of septic shock by improving hemodynamic parameters when initiated early. High doses are recommended initially with a continuous drip thereafter. Empirically, one suggested regimen provides an IV bolus of 0.03 mg/kg followed by a continuous IV infusion of 0.03 mg/kg/hr (adult: 0.4 mg/hr).
7. Human antiserum to mutant *Escherichia coli* has been used successfully in the treatment of gram-negative bacteremia in adults on an experimental basis.
8. Treatment of anaphylactic shock is discussed in Chapter 12.
9. Patients failing to respond to resuscitation efforts must be rapidly reevaluated to ascertain if other etiologic conditions may concurrently exist. Consultation is mandatory. Factors that must be considered include:
   a. Multiple organ failure
   b. Myocardial injury, ischemia, or other damage, as well as coronary artery disease
   c. Outflow or filling obstruction, such as tension pneumothorax or pericardial tamponade
   d. Coagulopathy and disseminated intravascular coagulation
   e. Renal failure
   f. Respiratory failure
   g. Uncontrolled sepsis
   h. Ongoing blood loss

DISPOSITION

All patients require immediate admission to an ICU. Cardiac, pulmonary, and infectious disease consultations should be requested immediately.

REFERENCES

Chen, H.L.: Naloxone in shock and toxic coma, Am. J. Emerg. Med. **2**:444, 1984.

Goldenheim, P.D., and Kazemi, H.: Cardiopulmonary monitoring of critically ill patients, N. Engl. J. Med. **311**:717, 776, 1984.

Rock, P., Silverman, H., Plump, D., et al.: Efficacy and safety of naloxone in septic shock, Crit. Care Med. **13**:28, 1985.

Smith, J.A.R., and Normal, J.N.: The fluid of choice for resuscitation of severe shock, Br. J. Surg. **69**:702, 1982.

Sprung, C.L., Caralis, P.V., and Marcial, E.H.: The effects of high-dose corticosteroids in patients with septic shock, N. Engl. J. Med. **311**:1137, 1984.

6 Dysrhythmias

Dysrhythmias are uncommon in the pediatric population. Because of the differences in etiologies, particularly in infants and children, and the absence of ischemic heart disease, only a few types of disturbances are seen with any frequency.

Cardiac stimuli arise in specialized neuromuscular tissues within the heart, consisting of the sinus (sinoatrial, or SA) node, AV (atrioventricular) junction, bundle of His, right and left branches, and Purkinje fibers. The primary pacemaker is the sinus node. When this node is depressed or fails to propagate impulses, a secondary pacemaker sets the cardiac rate. The stimuli become progressively slower as the site becomes more distal.

The sympathetic and vagal fibers modify stimuli through the sinus node and AV junction. The sympathetic nervous system stimulates the heart, and the vagal or parasympathetic system has a depressive effect, mostly on the sinus node and AV junction. Increased heart rate may result from increased sympathetic activity or decreased vagal tone; bradycardia is commonly caused by increased vagal tone, often secondary to myocardial hypoxia.

Dysrhythmias occur because of abnormal impulse formation or conduction, or a combined mechanism. *Tachyrhythmias* in children result from ectopic pacemakers or reentrant pathways that often involve abnormal or accessory pathways. Accessory pathways produce preexcitation syndromes such as Wolff-Parkinson-White (WPW), which predisposes to paroxysmal atrial tachycardia (PAT) or paroxysmal supraventricular tachycardia (PSVT). Therapy is focused on interruption of the reentry or prevention of premature beats that trigger the cycle. Ectopic pacemakers are treated by suppression of the focus.

Bradyrhythmias usually are caused by slowing of the intrinsic pacemaker or a conduction abnormality. The block in conduction may be complete, in which circumstance a more distal, slower pacemaker controls the rate, or it may be incomplete, allowing only a few impulses to pass (Tables 6-1 and 6-2).

Children at risk of dysrrhythmias may have congenital or acquired heart disease, systemic disease, intoxication, or acute hemodynamic alterations.

Assessment requires a careful history and physical examination, focusing on the vital signs, cardiac evaluation, and evidence of systemic disease. Prompt analysis of the ECG and hemodynamic parameters is imperative. Symptomatic patients may show evidence of congestive heart failure (Chapter 16), including pallor, irritability, poor eating, dyspnea, decreased cerebral blood flow associated with syncope and altered behavior, decreased coronary blood flow and anginal pain, or a perception of a rhythm disturbance marked by palpitations or missed beats.

ANALYSIS OF ELECTROCARDIOGRAM
(Appendix C-3, p. 652)

1. Rate
   a. Rate is age dependent (newborn: 100-160,

TABLE 6-1. Characteristics of common dysrhythmias

Dysrhythmia	Rate/min (>6 yr old)	Rhythm	P wave (atrial)	QRS complex
BRADYRHYTHMIAS				
Sinus bradycardia	<60	Regular	Upright I, II, aV$_F$	WNL
Sinus dysrhythmia	60-120	Irregular	Upright I, II, aV$_F$	WNL
SUPRAVENTRICULAR TACHYRHYTHMIAS				
Sinus tachycardia	120-200	Regular	Upright I, II, aV$_F$	WNL
Premature atrial complex (PAC)	60-120	Irregular	Variable	WNL
Paroxysmal supraventricular (atrial) tachycardia (PAT or PSVT)	150-250	Regular	Buried; nonsinus, variably retrograde	WNL
Junctional premature contraction	NA	Irregular	Retrograde, often obscured	WNL or aberrant
Atrial flutter	100-300 (atrial: 200-300)	Regular	Flutter (saw-toothed) waves II, III, aV$_F$	WNL
Atrial fibrillation	60-190 (atrial: 400-700)	Irregularly irregular	No P waves; fibrillation waves	WNL
VENTRICULAR TACHYRHYTHMIAS				
Premature ventricular complex (PVC)	NA	Irregular	Usually obscured	≥0.12 sec, premature, bizarre
Ventricular tachycardia	150-220	Regular or slightly irregular	Usually not recognizable	≥0.12 sec, bizarre
Ventricular fibrillation	Indeterminate	None	Not recognizable	Irregular undulation

*WNL, Within normal limits; NA, not applicable.

AV conduction	Response to vagotonic maneuver	Comments
WNL	None	Found in athletes, hypothyroidism, increased intracranial pressure, with drugs (propranolol or digitalis); if no symptoms, no treatment; If serious, use atropine, pacemaker; rate is age specific
WNL	Transient slowing	Normal variation with respiration and varying vagal tone; reassurance needed
WNL	Transient slowing	Secondary to fever, exercise, anemia, shock, hyperthyroidism; treat condition
WNL, may be first-degree block	Slows	Stimulants (caffeine, smoking, alcohol), digitalis toxicity, early CHF, hypoxia; if infrequent, no treatment; avoid stimulants; if frequent, treat condition; rarely need propranolol or quinidine
WNL	None or converts	Most common significant dysrhythmia (reentry); children <5 yr: infection, fever, congenital heart disease; older children: WPW (short PR segment, ±prolonged QRS complex, delta wave); may cause cardiac decompensation secondary to inadequate filling time; occurs with digitalis toxicity, particularly with block
Variable	None	Same as PAC
Variable block	None	Heart disease, thyrotoxicosis, pulmonary embolism, myocarditis, chest trauma
Variable block	Transient slowing	As above (atrial flutter); severe valvular disease (mitral stenosis, tricuspid insufficiency, aortic stenosis), WPW and without heart disease
Compensatory pause, variably retrograde	None	ST segment and T wave opposite in polarity to QRS complex: variably significant if >6/min, multifocal, occurs near T wave, increases with exercise, or occurs in bigeminy or trigeminy; associated with cardiac ischemia, digitalis toxicity, ↓ K+, hypoxia, alkalosis
None	None	ST segment and T wave opposite in polarity to QRS complex; may cause hemodynamic compromise requiring immediate treatment
None	None	Disorganized, ineffective cardiac activity without pulse or blood pressure; medical emergency: defibrillate

TABLE 6-2. Characteristics of conduction disturbances*

Type	Atrial rate	Ventricle rate	PR interval	Ventricular rhythm	P-QRS relation	QRS complex	Comments
First degree	Unaffected	Same as atrial	Prolonged for age	Same as atrial	Consistent 1:1	Unaffected	Block anywhere from AV node to bundle branches; may be caused by digitalis; no therapy necessary
Second degree (Wenckebach period)	Unaffected	Slower than atrial	Progressive increase until P wave is dropped	Irregular	Variable (recurring)	Narrow	Block at AV node; may be caused by digitalis or quinidine; therapy rarely needed; do not give potassium
Second degree	Unaffected	Slower than atrial	Normal or prolonged; constant	Irregular or regular	Fixed	Usually wide	Block at His bundle or below; may be precursor to complete block; pacemaker needed; temporize with atropine or isoproterenol
Third degree	Unaffected	Slower than atrial	Variable	Regular	None	Variable with site	Block is anywhere from the AV node to bundle branches; life-threatening; pacemaker; temporize with atropine and isoproterenol

Modified from McIntyre, K.M., and Lewis, A.J., editors: Textbook of advanced cardiac life suport, Dallas, 1981, American Heart Association, pp. VI-27.

*May be idiopathic, acquired (nonsurgical), postoperative, or congenital.

infant: 120-160, toddler: 80-150, child >6 yr: 60-120).

    b. Each small box is 0.04 sec, and time between vertical lines at top of strip is 3 sec. Determine rate by multiplying number of complexes between vertical lines by 20.

2. Axis: Axis is age specific, also reflecting hypertrophy or conduction defects.

3. Rhythm
    a. Regular or irregular
    b. Voltage (myocarditis, effusion)

4. P wave
    a. Presence implies atrial activity, although it may be buried in QRS interval, ST segment, or T wave. Seen best in leads II, III, and aV_F
    b. Enlarged or biphasic (V_1) (atrial hypertrophy); normal: 0.08-0.10 sec
    c. Configuration (normal vs ectopic foci)

5. PR interval
    a. A fixed relationship between the P wave and QRS interval implies that the rhythm is supraventricular in origin.
    b. Interval is age- and rate-dependent, ranging from 0.10-0.20 sec.
    c. Prolongation occurs with first-degree block, hyperkalemia, digitalis, propranolol, verapamil, and carditis (acute rheumatic fever)
    d. Short in WPW syndrome, it also has delta wave.

6. QRS complex
    a. Duration is normally ≤0.10 sec.
    b. Prolongation occurs with conduction defect, ventricular focus, severe hyperkalemia, quinidine.
    c. Abnormal configuration demonstrates that the focus is ventricular in origin or that there is a conduction defect.
    d. High voltage implies hypertrophy or overload pattern.

7. ST segment
    a. Elevated with transmural injury, pericarditis, ventricular aneurysm

    b. Depressed with subendocardial injury, digitalis, systolic overload, and strain

8. T wave
    a. Peaks in hyperkalemia (if severe, also has widened QRS interval); flat with hypokalemia
    b. Inverted with conduction defect or ischemia

9. QT segment
    a. Duration is rate dependent, but correction (QT_c) should be ≤0.42 sec.
    b. Prolonged with quinidine, procainamide, tricyclic antidepressant overdose, hypokalemia, hypocalcemia, and hypothermia.

ANCILLARY DATA

1. The patient's response to *vagotonic maneuvers* should be evaluated. Vagotonic maneuvers include massage of the carotid (unilateral), Valsalva, cold water applied to face briskly, deep inspiration, coughing, drinking cold water, and gagging. The resulting increased vagal tone should result in at least a transient slowing of the heart rate if the rhythm is supraventricular. Do not perform eyeball compression or simultaneous, bilateral carotid massage.

2. Monitoring on an ongoing basis is essential. In the hospital setting this should be done in a monitored unit. Following discharge, transtelephonic electrocardiography has been useful in defining dysrhythmias and monitoring the efficacy of drug and pacemaker therapy.

3. Electrophysiologic studies may be indicated.
    a. Tachyrhythmias. Supraventricular (preexcitation WPW) with syncope and frequent episodes of PAT unresponsive to vagotonic maneuvers or medication. Ventricular dysrhythmias requiring study include patients with associated heart disease and those with cardiac tumors, myocarditis, or metabolic disorders.
    b. Bradyrhythmias requiring investigation include sick sinus syndrome and AV conduction defects.

MANAGEMENT (Tables 6-3 and 6-4)

Once a dysrhythmia has been identified, it is imperative to determine if there is any compromise in cardiac output or hemodynamic parameters or if the rhythm is potentially life-threatening. Management must focus on prevention, control of the underlying condition, and specific therapy for the dysrhythmia.

1. Oxygen should be administered during sta-
bilization of the airway, ventilation, and circulation. Treatment of the underlying condition, which often causes hypoxia, may adequately resolve the dysrhythmia.

2. Usually, one medication is initiated until the therapeutic effect is achieved or toxicity is noted. If the agent fails, additional medications should be added.

3. *Electrical conversion* is used for the treat-

TABLE 6-3. Common antidysrhythmic drugs

Drug	ECG effect	Half-life	Blood level	
			Therapeutic	**Toxic**
Digoxin (Table 16-2)	Prolongs PR	24 hr	1-3.5 ng/ml	>3.5 ng/ml (variable)
Lidocaine	Shortens QT	5 hr	1-5 μg/ml	>10 μg/ml
Quinidine	Prolongs QRS, QT, ±PR	6 hr	2-6 μg/ml	>9 μg/ml
Procainamide	Prolongs QRS, QT, ±PR	3-4 hr	4-10 μg/ml	>10 μg/ml
Propranolol	Prolongs PR, shortens QT	2-4 hr	20-150 μg/ml	NA
Bretylium	No change	6-10 hr	0.5-1.5 μg/ml	NA
Verapamil	Shortens QT, prolongs PR	3-7 hr (variable		
Phenytoin (Dilantin)	Shortens QT	20-26 hr	10-20 μg/ml	>20 μg/ml
Atropine	Increases rate	<5 min	NA	NA
Isoproterenol	Increases rate	<5 min	NA	NA

±, Variable effect; NA, not applicable, TDD, total digitalizing dose.

ment of ventricular fibrillation and symptomatic tachyrhythmias that are unresponsive to pharmacologic therapy or for hemodynamic compromise. Children can usually tolerate tachyrhythmias for long periods of time before cardiac decompensation occurs.

a. Defibrillation is the untimed depolarization used to convert ventricular fibrillation. Cardioversion is a timed depolar-

ization that prevents stimulation of the heart during the vulnerable part of the cardiac cycle, thereby avoiding the initiation of lethal ventricular dysrhythmias. Cardioversion is useful in conversion of ventricular tachyrhythmias.

b. Direct current (DC) defibrillators are used; it is crucial that the low watt-second range be appropriately calibrated.

Dosage		Adverse reactions
Initial	Maintenance	
TDD premie: 0.01-0.02 mg/kg IV TDD 2 wk-2 yr: 0.03-0.05 mg/kg IV TDD newborn and >2 yr: 0.04 mg/kg IV; ½ TDD initially, then ¼ q 4-8 IV × 2	¼-⅓ TDD q 12-24 hr PO, or IV	Ventricular ectopy, tachycardia, fibrillation, atrial tachycardia, AV block, vomiting
1 mg/kg/dose IV (May repeat in 10 min) to max 5 mg/kg	20-50 μg/kg/min IV (adult: 2-4 mg/min)	Seizure, drowsiness, euphoria, muscle twitching; may give ET
15-60 mg/kg/24 hr q 6 hr PO (adult: 300-400 mg q 6 hr PO)	Same	GI symptoms, PVC, syncope, hypotension, anemia
2-6 mg/kg/dose IV slow (adult: 100 mg/dose IV q 10 min prn or 25-50 mg/min, and titrate up to total dose of 1 g)	20-80 μg/kg/min IV (adult: 1-3 mg/min IV) 15-50 mg/kg/24 hr q 4-6 hr PO (adult: 250-500 mg/dose q 4-6 hr PO up to 4 g/24 hr)	Hypotension, lupus-like syndrome, urticaria, GI symptoms
0.01-0.1 mg/kg/dose IV over 10 min (adult: 1 mg/dose IV q 5 min up to 5 mg)	0.5-1.0 mg/kg/24 hr q 6 hr PO (adult: 10-80 mg/dose q 6-8 hr PO)	Bradycardia, hypotension, cardiac failure, asthma, hypoglycemia; do not give to patient with asthma; overdose treated with glucagon 0.1 mg/kg/dose IV
5-10 mg/kg/dose IV over 10 min up to 30 mg/kg)	5 mg/kg/dose q 6-8 hr IV	Hypotension, initial increase of dysrhythmias, nausea
0.1 mg/kg/dose IV over 1-2 min repeated in 10-30 min prn (adult: 5-10 mg/dose IV)	NA	Bradycardia, hypotension, AV block, negative inotropic agent
5 mg/kg/dose IV over 5 min (<40 mg/min) (adult: 100 mg/dose IV q 5 min up to 1 g)	6 mg/kg/24 hr q 12 hr PO (adult: 300 mg/24 hr PO)	Ataxia, nystagmus, hypotension
0.01-0.03 mg/kg/dose IV; repeat q 2-5 min × 2 prn	NA	Tachycardia, mydriasis, dry mouth
0.05-1.5 μg/kg/min IV; begin 0.1 μg/kg/min and increase q 5-10 min (adult: 2-20 μg/min IV)	NA	Tachycardia, PVC

TABLE 6-4. Acute treatment of common dysrhythmias*

Dysrhythmia	Treatment	Comments
SUPRAVENTRICULAR TACHYRHYTHMIA		
Paroxysmal supraventricular (atrial) tachycardia (PAT or PSVT)	Vagotonic maneuvers	Attempt in all patients first: carotid sinus massage, Valsalva's maneuver
With critical hemodynamic compromise	Verapamil DC cardioversion (1-2 watt-sec/kg)	
Without critical hemodynamic compromise	Propranolol Verapamil Digoxin Edrophonium	Do not use digoxin if any question of WPW
Atrial flutter	Digoxin Verapamil DC cardioversion (1-2 watt-sec/kg)	Do not use digoxin with WPW; verapamil slows ventricular response; cardioversion if hemodynamic compromise occurs
Atrial fibrillation	Same as atrial flutter	Same as atrial flutter; considered anticoagulation with prolonged atrial fibrillation
VENTRICULAR TACHYRHYTHMIA		
Premature ventricular contractions (PVC)	Lidocaine Procainamide	Quinidine, procainamide, propranolol, or phenytoin for long-term suppression
Ventricular tachycardia With critical hemodynamic compromise	DC cardioversion (1-2 watt-sec/kg) Lidocaine Bretylium	Administer lidocaine bolus and infusion simultaneously with cardioversion; maintenance therapy includes quinidine or procainamide
Without critical hemodynamic compromise	Lidocaine Procainamide Bretylium DC cardioversion (1-2 watt/sec/kg)	Same as above
Ventricular fibrillation	DC defibrillation (2 watt-sec/kg) Lidocaine Bretylium	Initiate lidocaine infusion or bretylium simultaneously with conversion
DIGITALIS-INDUCED		
Paroxysmal atrial tachycardia (PAT) with block	Potassium chloride (40 mEq/L peripheral IV or 0.5-1.0 mEq/kg/hr central IV) Phenytoin	Stop drug, self-limited; avoid cardioversion, propranolol; worsened by $\downarrow K^+$, $\downarrow Mg^{++}$, $\uparrow Ca^{++}$
PVC or ventricular tachycardia	Potassium chloride Phenytoin Lidocaine	Avoid cardioversion, bretylium; see above
BRADYRHYTHMIA		
Atrioventricular block	Atropine Isoproterenol (temporary) Pacemaker	Be certain not digoxin induced

Modified from Abramowicz, M., editor: Med. Lett. Drugs Ther. **25**:21, 1983.
*CPR and other supportive treatment may be required. Cardiology consultation should be requested.

Paddle size should ensure full contact with the chest (infant: 4.5 cm; children: 8 cm; adult: 13 cm). Many models have a "quick-look" feature, allowing immediate assessment of the rhythm.

c. The paddles are placed on the anterior chest, one to the right of the sternum at the second intercostal space and the other to the left of the midclavicular line at the level of the xiphoid. Electrode cream or paste is applied to the paddles before they are placed on the chest.

d. Defibrillation employs 2 watt-sec/kg initially, which may be repeated if the first attempt is unsuccessful. If the second administration still is unsuccessful, epinephrine and sodium bicarbonate are administered with oxygen and correction of the acid-base status. Defibrillation is then repeated, if necessary.

e. Cardioversion is useful for tachyrhythmias. Commonly 1-2 watt-sec/kg is administered and, if unsuccessful, doubled.

4. Pacemakers, either temporary transvenous or permanent, are the definitive therapeutic modality in the treatment of bradyrhythmias and AV conduction abnormalities associated with hemodynamic compromise. External pacers are also available. Transesophageal pacing may be effective for cardioversion of atrial flutter and supraventricular tachycardias, but experience in children is limited.

DISPOSITION

Cardiology consultation is usually indicated in recurrent or unresponsive dysrhythmias, as well as those causing hemodynamic compromise. These parameters should also determine the need for hospitalization and the urgency of initiating therapy. It is imperative not only to treat the dysrhythmia but to institute a program to prevent recurrence. Caffeine and other stimulants should be avoided.

REFERENCES

Garson, A., Gillette, P.C., Titus, J.L., et al.: Surgical treatment of ventricular tachycardia in infants, N. Engl. J. Med. **310**:1443, 1984.

Goldberger, E.: Treatment of cardiac emergencies, ed. 4, St. Louis, 1985, The C.V. Mosby Co.

Guntheroth, W.G.: Disorders of heart rate and rhythm, Pediatr. Clin. North Am. **25**:869, 1978.

Ludmer, P.L., and Goldschlager, N.: Cardiac pacing in the 1980's, N. Engl. J. Med. **311**:1671, 1984.

Mahoney, L.T., Marvin, W.J., Atkins, D.L., et al.: Pacemaker management for acute onset of heart block in childhood, J. Pediatr. **107**:207, 1985.

McIntyre, K.M., and Lewis, A.J., editors: Textbook of advanced cardiac life support, Dallas, 1981, American Heart Association.

III FLUID AND ELECTROLYTE BALANCE

The management of the pediatric patient with fluid and electrolyte disturbance requires an understanding of maintenance requirements and sources of abnormal losses. It is imperative to correlate history, physical, and laboratory data in patient management.

7 Dehydration

DIAGNOSTIC FINDINGS

Clinical assessment with ancillary laboratory determines the urgency and type of therapy required.

Degree of dehydration

	Mild (<5%)	Moderate (10%)	Severe (15%)
Signs and symptoms			
Dry mucous membrane	±	+	+
Reduced skin turgor	−	±	+
Depressed anterior fontanel	−	+	+
Sunken eyeballs	−	+	+
Hyperpnea	−	±	+
Hypotension (orthostatic)	−	±	+
Increased pulse	−	+	+
Laboratory			
Urine			
Volume	Small	Oliguria	Oliguria/anuria
Specific gravity*	≤1.020[+]	>1.030	>1.035
Blood			
BUN	WNL[+]	Elevated	Very high
pH (arterial)	7.40-7.30[+]	7.30-7.00	<7.10

+, present; −, absent; ±, variable.
*Specific gravity can provide evidence that confirms the physical assessment.
[+]Not usually indicated in mild dehydration.

In the child with only very mild dehydration (2%-3%), a slight decrease in mucosal membrane moisture and the relative dryness and prominence of the papillae of the tongue may be all that is noted on physical examination. In the younger child it is important, as a guide to hydration status, to determine specifically the number of diapers changed and their dampness in the preceding 6-8 hr.

The amount of fluid deficit can be calculated by multiplying the percentage of dehydration by the weight of the child (e.g., a 10 kg child who is 10% dehydrated has a total deficit of 1,000 ml). The electrolyte composition of this fluid deficit is dependent on the rapidity of progression of dehydration (normally 60% extracellular fluid [ECF] and 40% intracellular fluid [ICF]). In general, the percentage of fluid lost from the ECF increases with a more acute progression and decreases with more chronic loss. The electrolyte composition of these compartments may be simplified as ECF: 140 mEq Na^+/L and ICF: 150 mEq K^+/L.

Types of dehydration

The types of dehydration are based on serum sodium reflecting osmolality in the moderately and severely dehydrated patient. Clinical assessment of the patient with hypernatremia tends to underestimate the degree of dehydration:

	Isotonic	Hypotonic	Hypertonic
Serum sodium			
(mEq/L)	130-150	<130	>150
Physical signs			
Skin			
Color	Gray	Gray	Gray
Temperature	Cold	Cold	Cold
Turgor	Poor	Very poor	Fair
Feel	Dry	Clammy	Thick, doughy
Mucous membrane	Dry	Dry	Parched
Sunken eyeballs	+	+	+
Depressed anterior fontanel	+	+	+
Mental status	Lethargic	Coma/seizure	Irritable/seizure
Increased pulse	+ +	+ +	+
Decreased blood pressure	+ +	+ + +	+

+, + +, + + +, relative prominence of finding.

Complications

Complications of dehydration are shock (Chapter 5) and acute tubular necrosis (p. 615).

Ancillary data

The following laboratory findings are indicated for all moderately and severely dehydrated children but rarely for mildly dehydrated youngsters:
1. Serum electrolytes and glucose
2. BUN: often elevated and, with appropriate rehydration, will decrease by 50% over first 24 hr. If fall does not occur, consider hemolytic-uremic syndrome (p. 608). If intake is poor or the child is malnourished, BUN may be low because of low protein
3. Specific gravity of urine to confirm physical findings
4. CBC to assess risk of infection

MANAGEMENT OF SEVERE AND MODERATE DEHYDRATION
Restoration of vascular volume: phase I

Patients require immediate infusion of fluids, particularly those with abnormal vital signs. If possible, orthostatic blood pressure and pulse should be obtained in the recumbent position on older patients with normal vital signs. While the patient goes from a lying to a standing (or sitting) position a decrease of 15 mm Hg in blood pressure or an increase of 20 beats/min in pulse after 2 to 3 min is considered significant. These changes may be seen in the absence of hypovolemia and therefore require clinical correlations.

Fluid therapy

1. D5.9%NS or D5WLR should be given at 20 ml/kg (adult = 1-2 L) over 20-30 min in the moderate or severely dehydrated child.
2. If a poor therapeutic response is noted, the initial infusion should be followed by 10 ml/kg (adult: 0.5-1.0 L) over 20-30 min, assuming normal renal and cardiac function.
3. Glucose should be omitted if diabetic ketoacidosis is the underlying etiology. It is not required if the patient is over 8 yr old and has a normal glucose and nutritional status or is in acute hypovolemic shock on the basis of blood loss.
4. If a poor therapeutic response is noted in the severely dehydrated child following two fluid pushes (i.e., no urine, continued abnormal vital signs, poor perfusion), with ongoing losses or with suspected cardiac or renal disease, central venous pressure or pulmonary capillary wedge pressure may need to be monitored.

Specific therapeutic plans

Case examples of the three major categories of dehydration (isotonic, hypotonic, and hypertonic) are listed below and provide a basis for fluid management. Ongoing abnormal losses need additional replacement therapy based either on approximations (Chapter 8) or by direct determination of the electrolyte composition of fluid losses. Vital signs, intake and output, and ancillary data (electrolytes, BUN, and glucose) must be constantly monitored. These patients require hospital admission.

Isotonic dehydration

1. Initial findings
   a. Preillness weight: 10.0 kg (a 1-yr-old)
   b. Degree of dehydration: moderate (10%)
   c. Body weight on admission: 9.0 kg
   d. Electrolytes:

Na^+ 135 mEq/L K^+ 5 mEq/L Cl^- 115 mEq/L HCO_3^- 12 mEq/L

2. Summary of fluids requirements

	H_2O (ml)	Na^+ (mEq)	K^+ (mEq)
Maintenance	1,000	30	20
	(100 ml/kg)	(3 mEq/kg)	(2 mEq/kg)
Deficit (100 ml/kg)			
ECF (60%)	600	84 (140 mEq × .6)	
ICF (40%)	400		30 (150 mEq × 0.4 × 50% correction)
TOTAL	1,000	84	30

3. Fluid schedule

| | Fluids | |
Phase	Calculation	Administered
I. 0-½ hr	20 ml/kg	200 ml D5W.9%NS or D5WLR over 45-60 min
II. ½-9 hr	½ deficit: 500 ml D5W with 42 mEq NaCl and 15 mEq KCl ⅓ maintenance: 333 ml D5W with 10 mEq NaCl and 7 mEq KCl Total: 833 ml with 52 mEq NaCl and 22 mEq KCl	833 ml (~100 ml/hr) of D5W.45%NS with 22 mEq KCl (~27 mEq/L) (this approximation facilitates care)
III. 9-25 hr	½ deficit ⅔ maintenance	1167 ml (~75 ml/hr) of D5W.45%NS with 28 mEq KCl (~24 mEq/L) (this approximation facilitates care)

NOTE: If patient is acidotic with HCO_3^- <11 mEq/L or pH <7.1 (on basis of metabolic acidosis), ⅓ of sodium should be administered as $NaHCO_3$.

Oral rehydration has been recommended in specific circumstances for children who can tolerate oral fluids and who are under the care of a physician experienced in this technique. Oral glucose facilitates the absorption of sodium and water across mucosal cells of the small intestine. Current recommendations in young children distinguish between fluids used for initial oral rehydration under close supervision and careful monitoring, followed by maintenance solutions:

Composition	Rehydration solution (treatment of acute dehydration)	Maintenance solution (maintenance of hydration)
Sodium	75-90 mEq/L	40-60 mEq/L
Potassium	20-30 mEq/L	20 mEq/L
Glucose	2-2.5 g/dl	2-2.5 g/dl

Hypotonic dehydration

In children the most common form of hyponatremia also is associated with hypovolemia (decreased total body water) (p. 53) caused by abnormal GI losses.
1. Initial findings
  a. Preillness weight: 10.0 kg (a 1 yr old)
  b. Degree of dehydration: moderate (10%)
  c. Body weight on admission: 9.0 kg
  d. Electrolytes:

Na^+ 110 mEq/L K^+ 5 mEq/L Cl^- 90 mEq/L HCO_3^- 12 mEq/L

2. Summary of fluid requirements

	H_2O (ml)	Na^+ (mEq)	K^+ (mEq)
Maintenance	1,000	30	20
	(100 ml/kg)	(3 mEq/kg)	(2 mEq/kg)
Deficit (100 ml/kg)			
ECF (60%)	600	84 (140 mEq $\times$ 0.6)	
ICF (40%)	400		30 (150 mEq $\times$ 0.4 $\times$ 50% correction)
Sodium		125	
TOTAL	1,000	209	30

A. Na^+ required to correct to 135 mEq/L = 135 mEq/L − 110 mEq/L (observed Na^+) = 25 mEq/L

B. Total body water (TBW) (L/kg) = 0.6 L/kg (preillness TBW) − 0.1 L/kg (water loss) = 0.5 L/kg

C. Preillness weight = 10 kg

Sodium deficit = A $\times$ B $\times$ C = 25 mEq/L $\times$ 0.5 L/kg $\times$ 10 kg = 125 mEq

3. Fluid schedule

	Fluids	
Phase	Calculation	Administered
I. 0-½ hr	20 ml/kg	200 ml D5W.9%NS or D5WLR over 45-60 min
II. ½-9 hr	½ deficit: 500 ml D5W with 104 mEq NaCl and 15 mEq KCl ⅓ maintenance: 333 ml D5W with 10 ml NaCl and 7 mEq KCl TOTAL: 833 ml with 114 mEq NaCl and 22 mEq KCl	833 (~100 ml/hr) of D5.9%NS with 22 mEq KCl (~27 mEq KCl/L) (this approximation facilitates care)
III. 9-25 hr	½ deficit ⅔ maintenance	1167 (~75 ml/kg) of D5W.9%NS with 28 mEq KCl (~24 mEq KCl/L) (this approximation facilitates care)

NOTE: If patient is acidotic with HCO_3^- <11 mEq/L or pH <7.1 (on basis of metabolic acidosis), ⅓ of sodium should be administered as $NaHCO_3$.

In the presence of severe hyponatremia with decreased total body water in symptomatic patients, hypertonic 3% saline may be given to raise the serum sodium to 125 mEq/L. A 3% saline solution contains approximately 0.5 mEq Na^+/ml. Patients may be given 3% saline 4 ml/kg IV over 10 min and the response monitored. Once seizures have stopped, one half of the deficit may be corrected over the next 8 hr as outlined in the fluid schedule.

In patients with increased total body water (TBW), whether associated with normal or slightly increased total body sodium, fluid restriction is usually necessary. Excess water may be calculated:

$$\text{Present TBW (L)} = \text{Weight(kg)} \times 0.6$$
$$\text{Desired TBW (L)} = \frac{\text{Weight(kg)} \times 0.6 \times \text{Measured } Na^+ \text{ (mEq/L)}}{\text{Desired } Na^+ \text{ (mEq/L)}}$$
$$\text{Water excess (L)} = \text{Present TBW} - \text{Desired TBW}$$

NOTE: Sodium is usually corrected to 125 mEq/L

In addition, in the moderately symptomatic patient furosemide (Lasix) 1 mg/kg/dose IV should be administered. During the subsequent diuresis, urinary sodium, potassium, and chloride should be measured and replaced milliequivalent for milliequivalent with 3% saline and supplemental potassium chloride (beginning with 20 mEq KCl/L).

Hypernatremic dehydration

Most patients have a deficit of free water, but rapid rehydration often results in serious neurologic complications, including seizures. The degree of hydration is difficult to assess.

If hypotension exists, phase I stabilization is used to expand the intravascular volume—initiating 20 ml/kg of D5W.9%NS or D5WLR over the first hour.

The underlying emphasis of therapy must be a *slow* and deliberate schedule designed to correct deficits over 48 hr. Guidelines include:

1. If the serum sodium is 175 mEq/L or greater, the deficit therapy should decrease serum sodium by 15 mEq/L/day.
2. If the serum sodium is less than 175 mEq/L, the deficit therapy should decrease the serum sodium half the way to normal in the first day of therapy.
3. If the loss is primarily water, some suggest that the water deficit is 50 ml/kg if the Na^+ is 150 mEq/L, 90 ml/kg if 160 mEq/L, and 140 ml/kg if 170 mEq/L. Other recommendations are that:

1. Fluids to be used should be D5W.2%NS. With altered mental status or seizures, higher sodium concentration may be needed.
2. The volume of free water needed to lower a serum sodium above 145 mEq/L by 1 mEq/L is approximately 4 ml/kg of free water, evenly over 48 hr
3. Maintenance fluids should be continued

Ongoing management: phases IV and V

1. Following parenteral hydration, oral fluids should be initiated slowly—initially with Lytren or Pedialyte—advancing the diet slowly in both volume and composition.
2. If the dehydration has followed an episode of acute gastroenteritis, a lactase deficiency is commonly present and a lactose-free formula should be used.
3. Following severe, prolonged diarrhea, an elemental formula such as Pregestimil or Vivonex may be necessary. Such patients require a deliberate, conservative approach, which may necessitate continuous NG feeding of dilute formula (¼-½ strength) and slow advancement to bolus feeding, with subsequent increase in volume and, finally, osmolality (p. 485).

Phases of response

Phase	Therapeutic plan	Pattern of response
I. Up to ½ hr Restoration of vascular volume	20 ml/kg D5W.9%NS or D5WLR over 20-30 min; may repeat 10 ml/kg	Improved vital signs Increased urine flow Improved state of consciousness
II. ½-9 hr Partial restoration of ECF deficit and acid-base status	⅓ maintenance fluids ½ deficit fluids	Gain in body weight Stabilization of vital signs Improved urine flow Partial restoration of normal acid-base status

III. 9-25 hr	⅔ maintenance fluids	Sustained gain in body weight
Restoration of ECF, ICF, and acid-base status	½ deficit fluids	Fall in BUN (50% in 24 hr)
		Sustained urine flow
		Improved electrolytes
IV. 25-48 hr	Ongoing parenteral ± oral hydration	Sustained gain in body weight
Total correction of acid-base and K$^+$ status		Normal electrolytes
	Maintenance fluids and replacement of ongoing losses	
V. 2-14 days	Ongoing oral support	Steady gain in body weight
Restoration of caloric and protein deficits		Plasma constituents normal

MANAGEMENT OF MILD DEHYDRATION (<5%)

1. Oral hydration is usually adequate in the child who is less than 5% dehydrated *if that patient can tolerate oral intake*.
2. If oral fluids are not retained, parenteral fluids should be given. Many children can tolerate fluids after initial phase I flush of 20 ml/kg of D5W.9%NS or D5WLR over 30-45 min. However, if fluids continue to be vomited, the patient then requires admission and calculation of fluids as outlined.
3. Patients require careful monitoring of intake, output, and weight. Laboratory data are rarely necessary.
4. Clear fluids (Table 7-1) should be pushed, although slowly in the child who is vomiting. Do not use rice water, tea, or boiled milk. Many fruit juices are hyperosmolar and may draw water into the intestinal lumen, worsening diarrhea.
5. In infants it is particularly important to provide adequate electrolytes while minimizing potential errors in formulation of solutions. Therefore Lytren, Pedialyte RS, or Infalyte is usually recommended.
6. Once ongoing losses have stopped, the diet may be advanced. Milk may be initiated slowly, although a lactose-free product usually is better tolerated in the child with prolonged (>7 days) gastroenteritis. Applesauce, strained carrots, and bananas have been found useful. Attention should be given to caloric intake to facilitate mucosal healing.

Disposition

If fluids are tolerated, patients with mild dehydration may be discharged if close follow-up and good compliance are ensured and there are no underlying medical conditions that necessitate early intervention (e.g., diabetes and sickle cell disease).

Parental education

1. Give only clear liquids; give as much as your child wants. The following may be used during the first 24 hr:
   a. Pedialyte RS, Lytren, or Infalyte (requires mixing)
   b. Jell-O water—one package strawberry per quart of water (twice as much as usual)

TABLE 7-1. Commonly acceptable clear liquids

Solution	Na$^+$ (mEq/L)	K$^+$ (mEq/L)	Cl$^-$ (mEq/L)	HCO$_3$/citrate (mEq/L)	Glucose (mg/100 mL)	Osmolality (mosm/kg H$_2$O)
Lytren	25	25	30	18	945	290
Pedialyte	45	20	35	30	2,500	250
Pedialyte RS	75	20	65	30	2,500	305
Infalyte	50	20	40	30	2,000	111
Gatorade	28	2			2,105	322
7-Up	4	0.2			3,095	525
Coca-Cola	3	0.1		13.4	1,495	600
Pepsi-Cola	2	0.9		7.3	4,900	672
Jello-O water (½ strength— strawberry)	10	0.1			118*	253

*Long-chain oligosaccharide subject to hydrolysis.

    c. Gatorade
    d. Defizzed, room-temperature soda for older children (>2 yr) if diarrhea is only mild
2. If child is vomiting, give clear liquids *slowly*. In younger children, start with 1 teaspoonful and slowly increase the amount. If vomiting occurs, let your child rest for a while and then try again. About 8 hr after vomiting has stopped, child can gradually return to a normal diet.
3. After 24 hr, your child's diet may be advanced if the diarrhea has improved. If child is taking only formula, mix the formula with twice as much water to make up half-strength formula, which should be given over the next 24 hr. Applesauce, bananas, and strained carrots may be given if child is eating solids.
    If this is tolerated, the child may be advanced to a regular diet over the next 2-3 days.
4. If child has had a prolonged course of diarrhea, it is helpful in the younger child to advance from clear liquids to a soy formula (Isomil, ProSobee, or Soyalac) for 1-2 wk. Children >1 yr should not have cow's milk products (milk, cheese, ice cream, or butter) for several days.
5. Do not use boiled milk. Kool-Aid and soda are not ideal liquids, particularly for younger infants, because they contain few electrolytes.
6. Call physician if:
    a. The diarrhea or vomiting is increasing in frequency or amount
    b. The diarrhea does not improve after 24 hr of clear liquids or does not resolve entirely after 3-4 days
    c. Vomiting continues for more than 24 hr
    d. The stool has blood or the vomited material contains blood or turns green
    e. Signs of dehydration develop, including decreased urination, less moisture in diapers, dry mouth, no tears, weight loss, lethargy, or irritability.

8 Maintenance requirements and abnormalities

MAINTENANCE FLUIDS AND ELECTROLYTES

Fluids

Normal maintenance fluids reflect the necessity to replace daily water and electrolyte losses from the skin and the respiratory, urinary, and gastrointestinal tracts. These may be divided into insensible, urinary, and fecal components; they amount to 100 ml/kg/24 hr up to age 1 yr and decrease thereafter.

Insensible losses (30 ml/kg/24 hr) occur through the skin and respiratory tract. Water loss is affected by humidity, body temperature, respiratory rate, and ambient temperature. Fever increases insensible water loss by 7 ml/kg/24 hr for each degree rise in temperature above 37.2° C (99° F).

Urinary losses (60 ml/kg/24 hr) reflect the solute load and obligate excretion and urine concentration. Normal *fecal* water losses (10 ml/kg/24 hr) are small and, in older children, insignificant.

Water requirements

Children <10 kg	100 ml/kg/24 hr
Children 11-20 kg	1,000 ml plus 50 ml/kg/24 hr for each kg over 10 kg
Children >20 kg	1,500 ml plus 20 ml/kg/24 hr for each kg over 20 kg
Adult	2,400 ml/24 hr

Beyond the newborn period, total body water comprises about 60% of body weight; 40% is intracellular fluid (ICF) and the remaining 20% is extracellular fluid (ECF). The intravascular volume represents 5% of the ECF in adults and is as much as 8% (80 ml/kg) in younger children.

Electrolytes

Cation	Requirement	Compartment
Sodium	3 mEq/kg/24 hr (adult: 80-100 mEq/24 hr)	ECF (includes intravascular)
Potassium	2 mEq/kg/24 hr (adult: 50 mEq/24 hr)	ICF

Osmolality

Because cell membranes are permeable to water and osmotic equilibrium is homeostatically maintained, the volume of ICF is determined by the tonicity of ECF. The osmolality of plasma and therefore ICF can be approximated:

$$\text{Plasma osmolality} = 2 \times (Na^+) + \frac{(Glucose)}{18} + \frac{BUN}{2.8}$$

Plasma osmolality normally ranges between 280-295 mOsm/kg water.

If the measured osmolality is normal but the calculated osmolality is low, the difference most likely is caused by a decrease in serum water content. This can occur in hyperglobulinemia, triglyceridemia, and hyperglycemia.

Acid-base balance

Compensatory mechanisms

The relationship between pH and bicarbonate-carbonic acid concentration is best expressed by the Henderson-Hasselbalch equation:

$$pH = pk + \text{Log}\, \frac{(HCO_3^-)}{(H_2CO_3)} \begin{matrix} \text{Renal} \\ \\ \text{Respiratory} \end{matrix}$$

$$H_2CO_3 = H_2O + \text{Dissolved}\,(CO_2)$$

The renal and respiratory compensatory systems determine acid-base balance.

1. *Respiratory* systems can provide a *rapid* alteration in pH by changing the respiratory rate and tidal volume. The classic example is Kussmaul's pattern breathing in diabetic ketoacidosis.
2. *Kidneys* provide a *slow* response, balancing the excretion of HCO_3^- and the secretion of H^+, primarily by the distal nephron.

   ### Anion gap
   In addition to determining pH, P_{CO_2}, and HCO_3^- as determinants of acid-base balance, the anion gap should be determined in considering potential etiologies:

$$\text{Anion gap} = Na^+ + K^+ - (Cl^- + HCO_3^-)$$

The normal anion gap is 8-12 mEq/L, comprised primarily of phosphates, sulfates, and organic acids. The gap is usually normal in metabolic acidosis secondary to diarrhea where there is a loss of bicarbonate ion through the GI tract and kidneys. It is increased with excessive production of organic acids (ketones), lactic acid (shock, sepsis, CHF), toxins (salicylates) or renal failure. A useful mnemonic for remembering entities that produce a metabolic acidosis with a large anion gap is MUDPIES: *m*ethanol, *u*remia, *di*abetes mellitus, *p*araldehyde overdose, *i*soniazid or *i*ron overdose, *e*thanol or *e*thylene glycol, and *s*alicylate overdose or *s*tarvation.

ELECTROLYTE AND ACID-BASE ABNORMALITIES

The two major cations, sodium and potassium, are the primary determinants of the distribution of water between the ECF and ICF spaces. These compartments are dependent on active transport of potassium into the cell and sodium out of cells by an energy-requiring process.

Sodium

Sodium regulation is a balance of intake, total body water, and excretion through urine, sweat, and feces. Disorders can result in hyponatremia or hypernatremia, both significantly affecting plasma osmolality.

1. *Hyponatremia.* Clinical presentation is variable, reflecting the rapidity of progression and severity of hyponatremia. Early signs may include apathy, difficulty in concentrating, and agitation, progressing to confusion, irritability, coma, and seizures. Nausea, vomiting, muscle weakness and cramps, myoclonus, and decreased deep tendon reflexes may be noted. Several mechanisms may produce hyponatremia, reflecting the balance between total body water and sodium:
   a. Decreased total body water and decreased total body sodium. Examples: renal salt loss (diuretics, adrenal insufficiency, renal tubular acidosis), extrarenal salt loss (severe sweating, cystic fibrosis, GI losses, vomiting, diarrhea), third spacing (burns, peritonitis, pancreatitis)
   b. Increased total body water and normal total body sodium. Examples: syndrome of inappropriate antidiuretic hormone (SIADH) (pulmonary disease, CNS trauma, drugs such as hypoglycemia agents, antineoplastic drugs, tricyclics, and thiazide diuretics), hypothyroidism, severe potassium depletion, psychogenic water drinking
   c. Increased total body water relatively greater than increased total body sodium. Examples: congestive heart failure, renal or hepatic failure, nephrosis, hypoproteinemia
   d. Pseudohyponatremia. Examples: hyperglycemia, hyperproteinemia, hyperlipidemia.
   NOTE: Serum sodium decreases 1.6 mEq/L for each increment of 100 mg/dl rise in serum glucose.
2. *Hypernatremia.* Patients may develop symp-

toms of altered mental status, irritability, seizures, and coma, with associated skeletal muscle rigidity and hyperactive reflexes. This may result from one of two mechanisms:

a. Decreased total body water and normal total body sodium (dehydration). Examples: increased insensible or renal water loss, excessive solute loss (mannitol, urea), abnormal water loss (diarrhea), diabetes insipidus

b. Normal total body water and increased total body sodium. Examples: salt poisoning, rehydration with boiled milk, CNS disease affecting hypothalamus

Potassium

Potassium is of central importance in the maintenance of ICF osmolality. Only 1.5%-2.0% of the total body potassium is ECF as reflected by serum measurements.

During metabolic acidosis, renal secretion of hydrogen ions is increased while that of potassium is decreased. For every 0.1 decrease in pH, serum potassium increases by about 0.5 mEq/L, with a similar reverse relationship.

To alkalinize the urine as required in treatment of barbiturate or aspirin ingestions, adequate amounts of potassium must be administered to facilitate renal excretion of sodium bicarbonate.

1. *Hypokalemia*. Patients may have muscle weakness, abdominal distension and decreased bowel sounds (ileus), impaired renal concentrating ability, and hypochloremic alkalosis. Delayed ventricular depolarization is noted with a relatively flat T wave on ECG. Decreased potassium commonly results from excessive loss of potassium from the GI tract, kidneys (diuretic, renal tubular acidosis), drug ingestion, and insulin or glucose therapy.

Significant hypokalemia (3.0-3.5 mEq/L), especially in patients taking digoxin or in those with myocarditis, should be treated cautiously. Such patients may receive 0.1-0.2 mEq/kg infusions of KCl every 4-6 hr while their serum levels are monitored. Larger boluses ideally should be given through a central line.

2. *Hyperkalemia*. The primary toxicity of cardiac conduction is common. A peaked T wave progresses to a widened QRS and ventricular dysrhythmias, and muscle weakness frequently is noted. Renal or metabolic disease may be present, as well as acidosis or excessive intake. Hemolysis of red blood cells during heelsticks or venipuncture may artificially elevate the measured serum potassium.

Acid base

Alterations in acid-base status, which represent a balance of compensatory mechanisms (p. 52), may be summarized as follows:

	pH	P_{CO_2}	HCO_3^-
Metabolic acidosis	↓ *	↓	↓
Metabolic alkalosis	↑ *	↑	↑
Respiratory acidosis	↓	↑ *	↑
Respiratory alkalosis	↑	↓ *	↓

*Indicates primary abnormality.

NOTE: Mixed metabolic and respiratory disorders are common. In a simple disturbance without compensatory reaction both the Pa_{CO_2} and HCO_3^- abnormalities are in the same direction.

Metabolic acidosis is initially accompanied by compensatory tachypnea and may be associated with cardiac dysrhythmias and cellular dysfunction. Initially, Pa_{CO_2} decreases, with a fall in Pa_{CO_2} of 1-1.5 times the reduction in HCO_3^-. Specific correction of the underlying condition requires treatment (often correction of intravascular volume); additionally, it may require supplemental HCO_3^- therapy. If the HCO_3^- is ≤10-11 mEq/L acutely, it should be corrected to at least the 12-15 mEq/L range. The initial correction should replace a maximum of half of the deficit:

Deficit mEq HCO_3^- = Weight (kg) × Base deficit
(mEq/L desired − mEq/L observed) × 0.6 × 0.5

Metabolic alkalosis may be accompanied by muscle cramps, weakness, paresthesias, seizures, hyperreflexia, tetany, and dysrhythmias. The $PaCO_2$ increases 0.5-1.0 mm Hg for each mEq/L increase in HCO_3^-. Primary treatment of the causative condition often requires restoration of intravascular volume or stopping diuretics, as appropriate. If alkalosis is severe, with a pH of 7.7 (lower if symptomatic), treatment options include:

1. Acetazolamide (Diamox) 5 mg/kg/24 hr q 6-24 hr (adult: 250-375 mg/24 hr) PO, IV. Use only if K^+ is normal: **or**
2. Ammonium chloride (NH_4Cl) 150-300 mg/kg/24 hr q 6 hr (adult: 8-12 g/24 hr) PO

ELECTROLYTE COMPOSITION OF BODY FLUIDS

Electrolyte composition of body fluids may be useful in delineating potential abnormalities associated with fluid loss.

ELECTROLYTE COMPOSITION OF BODY FLUIDS

Fluid	Na^+ (mEq/L)	K^+ (mEq/L)	Cl^- (mEq/L)	H^+ (mEq/L)	HCO_3^- (mEq/L)
Sweat	10-30	3-10	10-35		
Gastric	20-80	5-20	100-150	90	
Pancreas	120-140	5-40	50-120		90
Small intestine	100-140	15-40	90-130		25
Diarrhea	10-90	10-80	10-110		45

REFERENCES

American Academy of Pediatrics Committee on Nutrition: Use of oral fluid therapy and post-treatment feeding following enteritis in children in a developed country, Pediatrics **75**:358, 1985.

Finberg, L., Harper, P.A., Harrison, H.E., et al.: Oral rehydration for diarrhea, J. Pediatr. **101**:497, 1982.

Finberg, L., Kravath, R.E., and Fleischman, A.R.: Water and electrolytes in pediatrics: physiology, pathophysiology, and treatment, Philadelphia, 1982, W.B. Saunders Co.

Perkins, R.M., and Levin, D.L.: Common fluid and electrolyte problems in the pediatric intensive care unit, Pediatr. Clin. North Am. **27**:567, 1980.

Tamer, A.M., Friedman, L.B., Maxwell, S.R.W., et al.: Oral rehydration of infants in a large urban U.S. medical center, J. Pediatr. **107**:14, 1985.

Winter, R.W.: Principles of pediatric fluid therapy, ed. 2, Boston, 1982, Little, Brown & Co.

IV NEWBORN EMERGENCIES

ANTHONY F. PHILIPPS

The physician faced with a distressed newborn in the delivery room or emergency room may be forced to make rapid therapeutic decisions without an adequate data base. Under these conditions, basic guidelines for resuscitation, diagnosis, and management provide a basis for intervention.

9 Resuscitation in the delivery room

ANTICIPATION

Maternal factors associated with poor outcome for fetus are:

1. Diabetes, chronic hypertension, Rh sensitization, multifetal gestation, or history of oligohydramnios or polyhydramnios
2. Previous obstetric history: premature delivery or miscarriage, perinatal loss, previous growth retardation, or malformed neonate
3. Intrapartum disorders: toxemia of pregnancy, prolonged rupture of membranes, clinical chorioamnionitis, prolonged labor, breech or face presentation, abruptio placentae, or placenta previa

Fetal factors associated with poor outcome are:

1. Lack of fetal well-being: history of decreased fetal movement, heart rate abnormalities (particularly late or severe variable decelerations), meconium-stained amniotic fluid, or history of abnormal nonstress or stress test
2. Fetal immaturity: prematurity as estimated by dates, ultrasound, uterine size, or amniocentesis (lecithin/sphingomyelin [L/S] ratio <2.0 or absent phosphatidylglycerol suggests inadequate lung maturation).
3. Fetal growth: history of poor intrauterine growth or postdate delivery

PREPARATION
Equipment

Adequate preparation is essential.

1. Temperature: radiant warmer physically present and preheated. Special wraps (e.g., Thinsulate, manufactured by 3M) are specifically designed to function as an efficient insulating head wrap and bunting.
2. Airway and ventilation (Chapter 4): resuscitation bag with various face masks and ET tubes
3. Drugs (Table 9-1)
   NOTE: Parenteral fluids or drugs that contain benzoyl alcohol should not be used for neonates. In addition, vials should not contain this preservative.
4. Materials to initiate administration of parenteral fluids: normal equipment plus umbilical catheterization equipment, such as catheter (3.5 and 5.0 French [Fr]), three-way stopcock, and sterile umbilical artery catheterization tray containing towels, gauze pads, scissors, hemostats, curved iris forceps, scalpel, and umbilical tape
5. Warm dry towels to dry infant
6. Suctioning device such as DeLee with trap, wall suction, or bulb syringe

Personnel

A team approach is absolutely necessary in the resuscitation of a severely depressed neonate. This calls for close cooperation among physicians, nurses, and nurse practitioners. Practice drills are strongly recommended.

Optimally, the team should be familiar with principles of resuscitation and management of neonatal asphyxia, including bag and mask ventilation, ET intubation, chest massage and umbilical vein and artery catheterization.

TABLE 9-1. Drugs used in resuscitation of newborns

Drug	Availability	Indications	Dosage
Atropine	0.1 mg/ml	Bradycardia unresponsive to ventilation	0.01-0.03 mg/kg IV, ET
Epinephrine	1:10,000	Bradycardia	0.1 ml/kg IV, ET
Calcium gluconate	10% (100 mg/ml) 0.45 mEq Ca/ml)	Decreased cardiac output (controversial)	100 mg (1 ml)/kg IV
Calcium chloride	10% (100 mg/ml) 1.36 mEq Ca/ml	Decreased cardiac output (controversial)	33 mg (0.3 ml)/kg IV
Sodium bicarbonate	8.4% (1 mEq/ml)	Metabolic acidosis	1-2 mEq/kg (dilute 1:2 with sterile water to avoid hyperosmolarity)
Dextrose (glucose)	10%-25%	Hypoglycemia	4 ml (10%)/kg for term or preterm, given slowly over 10 min IV
Albumin	5%	Hypovolemic shock	10 ml/kg IV
Naloxone (Narcan)	0.02 mg/ml (neonatal)	Narcotic-induced respiratory depression	0.01 mg (0.5 ml)/kg IV (may go much higher)

TABLE 9-2. Apgar score

Sign	Score		
	0	**1**	**2**
Muscle tone (*Activity*)	Limp	Some flexion	Active, good flexion
Pulse	Absent	<100/min	>100/min
Reflex irritability* (*Grimace*)	No response	Some grimace or avoidance	Cough, cry, or sneeze
Color (*Appearance*)	Blue, pale	Pink body, blue hands/feet	Pink
Respirations	Absent	Slow, irregular, ineffective	Crying, rhythmic, effective

*Nasal or oral suction catheter stimulus.

MANAGEMENT

Immediately after delivery in high-risk situations if poor color or flaccidity are evident or if there is no cry:

1. Maintain temperature. Minimize heat loss by towel drying and placing infant under radiant warmer (avoid overheating) or in warm blankets.
2. Assess respiratory pattern and rate: heart rate by auscultation or cord palpation and by color. Determine presence of any major external anomalies (e.g., myelomeningocele, omphalocele).
3. Calculate Apgar score (Table 9-2) at 1 and 5 min, evaluating *a*ppearance (color), *p*ulse, *g*rimace (reflex irritability), *a*ctivity (muscle tone), and *r*espirations. The score is a useful indicator of neonatal depression.

GENERAL RESUSCITATIVE MEASURES
(Chapters 4 and 5 and Fig. 9-1)

Although intrapartum asphyxia may be the result of a variety of insults, apnea or hypoventilation with concomitant cyanosis and bradycardia is the most common symptom. If neonatal hypoxemia is not rapidly treated, tissue hypoxia,

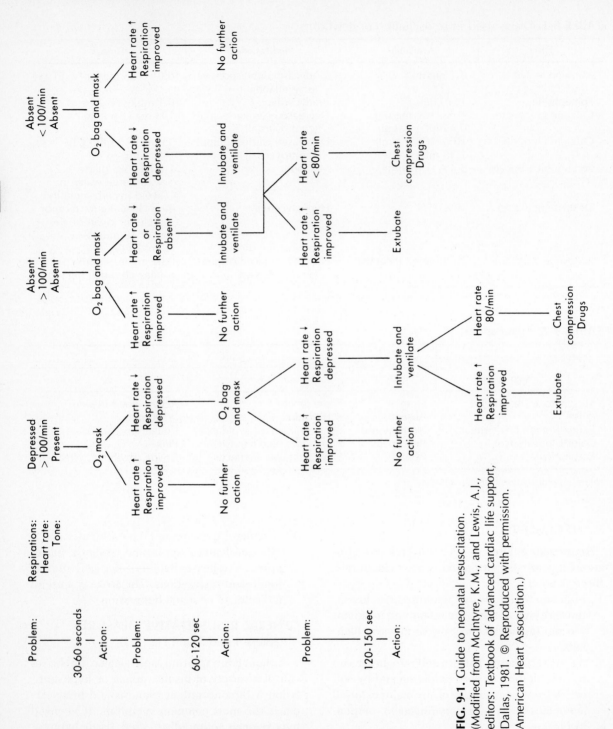

FIG. 9-1. Guide to neonatal resuscitation. (Modified from McIntyre, K.M., and Lewis, A.J., editors: Textbook of advanced cardiac life support, Dallas, 1981. © Reproduced with permission. American Heart Association.)

acidosis, and resultant organ damage (particularly to the CNS, heart, and kidneys) will occur.

1. Gently suction oropharynx and nares to remove amniotic fluid. Stimulate trunk and legs gently.
2. Place infant in Trendelenburg's position in the radiant warmer.
3. Use deep airway suction if apneic (not routinely done because of reflex bradycardia when performed within 5 min of delivery).
4. Assess airway and, with evidence of nasal obstruction or mandibular hypoplasia, insert oral airway.
   a. If infant is apneic with no response to stimulation, begin bag and mask inflation at 20-30/min. Insufflation bags should be able to deliver 100% oxygen. Positive pressure ventilation administered with a bag and mask is optimally achieved with the infant's head in the "sniffing" position. It is often helpful to place a towel under the infant's head to displace the coronal plane of the head slightly anteriorly from the coronal plane of the thorax.
   b. If poor response (no increase in heart rate or improvement in color) to previous measures, intubate and continue with bag to ET tube ventilation.
5. Assess heart rate and, if <80/min and not readily responsive to ventilation, initiate closed chest massage at midsternum. Heart rate is a good parameter in assessing the efficacy of resuscitation efforts.

Drugs are usually not necessary for the neonate with asphyxia unless there is vascular collapse or decreased cardiac output that is not responsive to previous resuscitative measures. In these situations, intravenous sodium bicarbonate and calcium as well as intravenous or intratracheal epinephrine may be warranted.

Volume resuscitation is infrequently indicated since most asphyxiated infants have normal or increased blood volume. Fluids may be appropriate if there are signs of inadequate blood volume (poor perfusion, metabolic acidosis, or

hypoperfusion). Hypovolemia most commonly occurs with placenta previa, placentae abruptio, and twin-twin or fetomaternal transfusions. Volume expansion with solutions such as Plasmanate (5% of albumin) or fresh frozen plasma is preferred.

Factors that should be considered when resuscitation efforts are unsuccessful include equipment failure, ET tube malposition, pneumothorax, or congenital anomalies such as diaphragmatic hernia and pulmonary hypoplasia.

Umbilical catheterization

In an emergency, the umbilical cord provides easy access for administration of intravascular drugs and fluid.

1. Restrain extremities, prepare abdomen and cord with antiseptic solution (surgical scrub), and drape lower abdomen and legs with sterile towels.
2. Trim umbilical cord to 1-2 cm above skin surface (vertical traction with hemostats will control venous bleeding).
3. Identify umbilical vein (single, thin wall, large-diameter lumen) and umbilical artery (paired, thick wall, small-diameter lumen).

Umbilical venous catheterization

This catheterization technique is easier and more practical in the delivery room. The vessel can be catheterized in the first 4-5 days after delivery as well.

1. Insert a 5 Fr end-hole type catheter (previously filled with saline solution and attached to a three-way stopcock and syringe) into the lumen. Gently pass the catheter cephalad in the direction of the liver for 5-8 cm or until blood return is noted. If resistance to passage is encountered once the catheter has gone beyond the peritoneal fascia, the tip is probably in a portal vein radical and the catheter should be pulled back until blood can be withdrawn smoothly.
2. Remove catheter when resuscitation is completed. Prolonged maintenance of indwelling umbilical venous catheters is associated with

neonatal bacteremia and portal vein thrombosis.

Umbilical arterial catheterization

This catheterization technique requires more time than umbilical venous catheterization and may not be appropriate for achieving vascular access in an emergency.

1. Gently dilate vessel with an iris forceps. Avoid trauma to the vessel wall.
2. Insert a 3.5 or 5.0 Fr end-hole catheter (previously filled with saline solution and attached to a three-way stopcock and syringe) into the lumen until blood return is noted, then advance an additional 2-3 cm. Catheter should be angled slightly caudad to conform with the direction of the umbilical arteries. Estimate length of catheter required for proper insertion, using markings on catheter and Fig. 9-2.
3. Resistance to passage is caused by vasoconstriction and usually can be overcome by gentle, steady pressure. Reposition or replace catheter if resistance persists. Observe the extremities and buttocks for evidence of arterial obstruction.
4. If the catheter is to be left in place after the resuscitation, check the position of the tip with abdominal roentgenography. Optimal position above the diaphragm is at T6-T9 and below the diaphragm at the aortic bifurcation (L4-L5). A catheter tip facing caudad is in the external iliac artery and must be removed. Secure catheter with 3-0 silk pursestring suture through the cord.

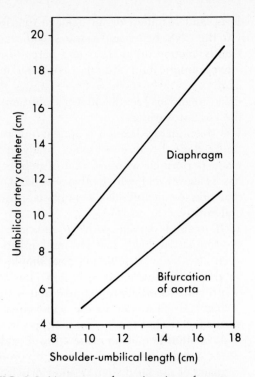

FIG. 9-2. Nomogram for estimation of proper length of umbilical artery catheter (distance from lateral end of clavicle to umbilicus vs. length of catheter to reach designated level). (From Dunn, P.M.: Arch. Dis. Child. **41**:69, 1966.)

5. Infuse parenteral solutions at a rate of at least 2-3 ml/hr IV. Heparinized saline (1 unit/ml) may be used but is usually unnecessary. Hyperosmolar solutions infused through the catheter may cause significant ischemic reactions.

10 Distress at birth

Several diagnostic entities cause distress of the newborn at birth.

INTRAPARTUM ASPHYXIA

1. **Etiology:** decreased transplacental gas exchange with resultant fetal hypoxemia, acidosis, and ischemia
2. **Diagnostic findings:** pallor or cyanosis, bradycardia, apnea, and flaccidity
3. **Management:** resuscitation as outlined

MECONIUM ASPIRATION (Chapter 11)

1. **Etiology:** occurs in 10% of patients with meconium-stained amniotic fluid caused by intrapartum asphyxia. Asphyxia promotes gasping, allowing meconium passage below the cords but probably not distally until after birth.
2. **Diagnostic findings:** meconium staining and other signs of asphyxia
3. **Management**
   a. Clear mouth and pharynx of meconium with DeLee suction or bulb before delivery of thorax from perineum or hysterotomy site.
   b. After delivery, perform laryngoscopy for further evidence of meconium. If meconium is present at cords or if newborn is severely asphyxiated, intubate, and use ET tube to suction out remaining aspirated meconium by mouth.
   c. Begin other measures of resuscitation involving support of ventilation and circulation only after *step b* is carried out.

MATERNAL DRUGS

Narcotics and magnesium sulfate may cause depression of the newborn.
1. **Etiology:** transplacental passage of agent with subsequent central or neuromuscular depression
2. **Diagnostic findings:** apnea, decreased muscle tone
3. **Management**
   a. If depression is believed to be the result of narcotics, administer naloxone (Narcan) 0.01 mg/kg/dose q 3-5 min prn IM or IV, and support. Larger doses may be required.
   b. If magnesium sulfate is suspected, give calcium gluconate 100 mg/kg/dose IV slowly with cardiac monitoring. In premature infants, temporary artificial ventilation may be required.

CONGENITAL ANOMALIES (Chapter 20)
Upper airway disorders

1. **Etiology:** choanal atresia, micrognathia, and macroglossia are most common. Less common causes include laryngeal atresia, cyst, or web; vascular ring; goiter; cystic hygroma; vocal cord paralysis; and tracheal anomalies.
2. **Diagnostic findings:** retraction and cyanosis, apnea, and inspiratory stridor. May note neck mass, hypoplastic mandible, etc. Passage of feeding tube or suction catheter through the nasopharynx is impossible in choanal atresia.

3. **Management**
   a. Oxygen and oral airway. Prone position, with micrognathia
   b. Intubation if obstruction unrelieved or apnea develops. Laryngoscopy may reveal cause of obstruction.
   c. Surgical consultation as needed

Lower airway and pulmonary disorders

1. **Etiology:** diaphragmatic hernia, tracheoesophageal fistula (TEF), or Potter's syndrome. Less commonly observed are neonatal chylothorax, congenital pneumonia, cystic adenomatoid malformation of the lung, and lobar emphysema.
2. **Diagnostic findings**
   a. Severe respiratory distress with poor air entry and cyanosis
      (1) Scaphoid abdomen prominent in diaphragmatic hernia
      (2) TEF suggested by excessive mucous production, crowing, hoarse cry, and inability to place NG tube in stomach. Usually associated with esophageal atresia
      (3) Potter's syndrome suggested by resistance to lung inflation, lung hypoplasia, early pneumothorax, flattened facies, redundant skin folds, renal dysgenesis, and oligohydramnios
   b. X-ray studies. Characteristic presentation in diaphragmatic hernia (unilateral lung hypoplasia with multiple bowel loops in chest), TEF (NG tube coiled in air-filled esophageal pouch), and Potter's syndrome (lung hypoplasia often with pneumothorax)
3. **Management:** high index of suspicion is important, particularly if oligohydramnios or scaphoid abdomen is present.
   a. Oxygen, intubation, and ventilatory support as indicated. Bag and mask ventilation in diaphragmatic hernia will inflate stomach that has already herniated and will compromise ventilation further.
   b. Early insertion of NG tube and suction for decompression
   c. Portable ultrasound to identify kidneys, cystic tumors, or pleural fluid (chylothorax)
   d. Appropriate surgical consultation

11 Postnatal emergencies

Cardiovascular disorders

DYSRHYTHMIAS (Chapter 6)

In the premature infant, the most common dysrhythmias are premature atrial and ventricular beats.

Paroxysmal atrial tachycardia (PAT) may require therapy if it persists over 1 hr or there is associated hemodynamic compromise. Management includes:

1. Propranolol 0.05-0.15 mg/kg/dose IV over 10 min. Maintenance of 0.2-0.5 mg/kg/24 hr q 6 hr PO
2. Use of digoxin (Table 16-3)
3. Avoidance of vagal stimulation
4. If condition deteriorates, synchronized cardioversion at 2 watt-sec/kg
5. Consultation with pediatric cardiologist

CYANOTIC CONGENITAL HEART DISEASE
(Table 16-2)

This condition results from fixed right-to-left shunt at any level. It is more common in infants of diabetic mothers and in those with chromosomal disorders. Most prevalent lesions in the neonate include transposition of the great vessels, tetralogy of Fallot, and pulmonary atresia.

Evaluation is outlined in Chapter 17, and consultation with a pediatric cardiologist is advised. Echocardiogram and catheterization may be indicated.

PERSISTENCE OF FETAL CIRCULATION (OR PERSISTENT PULMONARY HYPERTENSION)

Persistent fetal circulation (PFC) is more common than "fixed shunt" disorders, which it may mimic. It is commonly seen in term or near-term neonates, in those with significant intrapartum asphyxia, and in infants delivered postdate. PFC is occasionally associated with polycythemia or diaphragmatic hernias. PFC also may complicate pulmonary disease, such as hyaline membrane disease (HMD), meconium aspiration syndrome (MAS), or bacterial pneumonia. It is presumed to be caused by failure of the pulmonary arteriolar bed to vasodilate, with resultant continued pulmonary hypertension and right-to-left shunting through fetal channels (ductus arteriosus and foramen ovale).

Diagnostic findings

Cyanosis with quiet but persistent tachypnea in "pure" PFC occurs in the first 12 hr of life. If associated with pulmonary disease (e.g., MAS and diaphragmatic hernias), there may be significant dyspnea with retractions.

Ancillary data

1. X-ray films: usually normal with "pure" PFC. May be suggestive of decreased pulmonary vascularity. There may be associated findings in PFC with pulmonary disorders.
2. ECG: nonspecific right ventricular hypertrophy

3. ABG determinations show PaO$_2$ <50 mm Hg in room air without significant response to 100% oxygen (shunt steady). Radial artery PaO$_2$ is often 15 mm Hg above umbilical artery PaO$_2$, suggesting ductal shunting. Acidosis secondary to hypoxemia may be present. PaCO$_2$ is usually normal or decreased.

Management

1. Consultation with a tertiary care facility and with pediatric cardiologists should be obtained. A "fixed shunt" disorder cannot be excluded without further evaluation.
2. A minority of patients respond to increased ambient oxygen. Therapy using respiratory alkalosis achieved by curare and ventilator-assisted hyperventilation may be useful.
3. Other therapy (tolazoline or dopamine) may be useful but should not be administered with an uncertain diagnosis and without the support of a tertiary care center because of the lability of these patients and the systemic side effects encountered with drug therapy.

CONGESTIVE HEART FAILURE (Chapter 16)

Congestive heart failure (CHF) occurs most commonly as a result of a patent ductus arteriosus (PDA) in the premature neonate, often during recovery from hyaline membrane disease (HMD). Other causes include coarctation of the aorta, aortic stenosis or atresia, hypoplastic left ventricle, tachyrhythmias, viral myocarditis, arteriovenous fistula (CNS or liver), and structural cardiac lesions, with either a single large shunt or shunts at multiple levels. "Acyanotic" structural lesions (septal defects) rarely cause CHF in the first weeks.

Fetal echocardiography has made intrauterine diagnosis possible. CHF in the fetus may be demonstrated by scalp edema, pericardial effusion, ascites, and decreased fetal movement.

Shock may develop rapidly with closing of the PDA if there is a PDA-dependent lesion such as coarctation or critical pulmonary stenosis.

Patients should be transferred to a tertiary care facility after appropriate consultation and initial stabilization.

Endocrine/metabolic disorders

HYPOGLYCEMIA (Chapter 38)

Hypoglycemia is defined as <30 mg/dl in term infants and <20 mg/dl for premature infants.

Etiology

1. Most commonly caused by decreased availability of mobilizable substrates, such as in intrauterine growth retardation, postdate neonate, asphyxia, cold stress, sepsis, polycythemia, or prematurity
2. Less commonly caused by hypermetabolic states, usually a result of erythroblastosis or hyperinsulinism in infants of diabetic mothers

Diagnostic findings

1. Adrenergic: pallor, cool extremities, irritability
2. Central: jitteriness, poor feeding, seizures, apnea

NOTE: Hypoglycemia may not be accompanied by identifiable symptoms, particularly in the premature or asphyxiated newborn

Management

Anticipatory management is important, particularly in premature and high-risk infants.

1. In initial management, maintain a high index of suspicion with a history of maternal diabetes, asphyxia, sepsis, and other risk factors.
2. If stable condition and >34 wk, begin enteral feedings with 15-30 ml of D5W, and advance to formula or breast milk, as tolerated, with q 2-3 hr feedings. Perform serial Dextrostix or Chemstrip tests until three normal deter-

minations are recorded. At least one confirmatory serum glucose determination is indicated.

3. If unstable or premature <34 wk, begin D10W at 100-150 ml/kg/24 hr IV. Enteral feeding when stable
4. If symptomatic or serum glucose <20 mg/dl, administer D10W 4 ml/kg IV over 5 min. Follow by constant infusion of D10W 2-4 ml/kg/hr. Avoid high concentrations of glucose in hyperinsulinemic or premature neonates because of the risks of rebound hypoglycemia and hypertonicity.
5. If neither IV glucose solution nor infusion sites are available, give glucagon 0.1-0.2 mg/kg IM and consider cutdown. Glucagon will not be effective in states of limited substrate availability, such as prematurity and growth retardation.

HYPOCALCEMIA

Hypocalcemia is defined as serum calcium <7 mg/dl. It is a transient disorder in the neonate with asphyxia or prematurity or in infants of diabetic mothers.

Diagnostic findings

Findings may include jitteriness and irritability, occasional seizures in infants, low serum calcium, and ECG with prolonged QT interval.

Management

1. Calcium gluconate 100 mg (1 ml)/kg IV slowly. Watch for extravasation and bradycardia.
2. Begin maintenance calcium gluconate 200-300 mg/kg/24 hr q 6-8 hr IV or PO until full feedings are tolerated. Adjust diet.
3. If little response, obtain serum magnesium. If magnesium <1.5 mEq/L, treat with magnesium sulfate 20 mg/kg/dose q 12 hr IV.

OTHER DISORDERS

1. Hyponatremia (Chapter 8)
2. Hypernatremia (Chapter 8)
3. Hyperkalemia (Chapter 8)

Gastrointestinal disorders

A majority of significant gastrointestinal diseases in neonates are caused by obstruction, usually evident shortly after birth or in the first few weeks of life (Chapter 44).

ESOPHAGEAL ATRESIA AND TRACHEOESOPHAGEAL FISTULA

Tracheoesophageal fistula (TEF) symptoms may or may not be present at birth. The incidence of premature delivery increases with TEF and polyhydramnios. Esophageal atresia is associated with fistula between the trachea and distal esophagus in 85% of cases.

Diagnostic findings

Early respiratory distress in "mucousy" infant with hoarse cry or stridor. Vomiting and aspiration occur when infant is fed. NG tube will not pass. Small fistula causes coughing with feeding. Associated anomalies such as imperforate anus, limb defects, and vertebral or renal anomalies may be present.

Complications

Aspiration pneumonia

Ancillary data

1. X-ray studies. AP chest film shows tip of NG tube in air-filled upper esophageal pouch.
2. Contrast study should not be attempted without surgical consultation.

Management

1. Administer oxygen, keep NPO, and replace fluid deficits (Chapter 7) as required.
2. Elevate patient's head 15-20 degrees (may raise end of incubator or crib).
3. Perform intermittent low suction with double-lumen nasoesophageal tube (Replogle tube) or equivalent.
4. Arrange immediate surgical consultation.

OBSTRUCTIVE LESIONS

Obstructive lesions are most commonly congenital in origin, with an overall rate of 1:2,700 live births.

Etiology

1. Pyloric stenosis (p. 501)
2. Intestinal atresia: proximal jejunum and distal ileum most common sites. Duodenal atresia is common with Down's syndrome.
3. Meconium ileus: ileal obstruction is most commonly associated with cystic fibrosis
4. Volvulus (p. 502)
5. Imperforate anus: if associated with intestinal obstruction, perineal fistula is either absent or inadequate to permit elimination. Incidence of associated malformations (vertebral, cardiovascular, and tracheoesophageal) is as high as 50%.
6. Hirschsprung's disease (p. 496)

Diagnostic findings

1. High obstructions (mid-jejunum and above) are associated with less abdominal distension but persistent vomiting, which may be bilious if distal to the ampulla of Vater. Patients are hungry after emesis. They may have history of polyhydramnios.
2. Low obstructions are associated with more distension, less vomiting, and only occasionally a history of polyhydramnios. Palpable and visible bowel loops may be prominent. Respiratory distress or apnea as a result of elevated intraabdominal pressure and limited diaphragmatic excursion may be noted. High-pitched bowel sounds are often present.
3. Palpable mass, if present, is caused by volvulus or meconium ileus. Perforation may be accompanied by hypotension and sepsis.

Ancillary data

1. X-ray studies. Supine and upright abdominal films are often helpful, demonstrating air-fluid levels, distended bowel, and mass effects. Free air may be noted in the presence of a perforation.
2. Electrolytes and CBC

Management

1. Oxygen and fluid deficit replacement as required (Chapter 7); NPO

2. NG tube for drainage at atmospheric pressure or intermittent low suction
3. Immediate surgical and radiologic consultation as indicated by specific process

ABDOMINAL WALL DEFECTS

These occur in 1:2,500 live births.
1. Gastroschisis: abdominal wall defect lateral to umbilicus with herniation of abdominal viscera. Associated anomalies are rare.
2. Omphalocele: herniation of abdominal viscera through omphalomesenteric duct into umbilical cord. Sac may rupture. Associated congenital anomalies are common.

Diagnostic findings

A mass is noted at birth either in the cord itself (omphalocele) or paraumbilically (gastroschisis). The physician may visualize bowel loops, stomach, and, occasionally, the liver within the herniated mass. With the advent of intrauterine ultrasound, prenatal diagnosis is relatively common.

Management

1. Promptly prevent fluid loss. Cover herniated viscera loosely with saline-moistened gauze, and enclose mass and lower portion of patient in a plastic wrap or aluminum foil.
2. Avoid hypothermia via heated incubator. Radiant warmer accelerates water loss and should be avoided.
3. Promptly administer IV fluids: D5W.2%NS at 20-40 ml/kg over 2-6 hr.
4. Insert NG tube for drainage.
5. Monitor blood pressure, urine output, and serum electrolytes.
6. Arrange immediate surgical consultation.

NECROTIZING ENTEROCOLITIS

Ischemia of the bowel, with complicating bacterial invasion and consequent pneumatosis intestinalis, is the most likely cause of necrotizing enterocolitis (NEC) and may quickly progress to intestinal necrosis. NEC is commonly found in middle to distal ileum, but involvement of the stomach, as well as small and large intestines, has been reported. Prematurity, high tonicity of feedings, umbilical catheterization, hypoxic stress, polycythemia, and *Klebsiella* nosocomial infection have been implicated as risk factors. NEC occurs predominantly in preterm infants after the onset of feedings.

Diagnostic findings

Insidious onset of abdominal distension, with significant gastric residuals (often bile stained). Early nonspecific signs of lethargy and temperature instability may progress to hypotension, bloody stools, tachypnea, and apnea.

Ancillary data

1. X-ray studies. Early findings may include intestinal dilation with or without evidence of bowel-wall edema. The presence of pneumatosis intestinalis, with bubbly or linear air shadows in the bowel wall, confirms the diagnosis. Portal venous gas, which is occasionally seen, is a poor prognostic sign. Free air suggests intestinal perforation.
2. WBC is markedly elevated or depressed, with a shift to the left and presence of toxic granulations. Thrombocytopenia (platelet count <50,000/mm^3) is present in 50% of patients.
3. Serum electrolyte and glucose concentrations may demonstrate hyperglycemia and hyponatremia.
4. ABG often show a significant metabolic acidosis.
5. Cultures of blood and stool should be taken before antibiotic therapy.
6. Desseminated intravascular coagulation (DIC) may be demonstrated by coagulation studies.

Management

1. Intravenous hydration, with an initial bolus of D5W.2%NS or D5W.45%NS at 20-40 ml/kg over 2-3 hr if fluid deficit is present
2. NG tube for intermittent low suction
3. Antibiotics initiated after cultures are obtained:

   a. Ampicillin 100 mg/kg/24 hr q 12 hr IV **and**
   b. Gentamicin 5.0 mg/kg/24 hr q 12 hr IM or IV (if <7 days of age); 7.5 mg/kg/24 hr q 8 hr IM or IV (if 7-28 days of age) (if resistance is not a problem, kanamycin 15 mg/kg/24 hr q 12 hr IM may be substituted for gentamicin)
   c. If rapid development of symptoms and signs occur, *Clostridium* species must be considered as an etiologic agent. Initiation of chloramphenicol 25 mg/kg/24 hr q 12 hr IV is warranted. Blood levels must be monitored closely.
4. Surgical consultation

Hematologic disorders

ANEMIA (Chapter 26)

Normal hematocrit at birth is 45%-60%.

Etiology

1. Hemorrhage
   a. Prenatal or intrapartum hemorrhage or transfusion (e.g., abruptio placentae or fetomaternal transfusion)
   b. Internal hemorrhage caused by trauma or bleeding dyscrasia
2. Hemolysis
   a. Immune: erythroblastosis fetalis (EBF) caused by Rh, ABO, or minor blood incompatibilities
   b. Nonimmune: relatively uncommon; caused by RBC membrane defect (glucose-6-phosphate dehydrogenase [G6PD] deficiency, spherocytosis, etc.) or intravascular coagulation

Diagnostic findings

1. Pallor, tachypnea, weak pulse, hypotension (BP <30-40 mm Hg), and tachycardia if hemorrhage recent and significant (10% blood volume)
2. Hemolysis, usually chronic, often associated

with jaundice, hepatosplenomegaly, edema, and other signs of CHF

Ancillary data

Blood and cerebrospinal fluid (CSF) cultures if symptoms are vague and there is any suspicion of sepsis.

Management

1. Hemorrhagic, hypovolemic shock (Chapter 5)
2. Without shock but with hematocrit <30%: 10 ml/kg of packed RBC over 1-2 hr
3. If caused by EBF (Rh incompatibility), do immediate partial exchange transfusion via umbilical venous catheter if hematocrit is <30%. Exchange 20-25 ml/kg of patient's blood with O negative–packed RBC with a hematocrit of 70%-80%. This should be done, in the first hour of life without waiting for type-specific blood, in 5-10 ml increments to prevent asphyxial CNS damage. Follow serial serum bilirubins and hematocrit. Give phototherapy. Neonatology consultation is indicated for subsequent exchange transfusions for hyperbilirubinemia.
4. If immune hemolysis is a result of ABO or minor group incompatibility, follow serial serum bilirubins and hematocrits, and maintain adequate hydration. Use phototherapy. Patient may require exchange transfusion.

POLYCYTHEMIA

A venous hematocrit >65% is associated with increased blood viscosity and vascular resistance. There is increased incidence in infants with intrauterine growth retardation and in those with Down's syndrome and diabetic mothers.

Etiology

There is an absolute increase in fetal RBC mass with normal blood volume (chronic in utero hypoxemia) or an actual increase in blood volume (cord "milking").

Diagnostic findings

Most commonly, symptoms are absent. If pronounced hyperviscosity is present, infant may have plethora, tachypnea, respiratory distress, hypoglycemia, irritability, jitteriness, or seizures. Less common findings include frank CHF, oliguria, cyanosis, gangrene, or necrotizing enterocolitis.

Ancillary data

Peripheral venous hematocrit >65%. Capillary hematocrit usually 4%-7% above that in a peripheral or central vein

Management

Guidelines are controversial. One protocol that has been found useful follows:

1. With hematocrit of 65%-70%, observe if asymptomatic. If significant CNS, cardiopulmonary, or renal symptoms develop, treat with partial exchange transfusion via umbilical vein. Use fresh frozen plasma or 5% albumin in saline solution. Volume (ml) to be exchanged is

$$\frac{\text{Weight (kg)} \times 90 \times (\text{Initial Hct} - \text{Hct desired})}{\text{Initial Hct}}$$

   The volume is usually 15-25 ml/kg.
2. With venous hematocrit >70%, perform partial exchange as outlined above.
3. Monitor for hypoglycemia, and treat if present.

THROMBOCYTOPENIA (p. 530)

Thrombocytopenia may be a nonspecific sign of sepsis, anoxia, prematurity, or DIC. Maternal factors include toxemia of pregnancy, collagen vascular disease, idiopathic thrombocytopenic purpura (ITP), and platelet group incompatibilities.

Diagnostic findings

These reflect underlying cause.

Management

1. Treat underlying process, including sepsis, hypoxemia, or DIC if present.

2. Administer platelet transfusion: 10ml/kg/dose over 1-2 hr. Half-life of random donor platelets should be 2-4 days in peripheral blood.
3. With isoimmune thrombocytopenia, half-life of platelets is markedly reduced if random donors are used. Treat with maternal platelet concentrates 10 ml/kg over 1-2 hr.
4. Avoid intramuscular injections and other trauma.

DISSEMINATED INTRAVASCULAR COAGULATION (p. 522)
Etiology

Common initiating events (triggers) in neonate include:
1. Maternal factors of acute hemorrhage, amniotic fluid embolism, or dead fetal twin
2. Neonatal factors such as hypoxemia, bacterial or viral sepsis, erythroblastosis, necrotizing enterocolitis, and severe HMD

Diagnostic findings

These include petechiae, purpura, and evidence of underlying disease.

Management

1. Treatment of trigger with oxygen, ventilation, antibiotics, etc.
2. Transfusion of fresh frozen plasma 10 ml/kg over 1-2 hr
3. Blood platelet concentrate infusion if count <30,000/mm^3
4. Vitamin K 1 mg IV slowly
5. If DIC continues, particularly with accompanying hypotension, further therapy is controversial:
   a. Two-volume (neonatal blood volume 80-90 ml/kg) exchange transfusion with fresh heparinized blood or citrate-phosphate-dextrose (CPD) blood <72 hr old via umbilical vein in 5-10 ml increments. Alternatively, packed RBC reconstituted in fresh frozen plasma to a hematocrit of 50% is acceptable.
   b. Consideration of heparin infusion of 100 units/kg/dose q 4 hr IV, although it is rarely required

UNCONJUGATED HYPERBILIRUBINEMIA (NEWBORN JAUNDICE)

Physiologic jaundice in the newborn is common, self-limited, and without sequelae. However, jaundice in the first several days of life may be caused by an occult disease process and may require intervention. Peak bilirubin concentration (<12 mg/dl) occurs at day 3 in the term neonate; in premature infants the peak untreated concentration (<15 mg/dl) occurs by day 5.

Etiology

Most common disorders associated with unconjugated (indirect) hyperbilirubinemia in the first week of life include Rh or ABO incompatibility, prematurity, polycythemia, intestinal obstruction, sepsis, asphyxia, and hypothyroidism. Infants of diabetic mothers are also at high risk. Breast milk jaundice rarely occurs before 10 days of life and usually does not peak above 15 mg/dl. Conjugated hyperbilirubinemia must be excluded.

Diagnostic findings

1. Serial bilirubin determination. Clinically apparent jaundice usually indicates a serum bilirubin of ≥6 mg/dl.
2. Conjugated bilirubin usually <10% of total bilirubin
3. Blood type and Coombs' test, CBC, RBC morphology

Management

1. Adequate hydration. Treat sepsis, asphyxia, intestinal obstruction, or erythroblastosis as indicated.
2. Phototherapy indicated at given indirect bilirubin levels:
   a. Term neonate: >15 mg/dl
   b. Premature neonate: >10 mg/dl

c. Or in either group, if hemolysis and cord bilirubin is >5 mg/dl

d. Phototherapy is now possible at home in some communities. Children must be stable, parents compliant, and follow-up excellent.

3. Exchange transfusion indicated based on indirect bilirubin levels:
   a. Term neonate: >20 mg/dl
   b. Premature neonate: >10-15 mg/dl
   c. Or in either group, if bilirubin concentration reaches >10 mg/dl in the first 24 hr of life

4. At present, the risk of kernicterus from hyperbilirubinemia in a specific neonate cannot be assessed with accuracy. In general, management is dictated by consideration of the relative risk factors such as prematurity and acidosis, as well as the risks of active intervention.

Infectious disorders

CONGENITAL INFECTIONS

Congenital infectious disorders are commonly associated with TORCHS agents (*Toxoplasma gondii*, *r*ubella, *c*ytomegalovirus [CMV], *h*erpes, *s*yphilis). They may be associated with growth retardation, lethargy, thrombocytopenia, anemia, rash, and seizures. Although CMV is often silent, herpes infections may be life threatening. The previous signs and symptoms warrant an investigation to detect the etiologic agent. Initial data should include cord blood IgM, the Venereal Disease Research Laboratory test (VDRL), and titers for rubella, toxoplasmosis, CMV, and herpes. Urine cultures for CMV and both maternal and newborn convalescent titers also may be helpful. Treatment is usually of a supportive nature with three exceptions:

1. Proved congenital syphilis may be treated with benzathine penicillin G 50,000 units (U)/kg intramuscularly (IM) as a single dose. NOTE: Lumbar puncture should be performed before therapy. With increased CSF protein, cell count, and positive CSF and VDRL, treat with aqueous crystalline penicillin G 50,000 U/kg/24 hr q 12 hr IM or IV for a minimum of 10 days.

2. Isolation is suggested if any of these conditions are strongly suspected.

3. Perinatal acquisition of *Herpes simplex* virus (HSV-2) by the neonate is an increasing concern, because of rising rates of apparent and inapparent maternal genital infection, as well as high neonatal mortality and morbidity associated with neonatal infection. It is important to identify those children at risk early in life. Although treatment is controversial, the following guidelines may be helpful:
   a. With active maternal genital infection, infant isolation should be employed in most instances.
   b. A patient in labor with active genital lesions of HSV-2 and either intact membranes or those ruptured less than 4 hr should be delivered by cesarean section. Under these circumstances, most physicians would advocate performing surface cultures from the baby at delivery and observing the infant for 3-5 days in the hospital without specific chemotherapy.
   c. If active maternal lesions are present at the time of vaginal delivery and membranes were ruptured more than 4 hr before delivery, begin adenine arabinoside (Ara-a) 15 mg/kg IV over a 12 hr infusion period (dissolve Ara-a in D5W, not to exceed 0.7 mg Ara-a/ml) for a period of 10 days. Although acyclovir appears effective, it has not been extensively tested.
   d. In the absence of active genital lesions but with a positive past history, negative peripartum maternal cervical cultures would allow for protocol *b* to be used.

ACQUIRED NEONATAL BACTERIAL SEPSIS

This occurs in 3 to 5 newborns per 1,000 live births. Its incidence increases with prematurity, prolonged rupture of membranes (>24 hr), maternal history of recent fever, chorioamnionitis, urinary tract infection (UTI) or foul lochia, intrapartum asphyxia, and intravascular catheters in the neonate.

Etiology

Acquired neonatal bacterial sepsis is commonly caused by organisms present in maternal perineal flora, including *E. coli*, group B or D hemolytic streptococci, *Listeria monocytogenes*, *haemophilus* sp. and *Staphylococcus aureus*.

Diagnostic findings

1. Often subtle. Includes irritability, vomiting, poor feeding, temperature instability (usually hypothermia), and lethargy. May progress to more overt (but nonspecific) symptoms, including respiratory distress, apnea, poor peripheral perfusion, abdominal distension, jaundice, and excessive bleeding or bruising
2. Group B streptococci and *L. monocytogenes* commonly have an early (up to 3 days) form, with sepsis predominating and a late (4 to 14 days) form, with the primary presentation being meningitis.

Ancillary data
1. Severe neutropenia (<2,000 PMN*/mm³) or neutrophilia (>16,000 PMN/mm³), immature band forms, toxic granulations, thrombocytopenia, and coagulopathy may be present. Erythrocyte sedimentation rate (ESR) is elevated.
2. Cultures of blood, CSF, stool, urine, and, if available, gastric aspirate should be obtained once the diagnosis is suspected.
3. If patient's intrapartum course suggests high risk, gastric aspirate–Gram's stain may reveal the diagnosis of amnionitis with >5 PMN/

HPF* and the presence of a large number of organisms.
4. Chest x-ray films should be taken to exclude pneumonia.

Management
1. Treat under the following circumstances:
   a. If there are any of the overt signs discussed previously unless there are obvious etiologies (jaundice caused by incompatibility, etc.)
   b. In the presence of any symptoms noted previously and with an abnormal WBC, particularly neutropenia
   c. If the delivery is premature, with any overt symptoms or if risk factors (maternal fever, asphyxia, amnionitis, or foul smell) are present
2. Obtain cultures, particularly of blood and CSF
   a. Obtain before initiating antibiotics. If venipuncture is unsuccessful, heelstick blood culture (0.2 ml) is acceptable if the skin is properly cleansed with Betadine and alcohol.
   b. If conditions warrant, lumbar puncture may be delayed 6-12 hr. However, treatment should not be delayed nor should prolonged attempts be allowed to compromise the patient's clinical status.
3. Administer antibiotics
   a. Ampicillin 100 mg/kg/24 hr q 12 hr IV or IM **and**
   b. Gentamicin 5 mg/kg/24 hr q 12 hr IV or IM (if <7 days of age); 7.5 mg/kg/24 hr q 8 hr IV or IM (if 7-28 days of age). (If resistance is not a problem, kanamycin 15 mg/kg/24 hr q 12 hr IM may be substituted for gentamicin.)
   c. Chloramphenicol should not be used for neonatal sepsis unless specifically indicated by culture and sensitivity data and then

---

*Polymorphonuclear neutrophil (leukocytes).

*High power field.

only if serum concentrations can be assessed. Dose is 25 mg/kg/24 hr q 12 IV.

d. Specific therapy for resistant organisms should await full culture reports. However, if conditions or suspicions warrant or the patient continues to deteriorate, oxacillin (or equivalent) may be added: 75 mg/kg/24 hr q 12 hr IV or IM.

e. Decision regarding continuation of antibiotics should be made only after the cultures are 72 hr old. Treat for 7-10 days if the blood cultures are positive or if the patient is clinically precarious or markedly improved on initiating antibiotics, making sepsis likely. The last two situations may be associated with negative blood cultures.

f. The role of third-generation cephalosporins has not been fully defined.

BACTERIAL MENINGITIS (p. 549)

The most common organism is the group B streptococcus. Less commonly, *E. coli*, group D streptococcus, *Haemophilus* sp., and *Klebsiella* organisms are noted. High rate of significant neurologic sequelae and mortality (20%-40%) makes early diagnosis of paramount importance.

Intoxication

NEONATAL NARCOTIC WITHDRAWAL

This symptom complex is caused by withdrawal from passive addiction to maternal use of narcotics such as heroin, morphine, or methadone.

Diagnostic findings

Symptoms are voracious appetite, vomiting, sneezing, hypertonicity, diarrhea, jitteriness, and irritability. Seizures are relatively uncommon. Symptoms usually commence within 48 hr of delivery. Later manifestations (2-3 wk) may

occur in some patients, particularly with methadone withdrawal.

Management

1. Chlorpromazine (Thorazine) 0.5 mg/kg/dose q 6-8 hr IV, IM, or PO **or**
2. Phenobarbital 5 mg/kg/24 hr q 8-12 hr IV, IM, or PO
3. Treat for 1-3 wk while gradually tapering dose.
4. Monitoring for apnea and bradycardia is indicated until the patient is stable.

Neurologic disorders

SEIZURES (p. 559)
Etiology

1. Seizures result from widely divergent CNS insults. Time of appearance after birth and the history of pregnancy, delivery, drugs, and nutrition may be helpful in determining etiology.
2. Intrapartum complications: symptoms apparent at less than 24 hr of age
   a. Hypoxia and cerebral ischemia during labor. Increased incidence in intrauterine growth retardation, large-for-gestational-age infants, multifetal gestations, and after prolonged labor
   b. Hemorrhage. Subarachnoid and subdural hemorrhages are more common in term infants with breech extraction, forceps, asphyxia. Intraventricular or intracerebral bleeding occurs in premature infants under 34 wk, with increased risk if asphyxia or respiratory distress are present.
3. Infection
   a. Bacterial meningitis (group B streptococci and *E. coli* are most common), accounting for two thirds of cases. Increased incidence with prolonged rupture of membranes (PROM), chorioamnionitis, and maternal urinary tract infection

b. Viral and other infections: herpes, cytomegalovirus, and toxoplasmosis appear early. Echovirus and coxsackievirus B are seasonal and rarely seen in the first few days of life.
4. Metabolic
   a. Hypoglycemia (Chapter 38). Blood glucose less than 30 mg/dl. Increased risk in first day of life with intrauterine growth retardation, prematurity, postdate delivery of infant of diabetic mother, and polycythemia
   b. Hypocalcemia (<7 mg/dl). Peak incidence at less than 3 days related to prematurity or neonatal asphyxia or from 4 to 10 days because of elevated intake of phosphorus in certain milk
5. Narcotic addiction in mother

Diagnostic findings

1. Subtle evidence of seizures, including eye deviation, drooling, repetitive movements of mouth, and writhing movements of hips and shoulders are more common than classic tonic-clonic seizures seen in older patients.
2. Focal seizures are most commonly found during infections such as herpes; generalized disturbances are caused by asphyxia and metabolic problems.
3. There may be associated asphyxia, hemorrhage, or infection, with bulging fontanel, lethargy, pallor, or apnea.
   ### Ancillary data
1. Serum glucose, calcium concentrations, and lumbar puncture (cell count, protein, glucose, culture, and Gram's stain)
2. Ultrasound and CT scan for diagnosing hemorrhages
3. EEG

Management (Chapter 21 and p. 565)

1. Anticonvulsants
   a. Phenobarbital is the drug of choice. Loading dose: 15 mg/kg IV; maintenance: 5 mg/kg/24 hr q 12 hr PO or IV. Follow blood levels; 10-25 µg/ml adequate
   b. Phenytoin (Dilantin) is a useful adjunct to phenobarbital in the asphyxiated newborn who continues to have seizures. Poorly absorbed enterally by the newborn. Loading dose: 15 mg/kg IV; maintenance: 5 mg/kg/24 hr q 12 hr IV. Follow blood levels; maintain 10-20 µ/ml
   c. Paraldehyde, if control is not achieved with phenobarbital or phenytoin. Dose: 0.1-0.2 ml (100-200 mg)/kg/dose in 4 ml of 5% dextrose or normal saline q 4-6 hr PR prn
2. Supportive care, including maintenance of IV fluids, oxygen, incubator, and monitoring electrolytes, glucose, and calcium
3. Metabolic abnormalities (hypoglycemia, hypocalcemia) require immediate correction.
4. Consultation with neurologist for ongoing seizures
5. Serial head circumferences and ultrasound to exclude posthemorrhagic or postinfectious hydrocephalus
6. Long-term follow-up essential; many children require maintenance anticonvulsants and supervision to monitor for potential developmental delays

MYELOMENINGOCELE

This occurs in 1:500 live births. The posterior neuropore fails to close, leaving a spinal defect containing both neural and meningeal components. Distal limb and sphincter disturbances reflect the level of defect. Associated disorders include hydrocephalus, Arnold-Chiari malformation, or talipes equinovarus.

Diagnostic findings

There is a posterior midline deficit (with or without dural or epidermal covering), reflecting level of vertebral defect.

Management

1. Cover defect with saline-soaked gauze pads, and wrap lower trunk with plastic wrap or aluminum foil.
2. Consult with neurosurgeon. Although con-

troversy still clouds the issues of survival and quality of life, supportive care and early closure of defects are generally performed.

Pulmonary disorders

APNEA (Chapter 13)

Apnea is cessation of respiratory activity for more than 15-20 sec and is often associated with cyanosis and bradycardia (<100/min).

Etiology

1. Central: apnea of prematurity, particularly <34 wk or with a history of maternal narcotic or magnesium ingestion before delivery.
2. Metabolic: hypoglycemia, hypothermia
3. Infection: sepsis, pneumonia, meningitis
4. CNS damage: hemorrhage, hypoxic injury, seizures
5. Pulmonary: respiratory distress caused by hyaline membrane disease, pneumonia, obstruction

Diagnostic findings

Examination is indicated for rales, rhonchi, quality of air exchange, neurologic status, anterior fontanel tension, temperature, gestational age.

Ancillary data

Included are chest x-ray films, ABG, blood glucose, WBC with differential and, as indicated, lumbar puncture and blood cultures.

Management

1. Resuscitation, support, treatment for underlying disease, and ongoing cardiac and apnea monitoring
2. Apnea of prematurity: a diagnosis based on exclusion of other causes. All patients with this disorder require cardiac or apnea monitoring.
   a. Mild spells: require gentle stimulation and 22%-23% oxygen. Rocking water beds

are recommended by some clinicians.
   b. Frequent or severe spells: may require ventilation or constant positive airway pressure (CPAP). Pharmacologic approaches include theophylline (loading dose of 5 mg/kg/dose IV followed by 1-2 mg/kg/dose q 8 hr IV or PO for 2-3 wk, maintaining a plasma drug level of 5-10 μg/ml) or caffeine sodium citrate (20 mg/kg IM initially followed by maintenance of 5 mg/kg 24 hr q 24 hr PO, achieving plasma level of 8-16 μg/ml)
3. Neonatal and respiratory consultation

RESPIRATORY DISTRESS SYNDROME (OR HYALINE MEMBRANE DISEASE [HMD])

Risk of respiratory distress syndrome (RDS) increases in premature infants (<36 weeks gestation), particularly males, infants of diabetic mothers, and infants with intrapartum asphyxia.

Etiology

This respiratory disorder is caused by developmental deficiency of surfactant (surface active lecithins) with subsequent generalized microatelectasis.

Diagnostic findings

Tachypnea (respiratory rate >50-60/min), cyanosis in room air, dyspnea with xiphisternal and intercostal retractions, expiratory grunting, and flaring of alae nasi. Auscultation may reveal decreased air entry and fine rales within 2-4 hr after delivery. Peak of disease is 36-48 hr of age.

Ancillary data

1. Chest x-ray films: diffuse fine reticulogranular infiltrates, often with significant air bronchograms. May have loss of volume bilaterally
2. CBC, blood cultures to exclude sepsis, serial ABG

Management

1. Administer oxygen by hood with ongoing monitoring of ABG. Umbilical artery cathe-

ter should be placed if PaO_2 <50 mm Hg in 40% O_2. CPAP may be administered by special nasal prongs or by nasal or ET tubes. Normally, CPAP is begun at 4-6 cm H_2O. Ventilator support may be needed if unable to maintain PaO_2 >50 mm Hg or if $PaCO_2$ >55-60 mm Hg.

2. Increase ambient temperature (incubator or other device) to achieve core temperature of 37° C.

3. With significant distress, keep NPO, and begin D10W at 80-90 ml/kg/24 hr IV. Salt usually is not needed during the first 24 hr because of a postnatal physiologic contraction of the extracellular fluid compartment.

4. Consult neonatal specialists, with consideration of transfer to tertiary care nursery.

MECONIUM ASPIRATION SYNDROME
(Chapter 10)

Prenatal aspiration of meconium-stained amniotic fluid below the glottis causes meconium aspiration syndrome, MAS. After delivery, meconium progresses into bronchi and distally, with postnatal respiratory activity. Meconium causes intense tissue reaction and chemical pneumonitis, as well as mechanical obstruction.

Diagnostic findings

Early asphyxial syndrome (low Apgar, apnea, flaccidity). Meconium staining of the cords. Respiratory distress is often present within 1-2 hr of birth, with peak of severity at 24-48 hr. Dyspnea is present with retractions, tachypnea, and cyanosis in room air. Coarse rales and rhonchi, with alternating areas of decreased air entry, are auscultated.

Complications
Pneumothorax and pneumomediastinum in 15%-30% of cases

Ancillary data
1. X-ray films: patchy asymmetric infiltrates, often perihilar in nature with greater involvement of right middle and lower lobes. Hyperinflation evident on lateral views

2. CBC, glucose, and electrolytes. Blood cultures to exclude sepsis

Management

1. In delivery room, the obstetrician suctions oropharynx and nasopharynx with DeLee suction and bulb before delivery of thorax from perineum or from hysterotomy site in cesarean section. Postnatally, laryngoscopy should be performed. If meconium is seen at cords or if infant is apneic, intubation and ET suction with mouth must be done. Usual procedures of resuscitation are then carried out.

2. Patient with symptoms is treated as in HMD, with humidified oxygen by hood, serial blood gas determinations, and management of complications. Umbilical artery catheter may be necessary. As in HMD, patients with significant respiratory distress should be kept NPO and placed on D10W at 80-90 ml/kg/24 hr. Glucose should be monitored.

3. Neonatology consultation is advisable, with probable transfer to tertiary center if patient:
   a. Requires over 40% O_2 to maintain PaO_2 >50 mm Hg
   b. Has severe respiratory distress in first 24 hr of life
   c. Has $PaCO_2$ >50 mm Hg (exclude pneumothorax). Intubation may be required.
   d. Has recurrent apnea
   e. Has evidence of pneumothorax or pneumomediastinum

BACTERIAL PNEUMONIA (p. 601)

Bacterial pneumonia is generally associated with prematurity and with infants with prolonged rupture of membranes (>24 hr) or other signs of chorioamnionitis.

Etiology

Infection is caused most commonly by beta-hemolytic streptococci (particularly group B), *S. aureus* or *E. coli*, and other gram-negative organisms.

Diagnostic findings

Comparable to HMD, tachypnea, expiratory grunting, and sternal retractions. Fine rales and asymmetrically decreased breath sounds often are noted. Peripheral vasoconstriction with decreased pulses and hypothermia may suggest vascular collapse and sepsis. Cyanosis and vascular instability are often disproportionately great in relationship to the degree of respiratory distress.

Ancillary data

1. X-ray films: asymmetric patchy infiltrates often unilateral; a minority of patients will show pleural effusion. X-ray studies of infants with group B beta-hemolytic streptococcal pneumonia may mimic findings noted with HMD.
2. WBC may be increased or markedly decreased with a shift to the left and decreased platelets. Serial arterial blood gases may show hypoxemia and metabolic acidosis. Polymorphonuclear leukocytes and bacteria may be noted in tracheal effluent and gastric aspirate if obtained within 6 hr of delivery. Cultures of blood, spinal fluid, and urine should be obtained.
3. Gram's stain of tracheal secretions in newborn may demonstrate bacteria that is associated with congenital pneumonia.

Management

1. Oxygen, support of ventilation, and serial ABG as outlined for HMD. Umbilical artery catheter may be useful.
2. Antibiotics. Administer after appropriate specimens (blood, CSF, and urine) are obtained for culture:
   a. Ampicillin 100 mg/kg/24 hr q 12 hr IV **and**
   b. Gentamicin 5.0-7.5 mg/kg/24 hr q 12 hr IM or IV (if resistance is not a problem, kanamycin 15 mg/kg/24 hr q 12 hr IM may be substituted for gentamicin)
   c. If culture is positive for group B streptococcus, change to penicillin G 100,000 units/kg/24 hr q 12 hr IV.
   d. If *S. aureus* is a concern, add oxacillin 75 mg/kg/24 hr q 12 hr IV.
3. Neonatology consultation, particularly in presence of severe respiratory distress or vascular instability, is suggested. Treatment with exchange transfusion or granulocyte transfusion is advocated by some physicians.

TRANSIENT TACHYPNEA OF THE NEWBORN

Transient tachypnea of the newborn (TTN) also is called amniotic fluid aspiration. It is a self-limited disorder of term or near-term infants and is usually evident 2-4 hr postnatally. It is more frequent after cesarean sections or heavy maternal narcotic administration.

Diagnostic findings

Tachypnea with respiratory rate often at 80-100/min. Dyspnea is common but less prominent than in MAS or HMD. There is mild to moderate sternal retractions with coarse rales and rhonchi; increased anteroposterior diameter of the chest is possible. Maximum severity of distress occurs within 24-48 hr, with gradual resolution thereafter.

Ancillary data

1. X-ray films: nonspecific increase in perihilar markings with fluid in right minor fissure. Mild to moderate hyperinflation on lateral views
2. CBC, gastric aspirate, and blood cultures to exclude sepsis. Serial ABG to adjust oxygen delivery. Umbilical arterial catheterization usually unnecessary.

Management

1. Administer oxygen by hood with FIO_2 adjustment based on serial blood gases. Rarely requires over 40% O_2.
2. If respiratory rate >60/min, keep NPO, and give D10W 80-90 ml/kg/24 hr IV.
3. Consider consultation if:
   a. Respiratory distress with PaO_2 <50 mm Hg in 40% O_2 or $PaCO_2$ >50 mm Hg
   b. Apnea or increasing distress develops

PNEUMOTHORAX

Pneumothorax usually is associated with sudden deterioration of the patient with preexisting respiratory distress, particularly MAS or HMD. "Spontaneous" pneumothorax may be present at birth.

Diagnostic findings

1. Severe respiratory distress with deterioration and cyanosis. Tamponade and vascular collapse if under tension. Decreased breath sounds on the affected side. If on the left, the heart sounds may be heard in the right chest.
   #### Ancillary data
1. X-ray films: AP and lateral decubitus views are best for diagnosis. Clear shadow lateral to lung field with no lung markings present. Shift in carina from midline or depression of ipsilateral hemidiaphragm suggests tension pneumothorax. In pneumomediastinum (not life threatening and rarely requiring therapy), the air is noted lateral to the heart borders, with lung markings seen peripherally.
2. Asymmetric fiberoptic transillumination

Management

1. If distress is not severe and there is no evidence of tension pneumothorax, increase ambient oxygen to 40%-70%, monitor x-ray films, and ABG. This may be effective if pneumothorax is small (<10%-20%), and little underlying lung disease is present.
2. If large or tension pneumothorax is present, temporize by inserting a 14-gauge or a 16-gauge intravenous cannula ("over-the-needle" type) at the anterior axillary line, at the fourth to fifth interspace, with the tip angled anteromedially. Care should be taken to introduce the needle only far enough to enter the pleural space. Remove needle and advance the cannula 1 cm. Attach the cannula to IV extension tubing, connect to three-way stopcock and a 30 cc syringe. Tape in place and evacuate as needed until the chest tube is inserted, preferably by person experienced in newborn care. Attach the chest tube, once in place, to a neonatal water seal such as the Pleurovac (p. 615).
3. Transilluminate and repeat chest x-ray film to ensure adequate air evacuation.
4. Obtain neonatal or surgical consultation for decision to place chest tube.

Renal and genitourinary disorders

ACUTE RENAL FAILURE (p. 615)

Most neonates (95%) void before 36 hr of age. Failure to void should initiate a diagnostic evaluation, particularly if certain risk factors are present, including hypotension, sepsis, polycythemia, dehydration, or intrapartum asphyxia.

OBSTRUCTIVE UROPATHY

Obstructive uropathy must be considered if there is an early history of oliguria, with maternal history of oligohydramnios or abnormal in utero ultrasound and the presence of abdominal mass or spontaneous pneumothorax.

Etiology

1. Ureteropelvic or ureterovesicle obstruction, megaloureter (Hirschsprung's disease, prune belly syndrome), or urethral obstruction
2. Neurogenic bladder resulting from myelomeningocele or severe CNS insult

Diagnostic findings

1. Unilateral or bilateral flank mass, often cystic in nature. Palpable bladder may indicate urethral obstruction or neurogenic bladder. Poor feeding and emesis are common.
2. Ultrasonography may be diagnostic.

Management

1. Gentle bladder catheterization with 3.5-5 Fr feeding tube
2. Urologic consultation

REFERENCES

Britton, J.R.: Resuscitation of the newborn infant, J. Emerg. Med. **2**:95, 1984.

Brouard, C., Moriette, G., Murat, I., et al.: Comparative efficacy of theophylline and caffeine in the treatment of idiopathic apnea in premature infants, Am. J. Dis. Child. **139**:698, 1985.

Carson, B.S., Losey, R.W., Bowes, W.A., and Simmons, M.A.: Combined obstetric and pediatric approach to prevent meconium aspiration syndrome, Am. J. Obstet. Gynecol. **126**:712, 1976.

Cashore, W.J., and Stern, L.: Neonatal hyperbilirubinemia, Pediatr. Clin. North Am. **29**:1191, 1982.

Chameides, L., Melker, R., Raye, J.R., and Viles, P.: Resuscitation of the newborn. In McIntyre, K.M., and Lewis, A.J., editors: Textbook of advanced cardiac life support, Dallas, 1981, American Heart Association.

Gersony, W.M.: Neonatal pulmonary hypertension: pathophysiology, classification, and etiology, Clin. Perinatol. **11**:517, 1984.

Gill, F.M.: Thrombocytopenia in the newborn, Sem. Perinatol. **7**:201, 1983.

Kim, M.H., Yoon, J.J., Sher, J., and Brown, A.K.: Lack of predictive indices in kernicterus: a comparison of clinical and pathologic factors in infants with or without kernicterus, Pediatrics **66**:852, 1980.

Klaus, M.H., and Fanaroff, A.A.: Care of the high risk neonate, ed. 2, Philadelphia, 1979, W.B. Saunders Co.

Kosloske, A.: Pathogenesis and prevention of necrotizing enterocolitis, Pediatrics **74**:1068, 1984.

Manroe, B.L., Weinberg, A.G., Rosenfeld, C.R., et al.: The neonatal blood count in health and disease. I. Reference values for neutrophilic cells, J. Pediatr. **95**:89, 1979.

Mentzer, W.C.: Polycythemia and the hyperviscosity syndrome in newborn infants, Clin. Haematol. **7**:63, 1978.

Rahman, N., Boineau, F.G., and Lewy, J.E.: Renal failure in the perinatal period, Clin. Perinatol. **8**:241, 1981.

Siegel, J.D.: Neonatal sepsis, Sem. Perinatol. **9**:20, 1985.

Volpe, J.J.: Neonatal seizures, Clin. Perinatol. **4**:43, 1977.

Whiteley, R.J., and Alford, C.A.: Preventive and therapeutic approaches to the newborn infant with perinatal viral and toxoplasma infections, Clin. Perinatol. **8**:591, 1981.

Woodrum, D.E., editor: Hyaline membrane disease, Sem. Perinatol. **8**:245, 1984.

V EMERGENT COMPLAINTS

12 Anaphylaxis

ALERT: Acute respiratory distress from upper airway obstruction or lower airway broncho-spasm requires prompt intervention.

Anaphylaxis is a systemic allergic reaction mediated by IgE antibody, resulting from release of histamine, leukotrienes, and other vasoactive mediators.

ETIOLOGY

Antigens producing systemic reaction may be ingested, inhaled, or administered by injection. Although parenteral exposures have the highest risk, anaphylaxis may occur with oral ingestion.

Common agents responsible for anaphylaxis include:

1. Antigen extracts used for desensitization of skin testing
2. Antibiotics, particularly penicillin
3. Insect stings, including Hymenoptera order (bee, wasp, yellow jacket, hornet, and certain ants) (p. 232)
4. Foods, ranging from shellfish to nuts, eggs, milk, and legumes
5. Diagnostic agents (e.g., radiologic contrast media)
6. Local anesthetics
7. Aspirin
8. Narcotics such as morphine or codeine
9. Insulin and adrenocorticotropic hormone (ACTH)
10. Biologic agents, including foreign serum (usually horse), gamma globulin, and vaccines
11. Inhaled allergens such as dust, animal danders, and pollens

NOTE: Agents 5-8 are not IgE mediated and are called *anaphylactoid*.

DIAGNOSTIC FEATURES

There is a wide range of reaction to antigenic exposures, from mild distress, with a sense of anxiety, to true anaphylaxis, with respiratory distress and cardiovascular collapse. Patients often note a sense of "impending doom."

There may be upper and lower airway involvement of the respiratory tract. Patients may have rhinorrhea and initial sneezing that does not progress. Patients with significant distress will have dyspnea, tachypnea with retractions, respiratory compromise, and cyanosis.

1. Upper airway problems may cause stridor, laryngeal and epiglottic edema, and obstruction.
2. Lower airway bronchospasm may cause coughing, wheezing, and marked distress.

Circulatory collapse may develop. Patients will have mild hypotension or true vascular collapse and shock.

1. Initially, chest pain may be noted, sometimes secondary to myocardial ischemia.
2. Dysrhythmias and syncope are common.

Other diagnostic features

1. Urticaria, pruritus, and erythema are observed.
2. Nausea, vomiting, abdominal cramping, and diarrhea may occur.

Complications

The major life-threatening complications include:
1. Upper airway obstruction
2. Bronchospasm
3. Dysrhythmias and cardiac ischemia
4. Circulatory collapse and shock

Ancillary data

1. ABG for all patients with moderate or severe respiratory distress

Severity of airway obstruction	PaO_2	$PaCO_2$	pH
Mild	WNL	↑	↓
Moderate	↓↓	WNL/↓	WNL/↑
Severe	↓↓↓	↑	↓

2. ECG to assess for dysrhythmias, conduction abnormalities, and ischemic changes

DIFFERENTIAL DIAGNOSIS

The differential diagnosis is usually distinctly established by the clear temporal relationship of exposure to an antigenic agent. Special diagnostic considerations include:
1. Asthma
2. Infection—septic shock (Chapter 5)
3. Vasovagal reaction
4. Procaine reaction from inadvertent intravascular injection of penicillin (may cause confusion, syncope, or seizures)

MANAGEMENT

The management of the patient must reflect the severity of the illness.
1. Those with *mild* disease and no evidence of respiratory distress or cardiovascular compromise may be easily treated with antihistamines (diphenhydramine [Benadryl] 5 mg/kg/24 hr q 4-6 hr PO) and epinephrine.
2. Patients with *moderate* or *severe* distress present a potentially life-threatening emergency and require immediate stabilization and intervention (Chapter 5).
3. Attention must be directed to the airway and ventilation (assisted ventilation is rarely needed):

a. Oxygen administered at 3-6 L/min by mask or cannula
b. Intubation if there is airway obstruction
c. With significant bronchospasm, administration of bronchodilators:
   (1) *Epinephrine*. Administer 0.01 ml/kg subcutaneously (maximum 0.35 ml) of 1:1,000 dilution. With absent or partial response, repeat twice at 20 min intervals. Do not give until heart rate is 180 beats/min or below.
      (a) If the patient is in shock, epinephrine should be administered IV. With severe disease, many prefer administration by continuous infusion: start in child with 0.1 μg/kg/min, titrating response with increasing dose (prepare by adding 0.5 mg or 0.5 ml of 1:1,000 solution to 100 ml D5W to make concentration of 5 μg/ml). In adult administer bolus with 0.1 mg (0.1 ml of 1:1,000 solution mixed in 10 ml D5W to make dilution of 1:100,000), followed by infusion of 1 μg/min increased to 4 μg/min if needed (prepared by adding 1 mg or 1 ml of 1:1,000 epinephrine to 250 ml D5W to make solution of 4 μg/ml). The risk of dysrhythmias increases when infused at a rate >5 μg/kg/min.
      NOTE: 0.1 ml of 1:1000 solution contains 100 μg while 0.1 ml of 1:10,000 solution contains 10 μg.
      (b) Epinephrine may also be injected directly into the site of administration of the offending agent, if appropriate. After tourniquet is applied (in case of parenteral drugs), inject 0.05-0.2 ml of 1:1,000 solution.
   (2) **Theophylline.** Begin following initial administration of epinephrine, which provides a rapid beta-agonist bronchodilator.

(a) Parenteral therapy is indicated. The initial loading dose should be 6 mg/kg of aminophylline (5 mg/kg of theophylline) administered over 10-20 min.

(b) Most patients will require continuous aminophylline therapy over the next several hours (p. 584).

4. Antihistamines may be helpful. Administer diphenhydramine (Benadryl) in a dose of 2 mg/kg initially IV, followed by a maintenance dose of 5 mg/kg/24 hr divided in 4 doses and given IV, IM, or PO.

5. Steroids are usually indicated, although their benefit is delayed: hydrocortisone (Solu-Cortef) 4-5 mg/kg/dose q 6 hr IV.

6. For hypotension, a number of maneuvers is indicated.
   a. Keep the patient with legs raised in Trendelenburg position.
   b. Initiate appropriate fluids, initially infusing 20 ml/kg IV of 0.9%NS or LR over 30 min.
   c. If hypotension continues, initiate dopamine to be administered as a continuous IV infusion at a rate of 5-20 μg/kg/min. Metaraminol (Aramine) is preferred by some.

7. A tourniquet proximal to the site of injection of antibiotics, insulin, antigen extract, or insect sting may be useful.

DISPOSITION

1. Patients with only mild reactions may be observed for 4-6 hr and discharged to continue antihistamine therapy at home.

2. All patients with moderate or severe disease require admission to an ICU.

3. Prevention is an important aspect of management.
   a. Patients should be aware of allergies and avoid exposure. A Medic-Alert bracelet should be worn.
   b. Parenteral medications should be used only when appropriate. Patients should be observed at least 30 min after administration of such medications.
   NOTE: Prophylaxis with steroids and antihistamines may be indicated before exposure to radio-contrast media for patients with previous reactions.
   c. In settings where parenteral medications are administered, personnel should have access to emergency supplies, including epinephrine, oxygen and airway support, diphenhydramine (Benadryl), and aminophylline.
   d. Patients with a previous history of anaphylaxis, particularly to insect bites, should carry an emergency kit, including syringes, epinephrine, and diphenhydramine. Epinephrine is available as an autoinjectable premeasured kit (Anakit). Such patients should be considered for desensitization.

REFERENCES

Barach, E.M., Nowak, R.M., Lee, T.G., et al.: Epinephrine for treatment of anaphylactic shock, JAMA **251**:2118, 1984.

Foucard, T.: Acute anaphylaxis in children, Pediatrics **7**:176, 1978.

13 Apnea

ALERT: Apnea may be a nonspecific sign of a systemic illness.

Apnea occurs with the cessation of air flow for more than 20 sec or less than 20 sec if accompanied by bradycardia, cyanosis, pallor, or limpness. It must be distinguished from normal breathing irregularities during sleep, which may consist of alternating periods of regular breathing and respiratory pauses of 10 sec without color change in up to 3% of sleep time.

ETIOLOGY AND DIAGNOSTIC FINDINGS

Central apnea is marked by an absence of respiratory efforts, because of a lack of activation of the musculature that produces flow. This is particularly common in newborn infants, and the incidence in the preterm infant is inversely proportional to the gestational age and decreases with maturation. Other conditions that exacerbate the condition include infection, metabolic derangements, anemia, and hypoxic or vascular cerebral damage. Some premature infants have periodic breathing, and, rarely, some fail to maintain central ventilation during sleep (*Ondine's* curse) (Chapter 11).

Obstructive apnea occurs when airflow ceases but there is continued chest and abdominal breathing movement; that is, respiratory efforts continue. Airway patency is a reflection of airway constricting and dilating forces and the size of the upper airway lumen. Mixed mechanisms also may exist.

History is essential in the evaluation of the child with apnea. It is essential to determine the state of consciousness of the child (awake or asleep) during the episode, appearance (color and movement), tone (increased: seizures, choking, aspiration; decreased: prolonged seizure, hypoxia), precipitating events, duration, intervention required, and sequelae. Past medical information should focus on the prenatal and birth history, breathing patterns during sleep, medications, and family history of sudden infant death syndrome (SIDS). These data should help to determine what happened, the clinical significance of the episode, and the risk of potentially fatal apnea.

Infants may suffer apnea from a wide variety of clinical conditions, often reflecting a mixed pathophysiology involving components of central and obstructive mechanisms. Although near-SIDS is the most common and widely recognized, also encountered are seizures, trauma, breath holding, and problems with gastroesophageal reflux or feeding.

Children may suffer obstructive apnea, often related to sleep. They demonstrate restless sleep patterns and apnea. Tonsillar and adenoidal hypertrophy is most frequent, resulting in a relative upper airway obstruction. Pulmonary hypertension may be a secondary complication.

MANAGEMENT

Evaluation, as outlined on Table 13-1, must focus on the suspected pathophysiology and the underlying condition. Treatment after stabili-

TABLE 13-1. Apnea: diagnostic considerations

	Apnea in the infant	Obstructive apnea
HISTORY	Intercurrent illness Relationship to sleep, feeding, position (reflux) Prenatal, neonatal history Appearance (color, tone) Duration, sequelae Response to stimuli History of seizures	Sleeping: snoring, fitful, restless, hypersomnolence Irritability Obesity Mouth breathing Pattern of progression Response to stimuli
ETIOLOGY		
Infection	Viral: respiratory synctial virus (RSV), enterovirus, parainfluenza Bacterial: pertussis (p. 543)	**Tonsillitis, pharyngitis** (p. 459)
CNS	**Seizure** (p. 559) **Trauma** (p. 315) **Meningitis/encephalitis** (p. 549) Encephalopathy	Muscular dystrophy Cerebral hypotonia
Endocrine/ metabolic	Hyponatremia Hypoglycemia Hypocalcemia	Hypothyroidism (p. 475) Cushing's disease Obese: Prader Willi, pickwickian syndromes Mucopolysaccharides Pierre Robin syndrome
Congenital Vascular	Vascular ring Congenital heart disease: atrial septal defect (ASD), patent ductus arteriosus (PDA), ventricular septal defect (VSD) Dysrhythmia (Chapter 6)	
Miscellaneous	**Near-SIDS** (Chapter 22) Anemia (Chapter 26) **Gastroesophageal reflux** **Feeding problems** **Breath holding** (p. 549) **Overdose or ingestion** (Chapter 54)	**Tonsillar/adenoidal hypertrophy** **Laryngomalacia** Anemia (Chapter 26) Tumors
ANCILLARY DATA	CBC, electrolytes, glucose, Ca^{++}, ABG Chest x-ray films Cerebrospinal fluid (CSF) Cultures: bacterial, viral ECG EEG CT scan Barium swallow and manometry Transcutaneous O_2 monitoring and pneumogram	Lateral neck x-ray film ECG Chest x-ray film Laryngoscopy
MANAGEMENT	Admit if episode is within 2 days of contact, life threatening or follow-up difficult Treat underlying cause Consider continuous positive airway pressure (CPAP) or pharmacologic approach (p. 76) Close home monitoring	Admit as indicated Treat underlying problem Consider supplemental O_2, CPAP by nasal prongs Consider nasopharyngeal tube Consider tonsillectomy and adenoidectomy Tracheostomy only as last resort

zation must account for contributing pathology while being supportive. Patients normally require admission if the episode occurred within 2 days of contact, if it was clinically significant, if it was potentially fatal, or if follow-up and evaluation will be difficult. Consultation, monitoring, support, or pharmacologic (p. 76) intervention may be appropriate.

REFERENCES

Mathew, O.P.: Maintenance of upper airway patency, J. Pediatr. **106**:863, 1985.

McBride, J.T.: Infantile apnea, Pediatr. Rev. **5**:275, 1984.

Weinstein, S.L., and Steinschneider, A.: Prolonged infantile apnea: diagnostic and therapeutic dilemma, J. Respir. Dis. **1**:76, 1981.

14 Chest pain

ALERT: Potentially life-threatening conditions must be excluded by history, physical examination, and ancillary data.

Chest pain in children is usually not an ominous symptom and rarely suggests a serious underlying condition. Of those patients who have the problem for less than 6 mo, 65% have a definable etiology (Table 14-1). Somatic and visceral structures share sensory pathways. Visceral pathology may have somatic manifestations at the level of T1-T6. Abdominal pathology may cause chest pain because the posterior and lateral portions of the diaphragm are innervated by intercostal nerves and may be referred to the lower thorax and abdomen. The central and anterior portions are referred to the shoulder and neck regions.

In the history the focus is on past medical problems of the heart and lungs, family history of heart disease, presence of trauma, medications (particularly oral birth control pills), coagulopathies, sickle cell disease, and other predisposing factors. The pain should be characterized with respect to onset and progression, character, intensity, location, radiation, relationship to position, breathing, activity, reproducibility, ameliorating factors, and associated signs and symptoms. Other somatic complaints, sleep disturbances, syncope, shortness of breath, and exercise intolerance need specific questioning.

During physical examination, attention to vital signs is crucial, as is careful auscultation, percussion, and palpation of the lungs, heart, and abdomen.

A minimal workup should include a chest x-ray film. Other ancillary data, such as ECG, ABG, echocardiography, cardiac enzymes, $\dot{V}/\dot{Q}$ scan, or abdominal work-up rarely are needed unless there are specific indications. An exercise stress test or a Holter monitor may be helpful.

If the patient appears symptomatic on arrival or the pain is not obviously functional or musculoskeletal, oxygen and a cardiac monitor are appropriate. Treatment of the underlying pathology and reassurance are indicated.

REFERENCES

Brenner, J.I., Ringel, R.E., and Berman, M.A.: Cardiologic perspective of chest pain in childhood: a referral problem? to whom? Pediatr. Clin. North Am. **31:**1241, 1984.

Driscoll, D.J., Glicklich, L.B., and Gallen, W.J.: Chest pain in children: a prospective study, Pediatrics **57:**648, 1976.

Pantell, R.H., and Goodman, B.W.: Adolescent chain pain: a prospective study, Pediatrics **71:**881, 1983.

TABLE 14-1. Chest pain: diagnostic considerations

Condition	Diagnostic findings
TRAUMA (Chapter 62)	
Muscle strain	Point tenderness; pain reproducible with pressure or activity; often associated with new activity, particularly weight lifting; may also be secondary to prolonged coughing
Direct trauma to chest wall Fractured rib Contusion	History of trauma or hard, paroxysmal coughing; localized, point tenderness; may be associated with pneumothorax
Costochondritis (Tietze's syndrome)	Firm, painful, tender swelling over one or more costochondral or chondral-sternal junctions; localized; may be painful with deep inspiration or direct palpation
Pneumothorax	Acute onset of pain, often associated with shortness of breath, respiratory distress, and cyanosis; decreased breath sounds with hyperresonance; often no history of trauma
Abdominal trauma (Chapter 63) Splenic or liver laceration/bleed Diaphragmatic injury	Acute onset of abdominal or referred chest pain (often shoulder pain as well); abdominal exam and vital signs variable; possible anemia
INFECTION/INFLAMMATION	
Pneumonia (p. 601)	Cough, fever, tachypnea, variable respiratory distress, systemic illness; abnormal lung exam; possible shoulder pain
Pleurisy	Superficial, localized, sharp pain, and tenderness; accentuated with deep breathing, cough, and movement of arms
Pleurodynia	Sharp pain, tenderness; unilateral or bilateral; accentuated by movement, breathing, cough; may have fever and abdominal pain; etiology: coxsackievirus A-16
Pericarditis (p. 425) Viral Bacterial Tuberculosis Rheumatic fever Uremic	Sudden onset sharp pain, substernal over precordium, epigastrium, or entire thorax; friction rub; pulsus paradoxus; accentuated by deep breathing, cough, swallowing, twisting; may have associated myocarditis (p. 423)
Herpes zoster (Chapter 42)	May be prodrome before developing vesicles
Abdomen (Chapter 24) Peritonitis Appendicitis Hepatitis Pancreatitis Cholecystitis	Referred pain; symptoms specific for pathology
VASCULAR	
Angina, ischemia and infarct Sickle cell disease (p. 531) Pulmonary stenosis Aortic stenosis and left ventricular outflow obstruction Dysrhythmia (Chapter 6) Anomalous coronary artery	Crushing, sharp pain over left chest with radiation to left arm, neck, or jaw; associated shortness of breath, anxiety, and other signs of cardiac decompensation, including tachycardia, tachypnea, gallop, rales, edema, associated signs and symptoms; ECG indicated

Continued.

TABLE 14-1. Chest pain: diagnostic considerations—cont'd

Condition	Diagnostic findings
VASCULAR—cont'd	
Pulmonary embolism and infarct (p. 428)	Acute onset of dyspnea, tachypnea, tachycardia, hemoptysis and chest pain; V/Q scan indicated; exclude hyperventilation
Dissecting aortic aneurysm	Acute onset of sharp pain in chest, abdomen, or back; pulsating mass; asymmetric lower extremity blood pressures; murmur or bruit
Mitral valve prolapse	Usually asymptomatic but may have chest pain, palpitations, syncope; midsystolic click with late systolic murmur
INTRAPSYCHIC	
Functional (p. 578)	Acute stress, attention getting; story inconsistent; no effect on sleep or desired activity
Hyperventilation	Rapid and deep respirations; weakness, tingling; dyspnea; response to rebreathing; may mimic pulmonary embolism
CONGENITAL	
Hiatal hernia/esophagitis/reflux (Chapter 44)	Acute or chronic substernal pain and discomfort, vomiting, fullness after eating, and evidence of reflux; influenced by position and food; response to antacids
NEOPLASM	
Thoracic Mediastinal Spinal	May have organ involvement, pressure, or cord compression
MISCELLANEOUS	
Idiopathic	Most common category
Pneumothorax/pneumomediastinum (Chapters 20 and 62)	Acute onset of pain, often associated with tachypnea, respiratory distress, and cyanosis; may be spontaneous, traumatic, or associated with pulmonary disease (asthma, pneumonia, cystic fibrosis) or with forced inspiration (marijuana)

15 Coma

ALERT: The child with an altered level of consciousness requires evaluation of airway, breathing, and circulation and administration of oxygen, dextrose, and naloxone (Narcan). Diagnostic considerations need rapid evaluation.

ETIOLOGY

Coma in children is caused by a wide variety of pathologic processes. Physiologically, there is usually hypoxia, hypoglycemia, or direct tissue injury. Most patients suffer from meningitis, encephalitis, head trauma, or poisoning. Metabolic and endocrine abnormalities, prolonged seizures, and vascular accidents also must be considered. Tables 15-1 and 15-2 outline the common entities causing coma, primarily focusing on signs and symptoms noted with the deterioration of mental status from lethargy to stupor to coma. Common treatable causes of coma include infection (meningitis, empyema, abscess, encephalitis), trauma (subdural or epidural hematoma), intoxications (alcohol, barbiturates, opiates, carbon monoxide, and lead), endocrine/metabolic (hypoglycemia, uremia), vascular (shock, hypertension), and epilepsy. Intussusception, although not coma causing, does produce lethargy, with decreased response to environmental stimuli (p. 498). A useful mnemonic is I SPOUT A VEIN*: *i*nsulin (too much, too little), *s*hock, *p*sychogenic, *o*piates and other drugs, *u*remia and other metabolic abnormalities, *t*rauma, *a*lcohol, *v*ascular, *e*ncephalopathy, *i*nfection, and *n*eoplasm.

---

*Gottlieb, A.J., et al.: The whole internist catalogue, Philadelphia, 1980, W.B. Saunders Co., pp. 44-45.

DIAGNOSTIC FINDINGS

A thorough history should be obtained from friends or relatives and should focus on the progression of changes in mental status, past medical history, associated signs and symptoms, and localizing findings. A history of head trauma, medications, or possible ingestions (Table 54-3) is imperative in the assessment.

Physical examination is crucial not only in determining the patient's status but also in providing diagnostic information to ascertain the level of injury. A complete neurologic examination is imperative. Useful diagnostic clues are outlined on pp. 92-93. The Glasgow Coma Scale (p. 316) provides a means of serially monitoring patient responsiveness.

In examining the child and assessing responsiveness, a number of concurrent conditions may interfere with this assessment, potentially leading to an incorrect diagnosis of brain death. Other possible causes of findings that may be associated with brain death include:

1. Pupils fixed: anticholinergic drugs (systemic or topical), neuromuscular blockade, and preexisting eye disease
2. No oculovestibular reflex: ototoxic agent, vestibular suppressant, and preexisting disease
3. No respirations: posthyperventilation apnea and neuromuscular blockade

Text continued on p. 97.

DIAGNOSTIC SIGNS IN COMA

RESPIRATORY PATTERN

Cheynes-Stokes (alternating apnea and hypernoia)
1. Bilateral cerebral or diencephalic lesion
2. Metabolic abnormality
3. Incipient temporal lobe herniation

Hyperventilation
1. Lesion between low midbrain and midpons
2. Metabolic acidosis
   a. Diabetic ketoacidosis
   b. Uremia
   c. Intoxication—ethanol, salicylates
   d. Fluid or electrolyte abnormalities
3. Hypoxia

Ataxic breathing (irregular rate and depth): lesion of medulla

POSITION

Decorticate (arms flexed and abducted, legs extended): corticospinal tract lesion within or near the cerebral hemisphere

Decerebrate (arms extended and internally rotated against the chest, legs extended)
1. Midbrain—midpons lesion
2. Metabolic abnormality (hypoxia, hypoglycemia)
3. Bilateral hemispheric lesion

PUPILS

Pinpoint (1-2 mm), fixed
1. Pontine lesions
2. Metabolic abnormality
3. Intoxication—opiates, barbiturates (not fixed)

Small (2-3 mm), reactive
1. Medullary lesion
2. Metabolic abnormality

Midsize (4-5 mm), fixed: midbrain lesion

Dilated, fixed
1. *Bilateral*
   a. Irreversible brain damage (shock, massive hemorrhage, encephalitis)
   b. Anticholinergic (atropine-like) drugs
   c. Barbiturates (late, secondary to hypoxia)
   d. Hypothermia
   e. Seizures
2. *Unilateral*
   a. Rapidly expanding lesion on ipsilateral side (subdural hemorrhage, tumor)
   b. Tentorial herniation
   c. Lesion of III nerve nucleus
   d. Anticholinergic eye drops
   e. Seizures

DIAGNOSTIC SIGNS IN COMA—cont'd.

Dilated, reactive
1. Postictal
2. Anticholinergic drugs

BLOOD PRESSURE

Hypertension
1. Increased intracranial pressure
2. Subarachnoid hemorrhage
3. Intoxication

Hypotension
1. Associated injury with hypovolemia, spinal shock, or hypoxemia
2. Adrenal failure

NUCHAL RIGIDITY

1. Meningitis/encephalitis
2. Subarachnoid hemorrhage
3. Posterior fossa tumor

EYE MOVEMENT

Oculocephalic reflex (doll's eye): with the eyes held open, the head is turned quickly from side to side. Clear cervical spine first
1. Comatose patient with an intact brainstem will respond by the eyes moving in the direction opposite to that which the head is turned, as if still gazing ahead in initial position
2. Comatose patient with midbrain or pons lesions will have random eye movement

Oculovestibular reflex with caloric stimulation: with head elevated 30 degrees, ice water is injected through a small catheter lying in the ear canal (up to 200 ml is used in an adult)
1. Comatose patient with an intact brainstem will respond by conjugate deviation of the eyes toward the irrigated ear
2. Comatose patient with brainstem lesions will demonstrate no response

Conjugate deviation
1. Cerebral lesion
   a. Toward destructive lesion
   b. Away from irritative lesion
2. Brainstem lesion: away from destructive lesion

VI nerve palsy—eye(s) cannot move laterally
1. Increased intracranial pressure
2. Meningeal infection
3. Pontine lesion
4. Injury (e.g., trauma, neoplasm)

III nerve palsy—eyes point down and out
1. Tentorial herniation
2. III nerve entrapment (skull fracture)
3. Intrinsic III nerve lesion, e.g., diabetes
4. Compression (aneurysm, tumor)

TABLE 15-1. Coma: diagnostic considerations

Condition	Diagnostic findings	Ancillary data	Comments
INFECTION (p. 549)			
Meningitis	Fever, headache, nuchal rigidity, seizures, lethargy, irritability, usually no focal findings; may have otitis media or other infection	CSF: ↑ WBC, ↑ protein, ↓ glucose, ↑ pressure, culture positive	Viral or bacterial; consider in febrile patient with mental status change; antibiotics
Encephalitis	Fever, headache, variable nuchal rigidity, tremor, ataxia, hemiplegia, cranial nerve VI palsy, irritability or lethargy, variable focal findings; may have only minimal symptoms	CSF: ↑ WBC (mononuclear), ↑ protein, ↑ pressure, culture negative	Viral: measles, mumps, rubella, chickenpox, Epstein-Barr virus (infectious mononucleosis); bacterial: pertussis; immunization: pertussis, mumps
Intracranial abscess	Fever, headache, focal neuro signs, increased intracranial pressure	CT scan; CSF: ↑ WBC, ↑ protein, culture negative	Extension otitis media, mastoiditis; risks: congenital heart disease and polycythemia
Subdural empyema	Toxic, fever, focal neuro signs, increased intracranial pressure	CT scan; subdural tap; CSF: ↑ WBC, ↑ protein, ↑ pressure, culture negative	Follows trauma or complication of meningitis
TRAUMA (Chapter 57)			
Cerebral concussion	Dizziness, nausea, vomiting, headache, lethargy, amnesia, ataxia, transient blindness, no focal findings	Variable CT scan, depending on course	Rule our mass lesions
Subdural hematoma	After trauma, immediate onset of altered mentation, headache, focal neuro findings, increased intracranial pressure	CT scan immediately	Symptoms usually progress immediately after injury although, rarely, delayed days to wk
Epidural hematoma	Patient often awakens from concussion and, after a brief period of lucidity, lapses into coma; focal findings, headache, increased intracranial pressure	CT scan immediately	Delayed onset unless injury very severe
Drowning (Chapter 47)	No focal findings, variable increased intracranial pressure	CSF normal, CT WNL or edema	Injury reflects hypoxia
Heat stroke (Chapter 50)	Febrile (>40° C), headache, anorexia, confusion, posturing, acidosis	CSF WNL; ABG, electrolytes variable	Complications can be life threatening

INTOXICATION (Chapters 54 and 55; Table 54-3)

Condition	Clinical findings	Laboratory	Treatment
Sedatives/hypnotics	Lethargy, stupor, possibly dilated pupils, no focal findings	Toxicology screen	Support; forced alkaline diuresis
Narcotics	Miotic, pinpoint pupils, depressed respiratory, GI, and GU activity, hypotensive; no focal findings	Narcotic screen	Support; Narcan 0.1 mg/kg/dose (0.8-2.0 mg/dose) IV, repeated prn
Ethanol	Lethargy, ataxia, slurred speech, visual hallucinations, poor coordination, seizures; no focal findings	Levels >500 mg/dl (depends on chronicity)	Support; metabolized at about 30 mg/dl/hr; glucose, K^+
Salicylates	Tachypnea, hyperthermia, vomiting, tinnitus, excitability; lethargy, seizures; no focal findings	Level >90 mg/dl at 6 hr, ABG, electrolytes, ↓glucose	Chronic ingestion—levels not helpful; metabolic acidosis with anion gap
Carbon monoxide	Throbbing headache, dizziness, nausea, vomiting, collapse, progressing with diminished brain stem function; no focal findings	Carboxyhemoglobin level >50 mg/dl	Emergency oxygen therapy; hyperbaric chamber
Lead	Weakness, irritability, weight loss, vomiting, personality change, ataxia, increased intracranial pressure, seizures; no focal findings	Urine lead levels; glycosuria, proteinuria, acidosis; LP: ↑WBC, ↑pressure	Dimercaprol, EDTA
EPILEPSY (p. 559)	Following prolonged seizures, postictal period; may have focal findings (Todd's paralysis)	Anticonvulsant levels; evaluation of etiology	Support, oxygen; need to evaluate cause of seizures

ENDOCRINE/METABOLIC

Condition	Clinical findings	Laboratory	Treatment
Hypoglycemia (Chapter 38)	Sweating, weakness, tachycardia, tachypnea, tremor, anxiety; no focal findings; seizures	Hypoglycemia; LP WNL	Administer 0.5-1.0 g/kg/dose IV of D25W—rapid improvement; maintain glucose
Diabetic ketoacidosis (p. 469)	Kussmaul's breathing, orthostatic BP changes, polydipsia, polyphagia, weight loss; no focal findings	Hyperglycemia, ketonemia, acidosis; LP WNL	Fluids, insulin; variable bicarbonate therapy
Hyponatremia/hypernatremia (Chapter 8)	Dehydration, edema, seizures, intracranial bleeding; no focal findings	Electrolytes abn; LP WNL	Treat multiple etiologies in addition to sodium imbalance
Renal failure (p. 615)	Decreased urine output, edema, lethargy, dysrhythmia (secondary to ↑K^+), CHF, tachypnea, hypertension; no focal findings	Electrolytes, BUN, creatinine, abn; LP WNL	Support; multiple etiologies; dialysis may be needed
Reye's syndrome (p. 492)	URI with vomiting followed by lethargy, stupor, hepatic dysfunction, delirium, increased intracranial pressure; no focal findings	Liver function tests abn, LP WNL, elevated ammonia, bilirubin WNL	Multiple etiologies; support; intracranial monitor

TABLE 15-1. Coma: diagnostic considerations—cont'd

Condition	Diagnostic findings	Ancillary data	Comments
ENDOCRINE/METABOLIC—cont'd			
Addison's disease (p. 467)	Muscle weakness, pigmentation of skin, lethargy, anorexia, hypotension, weight loss; no focal findings	Electrolytes: ↓ Na$^+$, ↑ K$^+$, ↓ glucose; LP WNL	May follow stress (trauma, infection); IV glucose, hydrocortisone (Solu-Cortef) 5 mg/kg/dose IV q 6 hr
Amino/organic acid abnormality	Deteriorating growth and development; mental status change; no new focal findings	Acidosis, LP WNL	Evaluation of inborn errors; infection often precipitates problem
VASCULAR (Chapter 18)			
Subarachnoid hemorrhage	Acute onset of severe headache, nuchal rigidity, listlessness; usually no focal findings	CT scan; LP bloody	May be caused by trauma, AV malformation
Hypertensive encephalopathy	Rapid rise in BP, headache, vomiting, seizures, hemiparesis, lethargy	LP WNL; evaluate potential causes	Responds rapidly to reducing diastolic BP to <100 mm Hg
Cerebral vascular accident	Usually focal findings; seizures, hemiplegia following dehydration (cerebral vein or sagittal sinus thrombosis); papilledema, proptosis, conjunctival hemorrhage, ophthalmoplegia (cavernous sinus thrombosis)	CT scan, LP variable	Support, anticoagulation
INTRAPSYCHIC (Chapter 83)			
Hysterical	Inconsistent findings, often focal; if arm is held up, when dropped it does not hit patient; history of depression, anxiety	LP WNL	Usually history of mental illness

TABLE 15-2. Differential diagnosis of coma

No focal signs: normal CSF*	No focal signs: abnormal CSF	Focal signs: normal CSF	Focal signs: abnormal CSF
Intoxication	CNS infection	Subdural hematoma	Subdural hematoma
Concussion	Meningitis	Epidural hematoma	Epidural hematoma
Metabolic/endocrine disorder	Subdural hematoma	Arterial occlusion	Infection:
Hypertensive encephalopathy	Epidural hematoma	Postictal paralysis	Brain abscess
Postictal state	Encephalitis	Hypertensive en-	Subdural empyema
Hysteria	Subarachnoid hemorrhage	cephalopathy	Encephalitis
Hyponatremia	Cerebral vein thrombosis		AV malformation
Hydrocephalus	Lead poisoning		Neoplasm
	Midline tumor		

Modified from McMillan, J.A., Nieburg, P.I., and Oski, F.A.: The whole pediatrician catalog, Philadelphia, 1977, W.B. Saunders Co., p. 334.
*Check for cells, protein, and pressure.

4. No motor activity: neuromuscular blockade and sedative drugs
5. Isoelectric EEG: sedative drugs, hypoxia, trauma, hypothermia, and encephalitis

MANAGEMENT

Management must initially focus on administering fluids and on support of cardiac and respiratory status. Active intervention may be required. All patients should receive, on first contact, oxygen, glucose (0.5-1.0 g/kg/dose IV), and naloxone (Narcan) 0.1 mg/kg/dose IV initially, up to 0.8 mg/dose but, lacking response, 2.0 mg/dose IV. A urinary catheter should be inserted and bloods sent for glucose, electrolytes, BUN, ABG, and toxicology screen. Following stabilization, a rapid approach to delineating etiologic conditions is imperative to initiating specific therapy.

REFERENCE

Plum, F., and Posner, J.B.: The diagnosis of stupor and coma, Philadelphia, 1982, F.A. Davis Co.

16 Congestive heart failure

ALERT: Infants may have feeding difficulty, poor weight gain, irritability, and labored respirations without rales. Older children often have fatigue and anorexia accompanied by tachycardia, cardiomegaly, tachypnea with rales, rhonchi and wheezing, cyanosis, and evidence of venous congestion.

Congestive heart failure (CHF) is caused by the inability of the heart to pump adequate blood volume to meet circulatory and metabolic needs. Heart failure may result from volume overload (increased preload), pressure overload (increased afterload), myocardial dysfunction, and dysrhythmias.

Of those children who develop CHF, 90% do so in the first year of life because of congenital heart disease. The younger the infant with initial signs and symptoms of heart failure, generally the worse the prognosis if the condition remains untreated. Although older children may develop CHF from congenital heart disease, they more commonly suffer acquired disease from cardiomyopathy, bacterial endocarditis, or rheumatic carditis. About 25% of children with congenital heart disease have associated extracardiac anomalies.

ETIOLOGY

See boxed material on opposite page and Table 16-1.

DIAGNOSTIC FINDINGS

Symptoms reflect cardiac decompensation, as well as the underlying pathology. The acuteness of the process and the nature of any anatomic lesions determine the pattern of progression. Patients may have right, left, or combined heart failure, and the clinical findings will reflect the chamber(s) involved.

A careful history is essential, focusing on preexisting cardiac disease or surgery; hematologic conditions (sickle cell anemia or thalassemia); pulmonary problems; decreased exercise tolerance or associated orthopnea; altered behavior; and weight loss and eating habits.

The cardiac examination demonstrates evidence of dysfunction, reflecting a physiologic response to the inadequate cardiac output and underlying pathology:

1. Tachycardia secondary to increased adrenergic tone and catecholamine release
2. Cardiomegaly by examination and x-ray study. The point of maximal impulse is usually lateral to the midclavicular line in the fifth or sixth intercostal space. Hypertrophy occurs first with pressure overload, but dilation is initially more common with volume overload.
3. Gallop rhythm with prominent third sound reflecting impaired ventricular compliance and increased resistance to filling
4. Tachypnea, often with rales, rhonchi, wheezing, retractions, and symptoms of orthopnea and dyspnea. Pulmonary edema (Chapter 19) commonly is present.

CAUSES OF CONGESTIVE HEART FAILURE

VOLUME OVERLOAD (increased preload)

1. Vascular-congenital heart disease (Table 16-1)
   Left to right shunt: ventricular septal defect (VSD)
   Anomalous pulmonary venous return
   Valvular regurgitation (aortic insufficiency)
   Patent ductus arteriosus (PDA)
   Arteriovenous fistula
2. Anemia
3. Hypervolemia (malnutrition, iatrogenic)

PRESSURE OVERLOAD (increased afterload)

1. Vascular-congenital heart disease (Table 16-2)
   Ventricular outflow obstruction (aortic stenosis, coarctation)
   Left ventricular inflow obstruction (cor triatriatum)
2. Hypertension (Chapter 18)

DYSRHYTHMIA (Chapter 6)

1. Vascular
   Atrial or ventricular: ectopic pacemaker or reentry pathway
   Conduction defect
2. Metabolic: electrolyte, Ca^{++}, Mg^{++} abnormalities
3. Intoxication: digitalis, tricyclic antidepressants, etc.

MYOCARDIAL DYSFUNCTION

1. Vascular
   Pulmonary embolism (p. 428)
   Endocardial fibroelastosis (endocardial fibrosis)
   Anomalous coronary artery
   Pulmonary hypertension (obesity, pickwickian)

2. Infection/inflammation
   Cardiomyopathy
      Viral: coxsackie, influenza
      Bacterial: diphtheria, meningococcus, sepsis, toxic shock syndrome
      Miscellaneous: toxoplasmosis, spirochetes, parasites
   Bacterial endocarditis (p. 420)
   Pericarditis: viral, bacterial, mycobacterial
   Pulmonary disease: chronic infection, aspiration, cystic fibrosis
3. Endocrine/metabolic
   Newborn: infant of diabetic mother, hypocalemia, hypomagnesemia
   Hypothyroidism or hyperthyroidism
   Hypoglycemia: glycogen storage disease, etc.
   Pheochromocytoma
   Alpha$_1$-antitrypsin deficiency
4. Trauma/environment (Chapter 62)
   Cardiac tamponade, contusion or rupture secondary to blunt or penetrating trauma (p. 362)
   Hyperthermia (Chapter 50)
5. Autoimmune/allergy
   Asthma
   Acute rheumatic fever (ARF) (p. 426)
   Systemic lupus erythematosis (SLE)
6. Deficiency/degeneration
   Anemia
   CNS disease: progressive or degenerative
   Malnutrition: kwashiorkor, beri beri (thiamine), etc.
7. Intoxication: alcohol abuse, heavy metals, cardiac toxins (digitalis, beta blockers)
8. Neoplasm: metastatic or infiltration, atrial myxoma
9. Postsurgical condition

TABLE 16-1. Congenital heart disease: differentiation by chest x-ray film and ECG

Cyanotic

Decreased pulmonary blood flow (right to left shunt)			Increased pulmonary blood flow (right to left or left to right shunt)	
RVH	**LVH**	**LVH, RVH, CVH**	**RVH**	**LVH, RVH, CVH**
Pulmonary stenosis: variable VSD: CHF	Tricuspid atresia	Transposition of great vessels with pulmonary stenosis: CHF	Total anomalous pulmonary venous return: CHF	Transposition and VSD: CHF
Tetralogy of Fallot: CHF	Pulmonary atresia with hypoplastic right ventricle: CHF	Truncus arteriosus with hypoplastic pulmonary artery: CHF	Hypoplastic left heart: CHF	Single ventricle
Pulmonary atresia with variable VSD				Truncus arteriosus: CHF
Ebstein's: CHF				Tricuspid atresia with transposition: CHF

Acyanotic

Normal pulmonary blood flow (no shunt)			Increased pulmonary blood flow (left to right shunt)	
RVH	**LVH**	**CVH**	**RVH**	**LVH or CVH**
Pulmonary stenosis (severe): CHF	Coarctation: CHF		Atrial septal defect: CHF	Patent ductus arteriosus: CHF
Mitral stenosis: CHF	Mitral regurgitation		Left to right shunt (increased pulmonary pressure) (PDA, VSD, ASD): CHF	Ventricular septal defect: CHF
	Aortic stenosis			Arteriovenous fistula: CHF
	Anomalous left coronary artery: CHF			

RVH, Right ventricular hypertrophy; LVH, Left ventricular hypertrophy; CVH, combined ventricular hypertrophy; VSD, ventricular septal defect; CHF, indicates lesion often associated with congestive heart failure; PDA, patent ductus arteriosus; ASD, atrial septal defect.

5. Venous congestion associated with hepato-megaly, jugular venous distension, and pe-ripheral edema, especially with right-sided failure

6. Peripheral pulses that often are weak with impaired perfusion. Extremities are cool. Peripheral edema may develop on the dor-sum of the hands and feet, over the sacrum, and in the periorbital region if right-sided failure is present.

7. Cyanosis resulting from pulmonary or car-diac causes. Primary cardiac cyanosis be-cause of significant shunting (Table 16-1) will not respond to 100% oxygen administration, in contrast to pulmonary disease (Chapter 17).

8. Growth failure, undernutrition, and feeding difficulties, which are common in infants. Older children may experience fatigue and anorexia.

9. Altered mental status, which may result from decreased cerebral perfusion. Infants are typically irritable.

10. Pulsus paradoxus, which may accompany pericardial tamponade, pneumothorax, or severe asthma. Its presence is determined by having the patient breath quietly and lowering the blood pressure cuff toward the systolic level. The pressure when the first sound is heard is noted. The pressure is further dropped until sounds can be heard throughout the respiratory cycle. A differ-ence of ≥15 mm Hg indicates the presence of a paradoxic pulse.

11. Pulsus alternans, which is evidence of left-sided failure. When it is present, the sys-tolic pressure rhythmically alternates be-tween high and low pressures.

Complications

1. Pulmonary edema (Chapter 19)
2. Dysrhythmias (Chapter 6)
3. Shock (Chapter 5)
4. Superimposed pulmonary infection (p. 601)

5. Renal failure secondary to decreased renal perfusion (p. 615)
6. Cardiac arrest and death (Chapter 4)

Ancillary data

Specific studies clarify cardiac and pulmonary status. Additional studies may be indicated to further evaluate the underlying cause of CHF.

1. Chest x-ray films: posteroanterior (PA) and lateral. Anteroposterior (AP) view may be sufficient for initial evaluation of the criti-cally ill patient.
   a. Cardiac silhouette will demonstrate car-diomegaly. Other findings reflect the na-ture of any anatomic or functional lesion and may be diagnostic of a specific con-genital defect.
   b. Pulmonary edema causes fluffy infil-trates with perihilar haziness, Kerley B lines, and, periodically, pleural effusion. Pneumonia, if present, must be distin-guished from pulmonary edema.
   c. Noncardiac etiologies may be partially excluded: aortic aneurysm (widened me-diastinum on PA film), signs of trauma (broken ribs, etc.), and chronic pulmo-nary disease.

2. ECG, which is useful in the evaluation of a number of entities:
   a. Congenital heart disease (ventricular en-largement, axis deviation, abnormalities of P, QRS, or T waves) (Table 16-1)
   b. Cardiac ischemia, infarction, or contu-sion
   c. Cardiomyopathy or pericardial disease
   d. Metabolic abnormalities (hypokalemia, hypocalcemia, etc.) (Chapter 8)
   e. Dysrhythmias (Chapter 6)

3. Arterial blood gas to determine acid-base abnormalities on the basis of respiratory, cir-culatory (perfusion), or metabolic inadequa-cies. The response to oxygen may assist in distinguishing primary cardiac from pul-monary disease. Ongoing monitoring is es-sential.

4. Chemistries: electrolytes, glucose, BUN, creatinine, calcium, and magnesium. This is particularly important for patients with dysrhythmias and for those receiving diuretic therapy and to evaluate renal status and exclude prerenal azotemia.

5. Hematology: CBC to evaluate for anemia or infection. Erythrocyte sedimentation rate (ESR) is often decreased in active CHF.

6. Measuring pulmonary artery end diastolic pressure or mean pulmonary capillary wedge pressure with a Swan-Ganz catheter often is essential in monitoring the patient. Patients with moderate or severe disease require careful measurement of these parameters to assess cardiac function and fluid balance. Since central venous pressure is usually inadequate, this becomes particularly important in trying to balance inotropic agents with volume administration. Consultation should be sought.

7. Cardiac enzymes: CPK-MB, SGOT, and LDH if perfusion abnormality, ischemia, or inflammatory response is suspected

8. Thoracentesis (Appendix A-8)

9. Pericardiocentesis (Appendix A-5)

10. Ultrasonography. Echocardiography is a safe, noninvasive technique that may be performed at the bedside with portable equipment. It is particularly useful in assessing cardiac function, pericardial thickening or effusion, cardiac valve vegetations, and atrial myxoma. It is essential in monitoring the response of the failing heart to inotropic drugs. In the fetus, heart disease may be associated with scalp edema, ascites, and pericardial effusion.

11. Nuclear scans. Useful in the assessment of ventricular contractility, myocardial perfusion, and cellular viability. The ejection fraction as a measure of function represents the percentage of end-diastolic volume that is ejected per stroke using ^{99m}Tc radioisotope. Experience with small infants is still limited.

DIFFERENTIAL DIAGNOSIS

1. Vascular
   a. Noncardiogenic pulmonary edema. Evaluation of heart will determine level of dysfunction, if any. History may be helpful in focusing on other etiologies (Chapter 19).
   b. Intrapulmonary hemorrhage
   c. Pulmonary embolism (p. 428)
2. Infection: pneumonia (p. 601)
3. Allergy: asthma (p. 581)

MANAGEMENT

Initial cardiac and respiratory stabilization must be achieved while evaluating and treating the underlying condition. General management focuses on improving cardiac contractility and reducing the work load. It is important to distinguish between pump and muscle function, because it is possible that abnormal loads imposed on the heart may result in failure of the heart as a pump in the absence of depression of intrinsic myocardial contractility. Myocardial contractility may be depressed, but favorable loading conditions may reduce the impact of this impairment on the contractile quality of the myocardial fibers as reflected in the Frank-Starling curve. Often this interaction requires careful titration in the management of inotropic and unloading agents with volume status.

Therapeutic goals must be to improve cardiac performance, augment peripheral perfusion, and decrease systemic and pulmonary venous congestion.

The airway, breathing, and circulation need immediate attention. Oxygen should be administered. When stabilized, the patient should be kept in a semirecumbent position with ongoing cardiac monitoring and oxygen administration. Temperature should be normalized.

Inotropic agents: digitalis (Table 16-2)

Digoxin is the drug of choice in improving the inotropic action of the heart, but it is contrain-

TABLE 16-2. Digoxin: total digitalizing dose (TDD)

Age	IV	PO
Premature	0.01-0.02 mg/kg	0.02-0.03 mg/kg
Newborn-2 wk	0.03-0.04 mg/kg	0.03-0.05 mg/kg
2 wk-2 yr	0.03-0.05 mg/kg	0.04-0.07 mg/kg
Over 2 yr	0.04 mg/kg	0.06 mg/kg
Adult	0.5-2.0 mg	1.0-1.5 mg

1,000 µg = 1 mg. IV dose is generally 75% of PO dose.

dicated in idiopathic hypertropic subaortic stenosis (IHSS) and tetralogy of Fallot. It should be used with caution in patients with myocarditis.

Digoxin
1. Onset of action: 5-30 min when administered IV (IM absorption erratic)
2. Renal excretion: 48-72 hr
3. Oral absorption: 66%-75%
4. Preparations:
   a. Vial—0.1 mg (100 µg)/ml; 0.25 mg (250 µg)/ml
   b. Elixir—0.05 mg/ml
   c. Tablet—0.125, 0.25, and 0.50 mg

Dosage
1. Give ½ of total digitalizing dose (TDD) initially, then ¼ of TDD in 4-8 hr, and last ¼ of TDD 4-12 hr later, depending on severitiy of CHF. Patients also may be digitalized slowly by beginning the maintenance dose of digoxin. Therapeutic levels are reached in 5-7 days by this latter approach.
2. Maintenance daily dose is ¼-⅓ of TDD divided into a morning and evening dose. Normal dose: 0.010-0.015 mg/kg/24 hr PO in two divided doses. Maximum maintenance: 0.25 mg/24 hr
3. Therapeutic level: 1-2.0 ng/ml
   a. Infants and children may not show toxicity until levels of 4 ng/ml are achieved, although some require this level for a therapeutic effect.

   b. Obtain levels 4 hr after IV dose and 8 hr after PO dose.
   c. Variability exists between laboratories and individual toxic level in specific patient.

Other considerations
1. Dose of digoxin should be reduced in presence of myocarditis, pulmonary hypertension, decreased renal function, electrolyte abnormalities, hypoxia, or acidosis. Digoxin is contradicted in IHSS and tetralogy of Fallot.
2. Pulse and rhythm strip should be obtained before each parenteral dose until therapeutic levels are achieved.

Normal ECG findings associated with therapeutic digoxin include:
1. T-wave depression
2. ST-segment depression (scooped)
3. Prolongation of PR interval

Digitalis toxicity
There is a relatively narrow range between optimal therapeutic dose and toxicity. Toxicity is intensified by hypokalemia, which may accompany diuretic therapy. Signs of toxicity are diverse:
1. Dysrhythmias (Chapter 6)
   a. Bradycardia (infant <80-90/min, child <60-70/min, and older child and adult <50-60/min)
   b. Atrioventricular (AV) dissociation with second- and third-degree block
   c. Premature ventricular complex (PVC)
   d. Ventricular bigeminy
   e. Paroxysmal atrial tachycardia (PAT) with block
2. Vomiting, nausea, and decreased intake
3. Blurring of vision (rare in children)
   Digitalis toxicity is treated as follows.
1. Discontinue drug, which has a half-life of 24-36 hr.
2. Give infusion of D5W with 40-80 mEq KCl/L at a rate of 0.3 mEq KCl/kg/hr IV with close monitoring. Do not use if second- or third-degree block is present.

3. Give atropine 0.01-0.02 mg/kg/dose (minimum: 0.1 mg/dose; maximum: 0.6 mg/dose) IV for severe bradycardia.
   Dysrhythmias (Chapter 6) are treated as follows.
1. Give phenytoin, 1 mg/kg/dose IV over 1-2 min, which may be repeated every 5 min up to a total dose of 5 mg/kg.
2. Lidocaine and propranolol are sometimes helpful.
   NOTE: These drugs depress the myocardium and aggravate failure and must be used carefully.
3. Although there is still limited experience in children, digoxin-specific Fab antibody fragments may be useful in life-threatening situations.

Inotropic agents: shock (Chapter 5)

CHF is often accompanied by cardiogenic shock and low output states requiring aggressive management. Evaluation of fluid status is mandatory before initiating therapy.
1. A *fluid* push may improve cardiac output by increasing filling pressure, particularly if the PCWP is ≤15-20 mm Hg. 0.9%NS at 5 ml/kg over 30 min may be administered with careful monitoring of response.
2. *Pressor* agents are usually necessary with an inadequate response to fluid challenge. The agents of choice (Table 5-2) are:
   a. Dopamine administered by continuous IV infusion at a rate of 5-20 μg/kg/min up to 40 μg/kg/min (the higher infusion), the latter only if an alpha-blocking agent is used simultaneously; **or**
   b. Dobutamine by continuous IV infusion at a rate of 1-15 μg/kg/min (usually 10-15 μg/kg/min). Patients may respond to a low dose of 0.5 μg/kg/min, but others require 40 μg/kg/min. Dobutamine is more effective in children over 12 months.
   c. Low dosage of dopamine (0.5-3 μg/kg/min) to maintain renal flow combined with inotropic dosage of dobutamine.

Pulmonary edema (Chapter 19)

1. Airway and ventilation require immediate attention.
   a. Administer oxygen at 3-6 L/min by mask or nasal cannula.
   b. Determine the need for intubation and mechanical ventilation. Intubation is indicated for the patient receiving supplemental oxygen with FIO_2 of 50% if PaO_2 is <50 mm Hg (sea level) and known cyanotic heart disease is not present. Other indications for intubation with ventilation include a $PaCO_2$ >50 mm Hg (without preexisting disease), decreasing vital capacity, severe acidosis, and progressive disease or fatigue.
   c. If intubation is indicated, initiate positive end-expiratory pressure (PEEP) at 4-6 cm H_2O if severe pulmonary edema is present. Titrate upward as necessary, monitoring arterial blood gases to maximize PaO_2 without decreasing cardiac output.
2. *Fluid* resuscitation. Fluids (D5W) should be used to maintain urine output, administered at 0.5 ml/kg/hr following stabilization of intravascular volume. Although fluids usually can be maintained at about 60% of normal maintenance, this must be individualized for each patient. Observe for renal failure (p. 615) and fluid overload.
3. *Diuretics* (Table 16-3). In the acute situation, use furosemide (Lasix) 1 mg/kg/dose up to 6 mg/kg/dose q 4-6 hr IV. May be repeated q 2 hr, if indicated. Do not use if anuria is present.
4. *Morphine* sulfate lowers the PCWP and relieves anxiety.
   a. In severe pulmonary edema with CHF, 0.1-0.2 mg/kg IV should be administered slowly.
   b. Respirations may be depressed. Do not give if there is evidence of unstable vital signs, intracranial hemorrhage, chronic pulmonary disease, asthma, or narcotic withdrawal.

TABLE 16-3. Diuretics

Drug	Availability	Route	Dosage			Onset of action	Comments
			Frequency	Initial	Maximum		
Chlorothiazide (Diuril)	Solution: 50 mg/ml Tablet: 250, 500 mg	PO	q 8-12 hr	10 mg/kg/24 hr	20 mg/kg/24 hr (2,000 mg/24 hr)	1-2 hr	↓K$^+$, ↓Na$^+$, alkalosis, hyperglycemia; distal tubule
Hydrochlorothiazide (HydroDiuril)	Tablet: 25, 50, 100 mg	PO	q 8-12 hr	1 mg/kg/24 hr	2 mg/kg/24 hr (200 mg/24 hr)	1-2 hr	↓K$^+$, ↓Na$^+$, alkalosis, hyperglycemia; distal tubule
Furosemide (Lasix)	Ampule: 10 mg/ml Solution: 10 mg/ml Tablet: 20, 40 mg	IV, IM PO	q 6-12 hr q 6-12 hr	1 mg/kg/dose 1-3 mg/kg/dose	6 mg/kg/dose 6 mg/kg/dose	5-15 min 30-60 min	↓K$^+$, ↓Na$^+$, alkalosis, deafness; may give more often; ascending loop of Henle
Spironolactone (Aldactone)	Tablet: 25 mg	PO	q 6-12 hr	1 mg/kg/24 hr	3 mg/kg/24 hr (200 mg/24 hr)	3-5 days	↑K$^+$, ↓Na$^+$; useful as adjunct, not alone; aldosterone antagonist; collecting tubule
Mannitol	Vial: (250 mg/ml) 25%	IV (slow)		0.5 g/kg/dose	2.0 g/kg/dose	10-30 min	Reduces intracranial pressure
Acetazolamide (Diamox)	Vial: 500 mg Tablet: 125, 250 mg	IV PO	q 6-24 hr	5 mg/kg/24 hr	8 mg/kg/24 hr	1-6 hr	Carbonic anhydrase inhibitor; hyperchloremic acidosis
Metolazone (Zaroxolyn)	Tablet: 2.5, 5, 10 mg	PO	q 24 hr	2.5 mg/24 hr (adult)	10 mg/24 hr (adult)	1-2 hr	Useful when marked ↓ glomerular filtration rate; no experience in children; renal tubule

5. *Aminophylline* is indicated if there is wheezing or evidence of bronchoconstriction (p. 584).

Volume overload

Reducing the volume and cardiac-preload may be beneficial if the PCWP and CVP can be maintained. Fluids and diuretics as outlined in the previous section must be cautiously monitored to provide the best balance between volume status and cardiac function. In patients with volume overload and renal failure, peritoneal dialysis has been used successfully.

Pressure overload

Afterload reduction may be useful if there is an inadequate response to digoxin, diuretics, pressors, and fluid management. Agents that diminish afterload by decreasing peripheral resistance may improve cardiac output. Pharmacologic reduction of afterload should be used only with indwelling arterial monitoring and a Swan-Ganz catheter in place; it usually is deferred until admission to the ICU.

1. Sodium nitroprusside (Nipride) dilates systemic veins.
   a. Dosage: 0.5-8 μg/kg/min IV by infusion. Begin with an infusion rate of 0.1 μg/kg/min, and increase until the desired response is achieved. Average therapeutic dose is about 3 μg/kg/min.
   b. The clinical response is noted in 1-2 min and lasts for 5-10 min after stopping the infusion. Do not use in presence of renal failure.
2. Nitroglycerine dilates the systemic veins and is occasionally useful for patients taking digoxin and diuretics who have severe CHF and pulmonary edema, particularly if these are secondary to aortic or mitral regurgitation.
   a. Dosage for sublingual administration has not been established for children (nor is there adequate experience); administration must be titrated against clinical re-

sponse. Adult dose is 0.15-0.6 mg q 5 min sublingually up to a maximum of 3 doses in a 15 min period. May be routinely repeated in 1-2 hr. Onset of action is 1-2 min, lasting 30 min.
   b. Intravenous nitroglycerine (Nitrostat) has been used effectively in adults. In adults the infusion is usually begun at 5 μg/min with increments of 5 μg/min q 3-5 min until a therapeutic response is noted. Suggested pediatric dose is not defined.
   c. Other pharmacologic options include captopril (Capoten), hydralazine (Apresoline), and prazosin (Minipress) (Table 18-2).

Dysrhythmias (Chapter 6)

Dysrhythmias require urgent attention. Bradyrhythmias are primarily secondary to slowing of the intrinsic pacemaker or a conduction defect; tachyrhythmias result from ectopic pacemakers or reentrant pathways.

OTHER CONSIDERATIONS

1. *Sedation* may be essential in the anxious patient. If morphine sulfate is not used because of concern for depression of respiration, chloral hydrate 10-20 mg/kg/dose PO or PR up to 50 mg/kg/24 hr **or** phenobarbital 2-3 mg/kg/dose PO, IV, or IM up to every 8 hr may be employed.
2. *Anemia* should be treated if significant (Hct <20%) to improve oxygenation. Give 5-10 ml/kg of packed RBC over 4-8 hr with careful monitoring. An exchange transfusion may need to be considered.
3. *Premature* infants with CHF secondary to large patent ductus arteriosus (PDA) may respond to indomethacin 0.1-0.2 mg/kg administered q 12 hr up to a maximum dose of 0.6 mg/kg IV after consultation with a cardiologist to exclude a ductal-dependent lesion.

   Closure of the PDA in the face of coarctation of the aorta or other ductal dependent lesion may produce severe CHF requiring immediate intervention. Dilation of the PDA to maintain patency may be achieved by prostaglandin E_1 0.05-0.1 µg/kg/min IV infusion in consultation with a cardiologist.

4. *Surgery* may occasionally be required on an emergent basis where the lesion is amenable to surgical correction and medical management is unsuccessful, such as PDA, total anomalous pulmonary venous return, transposition of the great vessels, pulmonic stenosis, aortic stenosis, ventricular septal defect, atrioventricular canal, and coarctation of the aorta.

5. Unresponsive patients should have immediate cardiology and cardiac surgery (if appropriate) consultations. Other entities that require consideration include:
   a. Reactivation of rheumatic heart disease or concurrent infection (endocarditis, pericarditis, pneumonia, urinary tract infection)
   b. Electrolyte abnormality: hypochloremic alkalosis, hypokalemia, hyponatremia
   c. Digitalis toxicity (p. 103)
   d. Dysrhythmias (Chapter 6)
   e. Pulmonary embolism (p. 428)

DISPOSITION

Patients with CHF should be admitted to the hospital for immediate therapy. Those with moderate or severe disease require monitoring in an ICU with appropriate expertise and equipment. Very rarely, patients with mild, slowly progressive or chronic CHF and pulmonary edema of known etiology may be relatively asymptomatic and respond to an oral digitalizing regimen over 5-7 days as outpatients, if compliance and appropriate follow-up can be arranged.

A cardiologist should be involved with all patients to ensure follow-up. Most patients require digoxin and diuretic therapy on a long-term basis.

REFERENCES

Colucci, W.S., Wright, R.F., and Braunwald, E.: New positive inotropic agents in the treatment of congestive heart failure: mechanisms of action and recent clinical developments, N. Engl. J. Med. 314:290-299; 349-358, 1986.

Friedman, W.F., and George, B.L.: New concepts and drugs in the treatment of congestive heart failure, Pediatr. Clin. North Am. 31:1197, 1984.

Friedman, W.F., and George, B.L.: Treatment of congestive heart failure by altering loading conditions of the heart, J. Pediatr. 106:697, 1985.

Park, M.K.: Pediatric cardiology for practitioners, Chicago, 1984, Year Book Medical Publishers, Inc.

Smith, T.W., Butler, V.P., Haber, E., et al.: Treatment of life-threatening digitalis intoxication with digoxin-specific Fab antibody fragments, N. Engl. J. Med. 307:1357, 1982.

17 Cyanosis

ALERT: Impaired ventilation or perfusion on the basis of cardiac or pulmonary pathology is very common. Pending evaluation, oxygen should be administered and airway and ventilation stabilized.

Cyanosis results from decreased oxygenation of the blood. For it to be clinically apparent, there must be at least 5 g of reduced Hb/dl. Because of the increased affinity of fetal hemoglobin for oxygen, the infant may have hypoxia without cyanosis. Cyanosis is most evident where the epidermis is relatively thin, pigmentation minimal, and capillaries abundant (tips of finger and toes, under the nail beds, and buccal mucosa).

Central cyanosis involves cyanosis of the tongue, mucosal membranes, and peripheral skin. It may be caused by:
1. Decreased pulmonary and alveolar ventilation with impaired oxygen intake
2. Decreased pulmonary perfusion
3. An abnormal hemoglobin. Methemoglobin produces cyanosis when it represents greater than 15% of the total hemoglobin. It should be considered when there is a history of exposure or of central cyanosis that does not respond to oxygen and congenital heart disease is not suspected.

Evaluation for central cyanosis should include an ABG analysis, chest x-ray film, and ECG, as well as other studies related to the differential possibilities. In addition, the response to 100% oxygen should be measured by comparing ABG in room air and during the administration of oxygen. This assists in differentiating primarily cardiac disease resulting from major shunting and decreased perfusion from pulmonary disease, which has primarily ventilation deficits (Table 17-1).

Text continued on p. 112.

	Pulmonary disease (ventilation)		Heart disease (perfusion)	
	Room air	100% O_2	Room air	100% O_2
Color	Blue	Pinker	Blue	Blue
Pao_2 (mm Hg)	35	120 (range: 60-250)	35 or less	Little change
Saturation	60%	99%	60%	62%

TABLE 17-1. Central cyanosis: diagnostic considerations

Condition	Mechanism	Respiratory pattern	Response to 100% O_2	Ancillary data	Comments
VASCULAR: Cardiac (Chapter 16)					
Congenital heart disease* ↓ *pulmonary blood flow (PBF)* Pulmonary vascular obstruction Pulmonary atresia Pulmonary stenosis Tetralogy of Fallot Tricuspid atresia Transposition with pulmonary stenosis	↓ perfusion	RR 20-50/min	Little	ABG: ↓ PaO_2, ⇅ pH CXR: ↓ PBF, ↑ heart ECG: Variable Hypoglycemia	R → L shunt; prostaglandin E_1 may be helpful
↑ *pulmonary blood flow* Transposition of great vessels Total anomalous venous return Truncus arteriosus Hypoplastic L heart		RR 30-60/min	Little	ABG: ↓ PaO_2, ⇅ pH CXR: ↑ PBF, ↑ heart ECG: Variable Hypoglycemia	R → L shunt
Congestive heart failure	↓ alveolar ventilation, perfusion	RR 40-120/min	Mod	ABG: ↓ PaO_2, ↓ pH, ⇅ $PaCO_2$ CXR: ↑ PBF, variable pulmonary edema, ↑ heart ECG: Variable	
Pulmonary edema (Chapter 19)	↓ alveolar ventilation	RR 40-120/min	Mod	ABG: ↓ PaO_2, ⇅ pH, ↑ $PaCO_2$ CXR: Interstitial infiltrate ECG: Variable	Variable associated CHF
Shock (Chapter 5)	↓ perfusion	RR 20-80/min	Good	ABG: ↓ PaO_2, ↓ pH, ⇅ $PaCO_2$ CXR: Variable	Associated conditions
VASCULAR: Pulmonary					
Pulmonary hemorrhage **Pulmonary embolism** (p. 428)	↓ alveolar perfusion	RR 30-60/min	Mod	ABG: ↓ PaO_2, ⇅ pH, ⇅ $PaCO_2$ CXR: Abn ECG: WNL or RVH	May shunt
Persistent fetal circulation (newborn) (Chapter 11)	↓ perfusion	RR 30-60/min	None	ABG: ↓ PaO_2, ⇅ pH, ↑ $PaCO_2$ CXR: Variable	R → L shunt

*Complex heart lesions may have variable pulmonary blood flow.
CXR, Chest x-ray.
RVH, Right ventricular hypertrophy.

Continued.

TABLE 17-1. Central cyanosis: diagnostic considerations—cont'd

Condition	Mechanism	Respiratory pattern	Response to 100% O_2	Ancillary data	Comments
VASCULAR: Pulmonary—cont'd					
Pulmonary AV fistula				ECG: Variable	
Pulmonary hypertension					
Vascular ring	↓ ventilation	Stridor, retraction	Good	ABG: ↓PaO_2, ↑$PaCO_2$; CXR: Hyperexpansion; ECG: WNL or RVH	Barium swallow or bronchoscopy may be useful; Catheterization
VASCULAR: CNS hemorrhage (Chapters 18 and 57)					
Subdural					
Intracranial	↓ ventilation	RR <20/min, apnea, seizures	Mod	ABG: ↓PaO_2, ↑$PaCO_2$; CXR, ECG: WNL	Associated CNS findings
INTOXICATION (Chapter 54)					
Nitrates } well water, Nitrites } vegetables	Methemoglobinemia	Little distress unless >50% with dyspnea	None	ABG, CXR, ECG: WNL; Methemoglobin high—blood: chocolate when exposed to air	Rx: Methylene blue 1-2 mg (0.1-0.2 ml)/kg/dose IV over 5-15 min
Aniline dyes					
Sulfonamides					
Carbon monoxide	Displacement of O_2 by CO	RR 30-60/min	Good	Carboxyhemoglobin level	May have CNS symptoms, pulmonary edema; Rx: 100% O_2
INFECTION/INFLAMMATION					
Lower airway disease (Chapter 20)	↓ alveolar ventilation, perfusion	RR 30-120/min, flaring, grunting, wheezing	Mod	ABG: ↓PaO_2, ↓pH, ↑$PaCO_2$; CXR: Abn; ECG: WNL or RVH	Some shunting
Pneumonia (p. 601)					
Emphysema					
Hyaline membrane disease (Chapter 11)					
Bronchopulmonary dysplasia (Chapter 11)					
Atelectasis					
Aspiration					
Cystic fibrosis					

Condition	Mechanism	Clinical	Response	Laboratory	Comments
Upper airway disease (Chapter 20) **Croup** (p. 591) Epiglottitis Retropharyngeal abscess (p. 491)	↓ ventilation	Stridor, retraction	Good	ABG: ↓ PaO_2, ↕ pH, ↑ $PaCO_2$	
Meningitis (p. 549)	↓ perfusion ↓ ventilation	RR 10–80/min	Good	ABG: ↓ PaO_2, ↓ pH, ↕ $PaCO_2$	
DEGENERATIVE					
CNS: Seizures Progressive disease	↓ ventilation	RR 10–30/min, apnea, seizures	Good	ABG: ↓ PaO_2, ↓ pH, ↑ $PaCO_2$	Associated CNS findings
ALLERGIC					
Asthma (p. 581) Anaphylaxis (Chapter 12)	↓ ventilation ↓ alveolar ventilation	RR 40–80/min, flaring, wheezing, coughing	Good	ABG: ↓ PaO_2, ↕ pH, ↕ $PaCO_2$ CXR: Variable	
TRAUMA (Chapter 62)					
Upper airway foreign body (p. 599)	↓ ventilation	Stridor, retraction	Good	ABG: ↓ PaO_2, ↕ pH, ↑ $PaCO_2$ CXR: Lateral neck positive	
Lower airway Pneumothorax Drowning (Chapter 47) Contusion	↓ ventilation ↓ alveolar ventilation	RR 30–120/min, flaring	Good	ABG: ↓ PaO_2, ↑ $PaCO_2$ CXR: Abn	
Cardiac	↓ perfusion	RR 20–80/min	Good	ABG: ↓ PaO_2, ↓ pH CXR: Variable ECG: Variable	
INTRAPSYCHIC					
Breath holding (p. 549)	↓ ventilation	RR 0–10/min	Mod	ABG: ↓ PaO_2, ↑ $PaCO_2$	Self-limited
CONGENITAL (Chapters 11 and 20)					
Hereditary hemoglobinemia	Methemoglobinemia	Little distress unless >50% with dyspnea	None	ABG, CXR, ECG: WNL Methemoglobin high—blood: chocolate when exposed to air	Rx: Methylene blue 1–2 mg (0.1–0.2 ml/kg/dose IV over 5–15 min
Diaphragmatic hernia Atresia nasal choanal Macroglossia Hypoplastic mandible Tracheolaryngomalacia	↓ ventilation	RR 30–80/min	Good	ABG: ↓ PaO_2, ↕ pH, ↑ $PaCO_2$ CXR: Abn ECG: WNL or RVH	Requires surgery

Tetralogy of Fallot hypoxemic spells may cause sudden onset or deepening of cyanosis, dyspnea, alterations in consciousness, and decreased intensity of the systolic murmur. These episodes usually begin in the neonatal period. Treatment consists of oxygen and placing the child in the knee-chest position. Morphine sulfate 0.1 mg/kg/dose IV or propranolol 0.1-0.2 mg/kg dose IV over 2-5 min (may repeat once in 15 min) are useful in management of the acute stage. Avoid digitalis preparations.

Peripheral cyanosis is accompanied by a bluish discoloration of the skin caused by increased arterial-venous oxygen differences, with normal arterial saturation. It has a vascular etiology:

1. Vasomotor instability

   a. Common in newborns, particularly with temperature changes, sepsis, or metabolic abnormalities

   b. May be related to sepsis in older chidren

2. Capillary stasis or venous pooling
3. Raynaud's phenomenon
4. Hematologic

   a. Polycythemia

     (1) Congenital heart disease or chronic hypoxia

     (2) Maternal-fetal transfusion or twin-twin transfusion

   b. Hyperviscosity

5. Harlequin color changes. Half of body becomes pale or acutely reddened. This lasts only a few minutes and is not physiologically significant.

18 Hypertension

The assessment of a child's blood pressure requires the use of an appropriately sized cuff—one that covers about two thirds of the child's upper arm, the inflatable bladder encircling the arm without overlapping. Too narrow a cuff will give a false elevation of blood pressure, and too wide a cuff will give a low reading. Measurements by auscultation, palpation, flush, and Doppler methods are useful, the last being particularly important for the young infant. Normal values for diastolic and systolic blood pressures vary with age (p. 650). Children are considered to be hypertensive if they are above the 95 percentile for their age.

Hypertension in children under 12 yr usually is associated with anatomic pathology; older children more commonly have essential hypertension. Hypertension in *neonates* most commonly is caused by coarctation of the aorta, renovascular disease, and intracranial hemorrhage; a wide variety of entities constitute the underlying conditions causing hypertension in infants up to 2 yr, including renovascular disease, intrinsic renal disease (cystic, hydronephrosis, pyelonephritis, and Wilm's tumor), coarctation of the aorta, and neuroblastoma. Children 2-8 yr may have renovascular or intrinsic renal (cystic, pyelonephritis) disease. Children over 8 yr most commonly have renovascular disease, intrinsic renal (cystic, pyelonephritis, glomerulonephritis, and collagen) disease, or essential hypertension. A methodical approach is required to achieve control. Many entities that cause mild hypertension on a chronic or transient basis are outlined in the box on p. 114.

However, when there is a sudden increase in diastolic blood pressure to ≥140 mm Hg, with a corresponding rise in systolic pressure to ≥250 mm Hg (values for adolescent or adult), the episode may be life threatening and a *hypertensive crisis* exists. There is secondary organ damage, commonly involving the CNS, eyes, kidneys, or heart. A hypertensive crisis in previously normotensive patients can occur from acute glomerulonephritis, head injury, drug reaction, pheochromocytoma, toxemia, or pregnancy, etc. It is most commonly an accelerated phase of poorly controlled chronic hypertension of any etiology.

ETIOLOGY AND DIAGNOSTIC FINDINGS
Malignant hypertension

Malignant (accelerated) hypertension is a subacute, accelerated phase of blood pressure elevation accompanied by retinopathy. Common underlying pathology includes acute glomerulonephritis, hemolytic-uremic syndrome, obstructive uropathy, pyelonephritis, as well as other causes of hypertension.

Blood pressure should be brought under control in hours to days to prevent complications, including encephalopathy, intracranial hemorrhage, acute left ventricular failure, or renal failure.

Diagnostic findings

Headaches are common, classically described as constant, occipital, and most severe in the morning. Blurred vision, dizziness, anorexia, nausea, vomiting, and weight loss are common. Retinal hemorrhages, exudate, and papilledema

113

COMMON CAUSES OF HYPERTENSION IN CHILDREN

RENAL PARENCHYMAL DISEASE

1. Glomerulonephritis
2. Pyelonephritis
3. Henoch-Schönlein purpura (nephritis)
4. Hemolytic-uremic syndrome
5. Polycystic kidney disease
6. Dysplastic kidney
7. Obstructive uropathy
8. Autoimmune process: systemic lupus erythematosis, other vasculitides

RENAL VASCULAR DISEASE

1. Arterial anomalies or thrombosis, especially in newborns
2. Venous anomalies or thrombosis

VASCULAR DISEASE

1. Coarctation of the aorta
2. Renal artery stenosis
3. Vasculitis
4. Aortic or mitral insufficiency

NEUROLOGIC DISEASE

1. Encephalitis
2. Brain tumor

ENDOCRINE DISEASE

1. Pheochromocytoma
2. Steroid therapy—Cushing's disease, congenital adrenal hyperplasia, birth control pills

INTOXICATION—lead, mercury, amphetamine, LSD, and licorice

ESSENTIAL HYPERTENSION

---

often are present. Cardiomegaly is frequent. Neurologically, patients are normal but may develop persistent focal deficits.

Ancillary data include:

1. Hematologic: hemolytic anemia, thrombocytopenia, elevated ESR
2. Chemistry: elevated BUN and creatinine; electrolytes and PO_4 consistent with renal function
3. Urinalysis: microscopic hematuria, proteinuria, RBC casts (Chapter 37)
4. Chest x-ray film: cardiomegaly and left ventricular hypertrophy; possibly pulmonary edema
5. ECG: left ventricular hypertrophy
6. Studies indicated to evaluate diagnostic considerations

Hypertensive cerebrovascular syndromes

Hypertension associated with mental status changes may be caused by a number of cerebrovascular events that have a pathognomonic presentation and require rapid control of blood pressure. The decision to lower blood pressure must be individualized and may be accomplished by indirect methods used for lowering intracranial pressure.

1. Hypertensive encephalopathy
   a. Associated with rapid increase of blood pressure
   b. Gradual onset over 24-48 hr
   c. Variable neurologic findings: confusion, apprehension, and lethargy, progressing to stupor and coma, seizures, and hemiparesis
   d. Headache, nausea, vomiting, and anorexia concomitantly with progression of mental status deterioration. Visual blurring with transient blindness may be accompanied by retinal hemorrhages, exudates, and papilledema.
   NOTE: Patients respond dramatically to a decrease in diastolic blood pressure below 100 mm Hg.
2. Intracerebral hemorrhage
   a. Rapid onset with loss of consciousness, hemiplegia, and sensory loss
   b. Often accompanied by headache, nausea, and vomiting
   c. Focal neurologic findings usually fixed
3. Subarachnoid hemorrhage
   a. Rapid onset of a violent headache, with initial pain localized. Most patients have a stiff neck and progress to loss of consciousness; often have unequal pupils and variable, transient focal neurologic findings
   b. Spinal fluid usually bloody
4. Trauma: head or neck (Chapter 57)
5. Neoplasm

Other causes of hypertension

1. Left ventricular failure with pulmonary edema (Chapters 16 and 19)
2. Dissection of leaking aortic aneurysm
3. Pheochromocytoma
4. MAO inhibitors. Patients taking MAO inhibitors should not use alcohol and ripened cheeses (Brie, cheddar, Camembert, and Stilton), since these contain tyramine, which might produce an acute catecholamine release.
5. Emergency surgery on individuals with uncontrolled hypertension. Anesthesia must be individualized for these patients.
6. Intoxication (Table 54-2): sympathomimetics (amphetamine), hallucinogens (PCP, LSD), heavy metals
7. Toxemia of pregnancy with maternal convulsions, left ventricular failure, or fetal distress

MANAGEMENT

All patients must have a rapid evaluation to consider the acuteness of the rise in blood pressure, preexisting medical problems, potential etiologic factors, clinical findings related to the blood pressure, and compliance with medications.

The patient's hemodynamic status must be evaluated by measuring orthostatic blood pressure changes and the potential impact on cardiac, cerebral, and renal perfusion.

Evaluation and treatment of underlying conditions must be initiated immediately.

Antihypertensive medications work best when combined with volume contraction. For acute cases, parenteral furosemide (Lasix) is used; thiazide diuretics (Table 16-3) and salt restriction are effective in the management of chronic hypertension.

Mild hypertension

For the patient with only mild hypertension without evidence of crisis, a slow, sequential approach is appropriate:

1. Salt restrictions ($1\frac{1}{2}$-2 mEq/kg/24 hr sodium), weight reduction, and exercise
2. Diuretics(Table 16-3)
   a. Hydrochlorothiazide (Hydrodiuril) 1 mg/kg/24 hr q 12 hr PO **or**
   b. Chlorothiazide (Diuril) 10 mg/kg/24 hr q 12 hr PO
   c. Furosemide, if renal function is decreased
   d. Addition of spironolactone (Aldactone) 1-

TABLE 18-1. Agent of choice in hypertensive crisis

Hypertensive crisis	Agent of choice	Alternative choice	Contraindicated agents
Malignant (accelerated) hypertension	Nitroprusside Diazoxide	Hydralazine Methyldopa	Reserpine (causes sedation)
Primary renal disease	Nitroprusside Diazoxide	Hydralazine Methyldopa	Trimethaphan (decreases renal flow)
Encephalopathy	Nitroprusside Diazoxide	Hydralazine	Trimethaphan (dilates pupils) Reserpine/methyldopa (causes sedation)
Head injury	Nitroprusside	Hydralazine	Reserpine/methyldopa (causes sedation) Trimethaphan (dilates pupils) Diazoxide (causes hypotension)
Acute left ventricular failure with pulmonary edema	Nitroprusside	Trimethaphan	Diazoxide/hydralazine (increases cardiac output)
Aortic dissection	Propranolol Nitroprusside*	Trimethaphan	Diazoxide/hydralazine (increases cardiac output)
Pheochromocytoma/MAO inhibitor	Phentolamine Nitroprusside	None	All others
Eclampsia	Nitroprusside Diazoxide Clonidine	Hydralazine	Trimethaphan (decreases uterine flow)

*Initiate propranolol first.

TABLE 18-2. Useful drugs in management of hypertensive emergencies

Drug	Availability	Action		Dose
		Onset	Duration	
DIURETICS	See Table 16-3			
PERIPHERAL VASODILATOR				
Sodium nitroprusside (Nipride) (arterioles and veins)	50 mg/vial for reconstitution	1-2 min	1-5 min	0.5-10 µg/kg/min IV; average: 3 µg/kg/min
Diazoxide (Hyperstat) (arterioles)	15 mg/ml (20 ml)	3-5 min	½-12 hr	1-3 mg/kg/dose rapid push
Hydralazine (Apresoline) (arterioles)	20 mg/ml (1 ml)	10-30 min (IV)	3-6 hr	0.1-0.2 mg/kg/dose (1.7-3.5 mg/kg/24 hr) (use with propranolol)
	10,25,50,100 mg			0.75-3.0 mg/kg/24 hr

NOTE: Experience with clonidine (Catapres) and nifedipine (Procardia) for children is limited at this time.

3 mg/kg/24 hr q 6-12 hr PO, if potassium losses are not compensated by supplements and diet and if additional diuresis is needed

3. Addition of beta blocker, if there are no contraindications (e.g., CHF, asthma) and further control beyond steps *1* and *2* is required:
   - Propranolol (Inderal) 0.5-1 mg/kg dose q 6 hr PO. Other beta blockers that are used extensively in *adults* include Nadolol (Corgard): initial dose 40 mg/24 hr up to daily maintenance of 80-320 mg/24 hr PO; timolol (Blocadren): initial dose 10 mg q 12 hr PO up to 60 mg/24 hr PO; metoprolol (Lopressor): initial dose 50 mg/24 hr of 12-24 hr PO up to daily maintenance of 100-200 mg/24 hr q 12-24 hr PO; and atenolol (Tenorin): 25-100 mg/24 hr PO.

4. Addition of vasodilator if further control beyond steps *1-3* is required:
   - Hydralazine (Apresoline) 0.75-3.0 mg/kg/24 hr q 6-12 hr PO

5. Referral
   a. When multiple drugs are required
   b. To provide continuity for all hypertensive patients

Hypertensive crisis

Hypertensive crisis requires more rapid control, reflecting the clinical presentation and the urgency of signs and symptoms. The level of control must reflect the hemodynamic status of the patient. *Usually, only a moderate reduction in pressure is needed in the acute situation, often to the range of 100 mg Hg diastolic pressure:*

1. Furosemide (Lasix) 1-3 mg/kg/dose q 6-12 hr IV. May be repeated every 2 hr. In most cases, the physician cannot wait for significant diuretic effect but must use specific antihypertensive drugs.

2. Antihypertensive drugs
   a. Agents are summarized in Tables 18-1 and 18-2. In general, nitroprusside is an excellent agent for initial control in most

Frequency/route	Adult dose (>12 yr)	Advantages	Disadvantages
Continuous light-shielded IV infusion	0.5-10 µg/kg/min	Precise control; protects myocardial perfusion	Constant monitoring; light sensitive; cyanide poisoning; fatigue, nausea, disorientation
q 4-24 hr IV (if first dose ineffective, repeat in 30 min)	75-300 mg/dose	Prompt; no reduction of renal or coronary perfusion	↑HR, ↑cardiac output, variable hypotension, hyperglycemia, sodium retention
q 4-6 hr IV or IM	10-20 mg/dose (maximum: 300 mg/24 hr)	Prompt; maintains cerebral, renal, coronary perfusion	↑HR, ↑cardiac output; tachyphylaxis, SLE reactions; if sole agent, need higher dose
q 6-12 hr PO	10-75 (maximum: 300 mg/24 hr)		

Continued.

TABLE 18-2. Useful drugs in management of hypertensive emergencies—cont'd

Drug	Availability	Action		Dose
		Onset	Duration	
GANGLIONIC BLOCKERS				
Trimethaphan (Arfonad)	50 mg/ml (10 ml)	5-10 min	5-10 min	50-150 μg/kg/min)
CENTRALLY ACTING				
Methyldopa (Aldomet)	50 mg/ml (5 ml)	2-3 hr	4-8 hr	2.5-5 mg/kg/dose (maximum: 20-40 mg/kg/24 hr)
	125,250,500 mg			10 mg/kg/24 hr (maximum: 40 mg/kg/24 hr)
Reserpine (Serpasil)	2.5 mg/ml (12 ml)	2-3 hr	4-8 hr	0.02-0.04 mg/kg/dose (maximum: 2.5 mg/24 hr with hydralazine)
	0.1,0.25 mg			0.01-0.02 mg/kg/dose
BETA-ADRENERGIC BLOCKER				
Propranolol (Inderal)	10,20,40,80 mg	1-2 min	12 hr	0.5-1 mg/kg/dose and increase (maximum: 320 mg/24 hr)
ALPHA-ADRENERGIC BLOCKER				
Phentolamine (Regitine)	5 mg/ml (1 ml)	1-2 min	5-20 min	0.05-0.1 mg/kg/dose (repeat q 5 min until control)
ANGIOTENSIN-CONVERTING ENZYME INHIBITOR				
Captopril (Capoten)	25,50,100 mg	15 min	4-6 hr	1-6 mg/kg/24 hr (newborn: 0.1-0.4 mg/kg/dose)

Frequency/route	Adult dose (>12 yr)	Advantages	Disadvantages
Continuous IV infusion	0.5-1 mg/min	Precise control	Constant monitoring; tachyphylaxis; autonomic blockage—paralysis, pupils, bladder, bowel
q 6-8 hr IV	500-1,000 mg/dose	Gradual decrease	Variably effective; somnolence; ulcerogenic; orthostatic hypotension; bradycardia
q 6-12 hr PO	250-750 mg/dose		
q 4-12 hr IM	0.25-4.0 mg/dose	Gradual decrease	Somnolence, depression, ulcerogenic, rarely used
q 12 hr PO	0.1-0.25 mg/24 hr		
q 6-12 hr PO	10-40 mg/dose (maximum: 320 mg/24 hr)		Dysrhythmias (monitor); fatigue; hypoglycemia; beta blocker; contraindicated: CHF, asthma
q 1-4 hr IV	2.5-5 mg/dose	Rapid onset; specific for pheochromocytoma and MAO inhibitor	Hypotension, dysrhythmia
q 8 hr PO	25-150 mg/dose	Rapid onset; oral; useful when other drug combinations fail, esp. if high plasma renin	Variable response, hypotension; proteinuria, neutropenia, azotemia; absorption falls if taken with food; not approved in children unless other drugs fail

conditions causing a hypertensive crisis.

b. Oral antihypertensive drugs lower blood pressure less rapidly than parenteral medications, but they have been used extensively in *adults* in hypertensive emergencies without encephalopathy or cardiac decompensation. The experience in children is limited at present.

  (1) Clonidine (Catapres): 0.2 mg PO initially, then 0.1 mg/hr PO up to a maximum dosage of 0.8 mg/24 hr. Onset: ½-2 hr; duration: 6-8 hr. Disadvantages: sedation, hypertension. Mechanism: central sympatholytic

  (2) Nifedipine (Procardia): 10-20 mg PO or sublingual. Onset: 5-15 min; duration: 3-5 min. Disadvantage: may cause tachycardia (beta blocker may be given concurrently); variable response. Mechanism: calcium channel blocker

c. Choice of agent depends on

  (1) Urgency of treatment

  (2) Knowledge of agents

  (3) Availability of monitoring equipment

  (4) Long-term follow-up and input from those responsible for continuing care

Careful monitoring of the patient is required.

DISPOSITION

A patient with only *mild* hypertension may be followed closely as an outpatient if compliance can be ensured.

A *hypertensive crisis* requires immediate hospitalization in the ICU.

REFERENCES

Abramowicz, M., editor: Drugs for hypertension, Med. Lett. Drug. Ther. **26**:107, 1984.

Abramowicz, M., editor: Drugs for hypertensive emergencies, Med. Lett. Drug. Ther. **27**:22, 1985.

Ingelfinger, J.R.: Pediatric hypertension: major problems in clinical pediatrics series, vol. 24, Philadelphia, 1982, W.B. Saunders Co.

Lauer, R.M., Burns, T.L., and Clarke, W.R.: Assessing children's blood pressure—considerations of age and body size: the Muscatine study, Pediatrics **75**:1981, 1985.

Mirkin, B.L., and Newman, T.J.: Efficacy and safety of captopril in the treatment of severe childhood hypertension: report of the international collaborative study group, Pediatrics **75**:1091, 1985.

Pruitt, A.W.: Pharmacologic approach to management of childhood hypertension, Pediatr. Clin. North Am. **28**: 135, 1981.

Ram, C.V.S.: Hypertensive encephalopathy: recognition and management, Arch. Intern. Med. **138**:1851, 1978.

19 Pulmonary edema

ALERT: Cardiac etiologies often are accompanied by congestive heart failure, but noncardiogenic causes result from a wide variety of clinical entities. The chest x-ray film is particularly helpful in making this differentiation. All patients require oxygen.

Pulmonary edema occurs when there is abnormal extravascular water storage in the lungs. The majority of patients have cardiogenic pulmonary edema resulting from an elevated left atrial pressure with increased pulmonary capillary hydrostatic pressure. Noncardiogenic pulmonary edema results from altered permeability, decreased oncotic pressure, lymphatic drainage, or a sudden increase in negative interstitial pressure.

ETIOLOGY

1. Vascular
   a. **Congestive heart failure** (Chapter 16)
   b. Pulmonary embolism (p. 428)
   c. Cerebral vascular accident
   d. Fat embolism
2. Trauma/physical agent
   a. CNS: cerebral anoxia, embolism, head trauma (Chapter 57)
   b. Near-drowning (Chapter 47)
   c. High altitude pulmonary edema (HAPE) (Chapter 49)
   d. Radiation exposure
   e. Upper airway foreign body or following removal of obstruction
3. Intoxication
   a. Inhaled toxins: smoke, CO, phosgene, ozone, etc.
   b. Circulating toxins: snake venom, endotoxin
   c. Drugs: sulfonamides, narcotics (methadone, heroin), naloxone, propoxyphene, salicylates, hydrocarbon, phenytoin, organophosphates, amphetamines, thiazides
4. Infection/inflammation
   a. Pneumonia and other pulmonary infections (p. 601)
   b. Pulmonary aspiration
   c. Pancreatitis (p. 490) or peritonitis
   d. Upper airway obstruction (croup, epiglottitis, markedly enlarged tonsils and adenoids) or following relief of obstruction
   e. Disseminated intravascular coagulation: infection, eclampsia (p. 522)
5. Iatrogenic
   a. Fluid overload
   b. Decompression of pneumothorax
6. Metabolic: decreased oncotic pressure from hypoalbuminemia, as in liver failure
7. Seizures
8. Allergy/autoimmune
   a. Asthma (p. 581)
   b. Systemic lupus erythematosis
9. Neoplasm: CNS, pulmonary

DIAGNOSTIC FINDINGS

Although there are specific findings with pulmonary edema, the majority of presenting signs and symptoms are related to the underlying etiology and must be evaluated systematically.

Historically, patients report progressive dyspnea with orthopnea, cough, and pink, frothy sputum.

Vital signs are variable. Blood pressure often is elevated with cardiac decompensation. It may be increased in noncardiogenic pulmonary edema secondary to anxiety and catecholamine release. Tachycardia is present. Patients have pale and clammy skin.

Tachypnea is uniformly apparent (unless decreased by narcotics). Cyanosis results from ventilation-perfusion abnormalities. Patients demonstrate rales, wheezing, and, occasionally, pleural effusions. Unilateral effusions, when present, are usually on the right.

Cardiac findings reflect the underlying pathology associated with congestive heart failure, demonstrating gallop rhythm, increased heart sounds, and elevated jugular venous pressure (Chapter 16).

Mental status may be decreased with associated anorexia, listlessness, and headache, and, occasionally, the patient may progress to coma, Cheynes-Stokes respirations, or apnea, which occurs with cerebral hypoxia.

Complications
1. Cardiac failure with left or right ventricular failure (Chapter 16)
2. Superimposed pulmonary infection (p. 601)
3. Acute respiratory failure with $PaO_2 < 50$ mm Hg and $PaCO_2 > 50$ mm Hg at room air, sea level, progressive disease or fatigue, and respiratory acidosis
4. Disseminated intravascular coagulation (p. 522)
5. Cardiopulmonary arrest and death

Ancillary data
Studies must reflect the primary etiology, in addition to those directly related to pulmonary status:
1. Chest x-ray studies
   a. Fluffy alveolar infiltrates, with diffuse perihilar haziness, Kerley-B lines, cardiomegaly, and possibly pleural effusions
   b. If cardiac in origin, findings usually are associated with underlying cardiac lesion(s). Cardiomegaly is usually present.
2. ABG: hypoxia with respiratory acidosis or alkalosis
3. ECG: reflects underlying heart disease, strain, or ischemia
4. Electrolytes: particularly with diuretics (hypokalemia; BUN, creatinine)
5. Thoracentesis: if patient has pleural fluid leading to respiratory decompensation (Appendix A-7)
   NOTE: Analysis should include protein, glucose, cell count, lactic dehydrogenase (LDH), culture, and Gram's stain.
6. Other studies, as indicated
   a. Swan-Ganz catheter to measure pulmonary wedge pressure when cardiac failure is severe. It is usually inserted in the ICU.
   b. Echocardiogram to evaluate pulmonary hypertension and cardiac function and to determine if effusion is present.

DIFFERENTIAL DIAGNOSIS
1. Infection: pneumonia (p. 601)
2. Vascular
   a. Intrapulmonary hemorrhage, accompanied by hemoptysis, chest pain, and infiltrate on chest x-ray film
   b. Pulmonary embolism (p. 428) with hemoptysis, pleuritic chest pain, and dyspnea
3. Allergy: asthma (p. 581)

MANAGEMENT
The pulmonary status initially may be stabilized during the treatment of the underlying condition. For treatment of specific entities, see appropriate chapter.

The patient should be kept in a semirecumbent position with cardiac monitor.
1. Airway and breathing
   a. Oxygenation a necessity. Humidified oxygen at 3-6 L/min by mask or nasal cannula (or 50%) should be administered.
   b. Intubation and initiation of positive end-

expiratory pressure if the PaO_2 < 50 mm Hg at an FIO_2 of 50%, beginning at 5 cm H_2O and increasing with close monitoring in ICU

c. Mechanical ventilation after intubation for respiratory failure (PaO_2 < 50 mm Hg and $PaCO_2$ > 50 mm Hg at room air, sea level) to protect airway, to avoid rapid progression of disease or fatigue, or to treat unresponsive metabolic acidosis

2. *Fluid* resuscitation
   a. Fluid therapy must be a balance between expanding the intravascular volume necessary to improve cardiac output and controlling the subsequent increased pulmonary flow and edema. This may require the insertion of a Swan-Ganz catheter and observation of patient for renal failure.
   b. Crystalloid is used to maintain urine output at 0.5 mg/kg/hr in cardiogenic pulmonary edema but must be individualized in noncardiogenic pulmonary edema. Patients in general are maintained with fluids at a rate well below maintenance, while urine output is monitored.
   c. Albumin (25% salt poor administered 1 g/kg/dose over 2-4 hr) is indicated if pulmonary edema is secondary to hypoalbuminemia.
   d. Fluid management for patients with cardiac tamponade requires pushing fluids and periocardiocentesis (Appendix A-4).

3. Diuretics to reduce volume overload (Table 16-3)
   a. Diuretics for pulmonary edema that is cardiogenic in origin. If noncardiogenic, diuretics should be used only if the underlying pathophysiology is associated with fluid overload.
   b. Furosemide (Lasix): 1 mg/kg/dose up to 6 mg/kg/dose q 6 hr. May be repeated every 2 hr, if indicated. Not to be used if patient is anuric.

4. Morphine sulfate. Lowers pulmonary wedge pressure and relieves anxiety.

a. In severe pulmonary edema 0.1-0.2 mg/kg IV should be administered slowly.
b. Morphine should not be given if there is evidence of unstable vital signs, intracranial hemorrhage, chronic pulmonary disease, asthma, or narcotic withdrawal.
c. Use with caution in patients with respiratory depression or progressive disease. Close monitoring is essential.
d. Nalbuphine (Nubain) may prove to be a useful substitute for morphine. The experience with children is still limited.

5. Shock. Cardiogenic shock or low output state may accompany pulmonary edema and must be treated aggressively. The adrenergic agents of choice (Chapter 5) are:
   a. Dopamine administered by continuous IV infusion at a rate of 5-20 μg/kg/min. May be used in higher dose if alpha-blocking agents are used. There is extensive experience with children.
   b. An alternative is dobutamine administered by continuous IV infusion at a rate of 1-15 μg/kg/min. Some patients may respond to a low dose of 0.5 μg/kg/min; others may require 40 μg/kg/min. It may be used with low-dose dopamine (0.5-3 μg/kg/min).

6. Afterload reduction to diminish pressure overload. If there is an inadequate response to these measures, agents that diminish afterload by decreasing peripheral resistance may improve cardiac output. These drugs should be used only with indwelling arterial monitoring and a Swan-Ganz catheter in place (p. 630).
   a. Sodium nitroprusside (Nipride). Dosage: 0.5-8 μg/kg/min IV by infusion. Begin with rate of infusion of 0.1 μg/kg/min, and increase until the desired response is achieved. Average therapeutic dose is about 3 μg/kg/min. The clinical response is noted in 1-2 min and lasts for 5-10 min after stopping the infusion. Do not use if renal failure is present.

b. Nitroglycerine has no established dosage in children. Sublingual administration in adults (0.15-0.6 mg q 5 min up to a maximum of three doses in a 15 min period) may be useful for acute treatment, particularly in the prehospital setting in the patient with obvious cardiac decompensation. Intravenous nitroglycerine (Nitrostat) similarly has been used in adults (5 μg/min with increments of 5 μg/min every 3-5 min titrated to response) in the hospital environment.

7. Other considerations:
   a. Dysrhythmias require urgent treatment (Chapter 6).
   b. Steroids are not useful unless they have efficacy for the underlying condition.
   c. Aminophylline is indicated if there is wheezing and evidence of bronchoconstriction (p. 584).

DISPOSITION

Patients require admission to an ICU for appropriate intervention, immediate treatment and monitoring of the pulmonary edema, and management of the underlying condition.

The rare patient with mild, slowly progressive pulmonary edema of known etiology may be managed on an ambulatory basis, if compliance and follow-up can be ensured.

A cardiologist should be involved immediately.

REFERENCE

Feinberg, A.N., and Shabino, C.L.: Acute pulmonary edema complicating tonsillectomy and adenoidectomy, Pediatrics **75**:112, 1985.

20 Respiratory distress (dyspnea)

ALERT: Note any of the following: the acuteness of onset; accompanying fever; voice changes; trauma; underlying heart, liver, or kidney disease; metabolic abnormalities; the presence of an abnormal upper airway examination; asymmetric findings; or wheezing assist in rapidly assessing potential etiologies. Airway and ventilation must be stabilized immediately. Never leave the patient unattended.

Dyspnea or labored, rapid respirations usually reflect an impairment in ventilation, perfusion, or a metabolic or CNS drive. Upper airway problems produce primarily ventilatory abnormalities; lower airway disease may interfere with both ventilation and perfusion.

ETIOLOGY

Stridor is the major complaint with significant upper airway disease. Inspiratory stridor is usually supraglottic, whereas expiratory stridor emanates from the trachea. Patients with inspiratory and expiratory stridor or expiratory stridor alone usually have more significant obstructions, demanding urgent intervention.

Supraglottic stridor is usually quiet and wet, and it is associated with a muffled voice, dysphagia, and a preference to sit; a patient with subglottic lesions producing a loud stridor often has a hoarse voice, barky cough, and possibly, facial edema.

Lower airway disease consists of a more diverse group of entities that inhibit the ability of

See also Chapter 84: Pulmonary Disorders.

oxygen to diffuse into the capillaries. The most common are pneumonia and asthma. Pulmonary pathology often is associated with exertional dyspnea; cardiac disease, on the other hand, causes orthopnea and paroxysmal nocturnal dyspnea.

Common causes of respiratory distress in children under 2 yr include pneumonia, asthma, croup, congenital heart disease, foreign body inhalation, congenital anomalies of the airway (tracheal web, cysts, lobar emphysema), and nasopharyngeal obstruction (large tonsils and adenoids). The underlying disease in older children more frequently is asthma, poisoning, drowning, trauma, cystic fibrosis, peripheral neuritis, or encephalitis.

In addition to those conditions enumerated in Table 20-1, oxygen demand may be increased (increased activity, fever, hyperthyroidism), oxygen transport may be deficient (anemia, methemoglobinemia, or shock), the respiratory system may be stimulated as a compensatory mechanism in metabolic acidosis (diabetes mellitus, uremia, drug ingestions), the ambient oxygen may be low, or there may be a central neurogenic stimulation.

Text continued on p. 131.

125

TABLE 20-1. Respiratory distress: diagnostic considerations

Disease	Etiology	Signs and symptoms	Ancillary data	Comments/management
INFECTION		**UPPER AIRWAY OBSTRUCTION**		
Epiglottitis (p. 591)	*H. influenzae*	Toxic, febrile, inspir stridor, cyanosis, muffled voice, drooling, labored resp, cherry-red epiglottis	↑ WBC (shift left), positive lateral neck x-ray	Visualization and intubation, optimally in operating room; antibiotics
Croup (laryngotracheal bronchitis) (p. 591)	Virus: parainfluenza, respiratory syncytial virus	Inspir stridor, hoarse voice, croupy cough, variably labored resp, epiglottis WNL	Variable WBC, negative lateral neck x-ray	Cool mist; nebulized racemic epinephrine if needed; steroids controversial
Peritonsillar abscess (p. 458)	Group A streptococci	Fever, severe throat pain, late inspir stridor, drooling, dysphagia, tonsil displaced, posterior pharyngeal mass	↑ WBC	Ampicillin, drainage
Retropharyngeal esophageal abscess (p. 462)	*S. aureus*, group A streptococci		↑ WBC, positive lateral neck x-ray	Nafcillin (or equiv), surgical incision and drainage; usually child <3 yr
Bacterial tracheitis	*S. aureus*	High temp, inspir stridor, brassy cough, fails to respond to croup therapy	↑ WBC (shift to left)	Nafcillin (or equiv); may require intubation to remove thick secretions
Diphtheria	*Corynebacterium diphtheriae*	Toxic, slight fever, membrane, hoarse	Culture	History of exposure, no immunization; antitoxin and penicillin
TRAUMA				
Foreign body (p. 599) Pharynx, larynx, trachea, esophagus	Aspiration of vegetable or inanimate matter	History reflects level of obstruction, inspir or expir stridor, cyanosis, labored resp, wheezing, variable resp arrest	Chest (inspir and expir) and lateral neck x-ray: foreign body, wide mediastinum; findings vary with location	Back blow, chest/abdominal thrust, mechanical removal, surgical airway
Neck injury (Chapter 61)		History and findings of trauma, instability or disruption of neck, larynx, variable stridor	Clear cervical spine, look for signs of laryngeal injury	Stabilization of airway and neck

Cord paralysis	Congenital, traumatic, iatrogenic	Acute or chronic, voice change, inspir stridor, resp distress	Direct laryngoscopy	If acute, intubation or surgical airway
Subglottic stenosis	Trauma to glottis such as intubation; rarely congenital	Resp distress, usually insidious; may be exacerbated by respiratory infection	Direct laryngoscopy	Surgical airway may be needed
CONGENITAL (Chapters 10 and 11)				
Vascular ring Laryngeal web or polyp Small mandible (Pierre Robin) Large tongue (hypothyroid)	Congenital or acquired	Chronic inspir or expir stridor, variable resp distress (or both), wheezing	Laryngoscopy/ bronchoscopy	Surgical or medical approach to underlying problem
Tracheomalacia	Abnormal collapse of supraglottic area	Expiratory stridor		Need oxygen until stable; usually resolves spontaneously; may have feeding problem
Laryngomalacia	Floppiness of trachea	Inspiratory stridor		
ALLERGIC				
Spasmodic croup (p. 599)	Exposure to irritant or sensitizing agent	Rapid onset inspir stridor, croupy cough, variable labored respiration		Cool mist; nebulized racemic epinephrine
Anaphylaxis (Chapter 12)	Allergic response	Rapid onset stridor, resp distress, wheezing		Removal of sensitizing agent; epinephrine, antihistamines, steroids
Angioneurotic edema	Allergic response, hereditary	Rapid onset after eating, bee sting, environmental exposure		Airway support, epinephrine, etc. (Chapter 12)
NEOPLASM				
Tracheal, laryngeal, esophageal, neck	Carcinoma, teratoma, hemangioma, polyp	Insidious progression of stridor, dysphagia, labored resp		Radiologic and surgical evaluation

Continued.

TABLE 20-1. Respiratory distress: diagnostic considerations—cont'd

Disease	Etiology	Signs and symptoms	Ancillary data	Comments/management
INFECTION		**LOWER AIRWAY DISEASE**		
Pneumonia (p. 601)	Viral Bacterial: *S. pneumoniae, H. influenzae* Other	Febrile, recent onset tachypnea, cough, unequal breath sounds or rhonchi, variable chest pain	Variable WBC; chest x-ray: infiltrate; blood culture (if toxic)	Antibiotics as indicated
Bronchiolitis (p. 588)	Viral: parainfluenza, respiratory syncytial virus	Variable fever, very tachypneic, nontoxic, wheezing, variable cyanosis	Chest x-ray: hyperexpanded, infiltrate variable	Support: hydration, oxygen; SQ epinephrine and bronchodilators, variably helpful
Pleural effusion	Infections (viral or bacterial), CHF, nephrosis, liver failure	No fever, tachypneic with unequal breath sounds, variable chest pain	Chest x-ray (include lateral decibitus)	May need to aspirate
Empyema	*S. aureus*	Fever, toxic, tachypneic, cough, variable pain, unequal breath sounds	Chest x-ray, fluid culture, blood culture	Thoracentesis for diagnosis, then closed drainage and antibiotics
VASCULAR				
Congestive heart failure (Chapter 16)	Congenital or acquired heart disease	Fatigue, anorexia, cough, orthopnea, basilar rales, edema	Chest x-ray, ECG, ABG	Diuretics, oxygen, digitalis, morphine, nitrates
Congenital heart disease	R → L shunt, pulmonary edema	Cyanosis	Chest x-ray, ECG, ABG	Cardiology consult
Pulmonary edema (Chapter 19)	Heart, liver, renal vascular disease	Tachypnea, basilar rales, fatigue, cough, orthopnea, wheezing	Chest x-ray, serum protein, BUN, SGOT, electrolytes, UA	Evaluate systems involved; diuretics
Pulmonary embolism (p. 428)	Abn clotting, trauma, birth control pills	Tachypnea, hemoptysis, chest pain, variable fever	Chest x-ray, ABG, ventilation-perfusion scan	Immediate anticoagulation

Condition	Etiology	Clinical findings	Laboratory	Treatment
Polycythemia	Heart, pulmonary, renal disease, abn Hb	Plethoric	CBC with indexes	Hematology consult; may require partial exchange
Anemia (Chapter 26)	↓ production or ↑ loss; high output failure	Pale, fatigue, poor exercise tolerance	CBC with indexes, reticulocyte count	Hematology consult; transfusion
ALLERGIC				
Asthma (p. 581)	Exposure to irritant or sensitizing agent; infection; emotional stress	Insidious or rapid onset of tachypnea, wheezing, cough		Oxygen, epinephrine, bronchodilator, and steroid if needed
Anaphylaxis (Chapter 12)	Exposure to sensitizing agent	Rapid onset wheezing, tachypnea	Chest x-ray, ABG	
TRAUMA				
Foreign body Bronchial (p. 599)	Vegetable or inanimate material	History, cough, wheezing, asymmetrical breath sounds	Chest x-ray: inspir and expir, fluoroscopy	Bronchoscopy
Pneumothorax (Chapter 62)	Chest wound, spontaneous	Tachypnea, chest pain, asymmetrical breath sounds	Chest x-ray	Needle aspiration, chest tube
CONGENITAL				
Cystic fibrosis	Autosomal recessive, Caucasians	Progressive pulmonary disease, poor growth, steatorrhea	Chest x-ray, sweat test	Pulmonary consult
NEOPLASM		Progressive pulmonary disease	Chest x-ray	Oncology consult
DEGENERATIVE				
Kyphoscoliosis Progressive CNS disease	Multiple	Progressive pulmonary disease, secondary hypoventilation	Chest x-ray, ABG, pulmonary function	Neurology, pulmonary, orthopedic consult

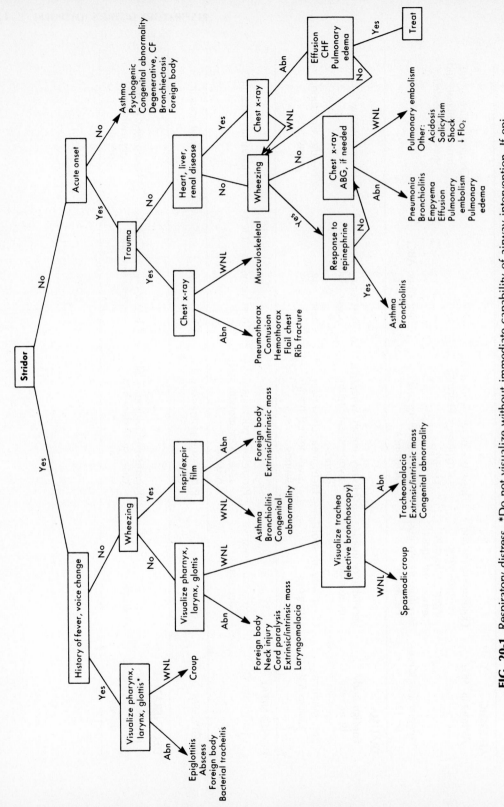

FIG. 20-1. Respiratory distress. *Do not visualize without immediate capability of airway intervention. If epiglottitis is suspected, procedure should be performed in operating room.

EVALUATION (Fig. 20-1)

The initial focus must be on the assessment of the airway and ventilatory status with intervention on an emergent basis as required. This often must occur before definitive diagnostic evaluation has been completed.

Airway integrity and ventilatory status can be rapidly assessed initially by evaluating for the presence of stridor and auscultating to determine the adequacy of air movement and the presence of wheezing, rales, or rhonchi.

1. *Upper airway obstruction.* Laboratory evaluation is usually ancillary to direct visualization, particularly in patients with respiratory distress. This must be done with great caution and anticipation. Specific measures are indicated for patients with potential foreign bodies (p. 599).
2. *Lower airway disease.* Chest x-ray films and ABG provide initial data. Specific tests for the suspected etiologies must be obtained (Table 20-1).

MANAGEMENT

Stabilization of the airway is central to any management plan and must not be delayed by obtaining excessive confirmatory data before instituting definitive therapy. All patients with respiratory distress require evaluation of the airway and ventilatory status and intervention as needed. Oxygen and cardiac monitoring should be initiated on arrival.

It is important to remember that upsetting the child should be avoided whenever possible. The degree of distress should never be underestimated, and the child should never be left unattended in the ED, x-ray department, or any other area of the hospital.

Specific intervention must reflect the status of the patient and conditions that may have caused that status.

REFERENCE

MacPherson, R.I., and Leithiser, R.E.: Upper airway obstruction in children: an update, RadioGraphics 5:339, 1985.

21 Status epilepticus

ALERT: Maintain airway; administer oxygen, dextrose, and naloxone (Narcan) (if appropriate) and then anticonvulsants. Consider diagnostic entities.

Patients are considered to be in status epilepticus when they experience continuous seizures for 20 min or have more than two seizures without a lucid period. Poor compliance is the most common explanation, although some patients may have lowered thresholds from fever and infection, head trauma, hypoglycemia and metabolic abnormalities, ingestions, drug interactions, hypertension, or an exacerbation of the underlying condition. It may be the first seizure in a child who goes on to have epilepsy (p. 559). Animal studies have shown that cellular ischemic changes begin within 10-15 min of onset of seizures and that irreversible damage may occur within 1-1½ hr.

DIAGNOSTIC FINDINGS

Grand mal seizures are most common, although other seizure categories may occur.

Patients experience seizure activity, loss of consciousness, and cyanosis. Temperature may be increased before the seizures because of meningitis or other infection or secondary to the increased muscle activity. Tachycardia and increased blood pressure are common.

Mydriasis and upward deviation of the eyes are present. The corneal reflex is decreased, and a positive Babinski's reflex is present. Fecal and urinary incontinence occur.

Complications

1. Death from anoxia, aspiration, or trauma secondary to the loss of consciousness
2. Encephalopathy from hypoxia
3. Acute renal failure associated with myoglobinuria and rhabdomyolysis
4. Respiratory arrest caused by medications

Ancillary data

Appropriate studies should be done:
1. A sample for blood glucose determination before infusion of D25W. Also rapid glucose approximation (Dextrostix/Chemstrip)
2. ABG for assessment of acidosis and hypoxia
3. Anticonvulsant levels, if patient has been taking medications
4. If the etiology is unknown: electrolytes, Ca^{++}, Mg^{++}, PO_4^-, CBC, and toxicologic screen. Consider lumbar puncture and CT scan as appropriate.

MANAGEMENT

Initial attention must be supportive, particularly to the airway and supplemental oxygen.
1. Intubation may be required to oxygenate the patient and minimize the risk of aspiration.
2. Traumatic injuries must be prevented by protecting the patient against self-injury.

Glucose has an immediate metabolic effect

and should be considered. A glucose level should be drawn before administration of glucose for later confirmation, if possible.

• Glucose D25W 0.5-1.0 g (2-4 ml)/kg/dose IV slowly; for preterm infant, D10W. For children >3 yr D50W may be used.

The following should be considered:

1. Naloxone (Narcan) 0.1 mg/kg/dose up to 0.8 mg IV. With no response and suspicion of opiates, give 2 mg IV. Available in vials of 0.4 mg/ml and 1.0 mg/ml. Very large doses may be required for propoxyphene (Darvon) and pentazocine (Talwin) overdoses.
2. Thiamine 100 mg/dose IV or IM initially and then twice every 24 hr PO for maintenance. Administer if alcoholism or malnutrition is suspected.
3. All *metabolic* abnormalities must be corrected. Rarely will anticonvulsants be totally effective in the presence of a significant metabolic abnormality.
   a. Hypoglycemia: D25W 0.5-1.0 g (2-4 ml)/kg/dose IV; then use extra glucose in maintenance fluids (at least D10W) (p. 200)
   b. Hyponatremia: 3% saline (0.5 mEq Na$^+$/ml) given at rate of 4 ml/kg IV over 10 min; then correct deficit over 16 hr
   c. Hypernatremia: correct over 48 hr
   d. Hypocalcemia: 10% CaCl$_2$ 20 mg (0.2 ml)/kg IV slowly; repeat as necessary
   e. Hypomagnesemia: MgSO$_4$ 25-50 mg/kg/dose q 4-6 hr for 3-4 doses IM or IV slowly (adult: 1 g 10% solution IV slowly)

Anticonvulsants (Table 81-6) should be considered, although the appropriate drug and the order of administration are controversial. Diazepam (Valium), phenobarbital, or phenytoin (Dilantin) may be used. Diazepam is usually preferred for acute termination but requires initiation of a second drug for long-term management. The risk of respiratory depression is thereby increased.

1. Diazepam (Valium)
   a. Dose: 0.2-0.3 mg/kg/dose IV over 2-3 min

at a rate not to exceed 1 mg/min. May have to repeat in 5-10 min if seizures continue. Maximum total dose: child, 10 mg; adult, 30 mg
   b. Although it is not preferred or fully substantiated, rectal administration has been successfully used. Undiluted commercial IV preparation is administered directly into the rectum using a plastic tube.
      • An initial dose of 0.5 mg/kg/dose PR is recommended.
   c. Intramuscular administration is unreliable, largely dependent on site and method of administration. In adults there have been good results when it is administered intramuscularly into the deltoid.
   d. Peak effect: 1-2 min, with an anticonvulsant effect for 20-30 min
   e. Toxicity: respiratory depression; synergistic with barbiturates
   f. Lorazepam (Ativan) may be a useful alternative with less respiratory depression and a longer half-life.
2. Phenobarbital
   a. Loading dose: 10-15 mg/kg/dose IV; infusion not to exceed 25-50 mg/min. Adult: 100 mg/dose IV q 20 min prn but not to exceed 3 doses. If more is given as load, be prepared to support blood pressure and ventilation. Although not preferred, it may be given deep IM (somewhat erratic absorption). If no response in status epilepticus, may give additional dose.
   b. Maintenance dose: 3-5 mg/kg/24 hr IV, IM, or PO
   c. Therapeutic level: 10-25 µg/ml
   d. Toxicity: respiratory depression; synergistic with diazepam
3. Phenytoin (Dilantin)
   a. Loading dose: 10-20 mg/kg/dose IV infusion (concentration of 6.7 mg/ml or less in saline, not water; not to exceed 40 mg/min. Maximum: 1,250 mg total dose
   b. Maintenance dose: 5 mg/kg/24 hr IV or PO

c. Peak effect in 15-20 min

d. Therapeutic level: 10-20 µg/ml

e. Toxicity: cardiac conduction block

4. Paraldehyde

a. Dose: 0.3 ml/kg (maximum: <10 yr: 5 ml; adult: 10 ml) mixed 1:1 in mineral or vegetable oil (1:3 in neonate) and given per rectum (PR).

IV administration (after consultation) may be done by mixing as a 4% solution (20 ml of paraldehyde 975 mg/ml added to 500 ml of 0.9%NS). Initially give 2.5-5 ml/kg (100-200 mg/kg) to yield a serum level of approximately 200 µg/ml. Follow by drip at 0.5 ml/kg/hr (20 mg/kg/hr) and titrate. Avoid plastic equipment.

b. Useful in intractable situations. Most commonly given rectally. Contraindicated in presence of hepatic, pulmonary, or renal disease.

If seizure control is difficult, a neurologist should be involved in the pharmacologic approach to the patient. A common practice is to use drugs in a sequential fashion until control is achieved. Although there is no agreement, many clinicians start with diazepam (Valium) and concurrently administer phenytoin (Dilantin) or phenobarbital. Another option is to omit diazepam and proceed directly to phenytoin or phenobarbital because of the marked respiratory depression noted in young children from diazepam, particularly when used in combination with phenobarbital. In children who have received diazepam, phenytoin has the advantage as the second drug because there is no synergistic respiratory depression.

Patients who continue to be resistant following loading with phenobarbital and phenytoin should receive paraldehyde. Another modality for resistant seizures following administration of the drugs outlined above (1-4) is general anesthesia (e.g., pentobarbital 5 mg/kg IV slowly followed by 1-3 mg/kg/hr infusion). Blood pressure must be monitored continuously. The barbiturate coma is followed with EEG, titrating to a burst suppression pattern.

Airway and ventilation must be monitored and maintained.

If patients previously have taken an anticonvulsant and the levels are subtherapeutic, maintenance dosage should be increased. If poor compliance is the basis for low levels, the patient should be reloaded (in full or part, depending on the level) and educated about the importance of taking the medication. Close follow-up with measurements of drug levels is necessary.

Concurrently, a therapeutic and diagnostic evaluation must be done to determine the potential etiologies while attempting to treat seizure activity with anticonvulsants. Metabolic causes require correction of the underlying abnormalities rather than additional anticonvulsants. Mass lesions and cerebral edema, for example, require specific therapeutic intervention. Infections should be treated expeditiously.

DISPOSITION

All patients should be admitted to the hospital to ensure ongoing control of seizure activity. Under circumstances where poor compliance was the causative factor, a period of observation (4 hr) after reloading may substitute for admission if intervention is possible in the home environment.

If seizures are refractory to normal medications, a neurologist should immediately be involved and the patient admitted to an ICU.

REFERENCES

Delgado-Escueta, A.V., Westerlain, C., Treiman, D.M., et al.: Management of status epilepticus, N. Engl. J. Med. **306**:1337, 1982.

Dulae, O., Aicardi, J., Rey, E., et al.: Blood levels of diazepam after single rectal administration in infants and children, J. Pediatr. **93**:1039, 1978.

Earnest, M.P., Marx, J.A., and Drury, L.R.: Complications of intravenous phenytoin for acute treatment of seizures, JAMA **249**:762, 1983.

Rothner, A.D., and Erenberg, G.: Status epilepticus, Pediatr. Clin. North Am. **27**:593, 1980.

Snead, O.C., and Miles, M.V.: Treatment of status epilepticus in children with rectal sodium valproate, J. Pediatr. **106**:323, 1985.

Vining, E.P.G., and Freeman, J.M.: Status epilepticus, Pediatr. Ann. **14**:765, 1985.

22 Sudden infant death syndrome

ALERT: The child who suffers near–sudden infant death syndrome (SIDS) requires aggressive resuscitation and support. Families who have lost a child from SIDS should receive immediate and ongoing support.

Sudden infant death syndrome is the sudden death of a young child between 1 mo and 1 yr of age, which is unexpected by history and in which a thorough postmortem examination fails to define an adequate cause of death. The peak incidence of SIDS is in infants between 2 and 4 mo of age. It commonly occurs in the fall and winter months. Many children experienced a recent respiratory infection.

ETIOLOGY

There are multiple contributing factors (such as infection, sleep, poor growth, aspiration, genetics), leading to respiratory obstruction and central apnea with associated hypoxia and death. Although infantile apnea (Chapter 13) may precede SIDS, there is no evidence to suggest that this occurs in most cases of SIDS.

DIAGNOSTIC FINDINGS

The child who has suffered a SIDS death experiences irreversible cardiac and respiratory arrest. The child who has experienced near-SIDS will have variable vital signs, depending on the duration of cardiac and respiratory arrest before intervention.

Complications of near–SIDS

1. Pulmonary edema (Chapter 19)
2. Aspiration pneumonia
3. Neurologic sequelae secondary to hypoxia

Ancillary data

1. An autopsy should be performed on all SIDS deaths by a competent and experienced pathologist.
2. Supportive data should be obtained in accordance with procedures for resuscitation (Chapter 4).

DIFFERENTIAL DIAGNOSIS

1. Trauma. Head trauma or child abuse may be difficult to distinguish in the absence of a reliable history.
2. Infection
   a. Overwhelming and acute infection may occur, but preceding signs and symptoms should be consistent with an infectious process.
   b. CNS infection (encephalopathy or meningitis) may have a similar presentation.
3. Congenital. Metabolic derangements, particularly those producing hypoglycemia (such as glycogen storage disease or severe acidosis) may result in apnea and seizures.
4. Vascular
   a. Subarachnoid bleeding may occur, with acute loss of consciousness and cardiac arrest.
   b. Cardiac dysrhythmias rarely occur in children.
5. Intoxication. Accidental or intentional poisoning can produce coma, with subsequent

135

hypoventilation, arrest, hypoxia, and death.
6. Infantile apnea (Chapter 13)

MANAGEMENT

The child with near-SIDS requires rapid evaluation and resuscitation efforts. Admission to the hospital for ongoing management is indicated, usually in the ICU.

Intense psychologic support for families and friends, both immediately and on a long-term basis, is required. Parents of children who die from SIDS normally demonstrate denial, anger, and then self-reproach and guilt. Verbalization of feelings, with reunion and ultimate separation from the child, are important. Assistance in arranging the funeral may be helpful.

Ongoing support must be ensured. Many communities have parents' groups. Where they are not available, the National Sudden Infant Death Syndrome Foundation, 2 Metro Plaza (#205), 8240 Professional Place, Landover, MD 20785 (301-459-3388), may be helpful.

DISPOSITION

After stabilization in the hospital, the child with near-SIDS may be discharged. Counseling must be provided. These patients should be placed on chalasia regimens with slow, careful feedings in an upright position for 30-60 min following meals.

When appropriate, apnea monitors are available for home use. Long-term follow-up provided by supportive health personnel is mandatory.

REFERENCES

Brooks, J.G.: Apnea of infancy and sudden infant death syndrome, Am. J. Dis. Child. 136:1012, 1982.
Gould, J.B., and James, O.: Management of the near-miss infant: a personal perspective, Pediatr. Clin. North Am. 26:857, 1979.
Shannon, D.C., and Kelly, D.H.: Sids and near-SIDS, N. Engl. J. Med. 306:959, 1022, 1982.

23 Syncope (fainting)

ALERT: Unless syncope is obviously self-limited, patients should be placed on a monitor and be given glucose and oxygen. The history is essential to determining potential etiologies.

Syncope is a transient, acute loss of consciousness. It is caused by relative cerebral hypoxia or hypoglycemia. Although it most commonly results from benign conditions, cardiac, vascular, and infectious etiologies should be excluded.

The history must focus on recent medications, past medical problems, intercurrent illness, metabolic abnormalities, social interactions, and family history. The episodes of syncope must be carefully described in regard to the precipitating factors and accompanying signs and symptoms (Table 23-1). History of syncope during exercise points toward cardiac disease such as aortic stenosis. Syncope should be characterized with regard to suddenness of onset and progression, duration, sequelae, and accompanying problems such as seizures.

The physician should focus on cardiac and pulmonary status, as well as performing a careful neurologic examination.

Ancillary data may include a chest x-ray study, ECG (Holter monitoring as indicated), glucose, CBC, and drug screen.

An ABG is sometimes helpful, but procedures such as EEG and CT scan are not routinely useful.

Distinguishing syncope from seizures is sometimes difficult. Seizures are usually prolonged (≥ 5 min) and accompanied by tonic-clonic movements and incontinence, followed by a period of confusion and sleepiness. In contrast, syncope usually lasts only seconds and there are no abnormal movements or incontinence. On awakening from an episode of syncope, patients usually are normal or only very mildly confused.

Since the episode is ordinarily self-limited, management involves a brief but appropriate evaluation and follow-up. Patients who have altered consciousness when they arrive at the ED should be administered dextrose, naloxone (Narcan), and oxygen and should be placed on a cardiac monitor pending evaluation.

TABLE 23-1. Syncope: diagnostic considerations

Condition	Diagnostic findings	Comments
INTRAPSYCHIC (Chapter 83)		
Vasomotor (vasovagal)	Rapid drop in BP, bradycardia; accompanying nausea, vomiting, sweating, pallor, numbness, blurred vision, weakness	Precipitated by fear, pain, anxiety, noxious stimuli; usually in hot, humid, closed space; common in adolescents
Hyperventilation	Rapid and deep respirations; secondary weakness, tingling, numbness of hands; feeling of dyspnea	Response to anxiety; common in adolescents, particularly females; responds to rebreathing
Breath holding (p. 549)	Cyanosis and frequent unconsciousness following vigorous crying	Usually self-limited; triggers usually easily defined (e.g., crying, anger)
Hysteria	No preceding nausea, vomiting, or somatic symptoms; no anxiety; avoids injury (falls while sitting)	Responds to environmental stimulus, unconscious; adolescents (females)
VASCULAR		
Postural hypotension (orthostatic)	Episode occurs following prolonged standing or on rising from a recumbent position; orthostatic changes variably present on exam	Poor cerebral perfusion initially; avoid rapid position changes; check Hct, BP standing and supine
Congenital or acquired heart disease (Chapter 16) Pulmonary stenosis Aortic stenosis Tetralogy of Fallot	Cardiac murmur, low output with poor perfusion, pallor, variable large pulse pressure	Poor cerebral perfusion
Congestive heart failure (Chapter 16)	Tachypnea, dyspnea, rales, wheezing, tachycardia, cardiomegaly, diaphoresis, cyanosis	Poor cerebral perfusion
Dysrhythmia (Chapter 6) Heart block Others Supraventricular tachycardia Ventricular tachycardia WPW	Bradycardia, irregular rhythm Abn rhythm, rate, poor perfusion; vital signs variable	Stokes-Adams attack: ECG required; if normal, Holter monitor and exercise evaluation; antiarrhythmics
Hypertension, malignant (Chapter 18)	Headache, dizziness, visual change, nausea, vomiting; variable change in mental status and focal neuro signs	May require treatment for encephalopathy
Posttussive cough	Episode following coughing	Caused by decreased venous return; may require cough suppressant

TABLE 23-1. Syncope: diagnostic considerations—cont'd

Condition	Diagnostic findings	Comments
INFECTION		
Upper airway obstruction (p. 591)		Secondary to cerebral hypoxia
Croup	Inspiratory stridor, cyanosis, labored resp, variably toxic, febrile	
Epiglottitis		
Lower airway disease		Secondary to cerebral hypoxia
Pneumonia (p. 601)	Fever, toxicity, tachypnea, rhonchi, rare chest pain	
Empyema		
TRAUMA		
Upper airway: foreign body (p. 599)	History, inspiratory or expiratory stridor, cyanosis, respiratory distress, wheezing, rare resp arrest	Secondary to cerebral hypoxia
ALLERGY		
Asthma (p. 581)	Wheezing, tachypnea, cough	Secondary to cerebral hypoxia
METABOLIC		
Hypoglycemia (Chapter 38)	Pallor, sweating, nausea, vomiting, tachycardia, tachypnea	Secondary to cerebral hypoglycemia
INTOXICATION (Chapter 54)	Hypotension, poor peripheral perfusion, dysrhythmia	Any drug that causes hypotension or hypoventilation (narcotics, sedatives, alcohol, diuretics, etc.) or dysrhythmias (digitalis)
MISCELLANEOUS		
Epilepsy (p. 559)	May be tonic-clonic (grand mal), transient lapse of consciousness (petit mal) or psychomotor	EEG required; may be difficult to differentiate
Anemia (Chapter 26)	Pale, tachycardia, light-headed	Decreased oxygen-carrying capacity and cerebral hypoxia
Dehydration (Chapter 7)	Hypotensive (orthostatic), poor perfusion, dry membrane	Secondary to poor cerebral perfusion

VI URGENT COMPLAINTS

24 Acute abdominal pain

ALERT: Severe abdominal pain lasting over 6 hr in a previously well patient usually requires surgery.

Acute abdominal pain in the child presents a diagnostic dilemma. The most common medical problem is acute gastroenteritis, although more serious etiologies must be excluded. Beyond this, the clinician must synthesize historical and physical data with anatomic and physiologic considerations.

ETIOLOGY

Diffuse abdominal pain results from one of several processes. A ruptured viscus produces peritonitis with rebound, guarding, and tenderness, commonly accompanied by sepsis and shock. Abdominal distension with high-pitched sounds and minimal rebound result from intestinal obstruction. Systemic disease may produce a diffuse pattern.

Pain is commonly referred. Diaphragmatic involvement from such entities as basilar pneumonia, subphrenic abscess, pleurisy, pancreatitis, peritonitis, or disease of the spleen, gall bladder, or liver may produce shoulder pain, which may be bilateral if the median segment of the diaphragm is irritated. Testicular pain may represent renal or appendiceal pathology. Complaints of back pain may be referred from a retroperitoneal hematoma, pancreatitis, or uterine or rectal disease. Pelvic abscesses may not produce diffuse peritonitis because of the relative absence of sensory innervation in that region.

Common diagnostic considerations vary with the age of the child. In the *infant*, acute gastroenteritis is most common, but it is essential to exclude intussusception, volvulus, perforated viscous, and Hirschsprung's disease. In *preschool* children, the most common underlying causes of acute abdominal pain are acute gastroenteritis, urinary tract infections, trauma, appendicitis, pneumonia, viral syndromes, and constipation. The *school-age* child frequently has acute gastroenteritis, urinary tract infection, trauma, appendicitis, gynecologic entities such as PID or ectopic pregnancy, inflammatory bowel disease, functional pain, constipation, or a viral syndrome associated with the pain.

DIAGNOSTIC FINDINGS

The history must define the onset of pain and its timing, quality, location, radiation, severity, course, and effect on activity. Associated vomiting, diarrhea, nausea, and other systemic signs and symptoms must be carefully delineated. Menstrual history should be defined.

Physical examination must include vital signs, temperature, and an overall assessment of the appearance and hydration status of the patient. The chest must be examined. The abdomen should be auscultated to assess bowel sounds and then palpated for masses and evidence of rebound, guarding, tenderness, and psoas or obturator signs. Hyperesthesia indicates parietal peritoneum inflammation. Rectal examination, with specimen testing for occult blood and polymorphonuclear leukocytes, is indicated in most patients. A pelvic examination should be done in all pubescent females with lower abdominal pain or any signs of pelvic disease.

Laboratory evaluation should include a urinalysis on all patients and, in those with severe pain, a CBC, ESR, and electrolytes and blood sugar analysis. Gonorrhea cultures and Pap smear should be done if a pelvic examination is performed. Abdominal (supine and upright) and posteroanterior and lateral chest x-ray films may be helpful. If there is a significant pathology and further diagnostic evaluation is indicated, other useful studies include amylase, liver function test (LFT), pregnancy test, peritoneal lavage, ultrasound, esophagoscopy, and contrast studies, including intravenous pyelogram (IVP), upper GI series, barium enema, and cholecystogram. See Table 24-1 for diagnostic considerations.

MANAGEMENT

The management of the patient with abdominal pain must reflect the severity, acuteness, and likely etiologies. Patients who must be seen immediately include those with prolonged, severe pain, high temperatures (>39° C), crying and doubling over with pain, associated trauma, potential dehydration, tachypnea or grunting; those with more prolonged fever (>2 days) with progression of pain made more comfortable by lying down should be seen on an urgent basis.

Many patients with prolonged pain, particularly those with nausea, vomiting, or diarrhea, have fluid deficits and benefit from intravenous hydration during the evaluation process (Chapter 7). Gastric decompression (NG tube) also may be useful. Surgical consultation should be sought for all patients with severe pain and significant abdominal examination.

REFERENCES

Hatch, E.I., Jr.: The acute abdomen in children, Pediatr. Clin. N. Am. **32**:1151, 1985.

Johnson, D.C., and Rice, R.P.: The acute abdomen: plain radiographic evaluation, RadioGraphics **5**:259, 1985.

Silen, W.: Cope's early diagnosis of the acute abdomen, New York, 1979, McGraw-Hill, Inc.

TABLE 24-1. Acute abdominal pain: diagnostic considerations

	Infection/inflammation	Congenital	Trauma	Endocrine/metabolic	Other
Systemic	**Influenza** Acute rheumatic fever	Sickle cell disease	Black widow spider bite	Diabetic ketoacidosis Porphyria Uremia Hyperparathyroidism Hypothyroidism	**Constipation, functional** Henoch-Schönlein purpura Neoplasm: leukemia, lymphoma, neuroblastoma Lead, heavy metal poisoning
Skin	Herpes zoster Cellulitis				
Abdominal wall		Hernia—inguinal, umbilical	Contusion Retroperitoneal hematoma		
Pulmonary	Pneumonia Pleurodynia				
Gastrointestinal	**Acute gastroenteritis** (virus, bacteria, parasite) **Mesenteric adenitis** **Appendicitis** Gastritis Hepatitis Cholecystitis, cholelithiasis Pancreatitis Esophagitis Diverticulitis Peptic ulcer Peritonitis	Meckel's diverticulum Volvulus Intussusception Hiatal hernia Hirschsprung's disease	Laceration: spleen, liver Perforation Intramural hematoma Pancreatic pseudocyst		**Colic** Mesenteric infarct Ulcerative colitis Regional enteritis Neoplasm
Urinary	**Pyelonephritis** **Cystitis**	Hydronephrosis	Renal contusion	Renal stone	Wilms' tumor
Genital	**Pelvic inflammatory disease** Salpingitis Tubo-ovarian abscess Epididymitis/oophoritis	Testicular torsion		**Mittelschmerz** **Dysmenorrhea** Hematocolpos Ovarian cyst Threatened abortion Ectopic pregnancy	
Other	Osteomyelitis Pelvic abscess		Pelvic or vertebral fracture Herniated disk		Lactose intolerance Dissecting aortic aneurysm Abdominal epilepsy

25 Abuse

ALERT: Suspicion is the key to recognition.

Child abuse: nonaccidental trauma

Children under 18 yr of age who suffer a non-accidental trauma (NAT) or physical injury that threatens their health or welfare are abused. This may take any one of several forms, including physical or emotional abuse, neglect (physical, emotional, medical, or educational), or sexual assault. A high index of suspicion is mandatory in evaluating children, particularly in settings that treat patients who are transient and whose care lacks continuity.

DIAGNOSTIC FINDINGS

Unique interpersonal dynamics form the basis for potential abuse and identify children who are at greatest risk.
1. The abused child
   a. Usually under 4 yr of age
   b. Often handicapped, retarded, hyperactive, or temperamental
   c. Premature birth or neonatal separation
   d. Multiple birth
2. The abusive parent
   a. Low self-esteem, depressed, a substance abuser
   b. Often abused as a child
   c. History of mental illness or criminal activity
   d. Violent temper outbursts toward child
   e. Rigid and unrealistic expectations of child
   f. Young maternal age
3. Family
   a. Monetary problems, often with unemployment
   b. Isolated and highly mobile
   c. Marital problems
   d. Pattern of husband/wife abuse
   e. Poor parent-child relationships
   f. Unwanted pregnancies, illegitimate children, youthful marriage

The introduction of one of the following triggers exacerbates the individual and family stresses, possibly resulting in child abuse: a family argument, discipline problem, substance abuse, loss of job, eviction, illness, or other environmental stresses. The child is often brought for care for a complaint other than the one associated with abuse or neglect ("somatic complaint").

Characteristics of history

1. Injury inconsistent with the history
2. Parents reluctant to give information, or they deny knowledge of how trauma might have occurred
3. Child developmentally incapable of specified self-injury (e.g., 9-mo-old falling off tricycle)
4. Inappropriate response to severity of injury
5. Delay in seeking health care

Physical examination (Table 25-1)

Bruises on the skin go through a typical evolutionary pattern that is useful in relating the objective findings to the history:

TABLE 25-1. Findings and differential diagnosis of child abuse

Physical findings	Differential diagnosis	Ancillary data
CUTANEOUS LESIONS		
Bruising (rope, tie, grab or slap marks, bites, cigarette burns; often different stages) (Chapter 29)	Trauma, accidental Hemophilia, Von Willebrand's Henoch-Schönlein purpura Purpura fulminans/meningo-coccemia	PT, PTT, bleeding time, platelets Rule out sepsis Rule out sepsis
Local erythema or bullae (abrasions or burns; burns may be immersion: doughnut shaped, slash burns, or outline object) (pp. 237 and 439)	Burn, accidental Staphylococcal impetigo Bacterial cellulitis Photosensitivity or contact dermatitis	Culture, Gram's stain Culture, Gram's stain History of sensitizing agent, orally or topically
OCULAR FINDINGS (Chapter 59 and p. 476)		
Retinal hemorrhage	Shaking or other trauma Bleeding disorder Resuscitation	Coagulation studies History
Conjunctival hemorrhage	Trauma, accidental Bacterial or viral conjunctivitis Severe coughing	Culture, Gram's stain History
Hyphema	Trauma, accidental	
ACUTE ABDOMEN (Chapters 24 and 63)		
Ruptured liver, spleen, or pancreas; intramural hematoma of bowel; retroperitoneal hematoma	Trauma, accidental Intrinsic gastrointestinal disease (e.g., peritonitis, obstruction, inflammatory bowel disease, Meckel's) Intrinsic urinary tract disease (infection, stone); trauma Genital problem (torsion of spermatic cord, ovarian cyst, etc.) Vascular accident Other (mesenteric adenitis, strangulated hernia, anaphylactoid purpura, pulmonary disease, pancreatitis, lead poisoning, diabetic ketoacidosis, etc.)	Rule out other disease X-rays, stool tests, etc. Urinalysis (hematuria), culture, IVP History, physical, technetium scan Angiography, sickle prep As appropriate

Modified from Bittner, S., and Newberger, E.H.: Pediatr. Rev. **2:**197, 1981. Copyright American Academy of Pediatrics, 1981.

TABLE 25-1. Findings and differential diagnosis of child abuse—cont'd

Physical findings	Differential diagnosis	Ancillary data
OSSEOUS LESIONS (Chapters 66-70)		
Fractures (multiple or in various stages of healing)	Trauma, accidental	
	Osteogenesis imperfecta	X-ray and blue sclera
	Rickets	Nutrition history
	Birth trauma	Birth history
	Leukemia	CBC, bone marrow
	Neuroblastoma	Bone marrow and biopsy
	S/P osteomyelitis or septic arthritis	History
		Physical examination
	Neurogenic sensory deficit	
Metaphyseal or epiphyseal lesions (particularly chip fractures)	Trauma, accidental	X-ray and nutrition
	Scurvy	History
	Syphilis	Serology
	Birth trauma	History
Subperiosteal ossification	Trauma, accidental	
	Osteogenic malignancy	X-ray and biopsy
	Syphilis	Serology
	Infantile cortical hyperostosis	No metaphyseal irregularity
	Osteoid osteoma	Response to aspirin
	Scurvy	Nutritional history
MENTAL STATUS CHANGE (Chapters 54 and 57, and p. 92)	Trauma: subdural, epidural, intracranial hemorrhage	CT scan
	Intoxication	Drug screen
	Infection: meningitis	Lumbar puncture
SUDDEN INFANT DEATH (Chapter 22)	Unexplained	Autopsy
	Trauma, accidental	Autopsy
	Asphyxia (aspiration, nasal obstruction, laryngospasm, sleep apnea)	"Near-miss" history
	Infection	Cultures: bacterial and viral
	Cardiac dysrhythmia?	Autopsy
	Hypoadrenalism?	Electrolytes
	Metabolic abnormality	Ca^{--}, Mg^{--}, Na^+, glucose

1. First 24 hr: bruise is reddish with some blue or purplish discoloration
2. 1-3 days: bruise turns blue to bluish-brown
3. 5-7 days: bruise develops a greenish coloration
4. 10 days: bruise becomes yellowish
5. 24 wk: normal

Mechanism of burns may be distinguished by physical findings. Splash burns are irregular and superficial, usually resulting from a toddler pulling over a container of hot liquid. An immersion burn often has a stocking/glove distribution with a sharp line of demarcation. It is even and deep and usually results from the infant being placed in hot water.

Behavioral signs that may either provoke or result from abuse or neglect include:
1. Anger, social isolation, or destructive patterns, with evidence of negativism
2. Difficulty in developing relationships
3. Evidence of developmental delays
4. Depression or suicidal signals
5. Repeated ingestions
6. Poor school attendance and poor performance
7. Poor self-esteem
8. Regressive behavior

Ancillary data (Table 25-1)

1. X-ray studies are indicated for all children under 5 yr to rule out unsuspected injuries in cases of physical abuse. For those over 5 yr, x-ray films are taken of areas of tenderness, deformity, etc. Skeletal or trauma series, including skull (AP and lateral), chest (AP), pelvis (AP), spine, and long bones (AP) should be obtained.
2. Bleeding screen (Chapter 29) is appropriate if there is a history of recurrent bruising and bruising is the predominant manifestation of abuse. May usually be done electively.

DIFFERENTIAL DIAGNOSIS

See Table 25-1 for differential diagnosis.

MANAGEMENT (Fig. 25-1)

The key to management is to maintain a high index of suspicion to permit recognition of actual and potential abuse situations. The immediate medical problems of course must receive attention.
1. Evaluate the family and the child's environment in a nonjudgmental and supportive fashion. A social worker should be involved in this phase.
2. Determine the extent of ongoing risk to the child.
3. Contact the appropriate protective services worker immediately. *In most states there is a legal obligation to report suspected abuse.* A representative of the agency will discuss the case and arrange for involvement of a staff member. A full written report is required within 24-48 hr (depending on the state). Each hospital should have its own routine for expediting this process. Usually a special form is completed and forwarded with the encounter form.

DISPOSITION

Hospitalization is indicated where it is medically appropriate, in the absence of an alternative placement facility, or if the child cannot return home because of ongoing danger. The child should not be discharged until the medical problems are receiving appropriate treatment, social and protective services have agreed on a temporary disposition, and the case is fully evaluated.

Optimally, a temporary crisis center is desirable if the patient is medically stable. If there is no ongoing risk, patient may be discharged and sent home, with close monitoring and ongoing evaluation. Follow-up for medical problems should be arranged before the patient is discharged.

Social services and protective services must arrange for ongoing evaluation and management of psychosocial problems.

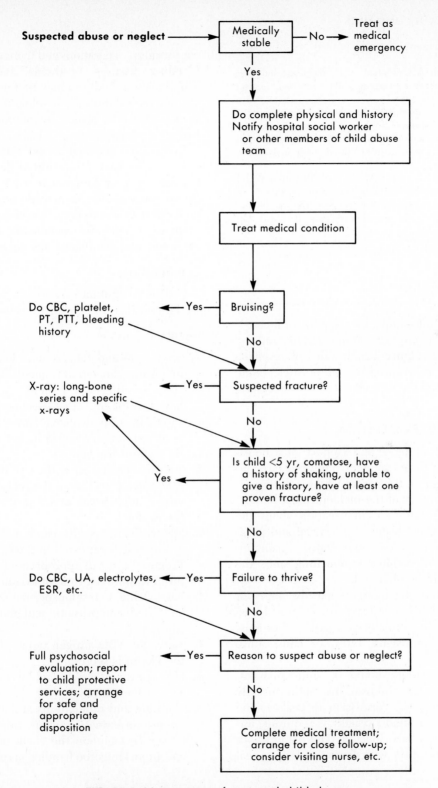

FIG. 25-1. Management of suspected child abuse.

REFERENCES

American Medical Association: AMA diagnostic and treatment guidelines concerning child abuse and neglect, JAMA **254**:796, 1985.

Bergman A.B., Larsen R.M., and Mueller B.A.: Changing spectrum of serious child abuse, Pediatrics **77**:113, 1986.

Ellerstein, N.S., and Norris, K.J.: Value of radiologic skeletal survey in assessment of abused children, Pediatrics **74**:1075, 1984.

Helfer, R.E., and Kempe, C.H., editors: The battered child, ed. 2, Chicago, 1974, University of Chicago Press.

Kempe, C.H., and Helfer, R.E., editors: Helping the battered child and his family, Philadelphia, 1971, J.B. Lippincott Co.

Sexual abuse

Sexual assault—rape, molestation, or incest—may occur in any age-group. Evaluation and management require a high index of suspicion and sensitivity. Appropriate authorities should be notified and the assessment must reflect local guidelines.

DIAGNOSTIC EVALUATION

Initially, confidence and rapport must be established. Where younger children are involved, it is often the parent who is most upset. A detailed history of the incident must be documented. In addition, information about the previous medical history, menstrual and pregnancy history, contraceptive status, recent intercourse, and bathing or douching since the assault should be obtained.

Acutely assaulted patients may be angry or withdrawn. The general appearance must be assessed and signs of external trauma, abrasions, lacerations, contusions, bites, or child abuse noted.

The examination should be individualized, and, with younger children, the mother usually should be present. Permission to perform the examination on minors usually is required, unless child abuse is suspected. The patient with acute trauma often will demonstrate perineal contusions or lacerations and hymenal tears with bleeding, fissures, erythema, and discharge. The uterus and adnexa may be tender. Signs of chronic molestation are residual findings of hymenal remnants, healed lacerations, a large introitus, and discharge (p. 514).

Beyond the neonatal period, nonsexual transmission of sexually transmitted diseases is uncommon in prepubescent females. In general, sexual abuse should be considered. This is particularly true in the presence of *Neisseria gonorrhoeae, Chlamydia trachomatis, Trichomonas vaginalis*, and *condyloma acuminatum*.

Complications

Emotional trauma varies with the age of the victim and the circumstances of the assault.

Ancillary data

1. Specimens and data are used to assist in documenting the circumstances and appropriately treating the patient. Many centers have kits for collecting specimens. Their use should be individualized. However, their value is minimal if over 48 hr has elapsed or if the patient has bathed.
2. Cultures are taken of the cervix for *N. gonorrhoeae*, as well as of the rectum and pharynx, if appropriate and repeated 2 wk after the assault.
3. Venereal Disease Research Laboratory test at the visit is repeated in 2 wk.
4. Pregnancy test (if appropriate) is used to determine status at time of assault.
5. Vaginal fluid to test for spermatozoa (wet prep and dried) and prostatic acid phosphatase are studied.
6. Saliva for ABO-antigen typing determines if the victim is secretor.
7. Hair specimen is obtained by combing pubic area of the victim.
8. Clothing and other items are submitted for forensic examination when appropriate.
   NOTE: To maintain the chain of custody all specimens must be handled carefully and re-

main in the physician's possession at all times until sealed. To ensure that the specimens are not altered before the introduction of the data in the courtroom, the "chain of evidence" must not be violated.

MANAGEMENT

The initial management of the patient must be supportive and understanding. The examination should proceed only after appropriate support services have assisted the patient and parents in dealing with the episode. Many institutions have specially trained individuals (often volunteers) to participate in this process. The examination must be individualized, reflecting the age of the child and the circumstances of the assault. If over 48 hr have elapsed, specimens will be of little value. The episode must be reported to the appropriate child protective services agency.

Pregnancy may be prevented and a number of options exist:

1. Diethylstilbestrol (DES) 25 mg 2 times/day for 5 days within 48 hr of the incident. It is associated with considerable nausea and vomiting. An antiemetic may be needed.

2. Ovral (norgestrel 0.5 mg and ethinyl estradiol 0.05 mg): 2 tablets taken within 72 hr of abuse and 2 more tablets 12 hr later

3. Do nothing and await next menses.

4. Recheck monoclonal antibody agglutination test to beta subunit of human chorionic gonadotropin (HCG) in urine or radioimmunoassay against beta subunit of HCG in blood in 7 days after incident. If negative, likelihood of pregnancy is low, but if positive, consider therapeutic abortion.

Follow-up with appropriate support groups and health care professionals is crucial. The patient should be seen in 2 wk to assess the reaction and repeat the cervical culture and VDRL test. If follow-up will be difficult, treatment for gonorrhea at the initial encounter should be considered (p. 515).

REFERENCES

Kobernick, M.E., Seifert, S., and Sanders, A.B.: Emergency department management of the sexual assault victim, J. Emerg. Med. 2:205, 1985.

Neinstein, L.S., Goldenring, J., and Carpenter, S.: Nonsexual transmission of sexually transmitted disease: an infrequent occurrence, Pediatrics 74:67, 1984.

26 Anemia

ROGER H. GILLER

ALERT: Anemia, which most commonly is caused by iron deficiency, requires a systematic evaluation of hematologic parameters.

Anemia is always a manifestation of a primary disease or nutritional deficiency. Because hemoglobin and hematocrits vary with age, anemia in children and adolescents is defined as that hemoglobin concentration which falls below the third percentile for a patient's age group (Fig. 26-1).

ETIOLOGY (Fig. 26-2)

Nutritional iron deficiency is the most common cause of anemia in children between 6 mo and 2 yr of age. It typically results from excessive cow's milk intake and inadequate consumption of iron-rich foods as the child outgrows inborn iron stores. Iron-deficiency anemia in those over 2 yr of age should prompt an investigation of causes of chronic blood loss.

Anemias unrelated to iron deficiency can be divided into two major categories:

1. Anemias caused by impaired red cell production, maturation, or release from the bone marrow

Disease	Mechanism
Malignancy, storage disease	Marrow infiltration
Fanconi's anemia, drugs, Blackfan-Diamond anemia, transient erythroblastopenia of childhood (TEC), aplastic anemia	Marrow aplasia/hypoplasia
Folate, B$_{12}$, B$_6$, copper deficiency	Impaired maturation of red cell precursors in bone marrow
Thalassemia syndromes, lead poisoning, sideroblastic anemia, pyridoxine deficiency	Impaired hemoglobin production, intramedullary hemolysis (thalassemias)
Chronic disease, inflammation, renal disease, hypothyroidism	Impaired erythropoiesis

2. Destruction, sequestration, or acute loss of circulating red cells

Disease	Mechanism
Sickle cell disease, vitamin E deficiency, autoimmune hemolytic anemia, RBC enzyme deficiency, RBC membrane defect, hemolytic uremic syndrome (HUS), disseminated intravascular coagulation (DIC), hemangioma, cardiac defect, prosthetic heart valve	Hemolysis
Portal hypertension, sickle cell disease	Splenic sequestration
Trauma, surgery, bleeding disorder, peptic ulcer disease	Hemorrhage

Term infants develop physiologic nadir of their hemoglobin levels in the 10.5 g/dl range at 2-3 mo of age. Levels may fall to 9 g/dl in normal preterm infants (Chapter 11).

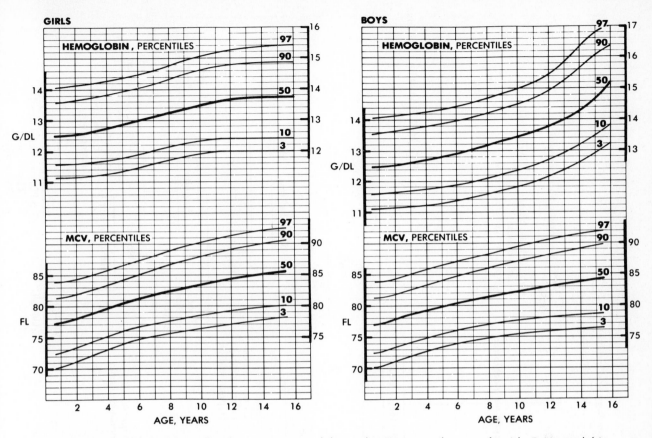

FIG. 26-1. Normal hemoglobin values by age. **A,** Hemoglobin and MCV percentile curves for girls. **B,** Hemoglobin and MCV percentile curves for boys. (From Dallman, P.R., and Siimes, M.A.: J. Pediatr. **94:**26, 1979.)

DIAGNOSTIC FINDINGS

Historically, it is important to consider age, sex, ethnic background, and dietary history; to determine the duration of symptoms; and to inquire about chronic illness or infection, bleeding, and pica. Family history must be reviewed in regard to history of anemia, jaundice, gallbladder disease, splenomegaly, or splenectomy.

The presenting signs and symptoms reflect the severity of the anemia, rapidity of onset, and underlying etiology.

1. With rapid onset of anemia (e.g., blood loss, sudden hemolysis), headache, dizziness, postural hypotension, tachycardia, hypovolemia, or high-output cardiac failure may be present (Chapters 5 and 16).

2. Insidious onset (e.g., nutritional deficiency, leukemia) is typically associated with pallor and decreased exercise tolerance.

3. Children with iron deficiency anemia may display behavioral disturbances, learning problems, and delayed motor development. Severe iron deficiency disrupts the integrity of the GI mucosa and may lead to a protein-losing enteropathy with blood in the stools.

4. Hemolytic anemia typically causes jaundice and splenomegaly. If chronic, symptomatic cholelithiasis may develop during childhood.

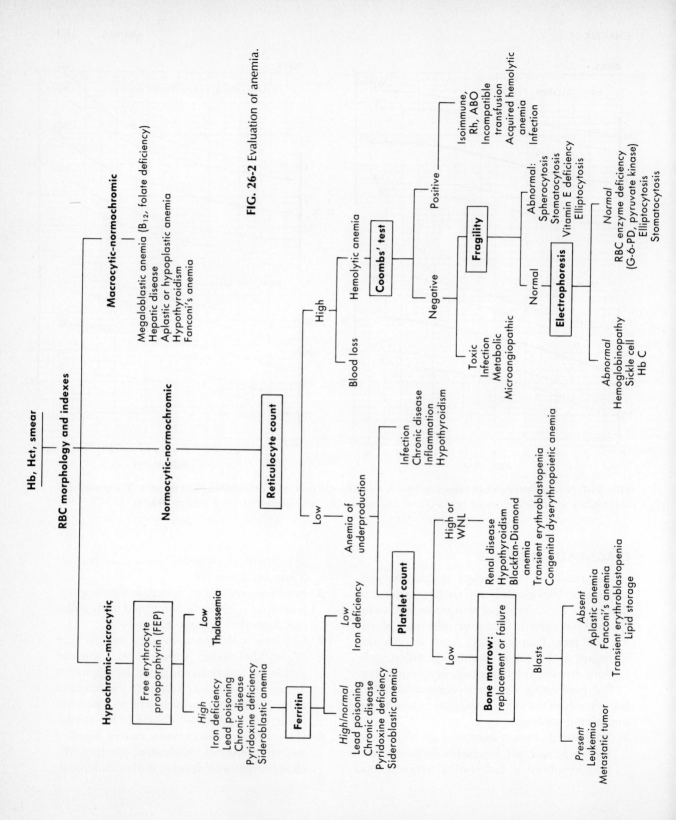

FIG. 26-2 Evaluation of anemia.

Underlying autoimmune disease (e.g., systemic lupus erythematosus) may be present.

Complications

Diminished oxygen-carrying capacity is generally well compensated for by increased cardiac output. However, severe tissue hypoxia can occur if the onset is rapid or there is concomitant high-output cardiac failure.

Ancillary data

1. Initial laboratory: CBC with Hb, Hct, RBC indexes, WBC, platelet count, peripheral smear, and reticulocyte count
2. Anemia in association with microcytosis. Strongly suggests iron deficiency. For further confirmation, determine the free-erythrocyte protoporphyrin (FEP) or serum ferritin. An FEP greater than 2.8 μg/g of Hb and a serum ferritin of less than 10 ng/ml are typical of iron deficiency. Iron saturation (serum iron/total iron-binding capacity × 100) of less than 20% also is indicative of iron deficiency but is subject to greater error because of diurnal and acute diet-related fluctuations in serum iron. An FEP of greater than 17.5 μg/g of Hb strongly suggests lead poisoning.
3. Stool for occult blood
4. Other studies, as indicated in Fig. 26-2

MANAGEMENT

In children 6 mo to 2 yr of age with no history of blood loss, a hypochromic, microcytic anemia is most likely caused by dietary iron deficiency anemia. It is appropriate to forego iron studies and initiate a therapeutic trial with careful follow-up. However, in children over 2 yr of age, where nutritional deficiency is less common, a more extensive evaluation to confirm iron deficiency and exclude chronic blood loss is indicated.

For initial treatment of suspected iron deficiency anemia:
1. Prescribe elemental iron 5 mg/kg/24 hr q 8 hr PO. Ferrous sulfate (Fer-in-Sol) 75 mg (15 mg elemental iron)/0.6 ml dropper is a useful formulation. The iron supplement should be continued for 2 mo after anemia is corrected to replenish iron stores.
   NOTE: With good compliance, normal absorption, and no ongoing iron losses, the reticulocyte count should increase in 3-5 days, and the hemoglobin should begin to rise during the first week of treatment.
2. Encourage iron rich foods.
3. Limit cow's milk intake to 24 oz/day.

A profound degree of anemia may produce life-threatening cardiovascular instability, requiring emergent intervention with blood products and fluids (Chapters 5 and 16). Other forms of anemia requiring specialized treatment should be handled on an individual basis in consultation with a hematologist.

DISPOSITION

Most children may be followed as outpatients. Admission is indicated for transfusion therapy if the Hct is below 20% (Hb < 7 mg/dl) or if there is evidence of cardiac decompensation, hypoxia, rapid ongoing blood loss, or hemolysis.

Parental education for iron deficiency anemia:
1. Give an iron supplement three times a day, preferably between meals. If there is any nausea, the iron may be given with foods. Keep the medication in a safe place, since accidental ingestion of a large amount can be dangerous.
2. Increase child's intake of iron-rich foods such as meat, eggs, green vegetables, and enriched cereals and breads. Limit milk intake to 24 oz/day.
3. Bring child back for recheck of blood counts in 1-2 wk and at 1 and 2 mo to be certain that youngster is no longer anemic.

REFERENCE

Oski, F.A., and Stockman, J.A. III: Anemia due to inadequate iron stores or poor iron utilization, Pediatr. Clin. North Am. 27:237, 1980.

27 Arthritis and joint pain

ALERT: Septic arthritis must be excluded in all patients.

Arthritis presents with joint swelling, limitation of motion, warmth, and pain or tenderness. Historically, patients must be questioned regarding the progression of signs and symptoms; the severity, duration, and type of pain, ameliorating factors; and family history. Relationship to trauma; infection; and systemic, vascular, and degenerative disease must be defined. Knowledge of previous medical problems and exposures and consideration of the patient's age may be helpful.

The patient must have a careful examination of the joint, with particular attention paid to the severity of involvement—defining objective parameters including warmth, tenderness, pain, the presence of fluid, and limitation of motion. Hip pain may be referred to the knee.

Ancillary data often are essential. If a fever or an elevated ESR (> 30 mm/hr) is present, an infectious or autoimmune process is eight times more likely than if both are absent. If both are present, only 7% of these patients lack a condition in either of these categories. CBC, blood culture, radiographs, bone scan, antinuclear antibody (ANA) tests, rheumatoid factor, and immunoglobulins may be selectively obtained.

If there is any question of the diagnosis and joint fluid is present, a joint aspirate should be obtained, usually after consultation with an orthopedist (Appendix A-2). The procedure usually is contraindicated if there is any overlying infection of the joint or if small joints only are involved. Typical findings are outlined in Tables 27-1 and 82-1.

REFERENCES

McCarthy, P.L., Wasserman, D., Spiesel, S.Z., et al.: Evaluation of arthritis and arthralgia in the pediatric patient, Clin. Pediatr. **19:**183, 1980.

Schaller, J., and Wedgwood, R.J.: Juvenile rheumatoid arthritis: a review, Pediatrics **50:**940, 1972.

See also Chapter 40: Limp.

TABLE 27-1. Arthritis and joint pain: diagnostic considerations and management

Condition	Diagnostic findings	Joints	Ancillary data	Comments/management
TRAUMA (Chapter 66)				
Sprain **Fracture**	History of trauma; joint tenderness, swelling; fracture may be occult	Usually monoarticular	X-ray variable	Orthopedic consult; consider child abuse (NAT)
"Little League elbow"	Swelling, tenderness; pitcher's elbow	Elbow on dominant arm	X-ray WNL	Restrict pitching
INFECTION				
Toxic synovitis of the hip (p. 569)	Preceding viral illness; nontoxic; often accompanied by limp; rarely warm, tender, limited range of motion	Hip	CBC, ESR: WNL; x-ray—variable effusion; aspirate if question of septic arthritis	Self-limited; common in 1½-7 yr-olds
Arthritis, septic (p. 569)	Acute onset, febrile; local swelling, warmth, tenderness	Monoarticular, large weight-bearing: knee, hip, wrist, elbow, shoulder; rarely polyarticular (gonococcal)	↑WBC, ↑ESR; x-ray; joint aspirate; may need bone scan	Requires urgent drainage and antibiotics
Arthritis, viral Rubella Rubella vaccine Hepatitis Epstein-Barr virus Chickenpox	Local swelling, warmth, tenderness; associated symptoms	Polyarticular; often large joints (knee)	CBC, viral titers, liver functions; x-ray—effusion; joint aspirate	Usually self-limited
Arthritis, uncommon Mycobacteria Fungi Syphilis	Often indolent with subacute progression; joint swelling, tenderness	Usually monoarticular, large joints	Joint aspirate; CBC; syphilis serology, PPD, as indicated	
Osteomyelitis	Fever, variable systemic toxicity, local swelling, tenderness, warmth	Monoarticular long bones (femur, tibia)	↑CBC, ↑ESR; x-ray; bone scan; joint and bone aspirate	May get arthritis and osteomyelitis concurrently; antibiotics
AUTOIMMUNE				
Juvenile rheumatoid arthritis (JRA) Acute febrile systemic (Still's) (20% JRA patients)	Irritable, listless, anorexic; hyperpyrexia (may precede arthritis); 90% have maculopapular rash; lymphadenopathy	Minimal or widespread; often only arthralgia; 25% severe arthritis	↑CBC, ↑ESR (70%); negative ANA, negative rheumatoid factor	Peak onset: 1-3 yr; ASA trial (100 mg/kg/24 hr q 4 hr PO) helpful; if fails: steroids; average age: 7½ yr

Continued.

TABLE 27-1. Arthritis and joint pain: diagnostic considerations and management—cont'd

Condition	Diagnostic findings	Joints	Ancillary data	Comments/management
Polyarticular (30% JRA patients)	Listless, anorexic; low-grade fevers, daily spike; rare maculopapular rash; rare iridocyclitis	≥4 joints (knee, ankle, wrist, elbow, hand); abrupt or insidious onset; swollen, red, tender; morning stiffness; severe arthritis associated with pos A-NA	↑ CBC, ↑ ESR (70%); positive ANA (25%), positive rheumatoid factor (10%-15%)	ASA trial; if fails: steroids
Monoarticular, pauciarticular (50% JRA patients)	Low-grade to no fever; rare rash; iridocyclitis (25%)	One or few joints—knee most common (others: ankle, elbow, wrist, fingers, sacroiliac); swollen, red, tender; morning stiffness	CBC, ESR: WNL; positive ANA (25%), positive rheumatoid factor rare; bone x-ray: accelerated maturation, periosteal proliferation; synovial fluid aspiration	Average age: 7½ yr; ASA trial; if fails: steroids
Rheumatic fever (p. 426)	Carditis, chorea, rheumatoid nodule, erythema marginatum, fever	Migratory, polyarticular, involving knee, ankle, wrist, elbow, shoulder; joints swollen, red, tender, hot, and painful	Variable CBC, ↑ ESR; ↑ streptozyme; throat culture variably positive	ASA trial; consider steroids; penicillin
Henoch-Schönlein purpura (anaphylactoid purpura) (p. 610)	Purpuric rash on ankles, buttock, elbow, beginning on lower extremity on extensor surface; abdominal pain, diarrhea, bleeding, intussusception; nephritis	Migratory polyarthritis of large joints	CBC, platelet: WNL; Hematest stool, urine; ↑ streptozyme, throat culture	Monitor for renal failure
Lupus erythematosus	Multisystem disease: weakness, fever, butterfly cheek eruption, hepatosplenomegaly, lymphadenopathy, nephritis; CNS: seizures, psychosis	Migratory; transient with arthralgia or redness, swelling, stiffness	↓ WBC, ↓ Hct, ↓ platelets; positive ANA; variable hematuria and proteinuria	Prednisone 1 mg/kg/ 24 hr PO; involve nephrologist
Serum sickness	Fever, rash, lymphadenopathy	Polyarthritis with redness, swelling, pain, stiffness, and large-joint effusion	↑↓ WBC; variable hematuria and proteinuria; reduced complement	Prevent exposure; antihistamine

Condition	History	Presentation	Diagnostic	Treatment/Comments
Inflammatory bowel disease / Ulcerative colitis / Regional ileitis	Diarrhea, variable rectal bleeding, abdominal pain	Polyarthritis, large joints	Sigmoidoscopy, barium swallow	Antiinflammatory agents, possibly surgery
Reiter's syndrome	Insidious onset; conjunctivitis, urethritis	Polyarticular, small joints	CBC, ESR: WNL; UA: WBC	Rare in children
CONGENITAL				
Hemophilia (p. 525)	Healthy male, variable history of trauma; history of hemophilia	Monoarticular; joint swollen, tender with hemarthrosis	X-ray; Abn bleeding screen	Factor replacement
Sickle cell disease (p. 531)	Systemic disease	Usually polyarticular; often insidious onset joint and bone pain	X-ray; Hct; positive Sickledex bone scan variable	May have concurrent infection; may be crisis or infarct
Dislocated hip	Normal newborn except for instability of joint; pos Ortolani's sign (abduction)	Abn placement and range of motion of hip	X-ray	Orthopedic consult; splint hip in flexion and abduction
VASCULAR				
Legg-Calvé-Perthes (avascular necrosis of proximal femoral head)		Insidious onset; pain of hip with limp or limitation of movement; pain may be referred to knee	X-ray: bulging capsule, widening joint space, decreased bone density around joint	Peak: males, 4-10 yr; orthopedic consult; treat hip in abduction and internal rotation
DEGENERATIVE				
Slipped capital femoral epiphysis	Usually obese child or tall, thin child with rapid growth	Unilateral or bilateral; knee pain (referred) on medial aspect thigh above knee; hip or knee pain made worse by activity; limp; limitation abduction and internal rotation	X-ray: widening of epiphyseal growth plate	Peak: 12-15 yr; orthopedic consult, surgical immobilization
OSTEOCHONDROSIS				
Osteochondritis dissecans	No systemic signs	Knee is painful, stiff with effusion	X-ray, tunnel view shows demineralization of medial femoral condyle	Teenagers; decreased activity; muscle strengthening
NEOPLASM				
Ewing's sarcoma / Osteogenic sarcoma / Leukemia / Neuroblastoma	Systemic signs often present	Local pain, effusion, with warmth and tenderness	CBC; x-ray; biopsy	Orthopedic consult

28 Ataxia

ALERT: Children with ataxia require attention to the diagnostic alternatives that permit early initiation of therapy when appropriate.

Infectious, inflammatory processes, and intoxication cause most incidents of acute ataxia in children. Hysteria, trauma, ear problems, migraines, and cerebellar and spinal cord tumors also may be causative (Table 28-1). A host of congenital (Freidreich's ataxia, ataxia telangiectasia) and metabolic conditions (Hartnup, maple syrup urine disease) have insidious onset of ataxia as a component of their presentations.

Cerebellar ataxia is associated with a wide-based, unsteady, and staggering gait, with difficulty turning. The patient cannot stand with the feet together whether the eyes are open or closed (Romberg's sign). Sensory ataxia from in-jury of the peripheral nerve or posterior column of the spinal cord also appears as a wide-based gait. However, the patient can stand with the feet together when the eyes are open but not when closed (positive Romberg's sign). This often is associated with lethargy, stupor, altered mental functioning, although ataxia may be the predominant finding.

Examination of the younger child must rely heavily on observation and cerebellar function demonstrated through play activities.

Ancillary data should usually include a spinal tap and drug levels, if indicated. Other tests must focus on potential etiologies.

TABLE 28-1. Acute ataxia: diagnostic considerations

Condition	Diagnostic findings	Ancillary data	Comments
INFECTION/INFLAMMATION			
Acute cerebellar ataxia	Prodrome of fever, respiratory or GI illness; abrupt onset; cerebellar ataxia; no evidence of intracranial pressure increase; normal mental function	CSF: WNL or slight lymphocytosis	2-6-yr-olds; resolves in 2-3 mo; usually viral
Postinfectious encephalitis	Preceding headache, exanthem, stiff neck, fever; changed mental status; cerebellar ataxia	CSF: ↑ protein, lymphocytosis	Usually viral; usually resolves
Bacterial: meningitis/encephalitis (p. 549)	Fever, toxic, stiff neck, changed mental status; cerebellar ataxia may be early symptom or postinfectious sequela	CSF: ↑ protein, ↑ WBC, ↓ glucose	Usually resolves following treatment
Cerebellar abscess	Fever, headache, cerebellar ataxia; may be signs of increased intracranial pressure	CT scan	Neurosurgical consult
Acute labyrinthitis	Cerebellar ataxia, vertigo, nystagmus, tinnitus, hearing loss, nausea, vomiting; may accompany otitis media		May also be traumatic
Multiple sclerosis	Cerebellar ataxia; spastic weakness; optic neuritis, diplopia; multiple neurologic deficits; relapsing	CSF: ↑ cells, ↑ protein, ↑ gamma globulin	Steroids (ACTH); physiotherapy
INTOXICATION (Chapter 54)			
Phenytoin	Cerebellar ataxia, nystagmus	Level >30 µg/ml	
Phenobarbital	Cerebellar ataxia, lethargy	Level >50 µg/ml	Tranquilizers also
Alcohol	Cerebellar ataxia, slurred speech, visual impairment, progressing to stupor and coma	Level dependent on whether acute or chronic use	
Carbon monoxide	Headache, confusion, cerebellar ataxia, seizures, stupor to coma	CO >30 mg%	Oxygen therapy, hyperbaric oxygen
Lead (also mercury and thallium)	Anorexia, vomiting, lethargy, cerebellar ataxia, increased intracranial pressure, papilledema, anemia; history of pica		Dimercaprol, EDTA
TRAUMA			
Head injury (Chapter 57)	Head trauma; headache; concussion; cerebellar ataxia	Variable skull x-ray	Close monitoring
Heat stroke/exhaustion (Chapter 50)	Fatigue, weakness, headache, cerebellar ataxia, seizures, psychosis, coma	Electrolytes; variable ABG and ECG	Treatment varies with condition
INTRAPSYCHIC (Chapter 83)			
Hysteria	Anxious, inconsistent findings		Psychiatric consult

29 Bleeding

ALERT: Patients with abnormal bleeding should be evaluated by an initial assessment that includes CBC, platelet count, PT, and PTT. Hemorrhage should be controlled when significant, usually by application of direct pressure. Resuscitation may be required with severe hemorrhage.

The evaluation of the patient with bleeding requires careful attention to the pattern of bleeding, its location, and whether it is spontaneous or in response to minor or major trauma. A positive family history of similar problems may indicate a hereditary basis for the bleeding disorder.

History and physical examination should classify the nature of the bleeding as well as ascertain its severity (Table 29-1).

Ancillary data that should be obtained on all patients with excessive or abnormal bleeding include:

1. CBC, peripheral blood smear, and platelet count
2. Bleeding time (BT)
3. Partial thromboplastin time (PTT)
4. Prothrombin time (PT)
5. Thrombin time (TT)
6. Fibrinogen

These tests assess various components of hemostasis (Fig. 29-1) and in combination with factor assays and platelet-function studies define most common bleeding abnormalities (Table 29-2).

Once classified, specific management can be initiated in consultation with a hematologist.

REFERENCE

Montgomery, R.R., and Hathaway, W.E.: Acute bleeding emergencies, Pediatr. Clin. North Am. 27:327, 1980.

TABLE 29-1. Patterns of bleeding

Diagnostic findings	Small-vessel hemostasis defect (platelet or capillary)	Intravascular defect (coagulation)
Bleeding pattern		
Spontaneous	Small, superficial, diffuse bleeding involving mucous membranes (epistaxis, GI, menorrhagia)	Major bleeding (musculoskeletal, CNS)
Superficial cut or abrasion	Profuse, prolonged	Minimal
Deep cut or tooth extraction	Immediate; good response to pressure	Delayed; poor response to pressure
Hemarthrosis	Rare	Common
Petechiae	Common	Rare
Ancillary data	Prolonged BT Abnormal platelets	Prolonged PTT, PT

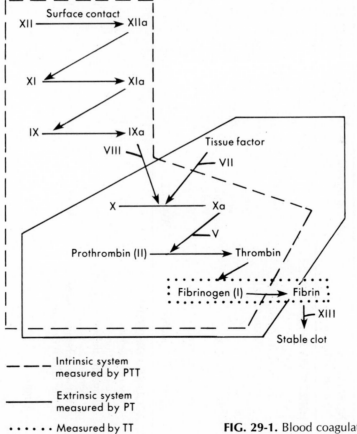

- - - - Intrinsic system
measured by PTT

———— Extrinsic system
measured by PT

• • • • • Measured by TT

FIG. 29-1. Blood coagulation scheme.

TABLE 29-2. Screening of the bleeding patient

Condition	Screening tests					Comments
	Platelet count	BT	PTT	PT	TT	
NORMAL (WNL) (varies with lab)	150-400,000/ml	4-9 min	25-35 sec	12-13 sec	8-10 sec	Fibrinogen 190-400 mg/100 ml
HEREDITARY DISORDERS						
Hemophilia						
Factor VIII (classic: A)	WNL	WNL	↑	WNL	WNL	Factor assay
Factor IX (Christmas: B)	WNL	WNL	↑	WNL	WNL	Factor assay
Factor XI	WNL	WNL	↑	WNL	WNL	Factor assay
Factor XII	WNL	WNL	↑	WNL	WNL	Factor assay
Factor II, V, X	WNL	WNL	↑	↑	WNL	Factor assay
Factor VII	WNL	WNL	WNL	↑	WNL	Factor assay
von Willebrand's (many variants)	WNL	↑	↑	WNL	WNL	VIII antigen, VIII cofactor, ristocetin cofactor
Platelet dysfunction	WNL/↓	↑	WNL	WNL	WNL	Platelet aggregation studies
ACQUIRED DISORDERS						
Disseminated intravascular coagulation	↓	↑	↑	↑	↑	↓ fibrinogen, ↑ fibrin split products
Idiopathic thrombocytopenic purpura	↓	↑	WNL	WNL	WNL	
Henoch-Schönlein purpura	WNL	WNL	WNL	WNL	WNL	
Liver failure (severe)	WNL/↓	WNL/↑	↑	↑	WNL/↑	↓ fibrinogen, ↑ fibrin split products
Uremia	WNL/↓	↑	WNL	WNL	WNL/↑	Secondary to hepatic dysfunction or protein loss
Anticoagulants						
Heparin	WNL	WNL	↑	WNL/↑	↑↑	Also lupus-like and inactivating anticoagulant
Coumadin	WNL	WNL/↑	WNL/↑	↑	WNL	
Aspirin	WNL	↑	WNL	WNL	WNL	

30 Constipation

ALERT: Constipation is commonly functional, although organic conditions must be excluded.

Constipation is present when children have difficulty with bowel movements because of an abnormality in the character of the stool rather than frequency. With persistent pain and discomfort, frequency will decrease. Elimination patterns reflect familial, cultural, and social factors. It is essential to determine if the stool pattern being described is actually normal. Constipation in the newborn often is associated with an anatomic problem, but in older children it is usually functional or dietary in origin.

ETIOLOGY

1. Dietary
   a. Lack of fecal bulk, causing an inadequate peristaltic stimulus; inadequate intake of roughage
   b. Excessive cow's milk intake and early introduction of solids such as cereals and yellow vegetables
2. Intrapsychic
   a. Abnormal or difficult toilet training, voluntary retention, or habit. There may be a history of prolonged, difficult toilet training, or constipation may begin with an anal fissure and be perpetuated.
   b. Psychogenic. Associated with parent-child and environmental problems and stresses. Fecal impaction, with secondary liquid stools soiling around the fecal mass, is common (encopresis).
3. Trauma. Anal fissures appear as small tears at the anus, often accompanied by blood streaking of the stools and pain.
4. Intoxication
   a. Excessive use of suppositories and enemas, causing the bowel to be insensitive to normal physiologic peristalsis
   b. Excessive use of antihistamine, diuretics, calcium channel blockers, diphenoxylate (Lomotil), or codeine-containing substances
5. Congenital (Chapter 11)
   a. Atresia of the colon or rectum
   b. Meconium plug syndrome in newborns, associated with cystic fibrosis and Hirschsprung's disease
   c. Hirschsprung's disease (p. 496)
   d. Myelomeningocele and other neurologic problems
6. Ileus secondary to infection or inflammatory bowel disease
7. Degenerative CNS diseases
8. Metabolic/endocrine
   a. Hypothyroidism
   b. Hypercalcemia
   c. Hypokalemia

DIAGNOSTIC FINDINGS

It is imperative to determine if the stool pattern is abnormal and if the constipation is an isolated finding or associated with systemic signs and symptoms. The characteristics of the stool must be assessed in regard to consistency, size, and frequency. Fecal soiling may occur.

Common complaints include anorexia, tenesmus, and abdominal pain. The pain may be crampy or constant and is usually recurrent. Occasionally, it may be severe enough to mimic a surgical abdomen.

Physical examination may demonstrate a palpable, cylindric mass. There is usually no distension, and the rectum is full of stool. Older children should have some evaluation of their adjustment, family and personal stresses, and maternal-child interactions.

Ancillary data

If the diagnosis is in doubt, a flat plate of the abdomen should be taken to demonstrate the extent of fecal retention.

MANAGEMENT
Simple constipation

Usually the elimination pattern is normal, and reassurance is all that is necessary after determining that there is no organic etiology. Generally, dietary manipulation is sufficient given the patient's age, severity of symptoms, and degree of parental anxiety. If constipation develops during bowel training, the pressure on training must be reduced.

1. For babies, add 1-2 tsp of Karo syrup to each bottle. If the child is over 4 mo of age, strained apricots, peaches, pears, and other fruits may be introduced. Avoid rectal stimulation with suppositories.
2. Older children should be encouraged to increase their intake of fruits and vegetables. These include prunes, figs, raisins, beans, celery, and lettuce. Prune juice is excellent and may be diluted with soda to improve the taste. Bran should be given in cereals, muffins, crackers, and other sources. Milk products may be constipating in some children. Push other fluids temporarily. Maltsupex ½-2 tbsp/day in 2 doses PO may be helpful. If necessary, docusate (Colace) 5-10 mg/kg/24 hr q 6-12 hr PO may be initiated for a short period (5-7 days).
3. Enemas and suppositories should not be given.

Anal fissures will usually disappear once the bowel movement pattern has been improved. Very rarely, chronic fissures may require surgical excision.

Long-standing constipation

Severe constipation in the older child, often with fecal impaction, requires a more aggressive approach after excluding organic considerations.

1. Fecal disimpaction by manual removal or by administration of hypertonic phosphate enema (Fleet pediatric) after overnight mineral oil. Often needs to be repeated once or twice. This frequently is followed by bisacodyl (Dulcolax) suppository twice a day for 2 days.
2. Continuing use of 15-60 ml mineral oil/dose two to four times per day PO
3. Referral for complete psychologic evaluation, support, and follow-up

REFERENCE

Fleisher, D.R.: Diagnosis and treatment of disorders of defecation in children, Pediatr. Ann. **5:**700, 1976.

31 Cough

ALERT: Upper and lower airway disease may produce coughing. Patients should be evaluated for respiratory distress (Chapter 20).

Coughing follows forceful expiration and opening of a closed glottis. The reflex, which is controlled in the medulla, receives vagal stimuli from the pharynx, larynx, trachea, and other large airways, as well as the ear. A number of different stimuli trigger the reflex, including mechanical, inflammatory, chemical, thermal, and psychogenic factors.

ETIOLOGY AND DIAGNOSTIC FINDINGS

The predominant cause of coughing is upper respiratory tract infections (Table 31-1). Other significant etiologies vary by age-group. In *infants*, structural abnormalities of the airway, gastroesophageal reflux, tracheoesophageal fistula, vascular rings, and physiologic mechanisms must be considered. *Toddlers* may have a foreign body, irritation of the airway (especially passive smoking), or asthma; *school-age* children often have asthma, sinusitis, or chronic rhinitis. *Adolescents* commonly have a cough caused by smoking or psychogenic factors. A chronic cough may be the only clinical presentation of reactive airway disease, but other entities to be considered with a prolonged cough include a foreign body, an unusual infection, or a congenital anomaly.

The type of cough may be useful in considering specific differential entities. Staccato, paroxysmal coughs accompany pertussis or chlamydia infections, but productive coughs imply that there is a lower airway or parenchymal infection. Purulent sputum is associated with bacterial pneumonia, lung abscess, bronchiectasis, and cystic fibrosis. Coughs that worsen at night usually are caused by posterior nasal drips from allergy or infection, and those coughs that improve during sleep often are psychogenic in origin.

Historically, it is imperative to determine the duration, frequency, quality, timing, and productivity of the cough. Inciting and ameliorating conditions should be defined, as well as associated signs and symptoms such as fever, shortness of breath, wheezing, allergies, and growth pattern. Family history should be obtained, focusing particularly on asthma, cystic fibrosis, tuberculosis, or any chronic pulmonary disease.

The physical examination must assess the patient's clinical condition, primarily based on a careful evaluation of the airway, lungs, and heart. Evidence of allergic disease or reactive airways should be sought.

Ancillary data must be individualized and may include a CBC, chest x-ray study (inspiratory and expiratory films if a foreign body is suspected), examination of sputum, pulmonary function tests, and specific studies such as a sweat chloride analysis to explore diagnostic considerations.

Hemoptysis, or coughing up blood often mixed with sputum (appearing red and frothy),

TABLE 31-1. Cough: diagnostic considerations

Condition	Diagnostic findings	Ancillary data	Comments
INFECTION/INFLAMMATION			
Upper respiratory infection (p. 463)	Acute onset, prolonged course; rhinorrhea, congestion, fever, pharyngitis, laryngitis, nonproductive cough	Throat cultures, if indicated	Self-limited; vagal stimulation; also croup (p. 591)
Pneumonia (p. 601)	Variable onset; fever, tachypnea, anorexia, irritability, productive cough, pleuritic pain; hemoptysis (group A streptococcus, TB)	Chest x-ray; CBC, ABG as needed	Viral, bacterial, mycoplasma, TB, fungal, chlamydial, pneumocystic; antibiotics, if needed
Bronchiolitis (p. 588)	Wheezing, tachypnea, unproductive cough, fever, relatively little respiratory distress early but may develop with cyanosis	Chest x-ray; ABG, if distressed	Viral; children <1 year; support, hydrate; inconsistent response to bronchodilator
Aspiration pneumonia	History of incident or patient with reduced level of consciousness; fever, productive cough; respiratory distress may be delayed 12-24 hr	Chest x-ray; serial ABG	May follow aspiration of gastric contents, bacteria, hydrocarbons; may be recurrent
Pulmonary abscess	Insidious; fever, malaise, anorexia, hemoptysis, productive cough; chest pain	Chest x-ray; culture of abscessed material	Aspiration of infected material or complication of pneumonia; drainage, antibiotics
Pertussis (whooping cough) (p. 543)	Catarrhal phase followed by paroxysmal cough with cyanosis and vomiting; prolonged cough	Chest x-ray; ↑ CBC (lymphocytes); fluorescent antibody	Hospitalize, support; erythromycin with catarrhal phase
Measles (Chapter 42)	Coryza, conjunctivitis, and productive cough, with generalized morbilliform rash, fever	Chest x-ray if significant and prolonged	Self-limited; complications of secondary infection
Pleurisy	Sharp, intense pain, worsens with inspiration; irritative, dry cough	Chest x-ray to exclude pneumonia, effusion	Self-limited; analgesia
Retropharyngeal abscess (p. 462)	Fever, difficulty swallowing, drooling, sore throat; irritative, dry cough	Lateral neck x-ray, CBC, culture material	Incision and drainage, antibiotics, analgesia
ALLERGIC			
Asthma (p. 581)	Wheezing, tachypnea, mild-to-moderate respiratory distress; nonproductive cough may be only symptom, unaccompanied by wheezing (may be induced by exercise); may be worse at night	Chest x-ray; ABG, pulmonary functions, as indicated	Responds to bronchodilators

	Clinical features	Diagnostic workup	Treatment
Posterior nasal drip (p. 463)	Prolonged, productive cough, often following respiratory infection, worse when lying down; rhinorrhea, bronchorrhea, congestion		Empiric treatment with decongestant before bedtime
TRAUMA			
Foreign body (p. 599)	If tracheal: partial or total obstruction of airway; bronchial: nonproductive cough, without accompanying illness, asymmetric wheezing	Chest x-ray: inspiration and expiration; direct visualization	Remove by bronchoscopy or if bronchial and less than 24 hr, postural drainage
Atelectasis	Fever, productive cough, hemoptysis; may have splinting; may be caused by trauma	Chest x-ray	Postural drainage, IPPB
VASCULAR			
Congestive heart failure (Chapter 16)	Tachypnea, tachycardia, murmur, rales, wheezing, cyanosis, cardiomegaly, productive cough	Chest x-ray; ABG; ECG	Diuretics, digitalis; evaluate underlying cause
Mitral stenosis	Dyspnea, cyanosis, pulmonary edema, CHF, hemoptysis	Chest x-ray; ABG; ECG	Congenital or rheumatic; cardiology consult
INTOXICATION			
Hydrocarbon ingestion (p. 292)	Initially asymptomatic, then in 12-24 hr tachypnea, fever; prolonged productive cough	Baseline and follow-up chest x-rays	Postural drainage; treat complications of secondary infection, CNS toxicity
CONGENITAL (Chapter 11)			
Cystic fibrosis	Chronic productive cough, recurrent pulmonary infection; frequent illness, poor weight gain; abnormal stools	Chest x-ray; ABG, pulmonary functions; positive sweat test	Postural drainage; antibiotics for acute exacerbations; dietary supplement
Tracheoesophageal fistula	Variable cough with feedings; poor weight gain, vomiting	Barium swallow	Surgery
Diaphragmatic hernia	As newborn, acute onset cyanosis, poor feeding, vomiting, nonproductive cough, respiratory distress	Chest x-ray; barium swallow	Surgery
NEOPLASM			
Pulmonary or mediastinal	Insidious onset, variable cough, hemoptysis, weight loss, chronically ill	Chest x-ray; nuclear scan, biopsy	Refer to oncologist

is an unusual pediatric condition, which may occur with a number of clinical entities.

1. Infection/inflammation
   a. Pneumonia: group A streptococci, tuberculosis
   b. Pertussis
   c. Pulmonary abscess
   d. Bronchiectasis, especially cystic fibrosis
   e. Viral infections: most common
2. Trauma: foreign body
3. Vascular: pulmonary hypertension, mitral stenosis
4. Neoplasm: mediastinal or pulmonary
5. Bleeding diathesis
6. Idiopathic pulmonary hemosiderosis
7. Following acute asthmatic attack

Most patients with coughing have only minimal signs and symptoms and may be discharged with an appropriate therapeutic regimen. Those with respiratory distress or significant hemoptysis should be hospitalized to define the underlying disease and facilitate treatment.

MANAGEMENT

The focus of management must be on determining the cause of the cough and instituting specific therapy for that condition. Beyond these specific steps, cough suppression may be necessary in older children if the cough is interfering significantly with activities, sleep, or eating or causing significant vomiting.

Therapeutic options for cough suppression include mixtures of honey (corn syrup in children under 1 yr), lemon concentrate, and liquor (for older children), medicines with dextromethorphan (DM), or antitussives with 10 mg codeine/5 ml and given as 1 mg codeine/kg/24 hr q 4-6 hr PO (adult: 10-20 mg codeine/dose PO).

Parental education

The following instructions apply to the child discharged with a cough, commonly following an upper respiratory tract infection.

1. Sucking on cough drops or hard candy may be useful for the older child. A good cough medicine can be made at home by mixing equal amounts of honey (corn syrup for children under 1 yr of age), lemon concentrate, and liquor such as Scotch or bourbon. You may omit the liquor for younger children.
2. Cough syrups are rarely useful. Stronger cough medicines containing dextromethorphan (DM) or codeine must be prescribed by a physician, but they have the danger of reducing the cough reflex that protects the lungs.
3. Humidifiers and pushing warm fluids may be helpful.
4. Call physician if
   a. Difficulty in breathing or shortness of breath develops
   b. Cough lasts over 2 wk
   c. Cough changes to croup ("barking-seal cough") or wheezing develops
   d. Child develops fever that lasts over 72 hr
   e. Cough spasms occur that cause choking, passing out, a bluish color of lips, or persistent vomiting
   f. There is blood in the mucus
   g. Chest pain develops

32 Acute diarrhea

ALERT: Initial evaluation of the child with diarrhea must include assessment of the hydration status. If there is evidence of dehydration, fluids should be administered to correct deficits.

ETIOLOGY AND DIAGNOSTIC FINDINGS

Acute diarrheal disease in childhood is primarily infectious in origin, resulting from a host of viral and bacterial agents delineated in Chapter 76. Acute gastroenteritis commonly leads to postinfectious malabsorption, secondary to lactose intolerance. Rarely do patients with peritoneal irritation, pneumonia, otitis media, or urinary tract infections have associated diarrhea. Antibiotics (such as ampicillin) are commonly prescribed for diarrhea (Table 32-1). When other obvious causes are ruled out, a patient probably has infectious diarrhea if there are unformed bowel movements at twice the normal rate, which are associated with one or more of the following: fever, nausea, vomiting, abdominal pain, cramps, blood or mucoid stools, or tenesmus.

Evaluation of more chronic diarrhea should account for inflammatory bowel disease, irritable bowel syndrome, malabsorption, secretory disorders, anatomic abnormality (especially Hirschsprung's disease), parasites, systemic disease, overfeeding, antibiotics, toxins, and secondary lactase deficiency.

The onset of symptoms and the characteristics of bowel movements are important, with partic-

ular attention to factors that increase (time, diet, etc.) or decrease (dietary elimination, withdrawal of drug, etc.) elimination. In addition, related symptoms and duration of illness must be assessed. The physical examination should focus on the state of hydration and associated findings.

Stool cultures and methylene blue smears should be done as well as cultures for ova and parasites, when appropriate. More exhaustive evaluations are rarely indicated unless the diarrhea has been prolonged. Sigmoidoscopy, barium enema, rectal biopsy, and other studies are done with severe disease in the absence of an infectious etiology.

MANAGEMENT

Management must focus on correcting any fluid deficits (Chapter 7) and treating the specific condition. Hospitalization should be considered when there is dehydration, intractable vomiting, young age (especially under 2-3 mo), underlying disease, systemic toxicity, and disrupted social or physical environment. Patients with severe abdominal pain associated with bloody stools require immediate evaluation and surgical consultation. The patient whose clinical status warrants it can usually be followed at home. Clear liquids usually should be given until there is some resolution of the diarrhea or specific therapy can be instituted.

See also Acute gastroenteritis, p. 480, and Vomiting, Chapter 44.

TABLE 32-1. Acute diarrhea: diagnostic considerations

Condition	Character of stool	Associated symptoms	Evaluation	Comments
INFECTION				
Acute gastroenteritis (p. 480)				
Virus	Loose; rare blood; rare WBC	Respiratory symptoms, vomiting	ELISA; electron microscopy	Acute onset
Bacteria	Loose/watery; variable blood; PMN	Vomiting; fever; seizure (*Shigella*); crampy abdominal pain	Culture; methylene blue for PMN	Acute onset; toxic; may be related to food poisoning
Parasite	Variable	Multisystem involvement; weight loss	Ova and parasite	May be insidious
Postinfectious malabsorption	Watery	Recovering from acute gastroenteritis	Reducing substance in stool (≥0.5%); pH <5.0	Usually lactose intolerance; may be primary
Food poisoning	Profuse	Abdominal pain, cramping, vomiting	Epidemiologic	Usually temporally related to food ingestion
Extraintestinal				
Acute appendicitis (p. 494) or peritonitis	Loose	Reflects associated problems	Abdominal x-ray; CBC	Surgical exploration
Respiratory infection (p. 601)			Chest x-ray, if needed	Antibiotics
Urinary tract infection (p. 620)			Urinalysis, urine culture	Antibiotics
INTOXICATION				
Antibiotics Iron (p. 294) Antimetabolites	Loose; fat (variable)	Vomiting, anorexia; adverse reactions of medication	Withdrawal of drug	Clindamycin causes pseudomembranous enterocolitis
AUTOIMMUNE/ALLERGIC				
Ulcerative colitis	Mucus; pus; blood; nocturnal	Urgency; tenesmus, abdominal pain, fever; weight loss; systemic signs (arthritis, etc.)	Sigmoidoscopy; barium enema	Insidious; age: 10-19 yr; treatment: sulfasalazine, steroids
Regional enteritis (Crohn's)	Loose; blood (variable); nocturnal	Abdominal pain; weight loss; fever; perianal disease	Sigmoidoscopy; barium enema	Insidious; teenagers; treatment: surgery, sulfasalazine, steroids

	Stool	Associated findings	Diagnosis	Comments
Milk allergy	Watery; blood (occult or gross)	Vomiting, anemia	Dietary elimination	May also be caused by soy formula
Gluten sensitivity (celiac disease)	Profuse; bulky; pale; frothy	Failure to thrive, anemia, vomiting, abdominal pain	Peroral intestinal biopsy, stool fat	Onset reflects age of introduction of gluten (wheat, rye, oats); eliminate gluten foods
IRRITABLE BOWEL SYNDROME	Watery; mucus	None; normal growth	Therapeutic response	Treatment: bland diet; reduce snacks; peak: 6-36 mo; multiple inciting causes
INTRAPSYCHIC				
Fear/anxiety	Loose	Anxiety	History helpful	Stress-reducing activities; needs long-term therapy
Fecal impaction (encopresis) (Chapter 30)	Watery	Variable abdominal pain	History; rectal exam; x-ray	Chronic constipation
CONGENITAL				
Cystic fibrosis	Fatty; bulky; foul-smelling	Respiratory infections; poor growth	Sweat test	Needs enzyme replacement; long-term follow-up
Hirschsprung's disease (p. 496)	Green, watery; foul-smelling	Abdominal distension; vomiting; fever; lethargy; poor growth	Barium enema; rectal biopsy	Surgical intervention
ENDOCRINE				
Hyperthyroid (p. 474)	Watery	Systemic signs	Thyroid studies	
NEOPLASM				
Lymphoma Carcinoma Neuroblastoma Zollinger-Ellison syndrome	Watery, variably severe	Associated problems	Variable	Important etiology to exclude

Parental education

1. Give only clear liquids; give as much as your child wants. The following may be used during the first 24 hr:
   a. Pedialyte RS, Lytren, or Infalyte (requires mixing)
   b. Jell-O water—one package strawberry/ quart water (twice as much as usual)
   c. Gatorade
   d. Defizzed, room-temperature soda for older children (>2 yr) if diarrhea is only mild
2. If child is vomiting, give clear liquids *slowly*. In younger children, start with 1 teaspoonful and slowly increase the amount. If vomiting occurs, let your child rest for a while and then try again. About 8 hr after vomiting has stopped, child can gradually return to a normal diet.
3. After 24 hr, your child's diet may be advanced if the diarrhea has improved. If child is taking only formula, mix the formula with twice as much water to make up half-strength formula, which should be given over the next 24 hr. Applesauce, bananas, and strained carrots may be given if child is eating solids. If this is tolerated, the child may be advanced to a regular diet over the next 2-3 days.
4. If child has had a prolonged course of diarrhea, it is helpful in the younger child to advance from clear liquids to a soy formula (Isomil, ProSobee, or Soyalac) for 1-2 wk. Children older than 1 yr should not receive cow's milk products (milk, cheese, ice cream, or butter) for several days.
5. Do not use boiled milk. Kool-Aid and soda are not ideal liquids, particularly in younger infants, because they contain few electrolytes.
6. Call physician if
   a. The diarrhea or vomiting is increasing in frequency or amount
   b. The diarrhea does not improve after 24 hr of clear liquids or resolve entirely after 3-4 days
   c. Vomiting continues for more than 24 hr
   d. The stool has blood or the vomited material contains blood or turns green
   e. Signs of dehydration develop, including decreased urination, less moisture in diapers, dry mouth, no tears, weight loss, lethargy, or irritability

33 Dysphagia

ALERT: After correcting hydration, diagnostic considerations should be evaluated before initiating definitive therapy.

Patients with dysphagia have difficulty swallowing because of pharyngeal, laryngeal, or esophageal lesions. Clinically, patients experience associated choking, regurgitation, pain and discomfort, and a sense of food sticking. When such symptoms are caused by esophageal lesions, the patient commonly has a subjective sensation of a bolus of food failing to pass, with accompanying pain and discomfort.

Dysphagia results from either anatomic obstruction or compression or a physiologic dysfunction of the neuromuscular process of swallowing; that is, swallowing requires coordination with sucking and breathing (Table 33-1). *Obstructive* or compressive lesions usually can be evaluated by careful physical examination and radiologic studies, including lateral neck film, barium swallow, or fluoroscopy. Such patients usually have difficulty only in swallowing solids. *Physiologic* dysfunction, often associated with systemic disease, is rarely isolated to the alimentary tract. Patients commonly have difficulty with both solids and liquids. The assessment of these patients must include defining the systemic problems (e.g., cultures, drug levels, edrophonium [Tensilon], cerebrospinal fluid, muscle biopsy, CT scan), as well as evaluating aspects of swallowing by fluoroscopy and manometric studies. It is imperative when evaluating the patient with dysphagia to obtain a careful history of the pattern of progression and associated signs and symptoms.

Management of the patient must focus initially on stabilization by ensuring adequate vital signs and hydration, followed by a diagnostic work-up.

TABLE 33-1. Dysphagia: diagnostic considerations

Condition	Primary mechanism: Obstruction/ compression (mechanical)	Primary mechanism: Physiologic dysfunction (motor)	Comments
INFECTION/INFLAMMATION			
Tonsillitis (p. 456)	Yes		Group A streptococci, diphtheria, infections, mononucleosis, etc.
Stomatitis (p. 465)	Yes		Herpes, aphthous
Peritonsillar abscess (p. 458)	Yes		Direct visualization
Retropharyngeal abscess (p. 462)	Yes		Lateral neck
Epiglottitis, croup (p. 591)	Yes		Direct visualization imperative
Botulism, rabies, polio (Chapter 80)		Yes	Cranial nerves affected
Guillain-Barré syndrome (Chapter 41)		Yes	Ascending paralysis
Monilia	Yes		
Esophagitis		Yes	Retrosternal discomfort (hiatal hernia, reflux, etc.)
Chalasia/gastroesophageal reflux	Yes	Yes	May be physiologic in infants
Pericarditis	Yes		Associated symptoms present
INTOXICATION			
Caustic ingestion (p. 282)	Yes	Yes	Requires immediate intervention to minimize injury
Phenothiazine overdose (p. 299)		Yes	Associated with dystonia
CONGENITAL (Chapter 11)			
Cleft palate	Yes	Yes	
Macroglossia	Yes		Consider hypothyroidism, Beckwith's syndrome
Esophageal web, atresia, stenosis	Yes		May be associated with tracheal anomaly (tracheal-esophageal fistula)
Riley-Day syndrome		Yes	

TABLE 33-1. Dysphagia: diagnostic considerations—cont'd

| Condition | Primary mechanism | | Comments |
	Obstruction/compression (mechanical)	Physiologic dysfunction (motor)	
DEGENERATIVE			
CNS disease		Yes	
Hypotonia		Yes	
Myasthenia gravis		Yes	Tensilon trial
INTRAPSYCHIC			
Globus hystericus		Yes	Psychiatry consult
TRAUMA			
Foreign body (p. 485)	Yes		History crucial
ENDOCRINE (p. 472)			
Goiter	Yes		Thyroid studies required
Hashimoto's thyroiditis	Yes		Thyroid studies required
NEOPLASM			
Carcinoma, Hodgkin's disease	Yes		Usually associated nodes, weight loss
VASCULAR			
Vascular ring	Yes		Chest x-ray, ECG, catheterization
Heart disease	Yes		Chest x-ray, ECG, catheterization
Aortic aneurysm	Yes		Chest x-ray, ECG, catheterization
AUTOIMMUNE			
Various collagen-vascular diseases (dermatomyositis)	Yes	Yes	Evaluate in detail

34 Fever in children under 2 years of age

ALERT: The acutely ill, febrile child under 2 yr requires a systematic approach to evaluation to exclude serious systemic disease. Following the initial evaluation and therapy, close follow-up is essential.

The febrile child, particularly under 2 yr of age, presents unique challenges to the clinician. Over 10% of visits in this age-group are for acute fevers. It is particularly difficult to determine the etiology in the young child because of problems in obtaining a specific history and defining physical findings. Children are considered febrile when their rectal temperatures are 38.0° C (100.4° F) or higher. Although axillary temperatures are easier to take, they are not totally reliable in mildly febrile children (38°-38.5° C). Fevers >42° C (107.6° F) usually are *not* infectious in origin (e.g., CNS involvement or heat stroke).*

ETIOLOGY AND DIAGNOSTIC FINDINGS

Historically, parents usually report nonspecific observations related to behavior and associated signs and symptoms rather than those that permit an early focus on the involved system. However, it is particularly important to define these alterations in behavior, activity, and eating habits and to determine if respiratory, gastrointestinal, musculoskeletal, and dermatologic

*Appendix C-5 contains centigrade and Fahrenheit conversions.

findings have developed. Urinary tract and CNS symptoms usually are reflected in changes in behavior, such as irritability and lethargy. Exposures to children with similar complaints are important to note as are recent events, such as DPT immunizations.

Early antipyretic therapy is imperative in facilitating observation. Many children who initially are irritable and disinterested in their environment will improve markedly with aggressive antipyretic management. Acetaminophen (10-15 mg/kg/dose PO) should be administered to all children with temperatures >38.5°-39.0° C (101.3°-102.2° F) on arrival in the clinic or ED to ensure optimal observation by reducing temperature and permitting a more accurate assessment of the child. Children with temperatures >39.5° C (103° F) should also be sponged with tepid water.

The physical examination to assess responsiveness must be done systematically, focusing on careful observation of the child at play and encouraging the youngster to follow lights, bright objects, or the mother. Components of this overall assessment that are useful and reassuring include:
1. Child looks and focuses on clinician and spontaneously explores the room

178

2. Child spontaneously makes sounds or talks in a playful manner
3. Child plays and reaches for objects
4. Child smiles and interacts with mother or practitioner
5. Child quiets easily when held by parent

While the child is distracted with play objects, obvious physical abnormalities such as limitation of limb movement, rashes, and points of tenderness or pain should be defined. The chest, heart, and abdomen require a gentle hand and patience. Tachypnea disproportionate to fever must be carefully evaluated, usually by chest x-ray film. Once these areas have been assessed, a full examination of ears, throat, neck, etc., is required.

In most children, this initial evaluation will define the cause of fever, and appropriate therapy can be initiated. With one group of children under 24 mo of age who had acute onset of temperatures of 40° C (104° F) or over, the diagnostic categories and their relative percentages* were:

Otitis media		36.9%
Nonspecific illness		25.5%
Pneumonia		15.5%
Recognizable viral illness		12.7%
Exanthem/enanthem	(5.8%)	
Meningitis/encephalitis	(3.6%)	
Gastroenteritis	(1.8%)	
Croup	(1.5%)	
Recognizable bacterial illness		9.4%
Bacteremia	(6.1%)	
Cellulitis	(0.9%)	
Meningitis	(1.2%)	
Urinary tract infection	(0.6%)	
Other	(0.6%)	

Although **bacteremia** occurs in association with a host of clinical entities, including meningitis, arthritis, epiglottitis, cellulitis, pneumonia, and kidney infections, about 6% of the febrile patients in this group had positive blood cultures,

---

*From McCarthy, P.L.: Controversies in pediatrics: what tests are indicated for the child under 2 with fever? Pediatr. Rev. **1**:51, 1979. Copyright American Academy of Pediatrics, 1979. Reproduced by permission of Pediatrics.

sometimes without localized findings. Occult bacteremia is a significant problem in children, who are at greatest risk with:

Age: ≤ 24 mo
Fever: ≥ 39.4° C (102.9° F)
WBC: ≥ 15,000 mm^3 (differential does not increase prognostic value)
ESR: ≥ 30 mm/hr (difficult to use because of length of time required to perform)

It is essential to evaluate such children carefully to be certain that there is no underlying disease such as pneumonia or meningitis. Although controversial, there is no conclusive evidence that performing a lumbar puncture on a bacteremic child significantly increases the risk of subsequently developing meningitis.

Organisms that are frequently cultured include *Streptococcus pneumoniae* and *Haemophilus influenzae*. *Staphylococcus aureus* and *Neisseria meningitidis* are less common pathogens.

MANAGEMENT

Fig. 34-1 outlines an approach for the child under 2 yr of age.

Children under 3 mo of age require more aggressive management. The risk factors are not predictive, and young children may develop systemic infections from enteric organisms, such as *Escherichia coli*, as well as those found in older children.

Parental education

Parental education is important in the management of the febrile infant. Obviously, instructions are indicated in the management of the specific diagnostic entity, but additional information about fever control must be provided. This is of utmost importance in the initial assessment of the child and may additionally make the child more comfortable throughout the duration of the illness. Fever is a means of fighting infection, and the degree of fever does not always reflect the severity of illness.

1. Fever is a temperature over 100° F (37.8° C)

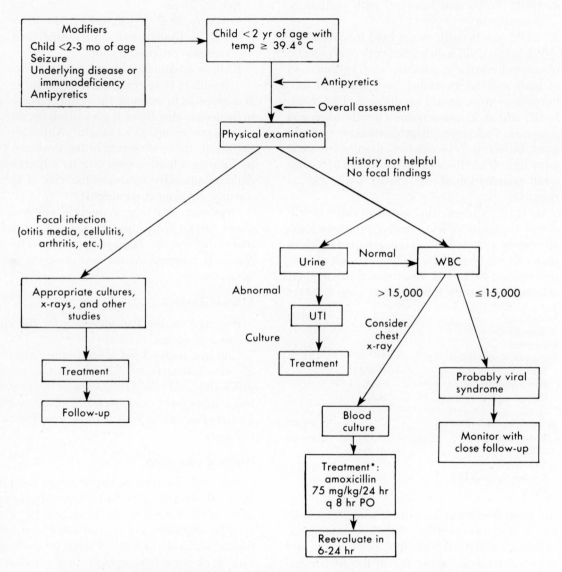

Fig. 34-1. Evaluation of the febrile child under 2 yr. For legend see opposite page.
*First dose (ampicillin 50-75 mg/kg) may be given parenterally.

Fig. 34-1.

1. *Children under 2-3 mo of age* require a more extensive evaluation because the height of fever and WBC are not predictive, and their risk for dissemination of infection is enhanced. The history is rarely more specific than the triad of fever, irritability, and poor feeding and the physical examination may fail to reveal specific focal findings despite the presence of systemic infections, which may be enteric, as well as the more common organisms infecting older children. Children under 3 mo with a temperature >38.5° C have a greater than 20-fold risk of having a serious infection than do older children with a similar temperature. Children under 2-3 mo with temperatures over 38° C (rectal) usually require blood cultures, urinalysis, and lumbar puncture unless they look remarkably well. Infants usually should be started on antibiotics (ampicillin 150 mg/kg/24 hours q 4-8 hr IV and gentamicin 5 mg/kg/24 hours q 8 hr IV) and admitted, particularly if the child appears ill or follow-up is difficult. Treatment should be modified if a specific focus is detected or if cultures are positive. Third-generation cephalosporins, such as cefotaxime (150 mg/kg/24 hr q 6 hr IV), ceftriaxone (50-100 mg/kg/24 hr q 12 hr IV), or cefuroxime (100-200 mg/kg/24 hr q 6-8 hr IV) may be substituted for gentamicin and administered in combination with ampicillin, the latter ensuring coverage of *L. monocytogenes.*

2. Meningitis must be considered in any febrile child who has a seizure. All children 12 mo of age and younger should have a spinal tap (p. 632).

3. A temperature of 41.1° C or higher is associated with a 10% incidence of meningitis in children under 2 yr of age.

4. Underlying cardiac, pulmonary, neurologic, and immunodeficiency (sickle cell, neoplasms, or taking steroids) diseases require early evaluation and treatment, regardless of age and the height of fever.

5. Previous antipyretic therapy requires a lower temperature threshold for initiating laboratory evaluation.

6. Children with WBC >15,000/mm³ from whom blood cultures have been obtained may be treated with antibiotics. Although controversial, such anticipatory therapy for at-risk children may facilitate clinical resolution.

7. Children with fever and petechiae may have a viral illness, Rocky Mountain spotted fever, or invasive bacterial disease. Those with fever and petechiae who have a normal LP, WBC count that is neither elevated nor decreased, normal absolute neutrophil and band count, and a temperature of less than 40° C probably do not have bacterial infection.

8. If the temperature has been present for less than 24 hr, if the child looks well on the basis of overall assessment and is over 3 mo old, and no helpful history or focal findings are detected, close follow-up for 6-12 hr may substitute for laboratory evaluation at the time of the first encounter. If the temperature remains elevated above 39.4° C at the follow-up appointment, evaluation should proceed.

9. If good follow-up is ensured, blood cultures may be delayed for 12-24 hr awaiting clinical resolution if the WBC is <20,000 cells/mm³. Otherwise, the 15,000 cells/mm³ cut-off should be used.

10. Follow-up is essential, usually in 6-24 hr, depending on clinical and logistic constraints.

    a. If the cultures remain negative, antibiotics may be stopped after 48 hr unless there was a specific focus initially or one develops. Follow-up until resolution of the illness is necessary.

    b. If the culture is positive, thereby documenting bacteremia, reexamination of the patient should determine treatment.

        (1) A patient who has a totally normal examination should continue taking the high-dose antibiotics as an outpatient if daily contact can be maintained or as an inpatient if compliance is questionable. A total 10-day course is necessary. Most patients who have been treated initially will be improved on follow-up, but this does not preclude the importance of continuing antibiotics.

        (2) Febrile or toxic patients who have no resolution of their illness or who develop a focus should be admitted for intravenous antibiotics and further evaluation. A total course of 10 days is necessary.

orally or 100.4° F (38.0° C) rectally (Fig. 34-2). If the fever is between 100° F and 101° F orally or rectally, the temperature should be taken again in 1 hr. Temperatures may be temporarily elevated from too much clothing or exercise. Oral temperatures can be raised by recently eaten warm food. Teething does not cause marked elevations of temperature.

2. Take the rectal temperature:

    a. Shake the thermometer down to below 97° F (36° C).

    b. Lubricate with Vaseline, cold cream, or cold water.

    c. Gently insert thermometer ½ inch into rectum. Often, holding the child stomach down on parent's lap is helpful.

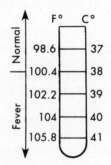

Fig. 34-2. Conversion scale.

d. Leave in 3 min or until silver line stops rising.

e. Do not leave child unattended. Hold child still.

f. Read by turning the sharp edge of the triangle toward you. Turn it slightly in each direction until you can see the end of the silver column.

g. On the centrigrade (Celsius) thermometer each line is 0.1° C; on the Fahrenheit thermometer each line is 0.2° F.

    NOTE: In unusual circumstances, axillary temperatures may be taken as a screen, holding the tip of thermometer under the dry armpit for 4 min. Elbow should be held against the chest. If the temperature is >99° F (37.2° C), recheck by taking a rectal temperature.

3. *Fever medicines* should be used if the temperature is above 101.5° F (38.6° C), if the child is very uncomfortable, or if any fever is present at bedtime. If your child is acting normally, fever medicines may be delayed until the temperature is 102.2° F (39.0° C).

    a. If your child is over 3 mo of age, give fever medicine if the temperature is over 101.5° F (38.6° C). Acetaminophen (Tylenol or equivalent) is recommended every 4-6 hr.

    b. If your child's temperature is 103° F (39.5°

				Dose of fever medicine				
Brand	0-3 mo	4-11 mo	12-23 mo	2-3 yr	4-5 yr	6-8 yr	9-10 yr	11-12 yr
Acetaminophen drops (80 mg/0.8 ml)	0.4 ml	0.8 ml	1.2 ml	1.6 ml	2.4 ml			
Acetaminophen elixir (160 mg/tsp)		½ tsp	¾ tsp	1 tsp	1½ tsp	2 tsp	2½	
Chewable tablet acetaminophen or aspirin (80 mg)			1½	2	3	4	5	6
Junior swallowable tablet (160 mg)				1	1½	2	2½	3
Adult tablet acetaminophen or aspirin (325 mg)						1	1	1½

C) or above, give the appropriate dose of acetaminophen *and* aspirin every 5-6 hr.

    c. Do not use aspirin if your child has chickenpox or an influenza-like illness, because of association of Reye's syndrome and aspirin.

4. *Sponging* is useful if the temperature remains over 104° F (40° C) after medicine. Sponge or partially submerge your undressed child in *lukewarm* water (96°-100° F). This can be done for 15-30 min as often as necessary. Some parents prefer laying the undressed child on a towel. Another towel or washcloth soaked in lukewarm water is placed on the child. The towel is changed every 1-2 min; this is done for 15-30 min.

5. Dress child lightly. Push fluids.

6. Call physician if

    a. The fever goes above 105° F (40.5° C)

    b. The fever lasts beyond 48-72 hr

    c. Your child is under 3 mo and has a rectal fever over 100.4° F (38° C)

    d. Your child has a seizure (convulsion) or abnormal movements of face, arms, or legs, stiff neck, purple spots, or fullness of the soft spot; looks sicker than expected; or develops difficulty breathing, burning on urination, decreased urination, abdominal pain, marked change in behavior; or level of consciousness or activity

REFERENCES

Carroll, W.L., Farrell, M.K., Singer, J.J., et al.: Treatment of occult bacteremia: a prospective randomized clinical trial, Pediatrics **72**:608, 1983.

DeAngelis, C., Joffe, A., Wilson, M., et al.: Inatrogenic risks and financial costs of hospitalization of febrile infants, Am. J. Dis. Child. **137**:1146, 1983.

Krober, M.S., Bass, J.W., Powell, J.M., et al.: Bacterial and viral pathogens causing fever in infants less than 3 months old, Am. J. Dis. Child. **139**:889, 1985.

McGarvey, A., Wise, P.H.: Evaluation of the febrile child under 2 years of age, J. Emerg. Med. **1**:299, 1984.

McCarthy, P.L., Cicchett, B.V., Stashwick, C.A., et al.: Diagnostic styles of attending pediatricians, residents and nurses in evaluating febrile children, Clin. Pediatrics **21**:534, 1982.

Nguyen, Q.V., Nguyen, E.A., and Weiner, L.B.: Incidence of invasive bacterial disease in children with fever and petechiae, Pediatrics **74**:77, 1984.

Yaffe, S.J.: Comparative efficacy of aspirin and acetaminophen in the reduction of fever in children, Arch. Intern. Med. **141**:286, 1981.

Gastrointestinal hemorrhage: hematemesis and rectal bleeding

ALERT: The initial focus must be on assessing the severity of bleeding, initiating necessary stabilization measures, and determining diagnostic considerations.

Gastrointestinal hemorrhage, whether it be manifested by vomiting (hematemesis) or rectal bleeding (melena), reflects infectious, inflammatory, or anatomic pathology (Tables 35-1 and 35-2). It must be differentiated from hemoptysis (p. 167), which presents as red, frothy material mixed with sputum.

ETIOLOGY

In the newborn, swallowed blood,* bleeding diathesis, and stress ulcers are the most common causes. Necrotizing enterocolitis (NEC) is occasionally noted in the nursery. During the first year of life, anal fissures and intussusception account for 70% of noninfectious gastrointestinal hemorrhage, with gangrenous bowel, peptic ulcers, and Meckel's diverticulum being less common. Lesions in older children include colonic polyps (50%), anal fissures (13%), peptic ulcers (13%), intussusception (9%), and esophageal varices (9%). Infectious diarrhea is a frequent cause.

---

*Apt test for maternal blood: mix 1 part bright red stool or vomitus with 5-10 parts water and centrifuge. Add 1 ml 0.2N NaOH to supernatant fluid. Pink color developing in 2-5 min indicates fetal hemoglobin and brown color adult hemoglobin.

DIAGNOSTIC FINDINGS

The diagnostic workup focuses on defining the site of hemorrhage with particular reference to whether it is proximal or distal to the ligament of Treitz after baseline laboratory data, including CBC, platelets, type and cross-match, and coagulation studies (platelets, PT, PTT), have been obtained (Fig. 35-1).

1. Lesions proximal to the ligament of Treitz will usually result in nasogastric (NG) aspirates positive for blood.
   a. Bright red hematemesis indicates that there is little or no contact with gastric juices; it results from an active bleeding site at or above the cardia. In children it is usually caused by varices or esophagitis and, rarely, Mallory-Weiss syndrome. Occasionally, duodenal or gastric bleeding may be so brisk that it is bright red.
   b. Coffee-ground aspirate indicates that it has been altered by the gastric juices.
   c. Evaluation should involve endoscopy and an upper GI series, depending on the stability of the patient and the likely cause.
2. If rectal bleeding is the primary presentation, the stool should be examined for stool leukocytes and a culture obtained. The color of

the blood in the stool reflects the amount and site of bleeding.

a. Hemorrhage proximal to the ileocecal valve produces tarry stools, but lower bleeding is red.

b. Depending on the suspected etiology and clinical status, other workup can include anal inspection, sigmoidoscopy, colonoscopy, technetium scan, and double-contrast barium enema.

Occult blood may be identified by guaiac test (most conveniently supplied as Hemoccult packets), which produces a blue discoloration when positive. Stools may appear black from ingestion of iron, large numbers of chocolate sandwich cookies, bismuth, Pepto-Bismol, lead, licorice, charcoal, or coal, or they may be red from gelatin. False positives may result from ingestion of iron, red fruit, and meats; false negatives occur when the fecal specimen is stored and dried

Text continued on p. 191.

TABLE 35-1. Gastrointestinal hemorrhage: diagnostic considerations by age

Infant (<3 mo)	Toddler (<2 yr)	Preschooler (<5 yr)	School-age child (>5 yr)
UPPER GASTROINTESTINAL BLEEDING			
Swallowed maternal blood	Esophagitis	Esophagitis	Esophagitis
Gastritis	Gastritis	Gastritis	Gastritis
Ulcer, stress	Ulcer	Ulcer	Ulcer
Bleeding diathesis	Pyloric stenosis	Esophageal varices	Esophageal varices
Foreign body (NG tube)	Mallory-Weiss syndrome	Foreign body	Mallory-Weiss syndrome
Vascular malformation	Vascular malformation	Mallory-Weiss syndrome	Inflammatory bowel disease*
Duplication	Duplication	Hemophilia	Hemophilia
		Vascular malformation	Vascular malformation
LOWER GASTROINTESTINAL BLEEDING			
Swallowed maternal blood	Anal fissure	Infectious colitis*	Infectious colitis*
Infectious colitis*	Infectious colitis*	Anal fissure	Inflammatory bowel disease*
Milk allergy	Milk allergy	Polyp	Pseudomembranous enterocolitis*
Bleeding diathesis*	Colitis	Intussusception*	Polyp
Intussusception*	Intussusception*	Meckel's diverticulum	Hemolytic uremic syndrome*
Midgut volvulus*	Meckel's diverticulum	Henoch-Schönlein purpura*	Hemorrhoid
Meckel's diverticulum	Polyp	Hemolytic uremic syndrome*	
Necrotizing enterocolitis (NEC)*	Duplication	Inflammatory bowel disease*	
	Hemolytic uremic syndrome*	Pseudomembranous enterocolitis*	
	Inflammatory bowel disease*		
	Pseudomembranous enterocolitis*		

*Commonly associated with systemic illness involving multiple organ systems either primarily or secondarily.

TABLE 35-2. Hematemesis and rectal bleeding: diagnostic considerations

Condition	Age	Character of bleeding	
		Gastric aspirate	Stool
INFECTION/INFLAMMATION			
Acute diarrhea (p. 480) Bacteria, virus, parasites	Any	—	Small (variable)
Gastritis (Chapter 44)	Any	Mild-moderate, coffee ground	Tarry
Ulcer			
Gastric	>6 yr	Small/large; red/coffee ground	Small/large; tarry
Duodenal	>6 yr	Small/large; red/coffee ground	Small/large; tarry
Stress	Any	Small/large; red/coffee ground	Small/large; tarry
Esophagitis	Any	Small	
Ulcerative colitis	Any	—	Small/large
Crohn's disease (regional enteritis)	10-19 yr	—	Variable, red
ANATOMIC			
Intussusception (p. 498)	<2 yr (5-12 mo)	—	"Currant jelly"
Volvulus (p. 502)	Neonate	—	Red/tarry
Rectal fissure (Chapter 30)	Infant	—	Blood-streaked stool
Polyps	2-10 yr	—	Small/moderate; red, intermittent
Meckel's diverticulum (p. 500)	4 mo-4 yr	—	Large; red and tarry
VASCULAR			
Esophageal varices	>2 yr (3-5)	Large; red	Large, tarry
Hemangioma/hematoma/ telangiectasia	Any	—	Occult/large

Signs and symptoms	Evaluation	Comments
Fever, diarrhea, polymorpho-nuclear cells (bacterial)	Stool leukocytes, culture, CBC, ova and parasites	Dietary manipulation useful
Vomiting		Acute gastroenteritis, ASA, alcohol
Vomiting, pain, anemia	Endoscopy, upper GI series; exclude Zollinger-Ellison syndrome; determine diet, family history	May be life threatening; cimetidine, ranitidine, or antacids (30 ml 1 and 3 hr after meals and before bed)
Vomiting, retrosternal pain	Upper GI, esophagoscopy	Hiatal hernia, chalasia; cimetidine
Insidious weight loss and pain	Proctoscopy, barium enema	Multiple complications
Insidious weight loss and pain	Proctoscopy, barium enema	
Acute onset, crampy, abdominal pain	Hydrostatic barium enema	Life threatening, requires immediate surgery
Bile-stained vomit, shock, abdominal distension	Barium enema	
Well child	Inspection of anus	Stool softener
Well, variable anemia	Proctoscopy, barium enema	Severe if Peutz-Jeghers syndrome; may be inflammatory, adenoma or hemartoma
Well with acute, massive bleeding	Pertechnetate scan	
Painless, cirrhosis, portal vein thrombosis	Esophagoscopy, barium swallow	
Painless, mucocutaneous lesions	Angiography, laparotomy	Familial (Peutz-Jeghers syndrome)

Continued.

TABLE 35-2. Hematemesis and rectal bleeding: diagnostic considerations—cont'd

Condition	Age	Character of bleeding	
		Gastric aspirate	Stool
TRAUMA			
Foreign body (p. 485)	2-6 yr	—	Variable, red
Mallory-Weiss syndrome		Large; red	
AUTOIMMUNE/ALLERGY			
Henoch-Schönlein purpura (p. 610)	3-10 yr		Small/large; red/tarry
Idiopathic thrombocytopenia purpura (p. 529)	Any		
Milk allergy (cow or soy)	<12 mo	—	Occult/small; red
CONGENITAL			
Hemophilia (p. 525)	Any (male)	Occult/large; red/coffee ground	Occult/large; red/tarry
DEGENERATIVE			
Vitamin K deficiency	1-2 days	Mild/large; red	Mild/large; red/tarry
ENDOCRINE			
Zollinger-Ellison syndrome	>7 yr	Small/large coffee ground	Tarry
NEOPLASM			
Esophageal/gastric carcinoma		Occult/large	Tarry; occult/large
MISCELLANEOUS			
Iron-deficiency anemia (Chapter 26)	<18 mo	—	Occult/small
Swallowed blood	Any	Small/large; coffee ground	Occult/small

Signs and symptoms	Evaluation	Comments
History, rectal pain History, vomiting	Digital exam, proctoscopy Esophagoscopy	
Abdominal pain, arthritis, hematuria, purpura	Physical exam, CBC, platelet count	Risk of intussusception
Recurrent vomiting, diarrhea, colic, failure to thrive; rarely fulminant enterocolitis	Dietary change	
History of bleeding diathesis	Coagulation screening	Factor replacement
Well or bleeding	PT	Vit K 1-2 mg (infant), 5-10 mg (child, adult)
Vomiting, pain, anemia	Endoscopy, upper GI series, gastric acid	Recurrent ulcers
Variable with location and histology	Endoscopy, barium contrast study	Rare in infants
Well, pale	CBC	Iron supplementation
Usually obvious source	CBC, Apt (newborn)	Newborn—maternal blood, epistaxis, etc.

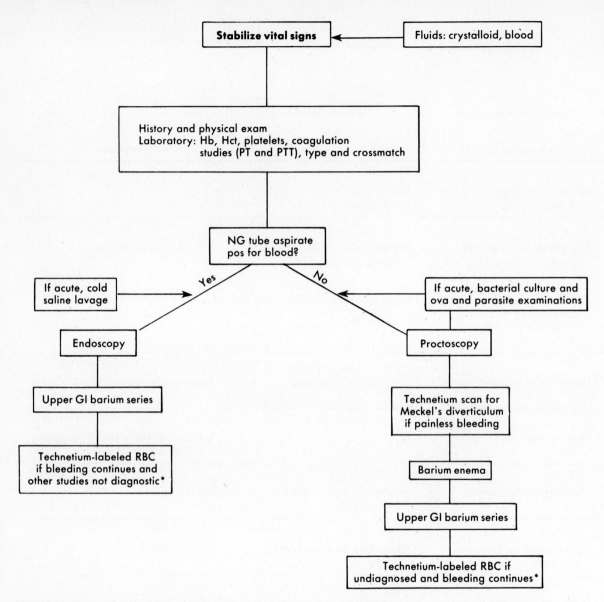

FIG. 35-1. Gastrointestinal hemorrhage. *Study may be useful in detecting and localizing sites of active bleeding. If nondiagnostic and bleeding continues, arteriogram may be indicated.

or there has been recent ingestion of ascorbic acid. Hemoccult testing is not useful for detecting gastric bleeding. Gastroccult testing should be used for detecting occult blood in gastric juice.

MANAGEMENT

Management of significant gastrointestinal bleeding involves stabilization of the patient, using crystalloid initially, followed by whole blood or packed red blood cells. Coagulopathies must be treated. Patients should be given oxygen, have intravenous line(s) started, and be monitored closely from the time they enter the ED. A hematocrit should be done immediately and blood sent for type and cross-matching. If upper gastrointestinal bleeding is present, a large-caliber nasogastric tube should be passed and the stomach lavaged with cooled saline to decrease mucosal blood flow while monitoring blood in the returned aspirate. Lavage is continued until the aspirate is clear. Consultation should usually be obtained, and if bleeding stops within 30-45 min, gastroduodenoscopy is often done to provide direct visualization. If the bleeding is massive or ongoing, endoscopy may not be useful and scanning or arteriography may be required. Vasopressin (Pitressin) may rarely be required with intractable variceal bleeding. After consultation, an initial bolus of 0.3 units/kg diluted in 2 ml/kg of D5W is given over 20 min followed by a continuous infusion of 0.2-0.4 units/1.73 m^2/min. If bleeding ceases, infusion is maintained at the initial dose for 12 hr and then is tapered over 24-36 hr. If it fails, sclerosing agents or a Sengstaken-Blakemore tube may be needed.

Surgical intervention is required if there is life-threatening hemorrhage, intussusception (if not reducible), volvulus, Meckel's diverticulum, ulcer (if perforated), or a neoplasm.

All patients require hospitalization for evaluation, monitoring, and intervention. Following stabilization and diagnostic evaluation, a long-term management plan must be developed. Mucosal lesions may be treated with antacids containing magnesium hydroxide and aluminum hydroxide (Maalox, Mylanta, etc.). During an acute episode, patients are given 0.5 ml/kg (maximum: 30 ml/dose) q 1-2 hr PO to maintain gastric pH $\geq$5. On a maintenance basis the same dose is given 1 and 3 hr after meals and before bedtime. Pharmacologic agents (H$_2$ receptor antagonist) that are equally effective include cimetidine (Tagamet) 20-30 mg/kg/24 hr q 6 hr PO (adult 600-1800 mg/24 hr PO) or 20-30 mg/kg/24 hr q 4 hr IV slowly as 15-min infusion, *or* ranitidine (Zantac) (adult: 150 mg q 12 hr PO or 50 mg q 6-8 hr IV). A pediatric dose for ranitidine has not been established but is expected to range from 2.5-3.8 mg/kg/24 hr q 12 hr PO.

REFERENCES

Cox, K., and Ament, M.E.: Upper gastrointestinal bleeding in children and adolescents, Pediatrics 63:408, 1979.

Hyams, J.S., Leichtner, A.M., and Schwartz, A.N.: Recent advances in diagnosis and treatment of gastrointestinal hemorrhage in infants and children, J. Pediatr. 106:1, 1985.

Oldham, K.T., and Lobe, T.E.: Gastrointestinal hemorrhage in children: a pragmatic update, Pediatr. Clin. North Am. 32:1247, 1985.

Steer, M.L., and Silen, W.: Diagnostic procedures in gastrointestinal hemorrhage, N. Engl. J. Med. 309:646, 1983.

36 Headache

ALERT: Children under 5 yr rarely have headaches and must be evaluated for an organic etiology.

TABLE 36-1. Differentiation of headache type by signs and symptoms

	Type of headache
ASSOCIATED EVENTS	
Abrupt onset	Convulsive
Afternoon	Muscle contraction
Present on arising	Convulsive (following nocturnal seizure), emotional depression, traction (tumor), vascular
Preceded by aura	Convulsive, vascular (migraine)
Exacerbated by coughing	Paranasal sinus, traction (tumor, increased intracranial pressure), vascular
Followed by lethargy	Convulsive, vascular
Followed by focal CNS deficit	Convulsive (Todd paresis), traction (tumor), vascular (hemiplegic migraine)
Related to posture	Posttraumatic, traction (tumor and following lumbar puncture)
Related to stress	Muscle contraction, vascular (migraine)
Nausea and vomiting	Migraine, convulsive, traction (tumor)
CHARACTER OF PAIN	
Steady	Emotional depression, muscle contraction, sinus, traction (tumor, increased intracranial pressure)
Throbbing	Convulsive, posttraumatic, traction (tumor, increased intracranial pressure), vascular (migraine, vasculitis, inflammatory)
LOCATION	
Frontal	Traction (supratentorial tumor), vascular
Occipital and neck	Muscle contraction, sinus (ethmoid), traction (posterior fossa tumor)
Unilateral	Traction (lateralized supratentorial tumor), vascular (migraine)

From Kriel, R.L.: Headache. In Swaiman, K.F., and Wright, F.S., editors: The practice of pediatric neurology, ed. 2, vol. 1, pp. 215-221, St. Louis, 1982, The C.V. Mosby Co.

Since the brain has no pain-sensitive structures, headaches secondary to intracranial disease arise from irritating pain fibers that innervate the dura or vessels of the pia-arachnoid. Headaches may also be extracranial involving muscles, blood vessels, epithelial tissue of the sinuses, orbit, and eye. The pain associated with headaches has several mechanisms:

1. Muscle contraction—tension
2. Vascular—migraine, cluster, hypertension
3. Traction—subarachnoid hemorrhage, mass lesion, postconcussive
4. Inflammatory—meningitis, sinusitis, arteritis
5. Secondary to extracranial structures—refractive error, sinusitis
6. Psychogenic—depression, conversion

DIAGNOSTIC FINDINGS

The initial evaluation of the patient with a headache who is otherwise stable must determine the characteristics with regard to location, nature of pain, age of onset, frequency, duration and progression, precipitating and ameliorating factors, pica, ingestions, exposures, associated signs and symptoms, medications, past medical history (especially hypertension, sinusitis, heart disease, ear infections, and seizures), and family history. The temporal pattern is particularly important to determine if the headache is acute (single event with no previous episodes), acute and recurrent, chronic and progressive (suggesting potential increased intracranial pressure with increasing severity and frequency), or chronic and nonprogressive (several times per day/wk, with no change in severity or signs and symptoms). Recent stresses and emotional stability should be delineated. A careful physical examination must be performed with a complete neurologic evaluation, including visual acuity and fields, cerebellar signs, and auscultation for bruits.

Since children under the age of 5 yr rarely have headaches, an organic etiology is highly likely. Increased intracranial pressure is suggested by a headache that awakens the patient from sleep, occurs in the morning, is associated with vomiting without nausea, or is related to a change in position from prone to supine or erect. Occipital pain is often associated with an anatomic abnormality. Presenting signs and symptoms are helpful in differentiating etiology of the headache (Tables 36-1 and 36-2).

Ancillary data

Ancillary data should reflect positive findings. Studies that may be useful under specific circumstances include skull x-ray studies, sinus series, CT scan (elevated intracranial pressure, progressive or new neurologic signs, focal EEG, meningismus, focal headache, or partial seizures), electroencephalography, and lumbar puncture.

MANAGEMENT

Management should focus on suitable analgesia and treatment of the underlying condition. An empiric trial is sometimes indicated. Hospitalization is indicated if there is any evidence of increased intracranial pressure, progressive or new neurologic signs, or intractable pain.

REFERENCES

Kerner, K.F.: Management of headaches in the emergency department, Top. Emerg. Med. 4:19, 1982.
Shinnar, S., and D'Souza, B.J.: Diagnosis and management of headache in children, Pediatr. Clin. North Am. **29**:79, 1981.

TABLE 36-2. Headache: diagnostic considerations

Condition	Diagnostic findings	Comments
INTRAPSYCHIC		
Tension	Common; anxiety, stress, recurrent headache; pain—occipital, neck, or generalized, although it can be bifrontal or frontotemporal; sense of pressure or constriction; no prodrome, aura; spasm of muscles of neck and shoulder	Attempt to reduce anxiety; analgesia, stress control
Conversion reaction (p. 575)	Inconsistent findings	
Depression	Inciting event	
INFECTION		
Meningitis/encephalitis (p. 549)	Acute onset, infectious prodrome and associated findings; pain on movement; diffuse headache; lumbar puncture diagnostic	Hospitalize; antibiotics; support
Abscess, cerebral	Low grade fever; focal neurologic findings; localized headache; meningism; lumbar puncture: variable WBC, neg culture; CT scan	Neurosurgical referral
Sinusitis (p. 463)	Unilateral or bilateral frontal headache; pain on percussion of sinus; if sphenoid, may be occipital; purulent rhinorrhea; sinus x-rays	Antibiotics; rare drainage and referral; other ENT infections can cause headache including otitis media, mastoiditis, and retropharyngeal abscess
Dental abscess (p. 447)	Insidious onset; local pain; dental x-rays	Dental referral
VASCULAR		
Migraine (p. 556)	Unilateral recurrent headache (young children—generalized); throbbing; associated visual, sensory, motor deficit; abdominal pain, nausea, vomiting, positive family history; 25%-50% of chronic headaches	Supportive; analgesia, ergotamine (Cafergot); prophylaxis if frequent
Cluster	Paroxysmal, unilateral, explosive retro- or periorbital or frontal headache; unilateral autonomic symptoms—nasal stuffiness, lacrimation, Horner's syndrome; cluster in short period of time separated by long pain-free interval; rare in children; lasts 30-120 min but extremely severe; may occur several times in 24 hr period	Propranolol, steroids, indomethacin, lithium
Subarachnoid or cerebral bleeding; AV malformation (Chapter 18)	Acute onset; intense headache; focal neurologic exam; obtundation; meningism; CT scan; lumbar puncture bloody	Predisposing factors: trauma, bleeding problem
Hypertensive encephalopathy	Diffuse headache, nausea, vomiting, confusion, seizure, focal neurologic finding; high BP	Associated illness: acute glomerulonephritis, etc.
TRAUMA (Chapter 57)		
Postconcussive	Diffuse headache, often occipital, neck, or generalized bifrontal; vertigo, dizziness, confusion, sensitivity to noise,	Observation; frequent exams; analgesia, muscle relaxants

TABLE 36-2. Headache: diagnostic considerations—cont'd

Condition	Diagnostic findings	Comments
TRAUMA—cont'd		
	movement, heat, light; emotional instability; normal neurologic finding	
Subdural	Acute or insidious onset headache; CT scan	Neurosurgical intervention, observation; frequent exams
Fracture	Local tenderness and swelling; skull x-ray	Neurosurgical consultation
INTOXICATION		
Carbon monoxide (p. 289)	Headache, weakness; dizziness; respiratory arrest, coma; carboxyhemoglobin level	Oxygen; hyperbaric chamber
Lead	Diffuse headache; weakness; irritability, personality change; ataxia; seizures, coma; pica; red cell δ-aminolevulinic acid dehydratase	Dimercaprol and EDTA; penicillamine
NEOPLASM		
Cerebral	Frontal unrelenting headache, unilateral or bilateral; usually worse on rising; papilledema; increased intracranial pressure	Neurosurgical consultation
Cerebellar	Occipital unrelenting headache; vomiting; ataxia	Neurosurgical consultation
Pseudotumor cerebri (p. 558)	Nausea, vomiting, diplopia, acute or insidious generalized headache; full fontanelle, variable papilledema, ↑ CSF pressure	Predisposing factors: viral illness, intoxication, head trauma, steroids, etc.
AUTOIMMUNE		
Temporal arteritis	Local headache with tenderness and pain over temporal artery	Steroids; rare; increased ESR
Trigeminal neuralgia	Unilateral, recurrent headache and pain over distribution of second branch, trigeminal nerve	Carbamazepine, phenytoin
MISCELLANEOUS		
Eye		
Glaucoma	Generalized headache; blurred vision, dilated pupil; tonometry	Miotic, osmotic, diuretic
Refractive error	Generalized headache	Glasses
Epilepsy (p. 559)	Paroxysmal onset of headache and abrupt termination; brief duration; loss of contact with environment; variable abdominal pain	Rare cause of headaches
High altitude (Chapter 49)	Diffuse headache; weakness	
Temporomandibular joint (TMJ) disease	Frontotemporal or temporal pain; bilateral or unilateral severe, steady ache; limited mandibular movement, tenderness in muscles of jaw and neck	Refer to dentist
S/P lumbar puncture	Diffuse headache following procedure; unusual in young children	Bed rest, supine

37 Hematuria and proteinuria

AILEEN B. SEDMAN

ALERT: Hematuria and proteinuria require a systematic evaluation to exclude glomerular or extraglomerular disease.

Hematuria is present when there are ≥5 RBC/HPF in a sediment of 10 ml of centrifuged urine. It can result from nonrenal as well as glomerular and extraglomerular pathology, which can often be clinically distinguished by urinalysis:

	Glomerular	Extra glomerular or nonrenal
Urine color	Brown, smoky	Red, pink, or bright-red blood
RBC casts	May be present	Absent
Blood clots	Absent	May be present

Hematuria in newborns results primarily from vascular disorders such as hypoxia, thrombosis, or circulatory compromise; in older children, urinary tract infections account for the majority of cases, followed by glomerulonephritis and trauma. Hypercalciuria and nephrolithiasis also can cause hematuria.

Hemoglobinuria and myoglobinuria can both cause false positive tests as can iodine. Obviously, a microscopic examination for RBC should be done. With myoglobinuria, the hematocrit is normal and the serum is clear (not pink). Common causes of hemoglobinurias and myoglobinurias include hemolytic anemia, incompatible blood transfusions, burns, exertion, crush injuries, cold, noctural and exertional hemoglobinuria, and drugs (carbon monoxide, sulfonamides, and snake venom). Drugs and other agents that cause a red or dark urine include aniline dyes, blackberries, phenolphthalein, phenazopyridine (Pyridium), rifampin, and urates (p. 277).

Proteinuria is clearly present when over 200 mg/m^2/24 hr of protein is excreted in the urine. It is usually transient, occurring with fever, exercise, seizures, pneumonia, CHF, or environmental stress. Orthostatic proteinuria occurs when an individual is in an upright position; it requires careful collection and comparison of standing and recumbent urines.

False positive dipstiks for protein can result from benzalkonium, which causes a highly alkaline urine.

The evaluation is outlined in Figs. 37-1 and 37-2 and Table 37-1.

REFERENCE

Dodge, W.F., West, E.F., and Smith, F.H., et al.: Proteinuria and hematuria in school children: epidemiology and early natural history, J. Pediatr. 88:327, 1976.

See also Chapter 85: Renal disorders.

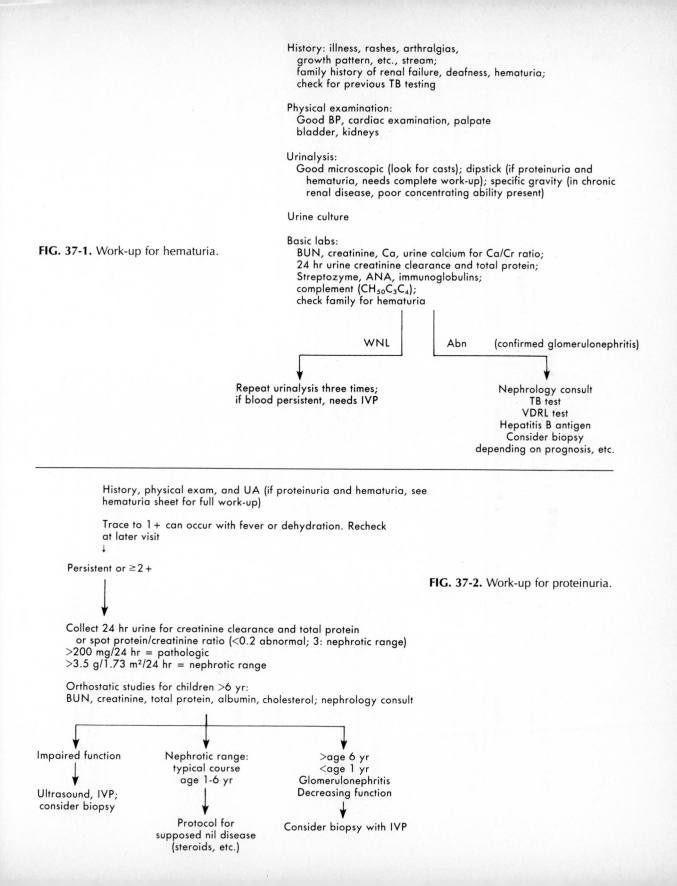

History: illness, rashes, arthralgias,
   growth pattern, etc., stream;
   family history of renal failure, deafness, hematuria;
   check for previous TB testing

Physical examination:
   Good BP, cardiac examination, palpate
   bladder, kidneys

Urinalysis:
   Good microscopic (look for casts); dipstick (if proteinuria and
     hematuria, needs complete work-up); specific gravity (in chronic
     renal disease, poor concentrating ability present)

Urine culture

Basic labs:
   BUN, creatinine, Ca, urine calcium for Ca/Cr ratio;
   24 hr urine creatinine clearance and total protein;
   Streptozyme, ANA, immunoglobulins;
   complement ($CH_{50}C_3C_4$);
   check family for hematuria

FIG. 37-1. Work-up for hematuria.

WNL

Repeat urinalysis three times;
if blood persistent, needs IVP

Abn   (confirmed glomerulonephritis)

Nephrology consult
TB test
VDRL test
Hepatitis B antigen
Consider biopsy
depending on prognosis, etc.

History, physical exam, and UA (if proteinuria and hematuria, see
hematuria sheet for full work-up)

Trace to 1+ can occur with fever or dehydration. Recheck
at later visit

Persistent or ≥2+

FIG. 37-2. Work-up for proteinuria.

Collect 24 hr urine for creatinine clearance and total protein
  or spot protein/creatinine ratio (<0.2 abnormal; 3: nephrotic range)
>200 mg/24 hr = pathologic
>3.5 g/1.73 m²/24 hr = nephrotic range

Orthostatic studies for children >6 yr:
BUN, creatinine, total protein, albumin, cholesterol; nephrology consult

Impaired function

Ultrasound, IVP;
consider biopsy

Nephrotic range:
typical course
age 1-6 yr

Protocol for
supposed nil disease
(steroids, etc.)

>age 6 yr
<age 1 yr
Glomerulonephritis
Decreasing function

Consider biopsy with IVP

TABLE 37-1. Hematuria and proteinuria: diagnostic considerations

Condition	Site of involvement	Diagnostic findings	Urinalysis		Comments
			Hematuria	Proteinuria	
INFECTION					
Urinary tract infection (p. 620)	Nonrenal/ex-traglomerular	Acute onset fever, dysuria, fre-quency, burning; if pyelone-phritis, may appear toxic, with CVA tenderness, WBC casts	Gross/micro	Positive	Cystitis or pyelone-phritis; bacterial, viral, TB, other; culture
AUTOIMMUNE					
Glomerulonephritis, acute (p. 607)	Glomerular	Malaise, headache, vomiting, fever, abdominal pain; oli-guria, edema, high BP	Gross/micro	Positive	Poststreptococci; high ASO titer; low complement
Membranoproliferative glomerulonephritis (p. 607)	Glomerular	Often insidious; malaise, headache, vomiting, edema, high BP	Gross/micro	Positive	Low complement; biopsy
Henoch-Schönlein pur-pura (p. 610)	Glomerular	Purpuric rash, arthritis, GI in-volvement	Micro	Variable	Variable involvement; may have elevated IgA
Lupus nephritis	Glomerular	Associated signs and symptoms	Micro	Positive	Variable involvement; pos ANA, low com-plement; biopsy
Nephritis Bacterial endocarditis (p. 420) Shunt	Glomerular	Acute illness, fever, toxicity, signs and symptoms of re-lated disease	Micro	Positive	Low complement
Nephrotic syndrome (p. 612)	Glomerular	Periorbital swelling and oligu-ria followed by edema, mal-aise, abdominal pain	Rare (25%)	Positive	Low albumin, high lipids; etiology un-known
TRAUMA (Chapter 64)					
Renal calculi	Nonrenal	Asymptomatic to severe back and abdominal pain, nau-sea, vomiting	Gross/micro	Negative	Idiopathic, UTI, ↑Ca^{++}, cystinosis, hyperuricemia; IVP indicated
Foreign body	Nonrenal	Frequency, urgency, pain	Micro	Negative	Usually experimenting or masturbating

Condition	Origin	Associated findings	Gross/micro	Proteinuria	Comments
Direct trauma (Chapter 64)	Variable	History of trauma with variable complaints	Gross/micro	Negative	Usually renal contusion; if gross, laceration or rupture; IVP
Exercise	Nonrenal	Follows heavy exercise	Micro	Variable	
Meatal excoriation (p. 379)	Nonrenal	Local lesion	Gross/micro	Negative	Local treatment
CONGENITAL					
Hydronephrosis	Extraglomerular	Abdominal mass	Micro	Positive	Most common UPJ
Polycystic kidney	Extraglomerular	Large kidney, other cystic anomalies	Micro	Positive	Infant, adult types
Hemangioma/telangiectasis	Extraglomerular	Hemangioma, telangiectasia	Micro	Negative	Rendu-Osler-Weber disease
Hemoglobinopathy Sickle cell trait, SC (p. 531)	Extraglomerular	Associated signs and symptoms	Micro	Negative	Difficulty concentrating urine
Coagulopathy, thrombocytopenia (p. 525)	Extraglomerular	Bleeding problems elsewhere	Gross/micro	Negative	Bleeding screen, platelets
Hereditary nephritis	Glomerular	Hearing deficit	Micro	Negative	Alport's syndrome
Benign familial hematuria	Glomerular	Intermittent or persistent	Micro	Negative	Benign
INTOXICATION					
Anticoagulants Aspirin Methicillin Sulfonamides	Extraglomerular	Nephritis or crystalluria	Gross/micro	Variable	Temporally related to drug use
NEOPLASM					
Wilms' tumor	Extraglomerular	Abdominal mass	Gross/micro	Negative	Surgical consult
Leukemia	Extraglomerular	Systemic disease	Micro	Variable	Oncology consult
OTHER					
Renal vein thrombosis	Extraglomerular		Gross/micro	Variable	Occurs in acutely ill children
Congestive heart failure (Chapter 16)	Extraglomerular	Dyspnea, tachycardia, tachypnea	Micro	Negative	Accompanies cardiac disease

38 Hypoglycemia

ALERT: If signs and symptoms are consistent, a therapeutic trial of glucose administration should be attempted after obtaining specimens for glucose determination.

Hypoglycemia is defined as a blood sugar of <40 mg/dl in the child, <30 mg/dl in the newborn, and <20 mg/dl in the preterm infant in the first 24 hr of life. These criteria are based on whole-blood determinations; serum and plasma levels are 15%-20% higher. Initial use of Dextrostix or Chemstrips is helpful for emergent approximations before confirmation by clinical analysis in the laboratory.

Fasting hypoglycemia, which is related to an imbalance between glucose production and use, is most common in thin male children between 18 mo and 5 yr. Reactive hypoglycemia produces a low glucose level within 5 hr after eating; it occurs with increased insulin and is usually severe. Drugs also can cause hypoglycemia.

ETIOLOGY

See Table 38-1.

DIAGNOSTIC FINDINGS

The patient's history may be helpful in focusing on the appropriate etiology. Onset, frequency, relationship to food (fruits and fructose intolerance, high protein–diet intolerance or leucine sensitive) and fasting, family history, and concurrent medical problems must be explored. Evidence of hepatic disease, endocrine deficiencies, and abnormalities in growth and development must be sought.

The systemic response primarily reflects excessive catecholamine release. Clinically, patients have sweating, weakness, tachycardia, tachypnea, variable elevations of blood pressure and temperature, anxiety, tremulousness, and hunger. Neonates may be asymptomatic.

If the hypoglycemia is not treated, cerebral dysfunction may progress, the presentation and complications paralleling those of hypoxia. Patients may have headaches, disturbed mental status with confusion, irritability and psychotic behavior, ataxia, seizures, and coma. The signs and symptoms of the underlying etiology may also be present.

1. **Complications:** permanent brain damage from frequent or prolonged hypoglycemia
2. **Ancillary data**
   a. Serum insulin and serum and urine glucose and ketones, phosphate and liver function tests
   b. Specific tolerance tests, response to ketogenic diet, enzymes in urine, liver biopsy, etc., may all need to be considered depending on the differential.

DIFFERENTIAL DIAGNOSIS

See Chapters 15 and 54.

MANAGEMENT

Concurrent with stabilization, the hypoglycemia must be treated.

1. In the newborn, early, frequent feedings are often adequate.
2. In the older child, if there are no vital sign

TABLE 38-1. Hypoglycemia: diagnostic considerations

Condition	Type	Hepatomegaly (variably abn liver function test)	Ketonuria/ketonemia
NEONATAL (TRANSIENT) (Chapter 11)			
Small-for-gestational-age infant	Fasting	No	No
Hyperinsulinism Infant of diabetic mother Erythroblastosis	Fasting	No	No
Perinatal insult Asphyxia, infection	Fasting	No	No
HEPATIC ENZYME DEFICIENCY			
Glycogen storage disease (I, III, VI)	Fasting	Yes	Variable
Disorder of gluconeogenesis	Fasting	Yes	No
LIMITED SUBSTRATE			
Ketotic hypoglycemia (onset 1½-5 yr; resolves by 9-10 yr)	Fasting	No	Yes
Endocrine (Chapter 74) Panhypopituitary Growth hormone deficiency ACTH deficiency Addison's disease Hypothyroid	Fasting	No	Yes
HYPERINSULINEMIA			
Beta-cell tumor, adenoma, hyperplasia	Fasting	No	No
Leucine sensitivity	Reactive	No	No
Extrapancreatic tumor	Fasting	No	No
Prediabetes	Fasting	No	No
INTOXICATION (Chapter 54)			
Salicylates		No	Yes
Ethanol		No	Variable
Propranolol		No	No
Insulin		No	No
MISCELLANEOUS			
Malnutrition	Fasting	Yes	Yes
Hepatic damage Reye's syndrome (p. 492) Hepatitis (p. 487)	Fasting	Variable	Variable
Fructose intolerance, galactosemia	Reactive	Yes	No
Amino acid abnormalities	Fasting	No	No

or CNS findings, oral sources of glucose may be attempted, with frequent feedings.

3. If the patient is unstable, with altered mental status, glucose should be administered parenterally:
   a. 0.5-1.0 g/kg/dose IV, usually administered as D25W (2-4 ml/kg/dose) given slowly; a rapid response is to be expected if hypoglycemia is the prominent cause. D50W (1-2 ml/kg/dose) may be used for children >3 year; D10W for preterm infants. D10W has 10 g glucose/dl.
   b. Thereafter, maintenance through adequate glucose homeostasis and fluid balance: 10%-20% glucose in 0.2NS at a rate of at least 5 mg dextrose/kg/min.

4. If glucose is unavailable, glucagon 0.03-0.1 mg/kg/dose IM, IV (1 mg may be given at any age) will provide transient elevation of glucose if there are adequate liver stores. Dose may be repeated in 20 min.

5. Sources of 20 g glucose available commonly include Kool-Aid with sugar (13.4 oz), Coca Cola (13.3 oz), orange soda (10 oz.), ginger ale (15.5 oz), Hershey's milk chocolate bar (2.5 oz bar), orange juice (12 oz), and apple juice (12 oz). Obviously these may vary because of variations in products or mixing technique.

6. In severe hyperinsulinemia, diazoxide 6-12 mg/kg/24 hr q 12 hr PO is usually required on an ongoing basis. Frequent feedings alone are often successful in avoiding fasting types of hypoglycemia. Underlying diseases must receive prompt treatment.

DISPOSITION

Most patients with suspected hyperinsulinemia or any vital-sign abnormalities or cerebral dysfunction should be admitted to the hospital until the etiology is clear and future episodes can be prevented. Patients with only minimal symptoms and a known etiology can, with adequate follow-up, often be monitored as outpatients.

REFERENCES

Bradows, R.G., Williams, C., and Amatruda, J.M.: Treatment of insulin reactions in diabetes, JAMA **252**:3378, 1984.

Pagliara, A.S., Karl, I.E., Haymond, M., et al.: Hypoglycemia in infancy and childhood, J. Pediatr. **82**:365, 558, 1973.

Senior, B., and Wolfsdorf, J.I.: Hypoglycemia in children, Pediatr. Clin. North Am. **26**:171, 1979.

39 Irritability

ALERT: Irritability may be the presenting complaint for a potentially life-threatening systemic disease. It is essential to consider such conditions in determining management.

Children tend to be irritable with acute infections, particularly those associated with fever. The febrile child needs careful evaluation to ensure that there is no underlying significant pathology associated with the behavioral change. Chronic illnesses, such as juvenile rheumatoid arthritis, may cause a child to be irritable.

Most children tend to have some period of the day when they are most irritable, usually toward the evening. When this becomes marked, it is known as colic and occurs in as many as 10% of children. Irritability from teething usually begins at 6 mo of age with the appearance of the first teeth. Since medications commonly cause irritability, this factor should be considered in prescribing drugs. Unrecognized trauma must also be excluded (Table 39-1).

Attempts must be made to make the child more comfortable while ensuring that there is no significant pathology and that the parents are dealing with the child's irritability with appropriate perspective. In addition to specific therapeutic interventions, support, empathy, and frequent follow-up are essential.

REFERENCES

Harley, L.M.: Fussing and crying in young infants, Clin. Pediatr. **8:**138, 1969.

Honig, P.J.: Teething: are today's pediatricians using yesterday's notions? J. Pediatr. **87:**415, 1975.

TABLE 39-1. Irritability: diagnostic considerations

Condition	Diagnostic findings	Comments
INFECTIONS		
Minor acute infections		
Upper respiratory infections (p. 463)	Rhinorrhea, cough, variable fever, decreased activity, nontoxic	Irritability decreases with antipyretic therapy; must rule out other pathology
Otitis media (p. 452)	Rhinorrhea, fever, ear pain	Irritability usually decreases with antipyretic therapy and local therapy (eardrops) if needed
Urinary tract infection (p. 463)	Fever, dysuria, frequency, burning	Irritability decreases in 24 hr with appropriate antibiotics
Other	Associated signs and symptoms	
Meningitis (p. 549) Encephalitis	Fever, anorexia, changed mental status, lethargy, variable stiff neck, headache	Important infection to consider in irritable child; may exist even in presence of other infection such as otitis media
Osteomyelitis (p. 571)	Bone pain, redness	Orthopedic consult
COLIC	Episodic, intense, persistent crying in an otherwise healthy child; usually occurs in late afternoon or evening	Usually begins at 2-3 wk and continues until 10-12 wk; must be certain no pathology exists; advise soothing, rhythmic activities (rocking, wind-up swing), avoiding stimulants (coffee, tea, cola) if breast feeding, and minimizing daytime sleeping; soy or hydrolyzed casein formula may be beneficial; make sure that mother gets adequate sleep and is handling stress; diagnosis of exclusion
TEETHING	Irritated, swollen gum; does *not* cause high fevers, significant diarrhea, or diaper rash	Advise teething ring, wet washcloth to chew on; rubbing gums with small amount of Scotch (or other liquor) or proprietary products; avoiding salty foods
INTRAPSYCHIC		
Maternal anxiety	Insecure, anxious parents; overly responsive, irritable well child	Unstable or changing home environment, inconsistent parenting; attempt to support parents
INTOXICATION (Chapter 54)		
Ephedrine Phenobarbital Aminophylline Amphetamines	In therapeutic dose may cause irritability as either a primary or paradoxical effect	May try different form of drug or substitute
Lead	Weakness, weight loss, vomiting, headache, abdominal pain, seizures, increased intracranial pressure	Dimercaprol, EDTA

TABLE 39-1. Irritability: diagnostic considerations—cont'd

Condition	Diagnostic findings	Comments
INTOXICATION—cont'd		
Narcotics withdrawal in newborn (Chapter 11)	Yawning, sneezing, jitteriness, tremor, constant movement, seizures, vomiting, dehydration, collapse	Symptoms begin in first 48 hr but may be delayed; support child: phenobarbital 5 mg/kg/24 hr q 8 hr IM or PO with slow tapering over 1-3 wk
TRAUMA		
Foreign body, fracture, tourniquet (hair around digit) (Chapter 66)	Local tenderness, swelling, often following injury; thread or cloth around digit or penis	Splinter or other foreign body, hairline fracture; contusion; tourniquet around digit or penis
Subdural hematoma (Chapter 57)	History of head trauma; progressively impaired mental status; vomiting, headache, seizures	May be acute or chronic; requires recognition, CT scan; neurosurgical consult
Epidural hematoma		
Corneal abrasion (p. 334)	May not have history; patch fluorescein positive	
DEFICIENCY		
Iron deficiency anemia (Chapter 26)	Pallor, learning deficit, anorexic, poor diet, microcytic, hypochromic anemia	Peaks at 9 and 18 mo of age; diet insufficient; elemental iron 5 mg/kg/24 hr q 8 hr PO
Malnutrition	Wasted, distended abdomen	May be caused by neglect or poverty
ENDOCRINE/METABOLIC		
Hyponatremia/hypernatremia (Chapter 8)	Dehydration, edema, seizures, intracranial bleeding	Multiple etiologies
Hypocalcemia	Tetany, seizure, diarrhea	Multiple etiologies
Hypercalcemia	Abdominal pain, polyuria, nephrocalcinosis, constipation, pancreatitis	Multiple etiologies
Hypoglycemia (Chapter 38)	Sweating, tachycardia, weakness, tachypnea, anxiety, tremor; cerebral dysfunction	Multiple etiologies; dextrose 0.5-1.0 g/kg/dose IV
Diabetes insipidus	Polydipsia, thirst, constipation, dehydration, collapse	May be hyponatremic; urine specific gravity <1.006; inability to concentrate urine on fluid restriction
VASCULAR		
Congenital heart disease	Cyanosis, other cardiac findings	Usually cyanotic
Congestive heart failure (Chapter 16)	Tachypnea, tachycardia, rales, pulmonary edema	Cardiac and noncardiogenic
Paroxysmal atrial tachycardia (Chapter 6)	Heart rate >180, restless, variably cyanotic, variable congestive heart failure	Irritability if prolonged
MISCELLANEOUS		
Incarcerated hernia	Specific abdominal findings	Surgical consult
Intussusception		
DTP reaction	Immunization within 48 hr	Analgesia

40 Limp

ALERT: Septic arthritis, osteomyelitis, and fracture must be considered. Hip pathology may appear as knee pain.

The child with a limp requires a systematic assessment of gait to determine the functional problem and etiology. In children it is often difficult to isolate pathology on clinical grounds alone because of the difficulty in eliciting specific signs and symptoms.

ETIOLOGY

By age-group, the following conditions are most commonly associated with limping (Table 40-1):

1-5 yr	5-10 yr
Toxic synovitis	Toxic synovitis
Occult fracture	Legg-Calvé-Perthes disease
Osteomyelitis	
Septic arthritis	**10-15 yr**
Juvenile rheumatoid arthritis	Slipped capital femoral epiphysis
	Osgood-Schlatter disease
	Osteochondroses

DIAGNOSTIC FINDINGS

The history is particularly important in helping to localize the exact site of pathology. The progression of signs and symptoms, precipitating factors, relationship to trauma, and infection and systemic disease are crucial in the initial evaluation. Previous medical problems, exposures, family history, and the patient's age are helpful in considering diagnostic entities.

In physically evaluating the child, it is important to watch the child walk, focusing on the components of gait. First, the hips, knees, and ankles should be examined for pain, warmth, effusion, asymmetry, and limitation of motion and then the femur, tibia, fibula, and foot and ankle bones. Length of legs from the anterior iliac crest to the medial malleolus should be compared. A complete neurologic examination of the lower extremities and examination of the abdomen and genitalia are required. Hip pain is often referred to the knee.

If the physical examination and history are not conclusive, CBC, ESR, and blood cultures may be useful in evaluating a potential infectious etiology. X-ray studies for infection, trauma, neoplasm, congenital abnormalities, and degenerative problems are often diagnostic. A technetium bone scan may be obtained for further clarification. When infectious arthritis or osteomyelitis is suspected, an aspirate may be useful, with appropriate stains and cultures (pp. 570 and 626). If the initial evaluation is unrevealing, serial examinations with close follow-up may be required, since an occult or stress fracture, osteomyelitis, infectious arthritis, or other condition may be delayed in developing objective signs and symptoms.

REFERENCES

Chung, S.M.K.: Identifying the cause of acute limp in childhood, Clin. Pediatr. 13:769, 1974.

Illingworth, C.M.: 128 limping children with no fracture, sprain or obvious cause, Clin. Pediatr. 17:139, 1978.

TABLE 40-1. Limp: diagnostic considerations

Condition	Diagnostic findings	Ancillary data	Comments/management
TRAUMA (Chapters 66-70)			
Sprain/contusion	History of trauma; local pain, tenderness, swelling, ecchymosis; variably unstable	X-ray negative	Support, restrict weight bearing
Fracture	Variable history of trauma; local pain, tenderness, swelling; may be occult	X-ray may be positive; if negative, do serial studies, looking for buckle fracture in the cortex of tibia, fibula, or femur; be certain x-ray includes all potentially involved areas; technetium bone scan rarely needed	Orthopedic consult; stress fracture may occur after repeated indirect trivial injuries; consider child abuse
Periostitis	Minor trauma to tibia, femur; local tenderness, fullness	X-ray for subperiosteal hemorrhage (may be delayed)	Periosteum is loosely attached, with minor trauma; may get periosteal hemorrhage
Foreign body/splinter in foot	Acute onset pain, local tenderness, variable erythema	X-ray rarely needed but foreign body may localize if radiopaque	Remove; location will dictate need for consult
Poorly fitting shoe	Limp disappears when shoe removed		
Vertebral disk injury	Motor defect—weakness, asymmetric reflexes; sensory defect	X-ray may show injury	Orthopedic and neurosurgical consultation
INFECTION/INFLAMMATION			
Toxic synovitis of hip (Chapter 69)	Preceding viral illness, nontoxic; hip rarely warm, tender, or limited range of motion	CBC, ESR: WNL; x-ray: variable effusion; aspirate if question of septic arthritis	Self-limited; common in 1½-7-yr-olds
Osteomyelitis (p. 571)	Fever, variable systemic toxicity; local swelling, tenderness, warmth, monoarticular, long bones (femur, tibia)	↑CBC, ↑ESR; x-ray; technetium bone scan; joint and bone aspirate	May get arthritis and osteomyelitis concurrently; antibiotics
Arthritis, septic (p. 569)	Febrile, monoarticular, large weight-bearing (knee, hip) joints; local swelling, warmth, tenderness	↑WBC, ↑ESR; x-ray; bone scan; joint aspirate	Requires urgent drainage and antibiotics
Arthritis, viral Rubella Rubella vaccine Hepatitis	Local swelling, warmth, tenderness; polyarticular, particularly large joints (knee); associated symptoms	CBC, viral titers, liver functions; x-ray: effusion; joint aspirate	Usually self-limited

TABLE 40-1. Limp: diagnostic considerations—cont'd

Condition	Diagnostic findings	Ancillary data	Comments/management
INFECTION/INFLAMMATION—cont'd			
Arthritis, viral—cont'd			
Chickenpox			
Arthritis, uncommon	Insidious, commonly hip with progression; leg is flexed, well abducted	Joint aspirate; CBC, variable syphilis serology, variable PPD	
Mycobacterium			
Fungal			
Appendicitis (p. 494)	RLQ pain, psoas/obturator sign, limited hip movement	↑WBC, variable pyuria	Important to consider in differential as well as other abdominal problems
Polio (Chapter 41)	Systemic disease with asymmetric flaccid paralysis, bulbar involvement	CSF pleocytosis; ↑WBC; positive viral culture	Decreased incidence
Guillain-Barré syndrome (Chapter 41)	Ascending symmetric paralysis with pain, paresthesias and paralysis; may involve cranial nerves; preceding viral illness	CSF: high protein	Danger of respiratory insufficiency; associated with viral infection, immunization (controversial)
VASCULAR			
Legg-Calvé-Perthes disease (Chapter 69)	Insidious onset pain of hip with limp or limitation of motion	X-ray: bulging capsule with widened joint space; technetium scan: ↓ uptake	Peak: males, 4-10 yr; orthopedic consult—treat hip in abduction and internal rotation
DEGENERATIVE			
Slipped capital femoral epiphysis (Chapter 69)	Unilateral or bilateral pain in knee (referred) or in medial aspect of thigh; hip or knee made worse by activity; limitation of abduction and internal rotation; child obese or tall and thin, with rapid growth spurt	X-ray: widening epiphyseal growth plate	Peak: 12-15 yr; orthopedic consult; surgical immobilization
Osgood-Schlatter disease (Chapter 69)	Pain in knee caused by patellar tendonitis at insertion into tibial tubercle	X-ray: fragmentation of tibial tuberosity	Peak: 11-15 yr; symptomatic treatment, decreased activity
Osteochondroses			
Chondromalacia patellae	Irregularity of patella, pain on compression of patellar at intercondylar notch with contraction of quadriceps	X-ray: WNL	Teenagers, female > males; symptomatic; treatment: quadriceps strengthening

	Signs and Symptoms	Diagnosis	Management/Comments
Osteochondritis dissecans	Pain, stiffness, swelling, clicking of knee	X-ray: tunnel view shows demineralization of medial femoral condyle	Teenagers; decreased activity, muscle strengthening
Neuromuscular disease	Associated motor and sensory findings		Often progressive
CONGENITAL			
Hemophilia (p. 525)	Variable history of trauma; muscle bleeding; monoarticular joint swollen, tender with hemarthrosis	X-ray; variable bleeding screen	Factor replacement
Sickle cell disease (p. 531)	Systemic disease; bone pain; polyarticular joint involvement	X-ray; Hct; positive sickle prep; variable technetium bone scan	May have concurrent infection; may be crisis or infarct
Dislocated hip	Normal newborn except for instability and range of motion of joint; pos hip click (abduction)	X-ray	Orthopedic consult, splint hip in flexion and abduction
Unequal leg length	Unequal length from anterior iliac crest to medial malleolus		Orthopedic consult
Testicular torsion (p. 506) Incarcerated hernia (p. 506)	Acute onset of scrotal or groin pain; mass, tender swollen		Surgical emergency
AUTOIMMUNE (Table 27-1)			
NEOPLASM			
Osteochondroma	Local pain with exostosis		
Leukemia Neuroblastoma Ewing Spinal cord tumor	Systemic disease with associated symptoms		
INTRAPSYCHIC			
Attention getting	Inconsistent signs and symptoms		May be functional habit following resolution of physical problem, particularly in children under 5 yr

41 Paralysis and hemiplegia

ALERT: Following assessment of respiratory status, the diagnostic work-up must quickly establish the underlying process to provide guidelines for support and therapy.

The acute onset of paralysis in children may be indicated by a youngster not wanting to walk. Infectious and inflammatory etiologies are most common (Table 41-1). In addition, spinal cord or central nervous system injury resulting from trauma can cause transient or permanent deficits. Heavy metal intoxications can induce paralysis. Hysterical conversion reactions may mimic paralysis, but usually the examination is inconsistent.

Central nervous system lesions generally are accompanied by a flaccid paralysis and loss of tone and deep tendon reflexes (DTR). After about a week, the patient may become spastic

TABLE 41-1. Paralysis: diagnostic considerations

	Guillain–Barré syndrome	Secondary polyneuropathy
Etiology	Unknown; role of viral, mycoplasma infections unknown	Infectious or inflammatory: viral, bacterial (diphtheria, botulism), immunizations; autoimmune; intoxication
Prodrome	Nonspecific respiratory or GI symptoms 5-14 days before onset	Low-grade fever and other signs and symptoms reflecting the underlying disease
Neurologic findings	Symmetric flaccid ascending paralysis; greater involvement of lower extremities, greater proximally; facial diplegia, cranial nerve, bulbar involved; muscle tenderness; sensory-distal hyperesthesia with impaired position, vibration	Variable involvement; flaccid paralysis with loss of DTR and position and vibration senses; ataxia; cranial nerve involvement with dysphagia; generalized weakness
Ancillary data	CSF: few WBC, high protein after 10 days	CSF: few monocytes with high protein; tests to determine underlying disease; nerve conduction velocity
Comments	Peaks in 5 to 9-yr-olds; usual recovery in 1-3 wk; supportive care	Major systemic illness reflects nature of underlying disease

with hyperactive reflexes. The evaluation should include a careful neurologic examination, as well as a check for associated symptoms. Spinal fluid should normally be examined.

The major complications encountered by these patients is respiratory failure (rarely requiring ventilatory support) and secondary bacterial infections. Treatment is generally supportive.

Rarely, patients have **acute hemiplegia,** secondary to emboli, thromboses, or intracerebral hemorrhage. Emboli produce a rapidly evolving clinical picture, but thromboses often evolve over hours to days. Predisposing factors include:

1. Infection
   a. Viral: herpes, coxsackievirus, encephalitis
   b. Bacterial meningitis
2. Vascular—embolic
   a. Congenital heart disease
   b. Endocarditis
   c. Dysrhythmias: atrial fibrillation
   d. Arteriovenous malformations
   e. Acute infantile hemiplegia: seizure followed by coma, hemiplegia, and fever caused by occlusion of the middle cerebral artery
3. Vascular
   a. Hemiplegic migraine
   b. Vasculitis
4. Trauma
   a. Blunt trauma to the neck (or intraoral trauma) may produce delayed onset of symptoms in 24-48 hr
   b. Penetrating trauma—may produce immediate loss or vascular foreign body emboli
5. Congenital
   a. Sickle cell disease (thrombosis, spasm)
   b. Hemophilia (hemorrhage)
6. Todd's paralysis: transient paralysis following seizures resolving without therapy

Fig. 41-1 provides a summary of the anatomic

Poliomyelitis	Tick-bite paralysis	Transverse myelitis/neuromyelitis optica
Poliovirus	Toxin release by tick	Unknown but may be inflammatory and related to multiple sclerosis
Fever, respiratory or GI symptoms; may have meningism	1 wk after tick bites and remains attached; fatigue, irritability	
Flaccid, asymmetric paralysis with maximum deficit 3-5 days after onset; lower extremities more involved than upper; bulbar involvement may occur very early; sensory exam normal; marked muscle tenderness, pain, fasciculations, and twitching	Rapid progression of muscle pain with ascending flaccid symmetric paralysis; pain and paresthesias	Rapid progression; may have ataxia, weakness, multiple neurologic deficits; optic neuritis; paralysis develops with sensory loss below lesion and hyperesthesia above; bowel and bladder problems
CSF: pleocytosis (initially PMN, then monocytes), elevated protein	CSF: normal	CSF: (not done routinely) pleocytosis, increased protein; myelogram if indicated
May be asymptomatic or nonparalytic; summer epidemic; unimmunized individuals	Tick usually attached to head or neck; rapid improvement with removal of tick (Table 45-1)	Steroids (ACTH) may be useful in treatment

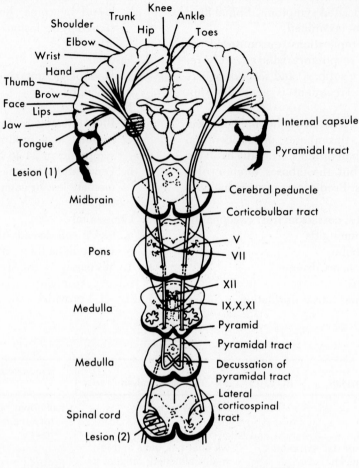

Lesion (1) | Lesion (2)

Upper motor neuron lesion | **Lower motor neuron lesion**

Contralateral hemiparesis
Postural flexion of arm, extension of leg
Muscles hypertonic
Tendon reflexes hyperactive
Atrophy not prominent
No muscle fasciculations
Pathologic reflexes present

Paresis limited to specific muscle groups
Gait depends on muscles affected; flail-like movements common
Muscles flaccid
Tendon reflexes absent or hypoactive
Atrophy prominent
Muscle fasciculations present
Contractures and skeletal deformities may develop

FIG. 41-1. The pyramidal system. (From Clark, R.G.: Essentials of clinical neuroanatomy and neurophysiology, Philadelphia, 1975, F.A. Davis Co.)

and functional correlations in upper and lower motor neuron disease. Treatment must focus on the underlying pathology as well as complicating conditions.

Bell's palsy is a seventh cranial nerve paralysis of sudden onset and unknown etiology. The patient has a flattened nasolabial fold on the affected side and is unable to close the eyelids, pucker the lips, or wrinkle the brow. Recovery usually occurs over 3-6 wk. Therapy should in-clude protection of the cornea with artificial tears. Steroids may be useful if initiated within 2 days of onset of symptoms. Prednisone 1 mg/kg/24 hr PO can be initiated and tapered over 7-10 days.

REFERENCES

Birse, G.S., and Strauss, R.W.: Acute childhood hemiplegia, Ann. Emerg. Med. **14:**74, 1985.

Gold, A.P., and Carter, S.: Acute hemiplegia of infancy and childhood, Pediatr. Clin. North Am. **23:**413, 1976.

42 Rash

ALERT: Lesions requiring emergent evaluation include petechiae, purpura, burns, cellulitis, or those with other evidence of systemic infection.

Although rash is a common presenting complaint, the term requires careful definition. The identification of a rash disease requires examination of the lesions, focusing on whether there are blisters or if solid, whether the lesions are red or scaling (Table 42-1). It is important to define the configuration and distribution of findings and relate the chronology of the evolution with the development of systemic signs and symptoms.

The majority of urgent encounters related to rashes have an infectious origin. Tables 42-2, 42-3, and 42-4 divide the common exanthems into categories based on morphology: maculopapular, vesicular, and petechial or purpuric.

See also Chapter 72: Dermatologic disorders.

Patients must be seen emergently if the lesions are purple or look like blood (purpura), do not blanch (petechiae), are burnlike (scalded skin), are red, blue, or tender to the touch (cellulitis), have red streaking, or are pustular. Lesions that are pruritic, have associated fever >24 hr, may be related to a medication, or are pustular with a red or cola-colored urine should also be seen.

Chapter 72 provides a more detailed summary of the common dermatologic problems that require evaluation and treatment.

REFERENCES

Kraemer, M.J., and Smith, A.C.: Rashes with ampicillin, Pediatr. Rev. 1:197, 1980.
Weston, W.L.: Practical pediatric dermatology, ed. 2, 1985, Boston, Little, Brown & Co.

TABLE 42-1. Rash: evaluation

Appearance	Diagnostic considerations
BLISTER (FLUID-FILLED)	
CLEAR	*Vesicular* (Tables 42-2 and 42-3): herpes simplex, varicella-zoster, scabies *Bullous:* bullous impetigo, erythema multiforme, burn, contact dermatitis, friction blister
PUSTULAR	Acne, folliculitis (bacterial, fungal), candidiasis, bacteremia (gonococcemia, meningococcemia)
SOLID (NON-RED)	
SKIN-COLORED	*Keratotic* (rough-surfaced lesion): wart, corn, callus *Nonkeratotic* (smooth lesion): wart, molluscum contagiosum, epidermoid (sebaceous) cyst, basal and squamous cell carcinoma, nevi
WHITE	Pityriasis alba, vitiligo, pityriasis versicolor, postinflammatory hypopigmentation, milia, molluscum contagiosum
BROWN	Café-au-lait patch, nevi, freckle, melanoma, hypopigmentation secondary to systemic disease, medication, or postinflammatory condition
YELLOW	Jaundice, nevi sebaceous
SOLID (RED, NONSCALING)	
INFLAMMATORY PAPULE/ NODULE	*Papule (maculopapular)* (Tables 42-2 and 42-4): viral exanthem, erythema multiforme, insect bite, scarlet fever, angioma *Nodule:* furuncle, erythema nodosum
VASCULAR (FLAT-TOPPED)	*Nonpurpuric:* toxic erythema (viral exanthem, medication, photosensitivity), urticaria (infection, medication), erythema multiforme, cellulitis (erysipelas) *Purpuric* (Table 42-2): vasculitis, petechiae, ecchymosis
SOLID (RED, SCALING)	
PAPULOSQUAMOUS DISEASE	No epithelial disruption: pityriasis rosea, tinea corporis, capitis, pedis or cruris, lupus erythematosus, syphilis
ECZEMATOUS DISEASE	Epithelial disruption: atopic (eczema); seborrheic, diaper, contact, or stasis dermatitis, tinea cruris, capitis or pedis, nummular eczema, impetigo, candidiasis

Modified from Lynch, P.J., and Edminister, S.C.: Ann. Emerg. Med. **13:**603, 1984; Weston, W.L.: Primary Care **11:**469, 1984.

TABLE 42-2. Acute exanthems

	Maculopapular	Vesicular	Petechial or purpuric

Infection	Viral
	  Measles
	  Rubella
	  Roseola } Table 42-4
	  Enterovirus
	  Infectious mononucleosis (p. 542)
	  Pityriasis rosea (p. 441)
	
	Other
	  Scarlet fever (Table 42-4)
	  Staphylococcal scalded skin (p. 443)
	  Toxic shock syndrome (p. 547)
	  Kawasaki disease (p. 538)
	  Meningococcemia (p. 542)
	  Mycoplasma pneumoniae
	  Tick diseases
	  Rocky Mountain spotted fever
	  Typhus
		Viral
		  Chickenpox
		  Herpes zoster Table 42-3
		  Herpes simplex
		  Enterovirus (Table 42-4)
		  Hand, foot, and mouth
		  Herpangina
		  Molluscum contagiosum
		    (p. 445)
		  Historical: smallpox
		
		Other
		  Impetigo (p. 439)
		  Rickettsialpox
		  Candidiasis
		  Staphylococcal scalded skin
		    syndrome (p. 443)
		  Erythema multiforme
		    (p. 435)
			Viral
			  Enterovirus
			  Hemorrhagic measles
			  Rubeola (atypical)
			  Chickenpox
			
			Other
			  Meningococcemia (p. 541)
			  H. influenzae
			  Pneumococcemia
			  Rocky Mountain spotted fever
			  Sepsis (with thrombocytopenia or
			    DIC)
			  Gonococcemia (p. 511
			  Endocarditis (p. 420)
			  Plague
			  Rare

Intoxication	Ampicillin Penicillin Barbiturates Anticonvulsants Sulfonamides	Rare	
Other	Sunburn (p. 444) Juvenile rheumatoid arthritis Serum sickness	Insect bites (p. 232)	Henoch-Schönlein purpura (p. 610) Idiopathic thrombocytopenia (p. 529) Coagulation disorder Trauma Tourniquet (distal) Coughing (head and neck) Leukemia Aplastic anemia

TABLE 42-3. Vesicular exanthems

	Varicella (chickenpox)	Herpes zoster (shingles)	Herpes simplex
Diagnostic findings	Rapid progression of erythematous macules, developing into papules and vesicles; vesicles are thin-walled and superficial, surrounded by an erythematous area; pruritic; distribution is central with relative sparing distally; marked variability in severity of exanthem—may only have a few lesions; usually febrile; enanthem—shallow mucosal ulcers; different ages of lesions; may initially resemble insect bites	Erythema followed by red papules that become vesicular in 12-24 hr, pustular in 72 hr, and crusts in 10-12 days; distribution is unilateral following peripheral dermatome or cranial nerve; preeruptive pain with hyperesthesia over involved skin	Multiple presentations **Gingivostomatitis:** fever, irritability, pain in mouth, throat, and with swallowing; shallow ulcers on mucosa (buccal, tonsillar, and pharyngeal); crusts on lips; cervical lymphadenopathy; lasts 1-14 days **Vulvovaginitis:** similar shallow ulcers on vagina and vulva; pain on urination **Keratoconjunctivitis:** corneal ulceration
Complications	Pneumonia Secondary bacterial infections 　Cellulitis 　Bacterial pneumonia Encephalitis, myelitis Hepatitis Reye's syndrome	Ophthalmic: neuralgia, corneal dendrites, iritis Postherpetic neuralgia and death	Ophthalmic: corneal ulceration Encephalitis Neonatal viremia with encephalitis
Management	Antipruritic agents Topical: calamine lotion; cold baths with small amount baking soda (⅓ tsp) in water Systemic: diphenhydramine Antipyretics—Do *not* use aspirin Treatment of complications Zoster-immune globulin for exposure in high-risk patient	Support, analgesia Eye involvement needs ophthalmology consultation	General support Gingival: topical analgesia—antacid or mixture of viscous lidocaine (Xylocaine), diphenhydramine, Kaopectate; Acyclovir (Zovirax); topical, IV, PO for initial and recurrent lesions
Comment	Incubation: 14-21 days Vaccine in high-risk populations Particularly dangerous in newborns, pregnant females, immunosuppressed or immunodeficient individuals	Common history of chickenpox	Sexual spread of vulvovaginitis Potentially life threatening to newborn, immunodeficient, or immunosuppressed; considers systemic agents (p. 72)

TABLE 42-4. Common maculopapular exanthems

	Measles (rubeola)	Rubella (German, 3-day measles)	Roseola (exanthema subitum)
Incubation	10-14 days	14-21 days	10-14 days
Prodrome	3 days high fever, cough, conjunctivitis, and coryza; child appears toxic, lethargic	May be none; lymphadenopathy (especially postauricular, suboccipital), malaise, variable low-grade fever	3-4 days high fever in otherwise well child, preceding rash
Exanthem	Reddish-brown; begins on face and progresses downward; generalized by third day; confluent on face, neck, upper trunk; lasts 7-10 days; desquamates; atypical measles: maculopapular, purpuric, petechial, or vesicular rash	Pink; begins on face and progresses rapidly downward; generalized by second day; discrete; lasts 2-3 days, fades in order of appearance	Appears after defervescence; rose, discrete; initially on chest, spreads to involve face and extremities; fades quickly
Enanthem	Koplik's spots (2 days before rash, on buccal mucosa opposite molars)	None	None
Complications	Pneumonia Encephalitis Otitis media Thrombocytopenia Hemorrhagic measles Pneumothorax Hepatitis Exacerbation of TB	Arthritis (common in women) beginning after 2-3 days' illness; knee, wrist, finger Congenital rubella syndrome Encephalitis Thrombocytopenia	Febrile seizure
Management	Supportive; may require hospitalization; active immunization of contacts; immune serum globulin (0.05 ml/kg) for children <1 yr; reportable	Supportive; isolate from pregnant women; active immunization of contacts; reportable	Supportive; good fever control
Comments	Rare with immunization	Rare with immunization; serologic diagnosis	Usually 1-4-yr-olds

Fifth disease (erythema infectiosum)	Enterovirus	Scarlet fever
7-14 days None	Variable (short) Variable; fever, malaise, vomiting, sore throat, rhinorrhea	2-4 days 1-2 days fever, vomiting, sore throat; often toxic
Erupts in 3 stages: (1) red-flushed cheeks with circumoral pallor (slapped cheek), (2) maculopapular eruption on extremities (lacelike), (3) may recur secondary to heat, sunlight, trauma	Maculopapular, discrete, nonpruritic, generalized; rubella-like; hand, foot, and mouth distribution	Erythematous, punctate, sandpaper texture; appears 1st in flexor areas, then generalized; most intense on neck, axilla, inguinal, popliteal skin fold; circumoral pallor; lasts 7 days, then desquamates
Variable	Variable	Red pharynx, tonsils; palatal petechiae; strawberry tongue
Transient arthritis	Aseptic meningitis Myocarditis Hepatitis	Rheumatic fever Acute glomerulonephritis
Rarely need care	Supportive	Penicillin
May be caused by human parvovirus	Concurrent family illness, gastroenteritis, herpangina	Group A streptococci (p. 459)

43 Vaginal bleeding

ALERT: Third-trimester bleeding requires immediate obstetric consultation. Dysfunctional uterine bleeding is most common in pubescent females; in younger girls the etiology is commonly trauma or foreign bodies. Hypotension may develop.

Vaginal bleeding is most commonly related to menstruation in the pubescent female. The most frequent problem associated with vaginal bleeding is dysfunctional uterine bleeding because of anovulatory cycles in which the bleeding is scanty, watery, and irregular. Most girls begin with anovulatory cycles, and it may be several years before ovulation occurs. Other etiologies must be considered, including complications of pregnancy, trauma, vulvovaginitis, and pelvic inflammatory disease (Table 43-1). A thorough pelvic examination must be performed (Chapter 78).

Pregnant women with third-trimester bleeding should be examined in the operating room, with preparations for a double setup whereby the baby can be delivered vaginally or by cesarean section. As appropriate, cultures of the cervical os and rectum (and pharynx), analysis of discharges, and a Pap smear should be done.

The prepubescent girl commonly has bleeding caused by foreign bodies or hymenal trauma. Vulvovaginitis may produce a bloody discharge. Tumors are uncommon unless the patient had an intrauterine exposure to diethylstilbestrol (DES). Vaginal bleeding may accompany endocrine and hematologic disorders.

REFERENCE

Emans, S.J.H., and Goldstein, D.P.: Pediatric and adolescent gynecology, ed. 2, Boston, 1982, Little, Brown & Co.

TABLE 43-1. Vaginal bleeding: diagnostic considerations

Condition	Signs and symptoms	Evaluation/comments
ENDOCRINE		
Uterine dysfunction (p. 508)	Irregular menses, flow too frequent, heavy, or prolonged	Diagnosis of exclusion; anovulatory cycle
Pregnancy complications (p. 518)		
Abortion	First trimester; cervix variably dilated; various products of conception	Treatment depends on type of abortion
Placenta previa	Third trimester; painless; may have profuse bleeding	Ultrasound; avoid pelvic exam in ED; double setup; fetal monitor
Abruptio placentae	Third trimester; abdominal pain, tender uterus; bleeding may be concealed	Ultrasound; avoid pelvic exam in ED; double setup; fetal monitor; common in blunt trauma
Ectopic pregnancy	Missed menses, pelvic pain, rebound, adnexal mass; low Hct, hypotension	Culdocentesis or ultrasound; rapid pregnancy test; potentially life-threatening
Following delivery	Bleeding without pain	Pharmacologic curettage (rarely mechanical); consider endometriosis
Thyroid disease (p. 472)	Associated signs and symptoms	Thyroid functions
Physiologic	Newborn may have bleeding at 5-10 days	Caused by withdrawal from maternal estrogens
TRAUMA		
Foreign body	Foul-smelling discharge	Peak is 5-9 yr (may occur at any age); forgotten tampon common in adolescent; also IUD
Laceration	Signs of trauma	Secondary trauma, intercourse, heavy exercise, molestation
INFLAMMATION		
Vulvovaginitis (p. 514)	Characteristic discharge and inflamed introitus	Culture, wet and KOH prep of discharge
Pelvic inflammatory disease (p. 510)	Abdominal, pelvic tenderness, fever, chills, nausea, vomiting	Elevated CBC and ESR, culture and Gram's stain
INTOXICATION		
Birth control pills	Irregular intake or acute overdose	
Anticoagulants	Bleeding sites elsewhere	Coagulation studies
DEFICIENCY		
Bleeding diathesis	Bleeding sites elsewhere	Coagulation studies
Idiopathic thrombocytopenic purpura (p. 529)	Bleeding elsewhere	Platelet count and coagulation studies
NEOPLASM		
Tumors, polyps, fibroids	Physical exam reveals mass, spotty bleeding	Unusual; may occur in children with DES exposure; Pap smear

44 Vomiting

ALERT: Assessment initially must determine the child's hydration status and correct any deficits, if present. Following stabilization, etiologic considerations must be determined.

Vomiting is the forceful ejection of the stomach contents into the esophagus and through the mouth. It may be caused by irritation of the peritoneum or mesentery, obstruction of the intestine, action of a toxin on the medulla, or primary CNS pathology.

ETIOLOGY

In children the most common cause of vomiting is acute gastroenteritis, as well as other infections including otitis media, urinary tract infections, and meningitis. Infants often vomit from faulty feeding techniques or chalasia. Other conditions that must be considered include congenital obstructions of the gastrointestinal tract, particularly pyloric stenosis, CNS lesions producing increased intracranial pressure, and a variety of endocrine, metabolic, and toxic problems. Newborns often have congenital obstructions (Table 44-1).

DIAGNOSTIC FINDINGS

The history must determine precipitating factors including trauma, recent illness, medications, poor feeding techniques, and instability in the environment leading to emotional upheaval. Associated symptoms and family history

---

See also Acute gastroenteritis, p. 480, and Chapter 32: Acute diarrhea.

are important. The nature of the vomiting must be determined: its color, composition, relationship to eating and position, onset, progression, and whether it was projectile. The expelled material should be examined.

1. Undigested food suggests an esophageal lesion at or above the cardia.
2. Nonbilious vomitus may result from lesions proximal to the pylorus.
3. Bile-containing material involves obstruction beyond the ampulla of Vater, or it may result from an adynamic ileus found in sepsis, significant other infections, or serious underlying disease. Bile turns green on exposure to air.
4. A fecal odor is consistent with peritonitis or a lower obstruction.

The physical examination should include inspection of the abdomen for trauma, distension, hyperactivity of the bowel, and congenital abnormalities as well as systemic illness.

MANAGEMENT

Management should focus on correction of fluid deficits (Chapter 7) as well as definitive treatment of underlying pathology. The well-hydrated patient with a self-limited problem can usually be discharged and sent home to follow a clear liquid regimen. Antiemetics are usually unnecessary for children. Otherwise, hospitalization is indicated.

Text continued on p. 227.

TABLE 44-1. Vomiting: diagnostic considerations

Condition	Diagnostic findings	Evaluation	Comments/management
INFECTIOUS/INFLAMMATORY			
Acute gastroenteritis (p. 480)	Acute onset with nausea, fever, diarrhea, and evidence of systemic illness	Fluid status, stool culture if needed	NPO, if indicated; clear liquids, advance slowly
Posttussive/posterior nasal drip	Follows vigorous coughing; may be greatest at night when recumbent; associated cough, rhinorrhea	Chest x-ray if needed	Therapeutic trial: cough suppressant or decongestant
Otitis media (p. 452)	Fever, irritability, painful ear		Antibiotics; topical therapy for extreme pain
Esophagitis/gastritis (Chapter 35)	Variably coffee ground, bloody; epigastric or substernal pain, discomfort; reflux	Endoscopy; upper GI series	Associated reflux, hiatal hernia; drugs; trial of antacids
Ulcer, peptic/duodenal (Chapter 35)	Usually coffee ground; epigastric, abdominal pain; may be chronic or acute; possible anemia	Endoscopy; upper GI series	May be life threatening
Hepatitis (p. 487)	Associated liver tenderness; icterus	Liver function tests	Usually infectious: viral, mononucleosis
Peritonitis Appendicitis (p. 494) Cholecystitis	Generalized or localized tenderness, guarding, rebound	WBC, x-rays, UA	Surgical exploration usually needed
Pancreatitis	Abdominal tenderness, pain, back pain	Amylase	GI rest, decompression; evaluate etiology
Cystitis Pyelonephritis (p. 620)	Associated fever, dysuria, frequency, burning, variable CVA tenderness	UA, urine culture	Initiate antibiotics, pending cultures
Meningitis (p. 549) CNS abscess Subdural effusion/empyema	Fever, systemic toxicity; changed mental status; local neuro signs, variable signs of increased intracerebral pressure	Lumbar puncture; CT scan if needed	Antibiotics; neurosurgical consult if indicated
CONGENITAL			
Pyloric stenosis (p. 501)	Regurgitation progressing to projectile vomiting; palpable olive-sized tumor in RUQ; vigorous gastric peristalsis present: variable dehydration, poor weight gain	Upper GI series—delayed gastric emptying, narrow pyloric channel ("string sign"); electrolytes to assess hydration	Usually male, 4-6 wk of age; treat fluid deficits, then surgery (pyloromyotomy)

Continued.

TABLE 44-1. Vomiting: diagnostic considerations

Condition	Diagnostic findings	Evaluation	Comments/management
CONGENITAL—cont'd			
Gastrointestinal obstruction (Chapter 11) Intestinal obstruction/ stenosis/bands Imperforate anus Malrotation Meconium ileus/plug	Obstructive pattern beginning in newborn period—greater than 20 ml in gastric aspirate; if proximal to ampulla of Vater: distension epigastrium or LUQ and gastric peristaltic wave; if distal to ampulla of Vater, vomitus contains bile, generalized distension	Abdominal x-ray with contrast studies if needed; electrolytes to assess fluid status	Immediate decompression; correction of fluid deficits; surgical consult Associated with cystic fibrosis Life threatening
Volvulus, sigmoid/midgut (p. 502) Intussusception (p. 498)			Life threatening
Hydrocephalus	Excessive growth of head circumference; irritability, lethargy, headache, bulging of fontanel	CT scan	May involve blockage of ventricular shunt; neurosurgical consult; urgent care
TRAUMA			
Concussion (Chapter 57)	Trauma: headache, minimally changed mental status; often projectile vomiting	Skull x-ray	Support; monitoring
Subdural hematoma (Chapter 57)	Marked change in mental status, signs of increased intracranial pressure: headache, ataxia, sixth-nerve palsy, seizures; focal neuro signs	CT scan	Immediate neurosurgical consult; support: intubate, hyperventilate, diuretics, etc.
Foreign body (p. 485)	History: may have dysphagia or total obstruction; may have respiratory distress	X-ray; esophagoscopy	If esophagus, attempt to remove by use of Foley catheter under fluoroscopy; if elsewhere, endoscopy or surgery, depending on foreign body
Intramural hematoma (Chapter 63)	Following even minimal blunt trauma: nausea, bilious vomiting, pain, tenderness, ileus; may have abdominal mass	Upper GI series	May be delay in symptom presentation
Ruptured viscus (Chapter 63)	Trauma followed by abdominal tenderness, rebound, guarding	Peritoneal lavage; x-ray for free air	Immediate surgical intervention; fluids, antibiotics

Condition	Clinical Features	Evaluation	Treatment
Subarachnoid hemorrhage (Chapter 18)	Headache, stiff neck, progressive loss of consciousness; focal neuro signs	CT scan: bloody spinal fluid	Neurosurgical consult; supportive care
Cerebral edema	Signs of increased intracranial pressure: headache, ataxia, sixth nerve palsy; altered mental status	CT scan	Diuretics, steroids, hyperventilation, elevation
INTOXICATION (Chapter 54)			
Alkali burns	Associated mouth burns, difficulty swallowing	Endoscopy	Lye, bleaches most common; surgery consult
Aspirin	Nausea, vomiting, tinnitus	Aspirin level	Stop medication; antacids, fluids
Iron	Hematemesis, shock, acidosis	Iron level, ABG, CBC	Urgent treatment with deferoxamine
Lead	Usually chronic exposure; signs of increased intracranial pressure	Lead level	Dimercaprol, EDTA
Digitalis	Underlying heart disease; nausea, arrhythmias	Digitalis level; ECG	Stop digitalis; institute active treatment of dysrhythmia, etc.
VASCULAR			
Migraine (p. 256)	Unilateral, throbbing headache; aura; family history		Consider therapeutic trial of ergotamine
Hypertensive encephalopathy (Chapter 18)	Rapid increase in BP; changed mental status; headache, nausea, anorexia	Evaluation of underlying disease	Rapid response when diastolic BP brought below 100 mm Hg
ENDOCRINE/METABOLIC			
Acidosis (Chapter 8)	Underlying etiology; rapid, deep breathing	ABG	Correction
Diabetic ketoacidosis (p. 469)	Kussmaul's breathing; history of diabetes; nausea, abdominal pain; ketones on breath	Electrolytes; ABG; glucose; ketones	Hydration, insulin, K^+
Uremia (p. 615)	Oliguria, often predisposing cause	BUN, creatinine, tests for underlying conditions	Evaluate and treat underlying etiology
Inborn errors of metabolism Amino/organic acids	Associated acute-onset vomiting and acidosis, progressive deterioration or poor growth and development	Urine and blood for amino and organic acids; electrolytes, ABG: acidosis	Exacerbation precipitated by acute illness
Fructose intolerance	Associated with ingestion of sugar or fruits	Challenge test under controlled conditions	
Addison's disease (p. 467)	Dehydration, circulatory collapse; if chronic: weakness, fatigue, pallor, diarrhea, increased pigmentation	Serum Na^+, K^+; urine adrenocorticoids low	Adrenal genital syndrome in newborns

Continued.

TABLE 44-1. Vomiting: diagnostic considerations—cont'd

Condition	Diagnostic findings	Evaluation	Comments/management
ENDOCRINE/METABOLIC—cont'd			
Reye's syndrome (p. 492)	Associated liver failure, with marked change in mental status (often combative)	Liver function tests and ammonia elevated	
INTRAPSYCHIC			
Attention getting	Inconsistent history; times usually related to getting attention	Psychiatric evaluation	Organic causes must be ruled out
Hysteria/hyperventilation	Anxiety, nausea, and other psychosomatic symptoms; may hyperventilate	Psychiatric evaluation	Exclude organic causes
NEOPLASM			
Gastrointestinal Intracerebral	Related to location, type, and extent of neoplasm; insidious onset of symptoms	Specific for tissue considerations	Rare in children
MISCELLANEOUS			
Improper feeding techniques	Often regurgitation; bad nipple; improper position; usually occurs shortly after feeding; usually vomited material is undigested	Rarely need upper GI series to rule out pathology	Implement support system; make sure child not overfed
Chalasia	May be small amounts; associated with feeding, usually within 30-45 min of feeding; child well, good growth	Upper GI series if needed	Trial of slow, careful, prone, upright feedings; child usually under 6 mo; avoid overfeeding
Pregnancy	Increased intraabdominal pressure; usually first trimester		
Epilepsy (p. 559)	Aura or seizure may involve vomiting	EEG	Requires good neurologic follow-up
Ascites	Increased intraabdominal pressure	As related to etiology; total serum protein, albumin	
Environmental Heat illness (hyperthermia) (Chapter 50)	Abnormal mental status; variably febrile, leg cramps, dehydrated	Electrolytes	Fluids, cooling
Superior mesenteric artery syndrome	Compression of duodenum in child (adolescent female) leading to obstruction; usually recent marked weight loss	Upper GI series	Usually requires psychiatric therapy for underlying problems; support

Parental education (p. 645)

1. Give only clear liquids *slowly:* Pedialyte, Lytren, Gatorade, defizzed soda pop (cola, ginger ale), etc. With younger children, start with a teaspoon and slowly advance the amount. If vomiting occurs, let your child rest for a while and then try again.
2. About 8 hr after vomiting has stopped, your child can gradually return to a normal diet. With older infants and children, give bland items (toast, crackers, clear soup) slowly.
3. Call physician if
   a. Vomiting continues for more than 24 hr or increases in frequency or amount
   b. Child develops signs of dehydration, including decreased urine, less moisture in diapers, dry mouth, no tears, or weight loss
   c. Child becomes sleepy, difficult to awaken, or irritable
   d. Vomited material contains blood or turns green

Many children will spit up *(regurgitate)* food, particularly during the first few months of life. This is normal in most children but may be exaggerated by faulty feeding techniques or gastroesophageal reflux **(chalasia)**. If the child is well and growing normally, the problem may be reduced by careful attention to feeding techniques. Suggestions that may be useful include:

1. Keep your child in an upright position during feeding and prone for 30-45 min following feeding.
2. Feed your baby smaller amounts more often.
3. Burp your baby frequently.
4. Thickened liquids may be helpful.

REFERENCES

Fomon, S.J., Filer, L.J., Anderson, T.A., et al.: Recommendation for feeding normal infants, Pediatrics 63:52, 1979.

Orenstein, S.R., Whittington, P.F., and Orenstein, D.M.: The infant seat as treatment for gastroesophageal reflux, N. Engl. J. Med. 309:760, 1983.

VII ENVIRONMENTAL EMERGENCIES

45 Bites

ALERT: Bites must be evaluated to determine the extent of local tissue injury and potential immediate and long-term systemic or local reactions of an infectious nature.

Animal and human bites

Children commonly experience animal bites, as many as 20% of which are dog bites. The peak age is 5-14 yr with the highest incidence occurring to males during the spring and summer. Management involves minimizing skin and soft tissue injury to achieve a good cosmetic and functional result, while providing prophylaxis against infection in the initial encounter and adequate follow-up to ensure prompt treatment of delayed infection.

DOG AND CAT BITES

Large dogs are responsible for the majority of animal bites, although smaller dogs and cats may bite and scratch. Up to 5% of dog bites and 20%-50% of cat bites become infected.

Etiology

1. *Pasteurella multocida* is often involved, with *Staphylococcus aureus* usually a secondary infection. Mixed infections are probably most common.
2. Rabies virus is an unusual pathogen but must be considered. Rodents (rats, mice, gerbils, hamsters, squirrels, etc.) do not carry rabies (p. 544).

Diagnostic findings

Patients commonly have soft tissue injuries, which are usually a combination of crush injury with lacerations.

Complications

Cellulitis may develop with onset of erythema, swelling, or tenderness. Lymphadenitis also may develop. If no signs of infection are present within 3 days of trauma, infection is unlikely to occur.

Other complications include:
1. Crush injuries
2. Osteomyelitis (p. 531)
3. Septic arthritis (p. 569)
4. Tenosynovitis

Ancillary data

Cultures and Gram's stain are not necessary with routine animal bites. However, if a wound becomes infected, cultures should be obtained, particularly if the infection has been unresponsive to previous therapy or if the patient is either taking prophylactic antibiotics or is immunosuppressed.

Management (Chapter 65)

1. Mechanical irrigation and debridement are crucial to the treatment of animal bites.
   a. Adequate cleansing may require local or regional anesthesia.
   b. Irrigation should be done extensively with 1% povidone-iodine solution (Betadine). Some prefer to use sterile saline. This is most efficiently done using an 18-gauge or larger flexible plastic catheter. The high pressure is directed at various angles so that all surfaces are cleansed.

c. Debridement of wound edges and devitalized tissues is essential.

d. Scrubbing (except with rabies potential) is usually harmful to tissues.

e. Wounds with extensive damage require particular attention to irrigation.

2. Suturing is indicated for cosmetic or functional reasons.

   a. It should only be done after thorough irrigation.

   b. Hand injuries, wounds involving extensive soft tissue injury or damage to deep tissues, puncture wounds, and those older than 24 hr should not be sutured. The wound should also be left open if there is any question about the extent of the wound, the adequacy of irrigation, or follow-up. Steri-strips may be useful.

3. Wounds that have a high risk of becoming infected include:

   a. Bites of the hand or foot

   b. Extensive wounds, where devitalized tissue cannot be entirely debrided

   c. Wounds that are sutured

   d. Those of patients with peripheral vascular insufficiency (e.g., diabetes)

   e. Puncture wounds

4. Antibiotics may be considered prophylactically with high-risk injuries (as defined above)

   a. Cephalexin (Keflex) or cephradine (Velosef) 25-50 mg/kg/24 hr q 6 hr PO **or** penicillin V 50,000 units (30 mg)/kg/24 hr q 6 hr PO

   b. Wounds that become infected, particularly those located in high-risk locations, require parenteral therapy:

      • Penicillin G 100,000 units/kg/24 hr q 4 hr IV **and** nafcillin (or equivalent) 100 mg/kg/24 hr q 4 hr IV

5. Other considerations

   a. Tetanus toxoid should be administered as indicated (p. 546).

   b. Wounds with great soft tissue injury should be immobilized and, if on an extremity, elevated.

c. If an abscess forms, surgical drainage is required.

d. Sutured wounds that become infected should have the suture material removed.

e. Rabies should be considered in some geographic areas, depending on the animal inflicting the scratch or bite, the location of the injury, and other factors outlined on p. 544.

Disposition

Patients with uncomplicated animal bites may be discharged, with careful instructions to monitor for infection. Those with high-risk bites should take antibiotics. Careful follow-up is essential. If a bite is sutured, it should be reexamined within 24 hr. Patients with high-risk category bites that become infected may require hospitalization for parenteral therapy.

Parental education

1. Instruct children about playing with unfamiliar animals. Do not allow children to place face near dog; do not leave children unattended with dogs. Obey leash laws and be particularly careful with large dogs.

2. Call physician if:

   a. The wound gets red, tender, swollen, or develops a discharge

   b. The child gets a fever

REFERENCE

Marcy, S.M.: Infections due to dog and cat bites, Pediatr. Infect. Dis. 1:351, 1982.

HUMAN BITES

Human bites have a greater risk of tissue damage and infection than do those inflicted by dogs and cats.

Etiology of bacterial infection

Over 40 organisms have been identified as mouth flora and may be potential pathogens.

Diagnostic findings

The most common injury involves a clenched fist striking an opponent's mouth, with potentially great tissue damage. Examination of damage to soft tissues and tendons must include repositioning of the hand in the clenched position. Other tissues may be involved.

Infection produces cellulitis with potential closed-space infections and abscess formation, as well as osteomyelitis and septic arthritis.

Management

Irrigation and debridement are similar to treatment given animal bites (p. 230) and must be done with meticulous care. These wounds should *never* be sutured.
1. Antibiotics should be administered:
   • Cephalexin (Keflex) or cephradine (Velosef) 25-50 mg/kg/24 hr 6 hr PO
   • Tetanus toxoid as indicated (p. 546)
2. Patients developing infections associated with human bites should usually be admitted to the hospital for parenteral therapy:
   • Ampicillin 100 mg/kg/24 hr q 4 hr IV **and** nafcillin (or equivalent) 100 mg/kg/24 hr q 4 hr IV

Disposition

Patients with uncomplicated human bites may be discharged with antibiotics and good follow-up. Patients with bites that are infected should be admitted to the hospital.

Arthropod (insect) bites

BROWN RECLUSE SPIDER

The brown recluse spider *(Loxosceles reclusa)* is ½-1 inch in length and is distinguished by violin-like markings on the dorsum of the thorax. The spider introduces a venom containing necrotizing, hemolytic, and spreading factors in the skin.

Diagnostic findings

Local pain and erythema at the site develop 2-8 hr after the bite, followed by bleb or blister formation, with a surrounding area of pallor. Over the ensuing 48-72 hr, central induration occurs and a dark violet color develops. The area then ulcerates, and a black eschar forms within a week.

Systemic signs develop in the initial 24-48 hr, including headache, fever, nausea, vomiting, joint pains, and, very rarely, cyanosis, hypotension, and seizures.

Complications
1. Hemolysis with hemoglobinemia, hemoglobinuria, and renal failure. Bites <1 cm in diameter rarely cause hemolysis. If bite enlarges on serial examinations, continue to monitor urine. Bites >1 cm require close monitoring of urine. If hemolysis occurs, hydrate and consider steroids.
2. Disseminated intravascular coagulation (DIC) (p. 522)
3. Seizures (Chapter 21)
4. Rarely, death

Management

1. Local care of the site of bite
2. Parenteral steroids. Hydrocortisone (Solu-Cortef) 5 mg/kg/dose every 6 hr IV given 4 times is indicated if any systemic signs develop.
3. Analgesia for pain
4. Excision, if the ulceration and necrotic area develop into an area >1 cm. Rarely needed
5. Specific treatment for complications
6. Experimental studies suggest the efficacy of dapsone (adult: 50-100 mg/24 hr PO) in reducing ulceration.

Disposition

Patients with evidence of systemic signs and symptoms should be admitted to the hospital; others may be followed closely as outpatients.

REFERENCE
King, L.E., and Rees, R.S.: Dapsone treatment of a brown recluse bite, JAMA **250:**648, 1983.

BLACK WIDOW SPIDER

The black widow spider (*Latrodectus mactans*) is identified by a shiny, black button-shaped body with a red hourglass marking on the underside.

Diagnostic findings

At the site of the bite, there is immediate pain with burning, swelling, and erythema. There are double fang markings at the site.

The degree of systemic signs and symptoms will reflect the number of bites, the amount of venom injected, and the toxicity of the spider's venom. Within 30 min of the bite, crampy abdominal pain, accompanied by dizziness, nausea, vomiting, headache, and sweating occur. The abdomen is characteristically boardlike, mimicking an acute abdomen. The patient's condition usually resolves in 24 hr, but the bite is associated with hypertension rather than hypotension.

Complications
1. Ascending motor paralysis (Chapter 41)
2. Seizures (Chapter 21)
3. Shock (Chapter 5)
4. Coma, respiratory arrest, death

Management

Supportive therapy should be instituted at the first sign of systemic symptoms:
1. Calcium gluconate (10%) 50-100 mg (0.5-1.0 ml)/kg/dose IV slowly
2. Muscle relaxant: diazepam (Valium) 0.1-0.3 mg/kg/dose IV
3. Analgesics: meperidine (Demerol) 1-2 mg/kg/dose q 4-6 hr IM, IV

An equine antivenin, ethacrynate (Lyovac)—in a vial containing 2.5 ml—is administered, according to package directions, after negative skin testing for horse serum sensitivity. It is particularly important for young children and individuals with hypertension and cardiac disease.

Disposition

All patients with known black widow spider bites require admission for observation and potential treatment.

HYMENOPTERA

Hymenoptera (honey bees, wasps, yellow jackets, and hornets) produce a variety of systemic effects, reflecting individual sensitivity and the number of bites inflicted by the offending insect.

Diagnostic findings

1. Local reactions commonly produce edema and pain.
2. Toxic reactions occur with multiple stings (10 or more): vomiting, diarrhea, dizziness, muscle spasms, and, rarely, convulsions.
3. Anaphylactic reactions, such as wheezing and urticaria (Chapter 12), occur in sensitive individuals.
4. Delayed serum-sickness reaction occurs 10-14 days after the sting, with morbilliform rash, urticaria, myalgia, arthralgia, and fever.

Management

1. Local attention to the point of sting—cleansing, removing the stinger, and cold compresses—may provide symptomatic relief. Local application of papain, found in meat tenderizer, is believed by some to relieve pain.
2. Diphenhydramine (Benadryl) 5 mg/kg/24 hr q 6-8 hr PO, IM, or IV may reduce local, as well as systemic, signs and symptoms.
3. Systemic signs of anaphylaxis are treated with epinephrine, theophylline, and steroids (Chapter 12).

Disposition

1. Patients with only local reactions can usually be discharged, with symptomatic treatment.
2. Those with severe reactions should be admitted for continuation of emergent care.

TABLE 45-1. Tick-transmitted diseases

	Tularemia	Relapsing fever	Rocky Mountain Spotted Fever (RMSF)	Colorado tick fever	Tick-bite paralysis (p. 235)
ETIOLOGY	Francisella tularemia	Borrelia	Rickettsia rickettsii	Colorado tick fever virus	Toxin
TICK VECTOR	Dermacentor	Orinthodoros	Dermacentor	Dermacentor	
INCUBATION	1-14 days	5-9 days	2-14 days	3-6 days	4-7 days
DIAGNOSTIC FINDINGS	Headache, persistent fever, malaise, anorexia, lymphadenopathy, conjunctivitis	Relapsing fever, occipital headache, malaise, myalgia, cough, meningismus, lymphadenopathy, leukocytosis	Resistant fever, headache, malaise, arthralgia, periorbital edema, conjunctivitis, meningismus, coma, centrifugal hemorrhagic rash, petechiae	Sudden onset of fever, retroorbital headache, myalgia, anorexia, myalgia, meningismus, rash, conjunctivitis, leukopenia	Ascending paralysis, ataxia, irritability
ANTIBIOTICS	Streptomycin, tetracycline,* chloramphenicol	Tetracycline,* penicillin, chloramphenicol	Tetracycline,* chloramphenicol	None (support)	None (support)

*Do not use in children <9 yr.

3. Following resolution of severe systemic and anaphylactic reactions, the patient should be referred to an allergist for hyposensitization.
4. A bee sting kit containing epinephrine and syringes should be carried by those who have experienced severe local or systemic reactions.

TICKS

The large majority of tick bites are benign and simply require removal. However, a number of diseases may be transmitted, with specific ticks serving as the vector (Table 45-1).

Imbedded ticks usually can be withdrawn by covering the tick with alcohol, mineral oil, nail polish, or an ointment. If these are unsuccessful, the body of the tick can be picked up with a forceps, applying gentle, steady traction. If this is not successful, the tick and superficial attached skin can then be easily cut away. Brief pressure will stop the bleeding.

Snake bites

ALERT: It is crucial to determine rapidly if a snake is potentially poisonous. If it is, urgent local treatment, support, and administration of antivenin are required.

Of the known species of snakes, only 5% are venomous. In the United States the most commonly encountered venomous snakes are Crotalidae (pit vipers, water moccasins, and copperheads) and Elapidae (coral snakes). Their venom consists of multiple poisonous proteins and enzymes that are absorbed through the lymphatic system following envenomation.

The severity of injury from poisonous snake bite reflects, among other factors, the amount of venom released and the size of the victim. The following factors should be considered:
1. Age, size, and health of the patient

2. The size of the snake. Larger snakes produce more venom.
3. The location of the injury. Peripheral injuries account for over 90% of bites and are usually less severe.

Distinguishing venomous from nonvenomous snakes is sometimes difficult. Venomous snakes usually have vertically elliptic pupils, facial pit between eye and nostril, rattle, fangs, and subcaudal plates behind oval plates—in pit vipers arranged in a single row. Nonvenomous snakes have round pupils; no pit, rattle, or fangs; and a double row of subcaudal plates.

DIAGNOSTIC FINDINGS

1. The site of the poisonous snake bite may display fang marks, with subsequent burning, pain or numbness, swelling, and erythema. This may progress rapidly to hemorrhage and necrosis.
2. Regional effects of extremity bites include edema of the arm or leg, ecchymoses, and lymphadenopathy.
3. Systemic signs and symptoms may develop within 15 min, depending on the severity of the injury.
   a. Nausea, vomiting, sweating, chills, numbness, paresthesias of the tongue and perioral region may occur.
   b. Fasciculations, dysphagia, bleeding, and hypotension are common.

Complications

1. Disseminated intravascular coagulation (DIC) and hemolysis (p. 522)
2. Respiratory failure
3. Renal failure (p. 615)
4. Seizures (Chapter 21)
5. Shock and death

Ancillary data

1. CBC, platelets, coagulation studies (PT, PTT, fibrinogen, fibrin split products [FSP])
2. Urinalysis, BUN, serial electrolytes, creatinine

3. Type and cross-match, which may be difficult once hemolysis occurs, should be done initially.

Nonpoisonous snake bites often leave the patient with major psychologic trauma, which may result in mild symptoms similar to those of actual envenomation.

MANAGEMENT

1. If possible, the snake should be killed and identified, with careful handling of the head since it can still deliver venom for as long as 1 hr after death.
2. Initially, a broad, firm, constrictive bandage should be applied proximal to the bitten area and around the limb.
3. The extremity should be splinted to reduce motion.
4. Activity of the patient should be minimized and cooling, which can cause further tissue damage, avoided.
5. Surgical excision of the wound site or fasciotomy is probably unnecessary.

Transport to the hospital should be expedited for support and administration of antivenin. First, skin tests for hypersensitivity to horse serum must be done. However, patients with serious bites must be given antivenin regardless of the sensitivity. Reactions can be managed by slowing down or temporarily stopping infusions and pretreatment with epinephrine and diphenhydramine (Benadryl) (Chapter 12).

Antivenin should be administered intravenously:

1. For rattlesnake, water moccasin, and copperhead bites: antivenin (Crotalidae) Polyvalent*
2. For coral snake bites: antivenin (Micrurus fulvius)*

NOTE: Antivenin for rare species may be obtained from Oklahoma Poison Control Center: (405) 271-5454.

With minimal symptoms (local swelling), administer 3-5 vials; with moderate or progressive symptoms (marked swelling, systemic signs), 6-8 vials; with severe symptoms (marked swelling, severe systemic symptoms, laboratory findings), 10-20 vials. Repeat infusion of 4-5 vials may be given q 1 hr if symptoms are progressing.

Complications

Complications include anaphylaxis shock, DIC, and serum sickness. Treatment of complications is essential to the ultimate outcome. Tetanus toxoids should also be given, if indicated.

DISPOSITION

All patients with poisonous snake bites should be admitted to the hospital for supportive care. Patients with unidentified snake bites may be discharged if no signs and symptoms develop in 4 hr of observation. Reassurance may be necessary.

REFERENCE

Abramowicz, M., editor: Treatment of snake bite in the USA, Med. Lett. **24**:87, 1982.

---

*Wyeth Laboratories: telephone (215) 688-4400.

46 Burns, thermal

ALERT: Rapid assessment of the depth, location, and extent of a burn should determine the severity of the injury. Airway and pulmonary status and associated trauma must be treated.

ETIOLOGY

The mechanism of heat transfer and injury influences the type of burn.

1. Scald burns result from contact with a hot object or hot liquid. They are most commonly seen in children under 3 yr of age and may be sharply demarcated and of partial thickness, except in young infants, where full-thickness injury may be noted.

2. Flame burns occur with direct-flame exposure resulting from ignition of clothing. They are commonly seen in children over 2 yr of age who play with matches, fires, and flammable materials. The borders are irregular and may be of full thickness.

3. Flashburns are caused by exposure to a explosion, resulting in a uniform, partial-thickness burn.

4. Electrical burns are discussed in Chapter 48.

DIAGNOSTIC FINDINGS

Initial evaluation must include information about the mechanism of injury, duration since the burn, patient's age and weight, underlying disease, past medical problems, and associated injuries.

Body surface area (BSA) in children may be estimated to determine the extent of burns (Fig. 46-1). In adults, the rule of 9 is easily used for estimating involved body surface: head and neck (9%); anterior trunk (18%), posterior trunk (18%), each leg (18%), each arm (9%), and anorectal area (1%).

The patient should be thoroughly examined to ascertain other associated traumatic injuries, as well as signs of smoke inhalation, including hoarseness, cough, singed nasal hairs, oral burns, carbonaceous sputum, wheezing, rhonchi, and cyanosis (Chapter 53).

Depth of burn is an important determinant of severity and potential complications.

1. Superficial partial-thickness (first-degree) burns involve only the epidermis and are characterized by erythema and local pain.

2. Partial-thickness (second-degree) burns involve the epidermis and corium.
   a. Partial-thickness burns produce erythema and blisters.
   b. Deep partial-thickness burns are white and dry and have reduced sensitivity to touch and pain. They blanch with pressure.

3. Full-thickness (third-degree) burns are numb, with a tough, brownish surface and a hard eschar. Spontaneous healing will not occur.

Severity of burns is determined by the depth of the burn, BSA involved, location of the injury, age and health of the patient, and associated injuries.

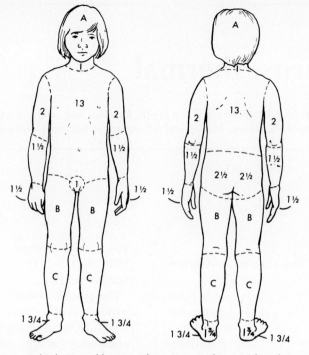

FIG. 46-1. Calculation of burn surface area. (After Lund and Browder.)

				Age			
Area percentage	<1 yr	1 yr	5 yr	10 yr	15 yr	Adult
A, ½ of head	9½	8½	6½	5½	4½	3½
B, ½ of one thigh	2¾	3¼	4	4¼	4½	4¾
C, ½ of one leg	2½	2½	2¾	3	3¼	3½

1. *Major* burn:
   a. Partial thickness: >25% BSA (adults); >20% BSA (children); or full thickness: >10% BSA
   b. Burns of the hands, face, eyes, ears, feet, or perineum
   c. Patients with inhalation injury, electrical burns, burns complicated by fractures or other major trauma
   d. Poor-risk patients, including those with underlying disease, associated major injuries, or suspicion of child abuse
2. *Moderate* uncomplicated burn: partial thickness: 15%-25% BSA (adults); 10%-20% BSA: (children); or full thickness: <10% BSA

3. *Minor* burn: partial thickness: <15% BSA (adults); <10% BSA (children); or full thickness <2% BSA

Complications

1. Smoke inhalation. Direct inhalation of toxic particles or exposure to hot smoke and air may produce respiratory distress on the basis of upper or lower respiratory pathology (Chapter 53).
2. Carbon monoxide poisoning (p. 289)
3. Dehydration and shock from fluid losses and inadequate fluid therapy
4. Renal failure secondary to myoglobinuria or dehydration

5. Sepsis and death

Ancillary data

1. Blood work for moderate or major burns should include, when appropriate, CBC, electrolytes, BUN, creatinine, arterial blood gas, type and cross-match, and carboxyhemoglobin level.
2. A chest x-ray film is useful for all patients with major burns and for those with any question of smoke inhalation. The initial film will be useful for comparison with later x-ray studies. Abnormal findings are often delayed up to 24 hr.
3. Urinalysis should be performed for specific gravity, sugar, protein, myoglobin, and hemoglobin.

MANAGEMENT OF MINOR AND SOME MODERATE BURNS

1. Burn wounds should initially be covered by a cloth cooled with saline. Minimize contact with nonsterile objects by placing patient on sterile sheets and using sterile gloves, gowns, and caps, if appropriate.
2. Intact blisters should be left unbroken unless they are at flexion creases. Ruptured vesicles should be debrided and the area cleansed gently with surgical soap such as diluted povidone-iodine (Betadine).
3. Superficial partial thickness burns require no topical therapy except for symptomatic relief.
4. Partial-thickness injuries may be treated with 1% silver sulfadiazine or by applying a fine-mesh gauze impregnated with a petroleum jelly (Xeroform, Adaptic, Vaseline). Very small burns, particularly those in difficult areas, may be left exposed.
5. The dressing should be changed in 24 hr and then every 2-3 days or sooner if an odor develops or if the area becomes painful.
6. Tetanus immunization should be given, if necessary.
7. Pain medication is rarely needed.
8. If the patient has evidence of group A strep-

tococcal disease, penicillin (50,000 units/kg/24 hr q 6 hr PO) should be given to prevent colonization of the burn.
9. Exclude child abuse in cases of inconsistent or suspicious injury.

Disposition

Patients with minor burns can routinely be sent home unless other medical problems, associated injuries, or suspicion of child abuse or lack of compliance preclude such management. Infants with over 10% BSA involvement and adults with 25% BSA burns or burns qualifying as major burns should be admitted.

Parental education

1. Keep the wound clean and dry.
2. Change the dressing in 24 hr and then every 2-3 days. Wash burn gently, apply cream, and dress as directed.
3. Call physician if
   a. Increasing redness or discolorations of the normal tissue around the burn site develop or if the area becomes odorous or painful
   b. Red streaks develop around the area
   c. Fever and chills are present
   d. Swelling or progressive inability to use fingers or toes (if extremities are involved) are noted
   e. Shortness of breath, increased cough, or difficulty in swallowing are present
   f. Blurred vision develops if face is involved

MANAGEMENT OF MAJOR AND MOST MODERATE BURNS

Assessment of airway and ventilation is crucial. Oxygen should be administered to all patients, and if respiratory distress or abnormal arterial blood gases are present, the patient should be intubated. Pulmonary disease may have a delayed onset of up to 24 hr, secondary to smoke inhalation or CO intoxication (Chapter 53 and p. 289).

Intravenous fluid resuscitation must be initiated immediately with 1-2 large-bore catheters.

Initial stabilization should include infusion of 20 ml/kg 0.9%NS or LR over 20-30 min. Although controversial, the following is then suggested:

1. *Day 1:* 4 ml lactated Ringer's with 5% dextrose × kg × (percentage of burn as number, e.g., 70% = 70) given over the first 24 hr, in addition to normal maintenance fluids (Chapter 8). Half of the total volume of fluids should be given during the first 8 hr following the burn and the remainder over 16 hr. For instance, a 10 kg child with 20% BSA burn would require the following fluid management, with adjustments as necessitated by urine output:
   a. Maintenance: 1,000 ml H_2O with 30 mEq NaCl and 20 mEq KCl—approximately D5W.2%NS with 20 mEq KCl/L.
   b. Replacement: 800 ml of D5WLR = 4 ml D5WLR × 10 (kg) × 20 (% BSA)
      • ½ of replacement and ⅓ of maintenance to be given during first 8 hr
2. *Day 2:* Crystalloid infused at about ½-¾ of the previous day's needs. In addition, colloid is useful at this time when administered as a 5% albumin solution at 0.5 g/kg/% BSA.

The following considerations should be kept in mind:

1. Potassium should not be added to the fluid.
2. If fluid management is difficult, a central venous pressure line should be inserted.
3. Urine output and vital signs are the most sensitive indicators of the adequacy of therapy. A Foley catheter should be inserted to monitor urine flow. Optimal flow output should be 2-3 ml/kg/hr, but a minimal level of 1 ml/kg/hr is acceptable.
4. A nasogastric tube should be inserted.

Wound management

1. Initially, the wound should be covered with a cloth cooled in saline. The patient should be placed on a sterile sheet, and those touching the patient should wear sterile gloves, gowns, and a cap.
2. The wound should be gently scrubbed, using povidone-iodine soap (Betadine) diluted in saline followed by irrigation. Cool saline or water may reduce pain.
3. Surgical consultation should be obtained.
4. All dead material should be debrided. Intact blisters should be left unbroken unless they are at flexion creases. Ruptured vesicles should be debrided.
5. Wounds should be dressed with a liberal application of a 1% silver sulfadiazine cream. An absorbent dressing of fine (36 × 44) mesh gauze or 4 × 4 fluffs is applied, using several layers and a role of gauze applied to hold the dressing.
6. The face and perineum should be left open after application of antibiotic cream.
7. Escharotomy is indicated with full-thickness, circumferential burns of the extremities accompanied by impaired neurovascular function. Eschars of the chest may impair ventilation and thus require surgical intervention.
8. Depending on the depth and severity of the wounds, dressings may be left on for 24 hr. At each change, the wound can be cleansed with warm water and debrided, often facilitated by a whirlpool. The burns may then be redressed after application of silver sulfadiazine and fine mesh gauze.
9. Skin grafting after early (3-5 days) burn excision is useful in some settings.

Other considerations

1. Pain medication may be used once vital signs have normalized. Optimally, drugs such as morphine or meperidine should be given intravenously.
2. Tetanus immunization should be updated, if appropriate.
3. Peptic ulcer (Curling's ulcer) prophylaxis—antacid therapy, using antacids or cimetidine (20-30 mg/kg/24 hr q 6 hr IV or PO)—should be initiated in the first 6 hr following burn.
4. Antibiotics should not be administered prophylactically but for specific signs and symp-

toms of infection after appropriate cultures. Penicillin should be given if there is evidence of a group A streptococcal infection.

5. Intravenous, tube, and oral nutrition should begin following the stabilization period.
6. Body temperature should be kept normal.
7. Psychologic support of the family in dealing with a major burn is imperative from the first encounter through the entire hospitalization. This is often complicated by concerns about potential child abuse.
8. Rehabilitation should be initiated following stabilization.
9. Exclude child abuse if cause of injury is suspicious.

DISPOSITION

All patients with moderate or major burns should be admitted to the surgical service with appropriate consultation as necessary.

Major burns can often best be cared for in burn centers where the burn team can deal with the total patient's needs on a more routine basis.

If transport is necessary, the initial stabilization should be achieved at the primary receiving hospital, often involving a surgical consultant at that time. The same level of care must be maintained throughout the transport process.

REFERENCES

Demling, R.H.: Burns, N. Engl. J. Med. **313**:1389, 1985.
Dimick, A.R.: Triage of burn patients. Top. Emerg. Med. **3**:17, 1981.
Moncrief, J.A.: Burns. I. Assessment; II. Initial treatment, JAMA **242**:72, 179, 1979.

47 Drowning and near-drowning

ALERT: After initial resuscitation, evaluate for associated injuries. Monitor patient for evolving pulmonary or cerebral edema.

The victim of a submersion episode may die immediately or within 24 hr from the hypoxic insult and its complications (drowning) or may survive the incident but require intensive support (near-drowning). The majority of accidents occur in swimming pools, ponds, lakes, and bathtubs, with a peak incidence in children at 4 yr and between 10-19 yr.

Although theoretically there are differences between fresh- and salt-water drownings, they do not appear to be clinically significant and the management is identical. Near-drowning in cold water is associated with a better prognosis after prolonged immersion.

ETIOLOGY: PRECIPITATING FACTORS

1. Trauma
   a. Head or neck (Chapters 57 and 61)
   b. Barotrauma: scuba diving
   c. Hypothermia (Chapter 51)
   d. Child abuse (Chapter 25)
2. Seizures (Chapter 21)
3. Intoxication: alcohol, sedatives, PCP, LSD (Chapter 54)
4. Exhaustion, boating accident, poor swimmer

DIAGNOSTIC FINDINGS

The signs and symptoms reflect pulmonary and cerebral hypoxic injury. The spectrum of illness may range from minimal or negative findings initially, with a delayed onset in 2-6 hr, to complete cardiac respiratory arrest. Vital signs and temperature must be determined. Hypothermia may be protective.

Pulmonary findings may include cyanosis, pallor with pulmonary edema, or aspiration pneumonitis often associated with intrapulmonary shunting. Patients may develop rales, frothy sputum, and rhonchi or wheezing and progress to respiratory failure or arrest. Seizures, changed mental status, and stupor or coma may be present with or without focal findings, reflecting hypoxia and cerebral edema. The patient may be postictal if a seizure precipitated the episode. Cardiac dysrhythmias and asystole are possible.

Evidence of trauma must be evaluated as possible precipitating factors, particularly head and neck injuries. Other unexplained signs may be indicative of child abuse.

Several researchers have defined factors that are unfavorable prognosticators in cases of pediatric near-drowning. Patients who are conscious or have only blunted levels of consciousness on arrival in the ED usually do well. However, many of these studies were done before recent advances in monitoring intracranial pressure objectively.

1. Ortowski (1979) reports the following indicators:
   a. Patient <3 yr of age
   b. Maximum submersion time over 5 min
   c. Resuscitation efforts not attempted for at least 10 min after rescue

d. Patient in coma on admission to hospital

e. Arterial pH ≤7.10

  NOTE: Mortality rate was 89% in those with ≥3 factors.

2. Peterson's (1979) unfavorable prognostic factors are:

  a. The need for cardiopulmonary resuscitation on arrival at hospital

  b. Seizures, fixed and dilated pupils, flaccid extremities, and lack of response to deep pain

  c. Submersion for 6 min or more

3. According to Dean and Kaufman (1981), a score on the Glasgow Coma Scale (Table 57-1) <5 was associated with an 80% mortality, but the group with scores ≥6 had no sequelae.

4. A recent study (1983) based on objective measures of intracranial pressure demonstrated that those children with an intracranial pressure (ICP) ≤20 mm Hg and a cerebral perfusion pressure (CPP) (difference between systemic arterial and intracranial pressure) ≥50 mm Hg had the best prognosis with only an 8% mortality rate.

Complications

1. Pulmonary edema, respiratory failure, adult respiratory distress syndrome (ARDS), and cardiorespiratory arrest (Chapters 4 and 19)

2. Hypoxic encephalopathy and seizures

3. Acute tubular necrosis and renal failure (p. 615)

4. Disseminated intravascular coagulation (DIC) (Chapter 79)

5. On-site resuscitation complications: pneumothorax, abdominal visceral tears, etc.

Ancillary data

1. Electrolytes: usually normal but when drowning occurs in water with high concentrations of electrolytes (i.e., Dead Sea), marked elevations of calcium and magnesium, as well as the more common electrolytes, may be noted.

2. CBC and coagulation screen: usually normal

3. ABG

4. Chest x-ray film: may be normal initially and have delayed onset of evidence of aspiration or pulmonary edema

5. Head, neck, and other x-ray studies as indicated by condition

6. Other studies, as indicated by possible precipitating factors

MANAGEMENT (Fig. 47-1)

In cases of significant near-drowning, initial management must focus on stabilization of airway, removal of foreign material, maintenance of ventilation, and administration of oxygen and fluids. Vital signs must be meticulously monitored. An NG tube and urinary catheter should be inserted. If the patient is febrile, antipyretics and a cooling mattress should be used. If patient is hypothermic, normalize aggressively (p. 252).

Consideration must be directed toward precipitating conditions, with particular attention to head trauma, neck injury, hypothermia, and barotrauma. Trauma requires neck immobilization until the lateral neck x-ray film and, ultimately, the full cervical spine series is cleared. Patients should be rewarmed in accordance with clinical protocol outlined in Chapter 51. Slow decompression* is required if the injury was secondary to barotrauma.

1. Pulmonary management

  a. Oxygenation is essential. Humidified oxygen at 3-6 L/min is given by mask or nasal cannula until stabilization and evaluation are completed. Continuous positive airway pressure (CPAP) should be considered if FIo_2 > 40% is needed. In the awake, cooperative patient, a CPAP of 10-12 cm H_2O can be administered by a tightly fitting face mask or other device. Otherwise, intubation may be required.

---

*Information about decompression chambers can be obtained from the Diver's Alert Network: telephone (919) 684-2948 or (919) 684-8111 (Emergencies).

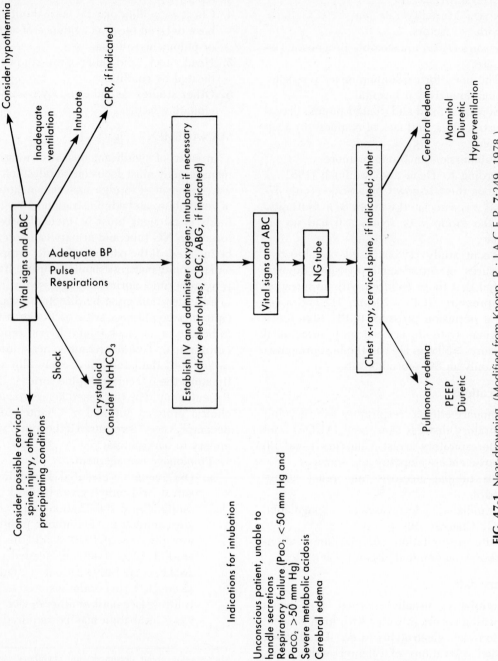

Indications for intubation

1. Unconscious patient, unable to handle secretions
2. Respiratory failure (PaO_2 <50 mm Hg and $PaCO_2$ >50 mm Hg)
3. Severe metabolic acidosis
4. Cerebral edema

FIG. 47-1. Near-drowning. (Modified from Knopp, R.: J.A.C.E.P. **7:**249, 1978.)

b. Intubation and initiation of positive end-expiratory pressure (PEEP) or CPAP are indicated if there is clear evidence of progressive pulmonary edema with an $FIO_2 > 40\%$ being required, particularly if CPAP delivered by mask has been unsuccessful. PEEP should be initiated at 5 cm H_2O and increased slowly, monitoring oxygenation and cardiac output. If the cardiac output decreases, increasing the intravascular volume may be useful.

c. Intubation and mechanical ventilation are indicated if the patient is unable to handle secretions, if respiratory failure (PaO_2 <50 mm Hg and $PaCO_2$ >50 mm Hg at room air at sea level) is present, if there is a severe metabolic acidosis, or if the patient has developed evidence of cerebral edema.

d. Monitor arterial blood gases.

2. Cerebral edema secondary to hypoxic injury (or head trauma): ICP monitor may be useful in measuring the therapeutic effect (p. 319). Optimally maintain ICP ≤ 20 mm Hg and CPP ≥ 50 mm Hg. Measures to reduce ICP may include one or more of the following:

a. Hyperventilate the patient to maintain a $PaCO_2$ of about 20-25 mm Hg.

b. Elevate the head of bed 30 degrees if vital signs, cervical spine, and head injuries from trauma are stable.

c. Give dexamethasone (Decadron) 0.25 mg/kg/dose q 6 hr IV. Controversial, without evidence of efficacy.

d. Give furosemide (Lasix) 1 mg/kg/dose up to 3 mg/kg/dose q 6 hr, which may be repeated q 2 hr if indicated.

e. Give mannitol 0.5 g/kg/dose over 30 min q 3-4 hr prn IV. Effect lasts 2-3 hr and there may be rebound. Use only when patient is symptomatic.

f. Restrict fluids to 50%-60% of maintenance rate while keeping CVP in the low to normal range (8-10 mm Hg) and urine output between 0.5-1.0 ml/kg/hr. Initial resuscitation may require a fluid bolus.

g. Barbiturates: useful with significant edema and elevated (and unresponsive) ICP. Intracranial monitor necessary.

• Pentobarbital (Nembutal): initial dose of 3-20 mg/kg slow IV push while monitoring BP. Maintain infusion of 1-2 mg/kg/hr. Level should be maintained between 25-40 µg/ml. Levels above 30 µg/ml are associated with hypotension in as many as 60% of patients.

h. Muscle relaxants may be required if the patient is symptomatic and requires ventilation. Intubate. Pancuronium (Pavulon) 0.1 mg/kg/dose q 1 hr or prn IV.

3. Other considerations

a. Acidosis, if present, requires treatment. Sodium bicarbonate 1-2 mEq/kg/dose IV should be given. Subsequent doses may be required in response to changes in ABG.

b. Hypoxic seizures may be controlled by oxygen, ventilation, and diazepam (Valium) 0.2-0.3 mg/kg/dose IV, which may be repeated every 2-5 min until seizures cease. Control airway. Begin phenobarbital or phenytoin (Dilantin) (Chapter 21).

c. Antibiotics are administered only with specific indications.

d. Steroids have no proven value beyond their controversial role in the treatment of cerebral edema in near-drowning.

e. Fevers may indicate that a secondary infection exists such as pneumonitis. It should be treated aggressively with appropriate antibiotics and antipyretics.

f. Maintain normal electrolytes, glucose, etc.

g. Avoid procedures that may be poorly tolerated.

h. Emotional support for the family and friends is imperative.

DISPOSITION

All patients with significant episodes of near-drowning require admission to the hospital, particularly in view of the delayed onset of symptoms. Most require the monitoring available in an ICU. Cessation of treatment may be guided by the prognostic factors that have been defined.

Parental education

1. Teach swimming and water safety techniques at an early age but probably not <3 yr.
2. Define water areas the children cannot use. Fence them off.
3. Children require supervision near water and boats. Always have appropriate supervision. Keep rescue devices and first aid equipment near pools.
4. Children with seizure disorders may swim if they have been seizure free for 1-2 yr but then only with supervision.

REFERENCES

Bell, T.S., Ellenberg, L., McComb, J.G., et al.: Neuropsychological outcome after severe pediatric near-drowning, Neurosurgery 17:604, 1985.

Dean, J.M., and Kaufman, N.D.: Prognostic indicators in pediatric near-drowning: the Glasgow Coma Scale, Crit. Care Med. 9:536, 1981.

Frewen, T.C., Sumabat, W.O., and Han, V.K.: Cerebral resuscitation therapy in pediatric near-drowning, J. Pediatr. 106:615, 1985.

Karch, S.B.: Pathology of lung in near-drowning, Am. J. Emerg. Med. 4:4, 1986.

Martin, R.G.: Near-drowning and cold water immersion, Ann. Emerg. Med. 13:263, 1984.

Nussbaum, E.: Prognostic variables in nearly drowned, comatose children, Am. J. Dis. Child. 139:1058, 1985.

Nussbaum, E., and Galant, S.P.: Intracranial pressure monitoring as a guide to prognosis in the nearly drowned, severely comatose patient, J. Pediatr. 102:215, 1983.

Ortowski, J.P.: Prognostic factors in pediatric cases of drowning and near-drowning, J.A.C.E.P. 8:176, 1979.

Peterson, B.: Morbidity of childhood near-drowning, Pediatrics 59:364, 1977.

48 Electrical and lightning injuries

ALERT: Extent of burns does not reflect severity of injury.

Electrical and lightning injuries have similar clinical presentations, both affecting the electrical charge of functional cells, particularly conductive tissue of the nervous system and heart, and causing cell death by intense heat. Individuals may have direct contact with electrical sources such as high-tension wires or faulty wiring in a home, or they may be struck by lightning. The injury will reflect the resistance of the tissue, the path and type of current (alternating being more dangerous), the voltage, and the duration of contact.

DIAGNOSTIC FINDINGS

The patient may have only minor burns or undergo full cardiac respiratory arrest. Most patients have some evidence of burns.

1. Entry-exit burns. The entry wound is ischemic, with a well-circumscribed area of whitish-yellow material and charred center. The exit wound is extensive, often with indistinct margins.
2. Arc burns, usually across joints
3. Flame burn, resulting in direct thermal injury
4. Mouth burns. In children they may look innocuous initially but often involve the labial artery, which, after some delay, may result in significant hemorrhage.

The extent of the burns rarely reflects the potential severity of the injury.

Cardiac dysrhythmias and even infarction may occur. Lower voltages produce ventricular fibrillation; higher voltage may produce asystole.

Neurologically, most patients have impaired mental status, with associated paresthesias, headache, aphasia, and paralysis. There may be permanent damage.

Additional findings include:

1. Pulmonary contusion and chest pain
2. Retinal detachment and burns; cataracts (a delayed sequela)
3. Tinnitus, hearing loss, and perforated tympanic membranes
4. Nonspecific abdominal pain, with nausea, vomiting, splenic rupture, intestinal perforation, and pancreatitis (rarely noted)

Complications

Complications include:

1. Cardiac respiratory arrest caused by central respiratory apnea, dysrhythmias, or cardiac ischemia leading to death
2. Neurologic complications such as amnesia, headache, sensorineural deafness, visual blurring, sensory complaints, and cerebral edema with seizures
3. Fractures, dislocations, and amputations secondary to falls, sustained muscle contraction, or direct cell death and neurovascular compromise

4. Acute tubular necrosis resulting from crush injury and myoglobinuria
5. Complications related to extensive burns

Ancillary data

1. CBC with elevated WBC, platelets
2. Electrolytes to check on potassium, which may be elevated
3. BUN and creatinine
4. Urinalysis (myoglobinuria or hemoglobinuria)
5. Cardiac enzymes
6. ABG
7. ECG
8. X-ray films
   a. Chest—to check for pulmonary contusion, cardiac decompensation
   b. Bones, cervical spine, and others as indicated

MANAGEMENT

The key to outcome is the adequacy of prehospital care, which must involve the rapid removal of the individual from the source, the institution of appropriate resuscitation, and immobilization of the cervical spine.

Stabilization in the ED should focus on airway and cardiac status and ensure that the cervical spine is stable:

1. Oxygen, IV fluids, NG tube, and urinary catheters as indicated
2. ECG and cardiac monitoring
3. Careful physical examination to assess degree of immediate injury
4. Fluid resuscitation must be done empirically on the basis of vital signs and urinary output because of the extensive deep tissue injury that occurs.

Burn care (Chapter 46) should be initiated. *Lip burns* should not be debrided. These patients should be observed for hemorrhage in the hospital for 3-4 days. Bleeding is controlled by pressure, with the area kept clean. Special feeding devices and arm splints may be necessary.

The patient is at risk for bleeding for 5-10 days following injury.

In cases of cerebral edema and seizures (p. 319):

1. Hyperventilate to maintain $PaCO_2$ at 20-25 mm Hg
2. Elevate head of bed 30 degrees if possible
3. Give furosemide (Lasix) 1 mg/kg/dose q 4-6 hr IV
4. Give dexamethasone (Decadron) 0.25 mg/kg/dose q 6 hr IV. Controversial
5. Give mannitol 0.5 g/kg/dose q 3-4 hr prn IV if patient has neurologic symptoms or seizures
6. Control seizure initially with diazepam (Valium) 0.2-0.3 mg/kg/dose q 2-5 min prn IV. Initiate other anticonvulsants (Chapter 21).

Other management techniques include:

1. Careful monitoring of urine output
2. Insertion of NG tube
3. Treatment of associated complications
4. Tetanus immunization, if indicated

DISPOSITION

All patients with a high-voltage injury ($>1,000$ volts) or with any evidence of cardiac, pulmonary, gastrointestinal, or neurologic abnormalities should be hospitalized. Patients with lip burns or those with potential neurovascular compromise require observation. Neurologic, ophthalmologic, otolaryngologic, and plastic surgery consultations may be useful in the management of the patient.

Asymptomatic patients may be discharged after a minimum of 4 hr of observation and after arranging for follow-up.

Parental education

1. Instruct child about the dangers of electrical injury.
2. Decrease access to electrical plugs and wires.
3. In case of lightning, have child stay indoors or seek shelter in a building. If there is no shelter, instruct youngster to avoid the high-

est object in the area, hilltops, open spaces, metal clotheslines, and wire fences.

4. If lightning does strike, initiate CPR immediately. If contact with electrical source occurs, withdraw patient from it without exposing rescuer to potential injury. Initiate CPR.

REFERENCES

Dado, D.V., Polley, W., and Kernahan, D.A.: Splinting of oral commissure electrical burns in children, J. Pediatr. **107**:92, 1985.

Kobernick, M.: Electrical injuries: pathophysiology and emergency management, Ann. Emerg. Med. **11**:633, 1982.

McLoughlin, E., Joseph, M.P., and Crawford, J.D.: Epidemiology of high-tension electrical injuries in children, J. Pediatr. **89**:62, 1976.

Myers, G.J., Colgan, M.T., and VanDyke, D.H.: Lightning-strike disaster among children, JAMA **238**:1045, 1977.

Orgel, M.G., Brown, H.C., and Woolhouse, F.M.: Electrical burns of the mouth in children: a method for assessing results, J. Trauma **18**:285, 1975.

Thompson, J.C., and Ashwai, S.: Electrical injuries in children, Am. J. Dis. Child. **137**:231, 1983.

Wood, B.D., Quinn, R.M., and Forgey, J.E.: Treating electrical burns of the mouths of children, J. Am. Dent. Assoc. **97**:206, 1978.

49 High-altitude sickness

ALERT: Acute onset of fatigue, respiratory distress, headache, or confusion when adapting to a high altitude requires intervention.

Individuals frequently have difficulty making the physiologic adaptation to altitudes above 7,500 ft (2,500 m), particularly on initial exposure to the low oxygen content of the air at that height. Fifty percent of nonacclimated people who ascend rapidly to 10,000 ft develop acute mountain sickness within 6-8 hr and respond well to conservative therapy. Most symptoms of hypoxia occur within 48-96 hr of arrival at high altitudes and are characterized by one of three clinical presentations (Table 49-1).

Factors predisposing individuals to high-altitude sickness include:

1. Rapid ascent (airplane vs. car vs. walking)
2. Return of high-altitude resident after a period of being at a lower level
3. Exercise
4. Preexisting infection
5. Preexisting pulmonary disease
6. Previous episodes

The underlying pathogenesis is a response to relative or absolute hypoxia.

Prevention must be emphasized. Acclimatization is essential, with attention to rate of ascent and initiation of a graded exercise program. Acetazolamide (Diamox) is useful in preventing high-altitude sickness (5 mg/kg/24 hr PO q 12 hr or in adult 500-750 mg/24 hr). It should be taken 2-3 days before ascent (it is not useful once illness has commenced) and should be continued during ascent.

REFERENCES

Foulke, G.E.: Altitude-related illness, Am. J. Emerg. Med. **3**:217, 1985.

Green, M.K., Kerr, A.M., McIntosh, I.B., et al.: Acetazolamide in prevention of acute mountain sickness, Brit. Med. J. **283**:811, 1981.

Hultgren, H.N.: High altitude medical problems, West. J. Med. **131**:8, 1979.

Larson, E.B., Roach, R.C., Schoene, R.B., et al.: Acute mountain sickness and acetazolamide: clinical efficacy and effects on ventilation, JAMA **248**:328, 1982.

TABLE 49-1. High-altitude sickness

	Acute mountain sickness (AMS)	High-altitude pulmonary edema (HAPE)	High-altitude cerebral edema (HACE)
Diagnostic findings	Nausea, vomiting, headache, lethargy, sleep disturbance, tinnitus, vertigo	Shortness of breath, tachypnea, tachycardia, cough, variable cyanosis	Headache, mental confusion, delirium, ataxia, hallucination, seizure, focal neuro signs, coma
Laboratory (in addition to those indicated for diagnostic evaluation)		ABG Chest x-ray ECG Bleeding screen	
Differential diagnosis			
Trauma	Concussion	Pulmonary contusion	Head
Infection	Gastroenteritis	Pneumonia	Meningitis Encephalitis
Metabolic		Uremia	Diabetic ketoacidosis Uremia Encephalopathy $\Updownarrow Na^+$, $\uparrow Ca^{++}$
Intoxication	Salicylates	Multiple	Narcotics
Vascular		CHF	Subarachnoid hemorrhage
Management			
Admit	Variable	Yes	Yes
Oxygen	Yes	Yes	Yes
Diuretic			
Acetazolamide	Prophylactic	Prophylactic	Prophylactic
Bronchodilator	No	Yes	No
Steroids	No	No	Controversial
Ventilation with PEEP	No	Yes	Hyperventilation

50 Hyperthermia

ALERT: Prompt attention must be given to fluid management and cooling.

Exposure to environmental heat without appropriate acclimatization, equipment, or fluid replacement may lead to a variety of clinical presentations that are usually preventable. Particularly at risk are athletes, laborers, soldiers, the chronically ill, and the very young or old (Table 50-1).

HEAT CRAMPS
Etiology

Heat cramps are caused by prolonged or excessive exercise, accompanied by profuse sweating, in an environment with high temperature and low humidity. Thirst is relieved by fluids that do not contain salt.

Diagnostic findings

Patients are alert and oriented, with normal or slightly elevated temperatures. They experience severe cramps in those skeletal muscles subjected to intense exercise, most commonly the legs.

Ancillary data
Low serum sodium is indicative of heat cramps.

Differential diagnosis

1. Intrapsychic: hyperventilation
2. Metabolic: hypokalemia
3. Trauma: black widow spider bite

Management
1. Hydration
   a. If severe, 0.9%NS at 20 ml/kg/hr over 1-2 hr
   b. If mild, oral salt solution: 1 tsp NaCl (4 g) in 500 ml water administered at same rate as *a*
2. Rest

HEAT EXHAUSTION
Etiology

Heat exhaustion is caused by exposure to a high-temperature environment, with continuous sweating and lack of appropriate replenishment of water or salt.

Diagnostic findings

Many individuals have a combination of the following:
1. *Water depletion:* inadequate water replacement (see Chapter 7 for hypernatremic dehydration). Signs and symptoms of dehydration are thirst, irritability, fatigue, anxiety, and disorientation. Temperature is usually normal.
2. *Salt depletion:* inadequate salt replacement—the more common type of heat exhaustion. Signs and symptoms of salt depletion are fatigue, headache, nausea, vomiting, diarrhea, and muscle cramps. Temperature

TABLE 50-1. Environmental heat illnesses: clinical presentation

Condition	Predisposing cause	Central nervous system	Skin	Muscle cramps	Thirst	Rectal temperature	Blood pressure	Pulse	Management
Heat cramps	Muscle work, sodium depletion, drinking large quantities of water	WNL	Sweating	Severe	WNL	$<40°$ C	WNL	WNL	Replace salt
Heat exhaustion	Heat exposure: (1) without access to water, (2) with replacement of sweat loss with water only	Fatigue, weakness, headache, anxiety	Sweating	Variable	Variable	$<40°$ C	Tends to be low	Tends to be low	Replace salt or water
Heat stroke	Heat exposure, K^+-Na^+ depletion, impaired sweating, increased heat production	Headache, listlessness, confusion, seizure, psychosis, coma	Hot, dry	Variable	Abnormal	$>40°$ C	Abnormal (high or low)	Elevated	Cooling and support

is normal or slightly increased. Acclimatized individual will have a lower salt content of sweat.

Complications

1. Shock
2. Seizures and coma

Ancillary data

Serum sodium may be high (water depletion) or low (salt depletion).

Management

Necessary stabilization must be provided. Management must reflect the underlying cause. In patients with only modest elevations in body temperature, oral fluids and sprinkling water over the body to increase evaporative losses may be adequate. In severe disease with obtundation, intravenous fluid should be initiated. If water depletion is accompanied by hypernatremic dehydration, fluid should be instituted slowly in accordance with the protocol in Chapter 7. With salt depletion and isotonic or hypotonic dehydration:

• Initiate 20 ml/kg of 0.9%NS over 30 min: then follow protocol for dehydration (Chapter 7).

Disposition

Patient with significant dehydration should be admitted for fluid management and monitoring. Those with no metabolic abnormalities and only mild symptoms may be discharged after initial fluid push.

Prevention requires the availability and intake of appropriate fluids.

HEAT STROKE
Etiology

The body's heat dissipation system (sweating, radiation, and convection) is overwhelmed by production and absorption of heat. Underlying conditions may contribute to this imbalance.

1. Trauma/physical
   a. Environment: particularly in newborn who has immature thermoregulation and

is more dependent on the environment
   b. Burns (Chapter 46)
2. Congenital
   a. Cystic fibrosis—excessive sweating and salt loss
   b. Dermatologic: anhidrotic ectodermal dysplasia, ichthyosis
3. Intoxication (Table 54-1)
   a. Decreased sweating—antihistamines, phenothiazines, anticholinergics, and cardiac beta blockers
   b. Increased heat production and impaired sweating—amphetamines, LSD, PCP, and thyroid replacements
   c. Increased heat absorption—ethanol

Diagnostic findings

Heat stroke may be caused by:
1. Exertion, which has rapid course
2. A preexisting condition that has a slow onset (nonexertional)
3. Intoxication
Symptoms include:
1. Anorexia, nausea, vomiting, headache, fatigue, and confusion or disorientation, possibly progressing to coma and posturing
2. Skin that is red, hot, and dry
3. High temperatures ($> 40°$ C), accompanied by tachycardia and hypotension

Complications

1. Coma with permanent neurologic sequelae
2. Acute tubular necrosis (p. 615)
3. Acidosis
4. Dysrhythmias (Chapter 6)
5. Rhabdomyolysis and myoglobinuria
6. Hepatic damage
7. Coagulopathy with disseminated intravascular coagulation (DIC) and thrombocytopenia (Chapter 79)
8. Death

Ancillary data

1. Arterial blood gas. Changes in body temperature alter true values. For each degree $>37°$

C, the following adjustments to the measured value should be made:

pH	↓ 0.015
$PaCO_2$	↑ 4.4%
PaO_2	↑ 7.2%

NOTE: The opposite adjustment should be made for each degree $<37°$ C.
2. Electrolytes (hyperkalemia, hypokalemia, hyponatremia, hypernatremia), BUN (increased), and glucose (hyperglycemia)
3. CBC and platelets
4. ECG: S-T depression, nonspecific T-wave changes, PVC, supraventricular tachycardia
5. Bleeding and DIC screen, if appropriate
6. Other studies to evaluate nature of underlying condition

Differential diagnosis

1. Infection: meningitis or encephalitis; rickettsial disease: typhus, Rocky Mountain spotted fever; malaria
2. Endocrine: hypothalamic disorder

Management

Heat stroke is life threatening and requires rapid intervention. Initial stabilization in the field should include removing the patient from the heat and drenching or immersing the individual in cool water. Airway should be stabilized and oxygen administered. Circulatory status should be assessed and intravenous fluids initiated. Patients require ongoing cardiac and rectal temperature probe monitoring.

Other management techniques include:
1. Ice bath (if unavailable, fan patient while sprinkling water or use ice packs) until patient reaches 38.5° C. Simultaneously massage extremities.
2. Intravenous fluids appropriate to the patient's electrolytes and fluid balance. Initially, give 0.9%NS at 20 ml/kg over 45-60 min. If cardiac status is unstable, insert a central venous line.

3. Foley catheter, with NG tube to minimize aspiration
4. Diazepam 0.2-0.3 mg/kg/dose IV for treatment of shivering

Disposition

All patients should be admitted to ICU.

Prevention includes ensurance of adequate water and salt intake during heat exposure. Individuals with cystic fibrosis or a dermatologic problem should avoid prolonged exposure. Response to predisposing drugs should be monitored.

Runners in hot weather should drink 100-300 ml water 10-15 min before a race and drink about 250 ml water every 3-4 km. Fluid losses exceed electrolyte abnormalities.

REFERENCE

Stine, R.J.: Heat illness, J.A.C.E.P. 8:154, 1979.

51 Hypothermia

ALERT: Resuscitation must continue in the pulseless, apneic patient until the core temperature is at least 30° C.

Hypothermia exists when a patient's core temperature is ≤35° C. It results from prolonged exposure, conditions that secondarily contribute to hypothermia, or systemic diseases that interfere with thermoregulation.

Neonates are particularly at risk because of their relatively large surface area and small percentage of subcutaneous fat.

ETIOLOGY (AND ASSOCIATED CONDITIONS)

1. Trauma/physical
   a. Exposure
   b. Near-drowning (Chapter 47)
   c. Head or spinal cord injury (Chapter 57)
2. Infection
   a. Bacterial meningitis (p. 549)
   b. Encephalitis
   c. Respiratory infection (p. 601)
   d. Gram-negative septicemia
3. Endocrine/metabolic factors
   a. Hypoglycemia (Chapter 38)
   b. Diabetic ketoacidosis (p. 469)
   c. Hypopituitarism
   d. Myxedema (p. 475)
   e. Addison's disease (Chapter 74)
   f. Uremia (p. 615)
4. Intoxication (Table 54-1)
   a. Alcohol
   b. Barbiturates
   c. Carbon monoxide
   d. Narcotics
   e. Phenothiazines
   f. Anesthetics, general
   g. Tricyclic antidepressants
5. Degenerative/deficiencies
   a. CNS disease
   b. Malnutrition and kwashiorkor
6. Vascular factors
   a. Shock (Chapter 5)
   b. Subarachnoid hemorrhage (Chapter 18)
   c. Subdural hematoma (Chapter 57)
   d. Pulmonary embolism (p. 000)
   e. Cerebral vascular accident
7. Intrapsychic: anorexia nervosa
8. Neoplasm, intracranial

DIAGNOSTIC FINDINGS

The severity of the findings reflect the degree and duration of hypothermia and the nature of any underlying or predisposing condition. Special low-reading thermometers are required.

In general, the progression of signs and symptoms reflect the degree of hypothermia:

Core temperature	Common signs and symptoms
35° C	Slurred speech, lapse of memory
32° C	Diminished mental status: drowsy, amnesic, confused, disoriented
	Muscle rigidity, poor muscle coordination
	Skin cyanotic, edematous
30° C	Stuporous, irritable
	Progressive decline in basal metabolic rate
	Myocardial irritability, bradycar-

	dia. **J** (or Osborne) waves on ECG, decreased cardiac output and hypotension
	Decreased minute ventilation
28° C	Dysrhythmias common with progression to ventricular fibrillation and asystole. This is the cardiac fibrillatory threshold at which ventricular fibrillation can be induced by cardiac stimulation.
26° C	Loss of consciousness, areflexive
25° C	Respirations cease

General findings

1. Patients will initially have tachycardia, progressing to bradycardia associated with a decreased respiratory rate, tidal volume, and hypoxia at 30° C. Blood pressure will decline with decreased cardiac output. On rewarming, patients may exhibit shock secondary to the initial vasodilation.
2. Myocardial irritability and impaired pacemaker function lead to atrial and ventricular dysrhythmias and bradycardia. Asystole and electromechanical dissociation develop at 20° C.
3. Neurologic status progresses from slight ataxia, slurred speech, and hyperesthesias to frank coma.
4. Body heat is partially maintained by shivering, which ceases somewhere between 30°-33° C. Pallor and cyanosis are noted. Muscular rigidity develops.
5. Renal function is diminished with poor renal perfusion. Oliguria may be noted.
6. With profound hypothermia (often <25° C), the patient will appear apneic, rigid, pulseless, areflexive, and unresponsive, with fixed, dilated pupils.
7. Infants with hypothermia have decreased feeding, lethargy, edema of the limbs, and cold, erythematous, and scleremic (hardened) skin. Bradycardia and abdominal distension may be observed. Metabolic acidosis, hypoglycemia, and hyperkalemia are usually present.

Complications

Frostbite

1. Ice crystallization in the cells associated with vasoconstriction
2. Fingers, hands, feet, toes, ears, and nose most common sites
3. Severity of injury dependent on temperature, duration of exposure, wind-chill factor, immobility, tightness of clothing, and dampness of environment
4. Classification

Degree	Clinical presentation
First	Skin is mottled, edematous, hyperemic, with burning and tingling. Peaks in 24-48 hr and may persist for 1-2 wk.
Second	Blister formation with paresthesia and anesthesia
Third (deep)	Necrosis of skin with ulceration and edema. Involves subcutaneous tissue.
Fourth (deep)	Necrosis with gangrene. Vesicle followed by eschar and ulceration. Progression over 24-36 hr. Demarcation may take several weeks.

NOTE: Initial evaluation may be faulty since involvement is dynamic.

Other complications

1. Metabolic abnormalities: metabolic acidosis, hypoglycemia, hyperkalemia
2. Gastrointestinal bleeding (Chapter 35)
3. Acute renal failure (p. 615)
4. Pancreatitis (p. 490)
5. Hypovolemia secondary to shift of fluids into extracellular spaces
6. Deep vein thrombosis (p. 428)
7. Coagulopathy, DIC, thrombocytopenia, leukopenia (Chapter 79)
8. Pulmonary edema (Chapter 19)

Ancillary data

1. Arterial blood gas. Changes in body temperature alter true values. For each degree <37° C, the following adjustment to the measured value should be made.

pH	↑ 0.015
PCO_2 (mm Hg)	↓ 4.4%
PO_2 (mm Hg)	↓ 7.2%

NOTE: The opposite adjustment should be made for each degree >37° C.

2. ECG: Dysrhythmias are noted with progression—e.g., J (or Osborne) wave at about 30° C. It appears as a "camel-humped" deflection of the QRS-ST junction.

3. Chemistries
   a. Hyperkalemia secondary to metabolic acidosis, renal failure, or rhabdomyolysis
   b. BUN and creatinine increased
   c. Increased amylase
   d. Glucose increased when patient is cold and decreased during rewarming. Liver function tests elevated with hepatitis

4. Hematology
   a. Possible coagulopathy with DIC
   b. Thrombocytopenia and leukopenia secondary to sequestration; possible hemoconcentration

5. Studies to assess status of underlying conditions

MANAGEMENT

Initial management must stabilize the patient and treat underlying conditions. In addition to standard regimens, the patient should be moved to a warm environment and clothing removed. Handling of the patient should be minimized to avoid precipitating a dysrhythmia. Cardiac and rectal probe monitors are necessary. Hypoglycemia and hypoxia should be corrected with administration of oxygen, glucose, and warmed IV solutions. Underlying conditions need prompt attention. A low-reading thermometer is needed.

Temperatures >32° C

1. Initiate passive external rewarming by warming the patient in blankets.
2. Attempt to raise the temperature 0.5°-2.0° C/hr
3. If there is no increase in temperature in 2 hr, evaluate for underlying disease and initiate active rewarming.

Temperatures <32° C

1. Begin active rewarming at 0.5° C/hr. Patient may experience rewarming shock during treatment (vasodilation may cause transient fall in blood pressure).
2. Monitor at all times. Handle patient carefully.
3. Avoid inserting intracardiac monitors and administering adrenergic drugs, until >28° C, if possible. If necessary, preoxygenate patient before performing invasive procedures.
4. Administer oxygen, humidified and heated, if possible. If intubation is required, preoxygenate well.

If the cardiovascular system is *stable*, active external rewarming is appropriate, using warmed blankets and heated objects (water bottle, etc.) applied primarily to the trunk. With temperature <28° C, emergent intervention is needed.

If the cardiovascular system is *unstable*, the patient is in diabetic ketoacidosis (insulin inactive at <30° C), spinal cord injury exists, or external rewarming is ineffective, initiate active core rewarming, which may be used in conjunction with active external rewarming procedures. Techniques may be used individually or in combination:

1. Humidified oxygen delivered at about 40.5° C (105° F)-42° C (107.6° F) by either mask or endotracheal tube
2. Warmed intravenous fluids: D5W.9%NS without potassium is preferred.
3. Peritoneal dialysis using K^+-free dialysate heated to 40.5°-42.5° C
4. Hemodialysis and extracorporeal blood rewarming. These are controversial but may be attempted if other approaches are unsuccessful. It is clearly indicated in the arrested, unresponsive patient or the nonarrested, stable patient with concomitant significant drug overdose, infection, or trauma. It should be continued until a core temperature of 30°-32° C is achieved. It is logistically difficult and

may produce complications of bleeding, etc.

5. Active/rewarming should generally be discontinued when the core temperature reaches 32°-34° C to avoid overheating.

Dysrhythmias

Lidocaine and bretylium are useful in treatment of hypothermic ventricular dysrhythmias. Defibrillation of ventricular fibrillation will usually not be effective under 30° C.

Bradycardia and atrial fibrillation will usually revert with warming.

Frostbite

1. Initial treatment in the field must include careful handling with rewarming only if there is no chance of a second freezing during transport. Superficial first- and second-degree injuries of the hand may be treated in the field by holding the fingers in the armpits or blowing on them with hot air. Once warmed they should be covered with a dry, clean cloth.

2. Deep frostbite should be treated definitively by immersion of the extremity or part in tepid water (40.5°-43.3° C) for 20 min after core rewarming is well underway. Protect the involved tissue from further damage. After warming, apply sterile gauze and elevate for 40 min.

3. Amputation of fourth-degree injuries must be delayed until there is good demarcation of necrotic tissue. Gentle debridement may be done.

4. Analgesics may be required. Handle involved area gently.

DISPOSITION

Patients with hypothermia require hospitalization and those with core temperatures <32° C should be admitted to an ICU. Patients with only superficial frostbite may be sent home.

Patients should be informed about the importance of appropriate clothing.

REFERENCES

Reuler, J.B.: Hypothermia: pathophysiology, clinical setting and management, Ann. Intern. Med. **89**:519, 1978.

Zell, S.C., and Kurtz, K.J.: Severe exposure hypothermia: a resuscitation protocol, Ann. Emerg. Med. **14**:339, 1985.

52 Radiation injuries

Radiation injuries most commonly occur from transportation, nuclear facility, or industrial accidents. Ionizing radiation may consist of alpha (noninjurious), beta (minimal surface injury), or gamma (penetrates deeply, causing acute radiation injury) exposure. Injury depends on the amount of body surface exposed, the length of exposure, the distance from the source, the type of radiation, and shielding techniques.

The clinical presentation is delineated in relationship to dose in Table 52-1.

From the perspective of the receiving hospital, the following steps should be taken:

1. Advance notification of arrival should be received.
2. Treatment areas, with specific entrance, should be designated.
3. Personnel should wear operating room attire with gloves.
4. Life-saving functions should be performed first.
5. Open wounds should be covered and clothing removed.
6. Contamination should be defined with radiation detectors.
7. Wounds should be flushed.
8. Patient should be washed with washcloths, soap, and water.
9. After the patient is medically stable, internal and external radiation exposure should be evaluated.
   a. Nasal swabs, urine, and feces
   b. CBC and platelet count initially and then every 6 hr
10. Expert medical consultation is usually necessary to assist in management. Routine steps for symptomatic patients with significant exposure include isolation, fluids, bowel sterilization with antibiotics, RBC, platelet and granulocyte infusions, and infection control and monitoring.

REFERENCE

Mettler, F.D.: Emergency management of radiation accidents, J.A.C.E.P. 7:302, 1978.

TABLE 52-1. Dose-effect relationships following acute whole body irradiation (x- or gamma)

Whole body* dose (rad)	Clinical and laboratory findings
5-25	Asymptomatic. Conventional blood studies are normal. Chromosome aberrations detectable
50-75	Asymptomatic. Minor depressions of white cells and platelets detectable in a few persons, especially if baseline values established
75-125	Minimal acute doses that produce prodromal symptoms (anorexia, nausea, vomiting, fatigue) in about 10%-20% of persons within 2 days. Mild depressions of white cells and platelets in some persons
125-200	Symptomatic course with transient disability and clear hematologic changes in a majority of exposed persons. Lymphocyte depression of about 50% within 48 hr
240-340	Serious, disabling illness in most persons with about 50% mortality if untreated. Lymphocyte depression of about 75+% within 48 hr
500+	Accelerated version of acute radiation syndrome with GI complications within 2 wk, bleeding, and death in most exposed persons
5000+	Fulminating course with cardiovascular, GI, and CNS complications resulting in death within 24-72 hr

From Mettler, F.D.: Emergency management of radiation accidents, J.A.C.E.P. 7:302, 1978.
*Conversion of rad (midline) dose to radiation measurements in R can be made roughly by multiplying rad times 1.5, e.g., 200 rad (midline) is equal to about 300 R (200 × 1.5).

53 Smoke inhalation

ALERT: Airway stabilization is imperative.

Smoke inhalation most commonly accompanies major burns and is considered to be the major respiratory complication of thermal burns (Chapter 46).

ETIOLOGY

1. Direct thermal injury to respiratory tract, often associated with flame burns in a closed room
   a. Major burns
   b. Nasopharyngeal—circumoral burns
      (1) Singed nasal hairs
      (2) Singed eyelids and eyebrows
2. Inhalation of toxins, often secondary to noxious fumes that may be the products of combustion
   a. Acetic acid (petroleum products)
   b. Formic acid or aldehydes (wood, cotton, paper, petroleum products)
   c. Chlorine (polyvinylchloride)
   d. Hydrochloric acid or HCN (hydrocyanic acid) (plastics)
3. Carbon monoxide (CO) poisoning
4. Hypoxia, usually secondary to closed-space fire

DIAGNOSTIC FINDINGS

1. Patients usually demonstrate thermal burns (Chapter 46) and may have evidence of CO poisoning (p. 289).

2. Patients demonstrate evidence of direct damage to the upper respiratory tract (which may be delayed up to 24 hr), for example, stridor, hoarseness, and black or brown carbonaceous sputum.
3. Concurrently patients may have CO poisoning, hypoxia, and upper airway obstruction. The relative hypoxia may cause confusion and agitation, rarely progressing to coma.

Complications

1. Upper airway obstruction, secondary to mucosal injury, similar to croup
2. Pulmonary edema (Chapter 19), usually developing 1-4 days after injury: dyspnea, cough, wheezing, rales, and respiratory distress
3. Bacterial pneumonia about 1 wk after injury

Ancillary data

All patients require ABG, carboxyhemoglobin level, and chest x-ray film.

DIFFERENTIAL DIAGNOSIS

See Chapters 19 and 20.

MANAGEMENT

Humidified oxygen should be administered to all patients. This is appropriate treatment for CO poisoning (p. 289) and direct respiratory tract injury.

1. Airway management
   a. If patient is compromised, intubate and initiate active control. PEEP and CPAP improve oxygen exchange in the lungs. Indications include:
      (1) Respiratory failure ($PaO_2 < 50$ mm Hg and $PaCO_2 > 50$ mm Hg)
      (2) Severe acidosis
      (3) Laryngeal obstruction
      (4) Difficulty with secretions
   b. If bronchospasm is present, useful bronchodilators include epinephrine or inhaled bronchodilator and aminophylline (Chapter 84).
   c. Early bronchoscopy is indicated for significant secretions or direct evaluation of injury when pulmonary lesion is suspected.
2. Management of associated burn, if present (Chapter 46)
3. Corticosteroids, which increase the mortality rate, are not indicated.

DISPOSITION

All patients with the following findings should be hospitalized:
1. Respiratory failure
2. Carboxyhemoglobin level elevation requiring admission (p. 289)

3. High-risk category: major and most moderate burns, facial or nasal burn
4. Upper airway signs of involvement (hoarseness, stridor)
5. Lower airway involvement (bronchospasm, dyspnea)

Patients with none of these factors may be discharged if follow-up and observation can be ensured and there is no question of child abuse. Parents must watch for any changes in respiratory status.

Parental education

1. Call physician immediately if your child develops any of the following:
   a. Increasing difficulty in breathing
   b. Hoarseness, stridor, cough, or wheezing
   c. Lethargy, agitation, or other behavioral changes
   d. Fever
2. Read information about fire prevention.

REFERENCES

Achauer, B.M., Allyn, P.A., Furnas, D.W., and Bartlett, R.H.: Pulmonary complications of burns: the major threat to the burn patient, Ann. Surg. 177:311, 1973.

Cahalane, M., and Demling, R.H.: Early respiratory abnormalities from smoke inhalation, JAMA 251:771, 1984.

Mellins, R.B., and Park, S.: Respiratory complications of smoke inhalation in victims of fire, J. Pediatr. 87:1, 1975.

VIII POISONING AND OVERDOSE

ROGER M. BARKIN
KENNETH W. KULIG
BARRY H. RUMACK

54 Management principles

Poisoning is a significant cause of morbidity and mortality in the United States; it is the fourth most common cause of death in children. Approximately 80% of accidental ingestions occur in children under 5 yr of age, the peak incidence being between 1½ and 3 yr. In children under 1 yr, poisoning usually results from therapeutic misuse of drugs, while the preschooler is adventuresome and curious and will ingest any accessible household product or medication. The adolescent may experiment with mind-altering drugs, often with peers, and manipulative behavior and suicide become important motivators. Family turmoil is commonly present and the poisoning tends to be recurrent.

Children under 5 yr frequently ingest soaps, detergents, plants, vitamins, and their parents' medications. The most significant exposures commonly involve salicylates, alkaline corrosives, acetaminophen, iron, petroleum products, antihistamines, tricyclic antidepressants, benzodiazapines, barbiturates, pesticides, carbon monoxide, and opiates. Of childhood poisonings, 87% occur in the home.

INITIAL CONTACT WITH THE POISONED PATIENT

1. *Basic information* is essential. Obtain name, weight, and age. Address and telephone number provide a means for later contact.
2. *Type of ingestion*. Define the product name, ingredients, amount consumed, and any current symptoms. Always relate the amount taken to the patient's weight. If there is any question about the medication, ask for a prescription number, the dispensing pharmacy, or prescribing physician. Always request that the product be brought to the ED. The history is often inaccurate.

INITIATION OF THERAPY AT HOME

Many accidental ingestions may be treated at home if the substance or the amount ingested is nontoxic (see box on opposite page).
1. Be certain to cover the areas of poison prevention. Dangerous substances that are often found in the household include medications, dishwasher soap and cleaning supplies, drain-cleaning crystals or liquids, paints and thinners, automobile products, and garden sprays.
2. Regional poison control centers provide an effective means of disseminating information, providing medical consultation, and arranging for follow-up. Unnecessary hospital visits may therefore be decreased.
3. If specific social problems are noted, initiate referral to a public health nurse. Any non-accidental ingestions or potential child abuse must be seen in a health care facility despite the seemingly benign nature of the exposure.

Prevention of absorption

Techniques to prevent further absorption can be initiated before the patient arrives at the ED.
1. External
   a. Skin exposed to insecticides (organophosphates or carbamates), hydrocarbons, or acids or alkali agents should be flooded with water and washed well with soap and a soft washcloth or sponge. Remove clothing.

b. Eyes must be irrigated immediately, before any transport or other therapy is discussed. Have the patient hold head under the sink or shower, or pour water into the eye from a pitcher or glass. Irrigation should be continued for a steady 15-20 min.

2. Internal

a. Dilute any acid or alkali ingestions with milk or water; do *not* induce emesis.

b. For other agents, and if so advised by the regional poison control center, emesis with syrup of Ipecac should be induced in children over 6 mo, if indicated. Do not use for children under 6 mo of age. Give 10 ml (child under 1 yr); 15 ml (child 1-12 yr); or 30 ml (child over 12 yr), followed by 15 ml/kg (up to 250 ml or 8 oz of water). Do not use milk or heavily sugared liquids. Ambulate the patient and wait for vomiting, which usually occurs in the next 20 min. Pharyngeal stimulation may be useful. If the patient does not vomit, repeat dose in 20 min if child is over 12 mo.

NOTE: Contraindicated in the home setting if:

(1) Patient is comatose, stuporous, seizing, has no gag reflex, is less than 6 mo of age, or has a bleeding diathesis

(2) Ingestion involves acid or alkali substances (p. 282)

LOW-TOXICITY INGESTIONS*

Abrasives
Antacids
Antibiotics
Baby product cosmetics
Ballpoint pen inks
Bathtub floating toys
Calamine lotion
Candles (beeswax or paraffin)
Chalk (calcium carbonate)
Clay (modeling or Play Doh)
Contraceptives
Corticosteroids
Cosmetics (most, except perfumes)
Crayons marked AP or CP
Dehumidifying packets (silica)
Deodorants and deodorizers
Etch-A-Sketch
Fish bowl additives
Glues and pastes
Greases
Gums
Hair products (dyes, sprays, tonics)
Hand lotions and creams

Ink (black, blue, indelible, felt tip)
Kaolin
Lanolin
Linoleic acid
Linseed oil
Lubricants and lubricating oils
Newspapers
Paint (indoor and latex)
Pencil (graphite)
Petroleum jelly (Vaseline)
Polaroid picture coating fluid
Putty (less than 2 oz)
Sachets (essential oils, powder)
Shampoos and soap
Shoe polish (not containing aniline dyes)
Spackle
Suntan preparations
Sweetening agents (saccharin, cyclamate)
Teething rings
Thermometers (mercury)
Tooth paste (without fluoride)
Vitamins without iron
Zinc oxide

Modified from Rumack, B.H. editor: Poisindex, Denver, 1985 Micromedix.

*These materials generally do not produce significant toxicity except in large doses. Toxicity is altered if the patient is pregnant or has an underlying disease.

(3) Ingestion involves hydrocarbons that do not contain camphor, halogenated or aromatic products, heavy metals, or pesticides ("CHAMP") (p. 292)

(4) Ingestion involves rapid-acting CNS depressant

TRANSPORT TO HOSPITAL

All patients requiring evaluation or treatment should be transported. The ED to receive the patient should be notified and given information about the treatment plan initiated and the means of transport. The parent or patient should be reminded to bring the ingested material for identification.

OTHER CONSIDERATIONS

If there is potential toxicity of an ingestion that is treated at home, arrangements should be made for the patient to be called back. Asking the older patient to call back is risky because of the possibility of the patient becoming obtunded or confused. Poison control centers can often facilitate this follow-up. All suicidal patients must be sent to a health care facility.

Records of all poison calls should be kept, including basic information, the type of ingestion, and therapy initiated.

Treatment information is available from multiple sources. Poisindex is a comprehensive information system available on microfiche or computer in many EDs. Poison control centers are a further source of data and management advice.

MANAGEMENT IN THE EMERGENCY DEPARTMENT

There is often an associated ingestion that may change the clinical presentation and treatment plan. *Dilution* of acid and alkali ingestions with milk or water is of immediate priority, even before patient arrival in the ED. Patients are usually NPO following initial evaluation and must be managed as any other potentially critically ill patient.

Cardiopulmonary status

1. Airway, ventilation, and circulation must be adequate.
2. Intravenous lines should be established in potentially serious ingestions.
3. Any patient with altered mental status, seizures, or coma requires simultaneous administration of the following:
   a. Oxygen at 4-6 L/min
   b. Dextrose 0.5-1.0 g (1-2 ml D50W)/kg/dose IV
   c. Naloxone (Narcan) 0.8 mg (2 adult ampules) initially IV; if no response in suspected opiate overdose, 2 mg (5 ampules) IV (1 mg/ml [2 ml] ampules are also available).

Other considerations

1. Physical examination should focus particularly on the cardiopulmonary and neurologic status. A specific toxic syndrome may be identified.
2. Patients should be placed on a cardiac monitor and have an ECG if the ingested drug or chemical might precipitate dysrhythmias.
3. Electrolytes and acid-base status should be evaluated.

Toxicologic screen

Blood analysis provides quantitative levels of specific drugs. Urine content, which provides a qualitative determination, is particularly important in identifying drugs with large volumes of distribution, high lipid solubilities, or long half-lives.

The toxicology laboratory alone should not be relied on to make the diagnosis. Patient history and physical examination are far more important (Tables 54-1 and 54-2).

1. Always let the laboratory personnel know what drug(s) are suspected.
2. Since a negative toxicologic screen does not exclude a drug overdose, you must know which drugs the laboratory has screened for in its analysis.

TABLE 54-1. Clues to diagnosis of unknown poison: vital-sign changes

DYSRHYTHMIAS

Amphetamines
Anticholinergics
Beta-blockers (propranolol, etc.)
Carbon monoxide
Chloral hydrate
Digitalis
Phenothiazines
Sympathomimetics (cocaine, etc.)
Tricyclic antidepressants, theophylline

CYANOSIS (secondary to methemoglobinemia; does not respond to oxygen)

Anesthetics, local
Nitrates
Nitrites
Phenacetin
Sulfonamides

Increased	Decreased
BLOOD PRESSURE	
Amphetamines	Cyanide
Anticholinergics	Narcotics
Sympathomimetics	Sedative/hypnotics (see Table 54-3, Coma)
HEART RATE	
Alcohol	Barbiturates
Amphetamines	Digitalis
Anticholinergics	Narcotics
Sympathomimetics (caffeine, cocaine, etc.)	Sedatives/hypnotics
Theophylline	
RESPIRATORY RATE	
Amphetamines	Alcohols (ethanol, isopropyl, methanol)
Anticholinergics	Barbiturates
Hydrocarbons	Narcotics
Secondary to metabolic acidosis ("MUDPIES") (p. 277)	Sedatives/hypnotics
Secondary to noncardiogenic pulmonary edema	
Carbon monoxide	
Hydrocarbons	
Narcotics	
Organophosphates	
Salicylates	
Sedatives/hypnotics	
TEMPERATURE	
Amphetamines	Alcohol (ethanol)
Anticholinergics	Anesthetic, general
Atropine	Barbiturates
Beta-blockers	Carbon monoxide
Phenothiazines	Narcotics
Salicylates	Phenothiazines
Sympathomimetics (cocaine, etc.)	Sedatives/hypnotics
Tricyclic antidepressants	Tricyclic antidepressants

TABLE 54-2. Clues to diagnosis of unknown poison: neurologic alterations

	Findings associated with coma		
COMA	**Seizures, myoclonus, hyperreflexia**	**Hyporeflexia, hypotension**	**Pulmonary edema, hypotension**
Amphetamines	+		
Anticholinergics	+		
Barbiturates		+	+
Benzodiazepines		+	
Carbamazepine	+		
Carbon monoxide	+		+
Chloral hydrate		+	
Cocaine	+		
Ethanol, isopropyl		+	+
Haloperidol	+		
Narcotics		+	+
Phencyclidine (PCP)	+		
Phenothiazines	+		
Phenytoin	+		
Salicylates			+
Sedative/hypnotics			+
Tricyclic antidepressants	+		

SEIZURES ("CAP")

Camphor	Aminophylline	Pesticides (organophosphates)
Carbon monoxide	Amphetamines and sympathomimetics	Phencyclidine (PCP)
Cocaine	Anticholinergics	Phenol
Cyanide	Aspirin	Propoxyphene

Also lead, isoniazid, drug withdrawal, carbamazepine (Tegretol), lithium, strychnine, tricyclic antidepressants, sympathomimetics and many others

BEHAVIOR DISORDERS

Toxic psychosis: hallucinogens (LSD, phencyclidine), sympathomimetics (cocaine, amphetamines), anticholinergics, heavy metals

Paranoid, violent reactions: phencyclidine

Depression, paranoid hallucinations, emotional lability: sympathomimetics (cocaine, amphetamines)

Hallucinations, delirium, anxiety: anticholinergics, hallucinogens

MOVEMENT DISORDERS

Choreoathetosis, orofacial dyskinesis, nystagmus, ataxia: phenytoin

Extrapyramidal: anticholinergics, phenothiazines, haloperidol

Choreoathetoid movements: tricyclic antidepressants

Ataxia, choreiform movements: heavy metals

Ataxia, tremors: lithium

Nystagmus: phenytoin, carbamazepine, primidone, phencyclidine, carbon monoxide

PUPILS

Pinpoint (miosis)		**Dilated** (mydriasis)
Barbiturates (late)	Alcohol	Meperidine
Cholinergics	Anticholinergics	Phenytoin
Narcotics (except meperidine)	Antihistamines	Sympathomimetics (i.e., am-
Organophosphates	Barbiturates	phetamines, cocaine, ephedrine, LSD, PCP, etc.)

Prevention of absorption

1. External
   a. Skin—as described on p. 266
   b. Ocular exposures, particularly to caustic agents, require immediate irrigation before examination. Each eye should be washed with a minimum of 1 L of saline, with eversion of eyelids and cleaning of the fornices.
2. Internal. Emesis or lavage is unlikely to be of benefit unless it is performed within 1-2 hr of ingestion or the ingested drug delays gastric emptying.
   a. *Emesis* with syrup of ipecac, if indicated. Do *not* give if patient is comatose, stuporous, seizing, has no gag reflex, is under 6 mo old, has a bleeding diathesis, or the ingestion involves an acid, alkali, or a hydrocarbon that does not contain camphor, halogenated or aromatic products, heavy metal, or pesticides (p. 267).

Age	Amount of ipecac administered
Under 1 yr	10 ml (do not repeat)
1-12 yr	15 ml
>12 yr	30 ml

   b. *Lavage*
      (1) Indicated for patients who have ingested a potentially toxic substance and are seen within 1-2 hr of ingestion and are seizing, comatose, uncooperative or have lost their gag reflex; or have ingested a drug likely to rapidly cause seizures. The procedure also facilitates later administration of activated charcoal and cathartics.
      (2) Contraindicated for caustic or acid ingestions
      (3) 28-36 Fr tube (36-40 Fr in adults) is inserted orally. Saline or half-normal saline at 100-200 ml per pass in adult (proportionately smaller in child) is administered and repeated until the return is clear. Often a funnel or other device attached to the tube will facilitate the procedure.
      (4) In comatose patients or those who lack protective reflexes (gag, cough, swallow), intubation is usually indicated before insertion of lavage tube.
      (5) Procedure is performed with the patient on the left side in the Trendelenburg (head down) position.
   c. *Activated charcoal* should be given after lavage or emesis. If emesis has been induced, wait 30-60 min following vomiting; in patients who have been lavaged, charcoal can be administered through the tube. Although it is recommended that 10 times the ingested material be administered, commonly 1 g/kg is the dose. Adults usually receive 30-100 g and children 10-30 g orally. It is often helpful to mix the charcoal in 100-200 ml of water, adding 7-15 ml of flavored syrup. It can also be mixed in D50W with a few drops of flavoring or 70% sorbitol.

   The efficacy is greatest when given early. However ingestions that reduce gastric motility (i.e., anticholinergics) may continue to be absorbed up to 12-24 hr following ingestion.

   Multiple dose charcoal (adult: 20-50 g q 2-4 hr PO) increases the clearance of theophylline, phenobarbital, carbamazepine, phenylbutazone, and meprobamate. Recent evidence supports mixing every other dose with a cathartic and administering every 2 hr.

   Drugs adsorbed by activated charcoal include:
   (1) Analgesic/antiinflammatory agents: acetaminophen, aspirin, nonsteroidals, morphine, propoxyphene
   (2) Anticonvulsants/sedatives: barbiturates, carbamazepine, chlordiazepoxide, diazepam, phenytoin, sodium valproate
   (3) Other: amphetamines, atropine, chlorpheniramine, cocaine, digitalis,

quinine, theophylline, tricyclic anti-depressants

d. *Catharsis,* using magnesium sulfate 250 mg/kg dose PO (adults 20 g PO), should be given to increase transit time. It is contraindicated in patients with renal failure, severe diarrhea, adynamic ileus, or abdominal trauma. Sodium sulfate, sorbitol, or magnesium citrate also may serve as cathartics.

Enhancement of excretion (Table 54-3)

1. *Diuresis* can hasten the excretion of only a few substances—namely, those with small volumes of distribution that are excreted by the kidneys. When a drug is ionizable, intracellular and CNS drug levels may be reduced and renal excretion increased by ion-trapping. Ionizable drugs cross lipid membranes (cell wall or blood barrier) only in a nonionized state. Alkaline pH favors dissociation (ion-trapping) of weakly acidic drugs (phenobarbital, salicylates). Acid pH favors ion-trapping of weakly basic drugs (amphetamines, PCP). Potassium depletion may prevent excretion of salicylates. Substances whose excretion may be definitely enhanced by diuresis include phenobarbitol (alkaline) and salicylates (alkaline) (Table 54-3). The goal of diuresis is to increase urinary excretion from a normal of 0.5-2.0 ml/kg/hr to a diuresis of 3-6 ml/kg/hr. Initially, give 0.9%NS or LR at 20 ml/kg over 1 hr if patient is dehydrated and adjust to maintain diuresis.

a. Alkaline diuresis is achieved by giving $NaHCO_3$ 1-2 mEq/kg/dose IV over 1 hr, with K^+ supplement as necessary. Adding 2-3 adult ampules (44.5 mEq $NaHCO_3$ per ampule) to 1 L of D5W will result in solution that is not hypertonic and that facilitates alkalinization. Urine pH should be >7.5. Monitor electrolytes. Potassium usually must be given. Contraindicated if pulmonary or cerebral edema or renal failure exist.

b. Acid diuresis is no longer recommended.

TABLE 54-3. Volume of distribution and efficacy of diuresis and dialysis

Drug	Volume of distribution (L/kg)*	Diuresis	Dialysis
Acetaminophen	1.0	No	No
Amphetamine	0.6	No	No
Benzodiazepines	>10	No	No
Caffeine	0.9	No	No
Digoxin	7.5-15	No	No
Ethanol	0.6	No	No
Ethylene glycol	0.6	No	Yes
Methanol	0.6	No	Yes
Narcotics	>5	No	No
Phencyclidine	8.5	No	No
Phenobarbital	0.75	Alkaline	Yes
Phenothiazines	>30	No	No
Phenytoin	0.75	No	No
Salicylates	0.3-0.6	Alkaline	Yes
Theophylline	0.46	No	Yes†
Tricyclic antidepressants	>8	No	No

*Dose (mg/kg)/plasma concentration (mg/L).

†Theophylline overdoses of significance may be treated with hemoperfusion. Dialysis may be useful if hemoperfusion is unavailable or patient is small child.

2. *Dialysis*, usually considered after failure of conservative medical treatment, may be useful in only a few circumstances. It is indicated if life-threatening symptoms are present with markedly elevated serum levels of phenobarbital, salicylates, theophylline, methanol, ethylene glycol, and lithium. Immediate dialysis should be performed for unresponsive patients, significant acidosis, renal failure, visual symptoms, or peak levels >50 mg/dl following methanol ingestion.

3. *Hemoperfusion* with charcoal or resin-filled devices has become increasingly popular but is still controversial. Hemoperfusion appears particularly useful for significant theophylline overdoses, but because of the greater availability of hemodialysis, it is usually preferred.

Antidotes (Table 54-4)

Specific antidotes are useful when used appropriately. The heretofore universal antidote (burned toast, magnesium oxide, and tannic acid) has no place in modern therapy.

Disposition

1. Discharge from the ED must reflect the severity of the ingestion and potential life-threatening medical and psychiatric considerations.

2. Before discharging the patient, specific attention must be focused on *poison prevention*, with emphasis on discarding old medications and placing needed drugs and toxic household substances in locked cabinets.

3. Patients overdosing as suicide gestures or environmental manipulation should receive *psychiatric evaluation* before discharge (p. 579).

4. Incidents of child abuse must be referred to the appropriate child welfare authorities (Chapter 25).

TOXIC SYNDROMES

While a patient's history is being obtained and the physical examination performed, certain toxic syndromes may become evident. This can assist the physician by focusing on a class of toxins to which the patient may have been exposed.

Narcotics and sedative-hypnotics (p. 295)

These drugs, which cause associated cardiorespiratory depression, can result in coma.

Diagnostic findings

1. Narcotics produce miosis (except with meperidine), noncardiogenic pulmonary edema, and seizures, especially with propoxyphene or meperidine.
   a. Anticholinergic findings—diphenoxylate (Lomotil) and atropine
   b. Treatment: naloxone (Narcan) 0.8 mg (2 adult ampules) initially IV; if no response, 2 mg (5 ampules) IV (also available as 1 mg/ml ampule). Propoxyphene (Darvon) and pentazocine (Talwin) ingestion may require very large doses for reversal. The use of naloxone is both therapeutic and diagnostic. Occasionally, a continuous infusion may be required.

2. Sedative-hypnotics: benzodiazepines (diazepam, etc.), barbiturates, methaqualone (Quāālude), meprobamate (Miltown), glutethimide (Doriden), ethchlorvynol (Placidyl), and methyprylon (Noludar)
   • Treatment: prevention of absorption and supportive care (alkaline diuresis for phenobarbital)

Anticholinergics (p. 284)

Classes of drugs include:
1. Antihistamines
2. Antiparkinsonian—benztropine (Cogentin)
3. Belladonna alkaloids (atropine)
4. Butyrophenones (haloperidol)
5. GI and GU antispasmodics
6. Over-the-counter (OTC) analgesics (Midol, Excedrin)
7. Over-the-counter cold remedies
8. Over-the-counter sleeping preparations
9. Phenothiazines
10. Tricyclic antidepressants

Plants may also be sources, such as *Amanita muscaria*.

TABLE 54-4. Common antidotes

Drug	Diagnostic findings requiring treatment	Antidote
Acetaminophen	History of ingestion and serum level; hepatotoxicity	N-acetylcysteine
Anticholinergics Antihistamines Atropine Phenothiazines Tricyclic antide- pressants	Supraventricular tachycardia (hemodynamic compromise) Unresponsive ventricular dysrhythmia, seizures, pronounced hallucinations or agitation	Physostigmine
Cholinergics Physostigmine Insecticides	Cholinergic crisis: salivation, lacrimation, urination, defecation, convulsions, fasciculations	Atropine sulfate
Carbon monoxide	Headache, seizure, coma, dysrhythmias	Oxygen, hyperbaric oxygen
Cyanide	Cyanosis, seizures, cardiopulmonary arrest, coma	Amyl nitrite Sodium nitrite (3%) Sodium thiosulfate (25%) Also consider hyperbaric oxygen
Ethylene glycol	Metabolic acidosis, urine Ca oxalate crystals	Ethanol (100% absolute, 1 ml-790 mg)
Iron	Hypotension, shock, coma, serum iron >350 mg/dl (or greater than iron-binding capacity)	Deferoxamine
Phenothiazines Chlorpromazine Thioridazine	Extrapyramidal dyskinesis, oculogyric crisis	Diphenhydramine (Benadryl)
Methanol	Metabolic acidosis, blurred vision; level >20 mg/dl	Ethanol (100% absolute)
Methemoglobin Nitrate Nitrites Sulfonamide	Cyanosis, methemoglobin level >30%, dyspnea	Methylene blue (1% solution)
Narcotics Heroin Codeine Propoxyphene	Respiratory depression, hypotension, coma	Naloxone (Narcan)
Organophosphates Malathion Parathion	Cholinergic crisis: salivation, lacrimation, urination, defecation, convulsions, fasciculations	Atropine sulfate Pralidoxime

Adapted from Conner, C.S., Robertson, N.J., Murphrey, K.J., et al.: Rational use of emergency antidotes, permission of Aspen Publishers, Inc., ©, 1979.

Dosage

---

140 mg/kg/dose PO, then 70 mg/kg/
   dose q 4 hr PO × 17
Child: 0.5 mg IV slowly (over 3 min) q
   10 min prn (maximum: 2 mg)
Adult: 1-2 mg IV slowly q 10 min prn
   (maximum: 4 mg in 30 min)

0.05 mg/kg/dose (usual dose 1-5 mg;
   test dose for child 0.01 mg/kg) q 4-
   6 hr IV or more frequently prn
100% oxygen (half-life 40 min); consider hyperbaric chamber
Inhale 30 sec q 60 sec
0.27 ml (8.7 mg)/kg (adult: 300 mg) IV
   slowly (Hb 10 g)
1.35 ml (325 mg)/kg (adult: 12.5 g) IV
   slowly (Hb 10 g)

1 ml/kg in D5W IV over 15 min, then
   0.16 ml (125 mg)/kg/hr IV; maintain
   ethanol level of 100 mg/dl
Shock or coma: 15 mg/kg/hr IV for 8
   hr; if no shock or coma 90 mg/kg/
   dose IM q 8 hr
1-2 mg/kg/dose (maximum: 50 mg/
   dose) q 6 hr IV, PO

1 ml/kg in D5W over 15 min, then 0.16
   ml (125 mg)/kg/hr IV
1-2 mg (0.1-0.2 ml)/kg/dose IV; repeat
   in 4 hr if necessary

0.8 mg (2 adult ampules) initially IV, if
   no response give 2 mg (5 vials) IV

0.05 mg/kg/dose (usual dose 1-5 mg)
   IV prn or q 4-6 hr
After atropine, 20-50 mg/kg/dose (maximum: 2,000 mg) IV slowly (<50 mg/
   min) q 8 hr IV prn × 3

In Top. Emerg. Med. **1:**27, 1979. Reprinted with

Diagnostic findings

Peripheral signs include:
1. Tachycardia
2. Dry, flushed skin
3. Dry mucous membranes
4. Dilated pupils
5. Hyperpyrexia
6. Urinary retention
7. Decreased bowel sounds
8. Dysrhythmias
9. Hypertension
10. Hypotension (late)

Central anticholinergic syndrome causes:
1. Delirium—organic brain syndrome
   a. Disorientation
   b. Agitation
   c. Hallucinations
   d. Psychosis
   e. Loss of memory
2. Extrapyramidal movements
3. Ataxia
4. Picking or grasping movements
5. Seizures
6. Coma
7. Respiratory failure
8. Cardiovascular collapse

Phenothiazines may result in pronounced hypotension secondary to alpha-blocking action (p. 299).

Treatment

1. Seizures: diazepam (Valium) or phenobarbital; for the unresponsive or psychotic patient, physostigmine
2. Dysrhythmias (tricyclics): alkalinization, phenytoin, lidocaine; for the unresponsive or psychotic patient, physostigmine (p. 285)
3. Pronounced hallucinations and agitation (in which patient may be in danger of harming self or others): may require physostigmine
   • Physostigmine 0.5 mg IV (children) or 1-2 mg IV (adults) slowly

Cholinergics

These include organophosphates and carbamate pesticides (p. 297), physostigmine, neostigmine, pyridostigmine, and edrophonium (Tensilon).

Diagnostic findings

1. "SLUDGE": *s*alivation, *l*acrimation, *u*rination, *d*efecation, *G*I cramping and diarrhea, and *e*mesis. Patients appear "wet."
2. CNS effects: headache, restlessness, and anxiety progressing to confusion, coma, and seizures
3. Sweating, miosis, muscle fasciculations, muscle weakness, bradycardia, bronchorrhea, and bronchospasm

Treatment

1. Decontamination and support
2. Atropine (blocks acetylcholine) 0.05 mg/kg/dose (usual dose 1-5 mg) q 10 min prn or q 4-6 hr IV. The end point of atropinization should be drying of pulmonary secretions. Following pupil size is unsatisfactory, as the pupils may initially be dilated.
3. Pralidoxine 2-PAM (cholinesterase reactivator) 20-50 mg/kg/dose IV slowly q 8 hr IV prn (3 times) after atropine

Sympathomimetic (p. 300)

These include amphetamines, phenylpropanolamine, ephedrine, and cocaine.

Diagnostic findings

These are similar to anticholinergic syndrome:

1. Psychoses, hallucinations, delirium
2. Nausea, vomiting, and abdominal pain
3. Possibly prominent piloerection
4. Tachycardia and cardiac dysrhythmias
5. Severe hypertension

Treatment

1. Supportive care after gastric emptying
2. Propranolol 0.01-0.1 mg/kg/dose (up to 1 mg/dose) q 5 min prn IV slowly for tachyrhythmias if pulse rate also elevated
3. Diazepam (Valium) 0.1-0.2 mg/kg/dose q 4-6 hr IV or PO for sedation
4. Haloperidol (Haldol) 1-10 mg IM or IV q 15 min prn

Drug-induced psychosis requires a reassuring attitude and maintaining verbal contact with the patient. Physical restraints should be avoided.

Classic manifestations of toxicity

See Tables 54-1 and 54-2 and the box on the opposite page.

Although there is tremendous variability in clinical presentations, certain manifestations of toxicity are commonly recognized and are particularly helpful in identifying unknown poisons.

REFERENCES

Boehnert, M.T., Lewander, W.J., Gaudreault, P., et al.: Advances in clinical toxicology, Pediatr. Clin. North Am. **32:**193, 1985.

Chafee-Bahamon, C., Lacouture, P.G., and Lovejoy, F.H.: Risk assessment of ipecac in the home, Pediatrics **75:**1105, 1985.

Comstock, E.G., Faulkner, T.P., Boisaubin, E.V., et al.: Studies in the efficacy of gastric lavage as practiced in a large metropolitan hospital, Clin. Toxicol. **18:**581, 1981.

Fazen, L.E., Lovejoy, F.H., and Crone, R.K.: Acute poisoning in a children's hospital: a 2-year experience, Pediatrics **77:**144, 1986.

Gilman, A.G., Goodman, L.S., and Gilman, A.: The pharmacological basis of therapeutics, ed. 7, New York, 1985, Macmillan, Inc.

Goldfrank, L.R.: Toxicologic emergencies: a comprehensive handbook in problem solving, New York, 1982, Appleton-Century-Crofts.

Ingelfinger, J.A., Isakson, G., Shine, D., et al.: Reliability of the toxic screen in drug overdose, Clin. Pharm. Ther. **29:**570, 1981.

Kelley, M.T., Werman, H.A., and Rund, D.A.: Use of activated charcoal in the treatment of drug overdoses, Am. J. Emerg. Med. **3:**280, 1985.

Kulig, K., Bar-Or, D., Cantrill, S.V., et al.: Management of acutely poisoned patients without gastric emptying, Ann. Emerg. Med. **14:**562, 1985.

Kulig, K., and Rumack, B.H.: Management of acute poisoning and overdoses, Denver, 1985, Rocky Mountain Poison Center.

Thompson, D.F., Trammel, H.L., Robertson, N.J., et al.: Evaluation of regional and nonregional poison centers, N. Engl. J. Med. **308:**191, 1983.

CLUES TO DIAGNOSIS OF UNKNOWN POISONS: LABORATORY AND OTHER ALTERATIONS

METABOLIC ACIDOSIS ("MUDPIES")

Methanol	Isoniazid, iron
Uremia	Ethanol, ethylene glycol
Diabetes mellitus	Salicylates, starvation
Paraldehyde	

NOTE: Metabolic acidosis may be caused by the above drugs, all cellular poisons, and all drugs causing seizures.

GLUCOSE

Increased	Decreased
Salicylates	Acetaminophen
Isoniazid	Isoniazid
Iron	Salicylates
Isopropyl alcohol	Methanol
	Insulin
	Ethanol

URINE COLOR

Red: hematuria, hemoglobinuria, myoglobinuria, pyrvinium (Povan), phenytoin (Dilantin), phenothiazines, mercury, lead, iron, anthrocycan (food pigment in beets and blackberries)

Brown-black: hemoglobin pigments, melanin, methyldopa (Aldomet), cascara, rhubarb, methocarbamol (Robaxin)

Blue, blue-green, green: amitriptyline, methylene blue, indigo blue, triamterene (Dyazide), Clorets, *Pseudomonas*

Brown, red-brown: porphyria, urobilinogen, nitrofurantoin, furazolidone, metronidazole, aloe (seaweed)

Orange: dehydration, rifampin, phenazopyridine (Pyridium), sulfasalazine (Azulfidine)

X-RAY STUDY (radiopaque medications: "CHIPE", i.e., heavy metals and enteric-coated tablets)

Chloral hydrate	Phenothiazines
Heavy metals	Enteric coated tablets
Iron	

BREATH ODOR

Alcohol: ethanol, chloral hydrate, phenols
Acetone: acetone, salicylates, isopropyl alcohol, paraldehyde
Bitter almond: cyanide
Burned rope: marijuana
Garlic: arsenic, phosphorus, organophosphates
Oil of Wintergreen: methylsalicylates
Rotten egg: disulfiram

55 Specific ingestions

Acetaminophen

Acetaminophen is a widely used antipyretic and analgesic that is metabolized in the liver in part by conjugation with glutathione. After an acetaminophen overdose, the glutathione substrate can be overwhelmed, and a toxic metabolite is formed via an alternate pathway. The toxic metabolite may bind covalently to hepatic macromolecules, producing cellular necrosis.

In adults, 150 mg/kg is considered a toxic overdose, but the same dose may produce only minor changes in children under 10 yr; children appear less susceptible to injury. Simultaneous ingestion of alcohol, as well as malnutrition, appears to be hepatoprotective. Therapeutic levels are 10-20 μg/ml, whereas toxic levels are 150 μg/ml at 4 hr and 37.5 μg/ml at 12 hr.

DIAGNOSTIC FINDINGS

The history of ingestion is usually inadequate and bears little correlation to the blood levels. Patients may develop hepatic failure secondary to necrosis of the centrilobular type. Encephalopathy, coma, and death may follow. Children are unlikely to have toxic levels if they experienced early, spontaneous emesis.

1. Initially, patients may develop gastrointestinal symptoms and diaphoresis during the 7-14 hr following ingestion. Many remain asymptomatic.
2. An asymptomatic period follows for 24-48 hr, although hepatic enzymes begin to rise.
3. After about 72 hr evidence of liver injury becomes apparent, with markedly elevated hepatic enzymes, which subsequently normalize over the ensuing 4-7 days.

Ancillary data

1. Acetaminophen level obtained 4 hr after ingestion and plotted on nomogram (Fig. 55-1). Level is considered toxic if it is 25% below line on nomogram (4 hr: 150 μg/ml). At equal toxic blood levels, children under 10 yr are less likely to develop hepatic toxicity.
2. Liver function test, including SGOT, SGPT, bilirubin, and PT
3. ABG and other evaluations as indicated by CNS findings

DIFFERENTIAL DIAGNOSIS

1. Infection: acute gastroenteritis (Chapter 76) and hepatitis (p. 487)
2. Encephalopathy (p. 556)

MANAGEMENT

The decision regarding intervention is based on the presumed history of ingestion and, ideally, an acetaminophen level. Information regarding the treatment protocol can be obtained from the Rocky Mountain Poison Control Center at 1-800-525-6115.

1. Initial stabilization of patient. Emesis or lavage may be indicated. If charcoal is given in initial treatment, stomach should be lavaged if N-acetylcysteine is to be administered orally because charcoal theoretically

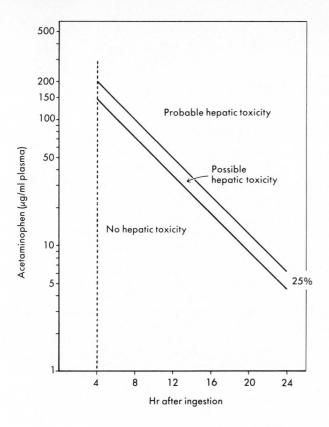

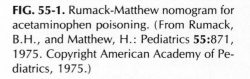

FIG. 55-1. Rumack-Matthew nomogram for acetaminophen poisoning. (From Rumack, B.H., and Matthew, H.: Pediatrics **55**:871, 1975. Copyright American Academy of Pediatrics, 1975.)

decreases the absorption of N-acetylcysteine.

2. N-Acetylcysteine 20% (Mucomyst): diluted fourfold to a 5% solution in grapefruit juice, water, or cola. An IV preparation also is available.

   a. Indicated if serum acetaminophen level is in the toxic range and less than 24 hr has elapsed since ingestion. Toxic levels are considered to be those levels 25% below the concentration known to cause hepatic toxicity in adults. Children appear to have more resistance to toxicity.

   b. If no levels are immediately available and the ingestion is considered to be toxic, therapy should be initiated and may be stopped if level comes back in safe range.

   c. Dosage. Load with 140 mg/kg/dose PO followed by 70 mg/kg/dose q 4 hr PO for 17 doses. An IV preparation also is available. Full regimen should be completed if initial level was toxic and subsequent ones return to normal during the treatment course.

DISPOSITION

All patients requiring treatment with N-acetylcysteine should be admitted for treatment and monitoring. Long-term follow-up will be required.

REFERENCE

Rumack, B.H., Peterson, R.C., Koch, G.G., et al.: Acetaminophen overdose: 622 cases with evaluation of oral acetylcysteine treatment, Arch. Intern. Med. **141**:380, 1981.

Alcohols: ethanol, isopropyl, methanol, ethylene glycol

Ethanol is becoming an increasingly popular drug among adolescents. The immediate medical problems, as well as the long-term psychiatric ones, must be treated.

DIAGNOSTIC FINDINGS (Table 55-1)

Classically, the progression of findings in nontolerant intoxicated individuals is related to the blood alcohol level (Table 55-2). There is a progressive change in mental status and sensory impairment, ultimately leading to respiratory failure and death.

1. *Ethanol* equivalents: 53.3 ml (about 2 oz) of absolute ethanol (100% or 200 proof) results in a peak blood level of about 100 mg/dl at 1 hr after ingestion in an adult.

2. *Isopropryl* alcohol is considered to be more of a CNS depressant and gastrointestinal irritant than ethanol. There may be a smell of

TABLE 55-2. Blood ethanol levels and clinical findings in the nontolerant adult

Blood ethanol level (mg/dl)	Clinical findings
≤99	Changes in mood, personality, behavior
	Progressive muscular incoordination
	Impaired sensory function
100-199	Marked mental and sensory impairment
	Incoordination, ataxia
	Prolonged reaction time
	Grossly intoxicated
200-299	Nausea, vomiting, diplopia, marked ataxia
300-399	Amnesia, dysarthria, hypothermia
400-700	Coma, respiratory failure, death

TABLE 55-1. Alcohol ingestion and overdose

Alcohol (uses)	Toxic level	CNS depression	Acidosis	Ketonemia	Increased osmolality at 50 mg/dl
Ethanol (beverages, mouthwash, perfumes)	3-5 g/kg (>100 mg/dl)	+	±	±	11.4 mOsm/kg H_2O
Isopropyl (rubbing alcohol, solvent)	2-3 g/kg (>50 mg/dl)	+	+	+ +	8.5 mOsm/kg H_2O
Methanol (canned heat, antifreeze, solvent, denaturant)	1-2 ml/kg (>20 mg/dl)		+ + +	±	11.4 mOsm/kg H_2O
Ethylene glycol (antifreeze, deicer)	1-2 ml/kg (>20 mg/dl)	+	+ + +	−	8.3 mOsm/kg H_2O

Modified from Goldfrank, L.R., and Starke, C.L.: Metabolic acidosis in the alcoholic. In Goldfrank, L.R.: Toxicologic emer

acetone on the breath following ingestion.

3. *Methanol* ingestion results in a nonintoxicated, acidotic patient with visual symptoms 3-24 hr after ingestion.
4. *Ethylene glycol* produces an intoxicated patient with severe acidosis, rapid progression of CNS signs, renal dysfunction frequently associated with calcium oxalate crystalluria, pulmonary edema, and shock.

There is frequently an associated ingestion of a drug or another alcohol and there are many alcohol drug interactions.

Ancillary data

1. Ethanol, methanol, ethylene glycol, and isopropanol levels
2. Blood glucose, electrolytes, osmolality (by freezing point depression), and ABG

DIFFERENTIAL DIAGNOSIS

Differentiation of the alcohols may be made on the basis of blood levels, acid-base status, breath odor, and diagnostic findings.

- Metabolic acidosis: "MUDPIES" (methanol, *u*remia, *d*iabetes mellitus, *p*araldehyde, *i*ron, *i*soniazide, *e*thanol, *e*thylene glycol, *s*alicylates, and *s*tarvation). Acidosis is caused by these agents, those that cause seizures, and all cellular poisons (e.g., iron, cyanide).

MANAGEMENT

1. *Supportive care* with particular attention to the airway and fluids. Treatment of acidosis, hypoglycemia, hypocalcemia, respiratory and renal failure, or pulmonary edema
2. *Gastric emptying* within 6 hr of ingestion or if there is any question of associated ingestion.
3. *Ethanol*, as outlined in Table 55-1, for methanol or ethylene glycol ingestions. Maintain ethanol level at $\geq$ 100 mg/dl.
4. *Dialysis* is indicated early in the treatment of methanol and ethylene glycol ingestions,

Diagnostic findings	Odor on breath	Treatment
Intoxication with nausea, vomiting, ataxia, uncoordination, slurred speech progressing to seizures, coma, hypothermia, respiratory failure, death	Ethanol	Gastric emptying, fluids, glucose support; blood level declines at 15-35 mg/dl/hr; consider dialysis if life threatening
Intoxication with significant CNS depression, hemorrhagic tracheobronchitis, gastritis; twice toxicity of ethanol	Acetone	Gastric emptying, fluids support; dialysis if life threatening
Not intoxicated; delayed onset; slight CNS depression initially may become severe; intractable acidosis; blurred vision with pink edema of optic disk in 12-24 hr; abdominal pain (pancreatitis)	None	Gastric emptying, fluids support; ethanol (100%) 1 ml/kg over 15 min, then 0.16 ml (125 mg)/kg/hr IV; dialysis if peak level >50 mg/dl, visual symptoms, or severe acidosis
Intoxicated—stupor, ataxia progressing to seizures, coma; severe acidosis; ocular—nystagmus; CHF and pulmonary edema; shock; renal failure—calcium oxalate crystalluria, oligura, hypocalcemia	None	Gastric emptying, fluids support; calcium prn; ethanol (100%) 1 ml/kg over 15 min, then 0.16 ml (125 mg)/kg/hr IV; dialysis if renal failue, severe acidosis or peak level >50 mg/dl

gencies, New York, 1982, Appleton-Century-Crofts.

with peak levels >50 mg/dl or accompanying severe acidosis, but only in life-threatening intoxication of ethanol and isopropyl alcohol. NOTE: Adolescents and adults undergoing alcohol withdrawal and the hyperkinetic state associated with chronic use of ethanol may be partially controlled with clorazepate (Tranxene) 15 mg q 6 hr PO, lorazepam (Ativan) 0.5-1.0 mg q 6 hr PO, *or* chlordiazepoxide (Librium) 50-100 mg IM or IV in adult. Diazepam (Valium) also may be useful.

DISPOSITION

All pediatric patients with significant methanol or ethylene glycol ingestions should be admitted, as well as those with toxic levels of ethanol and isopropyl alcohol.

Long-term psychiatric follow-up usually is indicated.

REFERENCE

Roth, A., Normann, S.A., Manoguerra, A.S., et al.: Short-term hemodialysis in childhood ethylene glycol poisoning, J. Pediatr. **108**:153, 1986.

Alkalis and acids

ALERT: Immediate dilution with milk or water should be initiated.

A large number of household products contain alkali or acid and may be ingested by the curious child. Accidental ingestions usually occur in children under 4 yr of age, whereas older individuals may be attempting suicide or self-mutilation.

ETIOLOGY

1. Common alkalis
   a. Sodium or potassium hydroxide (lye), washing powders, paint removers, drain pipe and toilet bowl cleaners, Clinitest tablets
   b. Liquids: drain (Liquid Plumber, Drāno) and oven cleaners

   c. Solid: Drāno (granular), Clinitest (tablets)
   d. Other: sodium hypochlorite bleach (if >5%), some detergents, electric dishwashing agents
   e. Button (disk) batteries
2. Common acid
   a. Hydrochloric acid: metal, swimming pool, and toilet bowl cleaners
   b. Sulfuric acid: battery acid, toilet bowl cleaners, industrial drain cleaners
   c. Other: slate cleaners, soldering flux

DIAGNOSTIC FINDINGS

The nature of the ingestion must be defined. Specific attention should be directed to the material ingested (solid or liquid, acid or alkali), to its volume, to the length of contact (when? was there emesis? was diluent used?), to the volume of liquids or solids in the stomach at the time of ingestion, and to the presence of pain, dysphagia, drooling, or other symptoms.

Physical examination should include a check for drooling, respiratory distress, oral or pharyngeal burns, evidence of chest pathology or mediastinitis, and abdominal pain, guarding, or tenderness.

1. *Alkalis* primarily produce liquefaction necrosis and thermal injury, with deep tissue penetration and a high risk of perforation. Skin burns and major ocular injury may occur (Chapters 46 and 59). Initially, esophageal burn is characterized by erythema followed by shallow ulceration within 24 hr. Edema may lead to narrowing in 48-72 hr and eventually scar tissue and strictures 4-6 wk after the initial injury.
   a. Oropharyngeal burns with associated drooling and dysphagia are common. Crystalline caustics tend to attach to the oral mucosa and produce severe burns of the mouth rather than the esophagus. Gulping caustic liquids may spare the oral and pharyngeal mucosa and cause severe burns of the esophagus. Solid alkali, particularly lye, may lodge in the oropharynx

or esophagus. Clinitest tablets have a high incidence of esophageal burns with stricture, intestinal perforation, and laryngeal edema.

b. The absence of oropharyngeal burns does not exclude esophageal injury. Esophageal injury is most commonly present if two or more of the following are present: vomiting, drooling, or stridor. Esophageal perforation may result in mediastinitis and shock. Stricture may develop as a delayed complication.

c. Soft tissue swelling of the upper airway caused by involvement of the larynx, epiglottis, or vocal cords or by tracheal aspiration may produce respiratory distress.

2. *Acid* substances cause coagulation necrosis and thermal injury. The skin may be burned by exposure, and a major ocular emergency results from acid exposure (Chapters 46 and 59). There may be associated soft-tissue swelling, with potential respiratory obstruction. Specific effects may include:

a. Oropharyngeal burns with significant ingestions; rare esophageal perforation

b. Perforation of the stomach or small intestine, acute peritonitis, and shock

3. Bleach in combination with acids (HCl) may produce chlorine gas, resulting in pulmonary damage if inhaled. Household bleach ingestion (about 3%), rarely causes esophageal burns.

Ancillary data

1. CBC, type and cross-match, and ABG with significant exposure

2. X-ray films. Lateral neck may be useful in evaluating upper respiratory edema; chest and abdominal films are needed if there are extensive complications.

MANAGEMENT

The first priority must be to assess the airway and ensure that any obstruction, if present, is relieved. If there are extensive burns of the oro-

pharynx, a cricothyrotomy may be indicated. Ventilation and circulatory insufficiency must be treated.

1. Administer oxygen, particularly if the exposure has been to chlorine gas.

2. Dilute ingested material with milk or water as soon as possible. This should optimally be initiated at home before leaving for ED. Do not use weak acids or alkalis for neutralization, since a tremendous amount of heat can be produced. If involved, the skin should be washed well and each eye irrigated with 1-2 L saline for at least 20 min (Chapter 59).
NOTE: Dilution of ingested material is contraindicated if perforation, shock, or upper airway compromise is present.

3. Do not initiate emesis, lavage, or catharsis or give charcoal.

Other considerations

1. Steroids may have a role in deep or circumferential esophageal burns, but their role is controversial. If used, they should be initiated as soon after injury as possible and continued for at least 3 wk.
   • Hydrocortisone (Solu-Cortef) 4-5 mg/kg/dose q 6 hr IV *or* methylprednisolone (Solu-Medrol) 2 mg/kg/dose q 6 hr IV

2. Antibiotics are not indicated prophylactically but may be required if mediastinitis or perforation develops.

3. A surgeon should be involved early in the evaluation. Surgery is immediately required if perforation or mediastinitis develops.

4. Esophagoscopy should be performed in the first 24-48 hr following ingestion in all patients with any oropharyngeal burns, symptomatology, or history of significant ingestion.

a. Should be performed only to the point of the burn and not beyond

b. Contraindicated with respiratory obstruction, perforation, shock, or third-degree burns of the oropharynx

5. Button (disk) batteries require special con-

siderations. Children with a history of ingestion should have radiographs performed to localize the battery. If it is lodged in the esophagus, removal should be done immediately. Batteries less than 18 mm (penny size) rarely are stopped in the esophagus. Beyond the esophagus, the patient should be followed and observed for symptoms; if symptoms develop, the battery requires removal. Cathartics may be helpful. Follow-up in 7 days is useful if the battery has not been found in the stools.

6. The timing of esophageal dilation and bougienage is controversial, most preferring to wait until several weeks after injury. Serial barium swallows may provide evidence of developing esophageal stricture; if present, discontinue steroids and begin dilation.

DISPOSITION

All patients with oropharyngeal burns should be admitted for fluid management and observation of respiratory and gastrointestinal complications, as well as for esophagoscopy. Nutrition must be maintained.

Long-term follow-up is essential to monitor the development of esophageal or gastric stenosis, with esohagoscopy or barium studies. Dilation and bougienage may be necessary. In patients who develop complete obliteration of the esophagus from stricture or who have not responded to dilation, colon interposition may be considered.

Psychiatric involvement is required in self-inflicted injuries, and poison-prevention counseling is essential.

REFERENCES

Crain, E.F., Gershel, J.C., and Mezey, A.P.: Caustic ingestions: symptoms as predictors of esophageal injury, Am. J. Dis. Child **138**:863, 1984.

Krenzelok, E.P.: Caustic esophageal and gastric erosion without evidence of oral burns following detergent ingestion, J.A.C.E.P. **8**:194, 1979.

Litovitz, T.L., Butterfield, A.B., Holloway, R.R., et al.: Button battery ingestion: assessment of therapeutic modalities and battery discharge state, J. Pediatr. **105**:868, 1984.

Rumack, B.H., and Rumack, C.M.: Disk battery ingestion, JAMA **249**:2509, 1983.

Wason, S.: The emergency management of caustic ingestions, J. Emerg. Med. **2**:175, 1985.

Wasserman, R.L., and Ginsburg, C.M.: Caustic substance injuries, J. Pediatr. **107**:169, 1985.

Anticholinergics

ALERT: Peripheral and central effects are prominent. Physostigmine is indicated for unresponsive seizures and dangerous psychoses.

A wide spectrum of drugs possess anticholinergic properties. For most of these agents, there is good GI absorption with a peak effect of 1-2 hr.

PHARMACEUTICS WITH ANTICHOLINERGIC PROPERTIES

1. Antihistamines: diphenhydramine (Benadryl), tripelennamine (Pyribenzamine)
2. Belladonna alkaloids and related synthetic compounds: atropine, scopolamine, glycopyrrolate
3. Phenothiazines: chlorpromazine (Thorazine), thioridazine (Mellaril), prochlorperazine (Compazine), trifluoperazine (Stelazine)
4. Butyrophenones: haloperidol (Haldol)
5. Thioxanthenes: chlorprothixene (Taractan), thiothixene (Navane)
6. Tricyclic antidepressants: amitriptyline (Elavil), nortriptyline (Pamelor), imipramine (Tofranil), desipramine (Norpramin), doxepin (Sinequan)
7. GI and GU antispasmodics: dicyclomine (Bentyl), propantheline bromide (Pro-Banthine)
8. Local mydriatics: tropicamide (Mydriacyl), cyclopentolate (Cyclogyl)
9. Over-the-counter (OTC) analgesics: pyrilamine (Excedrin P.M.), cinnamedrine (Midol)

10. OTC cold remedies
11. OTC sleep aids: pyrilamine (Sominex, Sleep-Eze), doxylamine (Unisom)
12. Antiparkinsonian medications: benztropine (Cogentin), trihexyphenidyl (Artane)

PLANTS CONTAINING ANTICHOLINERGIC ALKALOIDS

1. *Amanita muscaria* (fly agaric)
2. *Amanita pantherina* (panther mushroom)
3. *Datura stramonium* (jimsonweed)
4. *Myristica fragrans* (nutmeg)
5. *Solanum carolinense* (wild tomato)
6. *Solanum dulcamara* (bittersweet)
7. *Solan tuberosum* (potato)
8. *Lantana camara* (wild sage)

DIAGNOSTIC FINDINGS

Anticholinergics present a consistent clinical picture, although there is some variability in findings with specific drugs. Patients with diphenoxylate and atropine (Lomotil) overdoses primarily have anticholinergic (atropine) findings initially, but many hours after ingestion they may develop cardiopulmonary depression, miosis, hypotension, and coma consistent with a narcotic overdose.

1. *Peripheral* signs and symptoms of anticholinergic overdose result primarily from muscarinic blockage:
   a. Vital sign alterations: tachycardia, hyperpyrexia, hypertension. Hypotension may be a late finding (phenothiazines may cause hypotension because of their alpha-blocking action)
   b. Dry flushed skin and dry mucous membranes
   c. Dilated pupils (mydriasis)
   d. Urinary retention and decreased bowel sounds
   e. Dysrhythmias, primarily as a result of direct myocardial depressant effect. Only tricyclic antidepressants predictably cause ventricular dysrhythmias. Tricyclic antidepressants also prolong AV conduc-

tion and prevent reuptake of norepinephrine, leading to ventricular dysrhythmias and heart block. Thioridazine (Mellaril) may have a similar effect.
2. *Central* anticholinergic syndrome: a delirium characteristic of an evolving organic brain syndrome. Signs are:
   a. Disorientation, uncontrolled agitation, impaired long-term memory, and hallucinations. Patient is rarely violent or self-mutilating.
   b. Movement disorders
      (1) Phenothiazines and tricyclic antidepressants frequently cause extrapyramidal reactions, including myoclonus and choreoathetosis.
      (2) Picking and grasping movements are common with overdoses of most of the anticholinergics.
   c. Seizures, coma, respiratory failure, and cardiovascular collapse.

Ancillary data

1. Urine toxicology screen may be useful, but the laboratory should be notified which agents are suspected.
2. Glucose, ECG, and ABG as indicated.
3. X-ray films. Abdominal film taken before tablets dissolve may show phenothiazine.

MANAGEMENT

Supportive care (airway management and maintaining vital signs) is of highest priority. All comatose patients should receive 0.5-1.0 g/kg IV dextrose and 0.1 mg/kg (maximum 0.8 mg or 2 adult ampules) IV naloxone.

Physostigmine is a naturally occurring alkaloid that is a reversible cholinesterase inhibitor. Centrally, it crosses the blood-brain barrier and is capable of reversing coma, delirium, seizures, and extrapyramidal signs. Peripherally, it is effective in reversing the muscarinic blockade.

1. Indications for physostigmine
   a. Supraventricular dysrhythmias resulting in hemodynamic instability

b. Ventricular dysrhythmias unresponsive to standard antidysrhythmic therapy, including alkalinization and phenytoin in tricyclic antidepressant toxicity

c. Seizures unresponsive to standard anticonvulsants. Myoclonic jerking usually requires physostigmine.

d. Pronounced hallucinations and agitation in which the patient may be a danger to self or others

e. Coma caused by anticholinergic overdose. Physostigmine should be used as a diagnostic test and not given just "to wake the patient up."

NOTE: It is best to reserve physostigmine for life-threatening situations because there are safer agents for treatment of seizures (phenytoin, phenobarbital, and diazepam) and dysrhythmias (alkalinization, phenytoin, lidocaine).

2. Dosage (administer slowly)
   a. Children: 0.5 mg IV slowly over 3 min q 10 min up to 2 mg
   b. Adults: 1-2 mg IV slowly over 3 min q 10 min until cessation of life-threatening condition or until it appears ineffective. Maximum dose: 4 mg in 30 min
3. Side effects. Include seizures, bradyrhythmias, asystole, and cholinergic crisis (hypersalivation, bradycardia, and hypotension).
4. Contraindications. Patients with asthma, gangrene, cardiovascular disease, or obstruction of the GI or GU tracts
   Other management techniques include:
1. Initial treatment of seizures with diazepam (Valium) 0.2-0.3 mg/kg/dose IV, followed by phenobarbital (Chapter 21)
2. Treatment of tricyclic antidepressant overdoses. If the QRS is prolonged or there are ventricular dysrhythmias, treat with sodium bicarbonate 1-2 mEq/kg/dose q 10-20 min IV to achieve alkalinization (plasma pH >7.5), as well as phenytoin or lidocaine (p. 38)
3. Sedation. May usually be achieved by treatment with diazepam (Valium)

4. Large amounts of naloxone (Narcan) 0.8-2.0 mg prn IV with some cases of diphenoxylate (Lomotil) overdoses

DISPOSITION

All symptomatic patients require inpatient treatment and observation, usually in an ICU capable of cardiac and neurologic monitoring.

REFERENCES

Greenblatt, D.J., and Shader, R.I.: Anticholinergics, N. Engl. J. Med. **288**:1215, 1973.
Rumack, B.H.: Pharmacology for the pediatrician: anticholinergic poisoning, Pediatrics **52**:449, 1973.

Aspirin (salicylates)

ALERT: Consider if patient has tachypnea, hyperthermia, or metabolic acidosis.

Ingestion of salicylates is common but has decreased with the widespread use of safety lids on medication bottles and the popularity of acetaminophen-containing products. A wide variety of products contain salicylates, and an acute, single ingestion of 250 mg/kg may produce toxicity. Signs and symptoms are related to the salicylate levels diagrammed in the Done nomogram (Fig. 55-2). Therapeutic levels are 15-30 mg/dl in arthritic conditions. The Done nomogram cannot be used in cases in which chronic ingestion produces symptoms at levels below those normally considered to be toxic or for overdose of sustained release aspirin products. Methyl salicylate (Oil of Wintergreen) is particularly toxic, having 720 mg salicylate/ml.

DIAGNOSTIC FINDINGS

Patients with significant ingestions initially may have tachypnea and deep, labored respirations, hyperthermia, tinnitus, and vomiting. Mental status changes may develop with moderate ingestions, ranging from lethargy or excitability and progressing to seizures and coma.

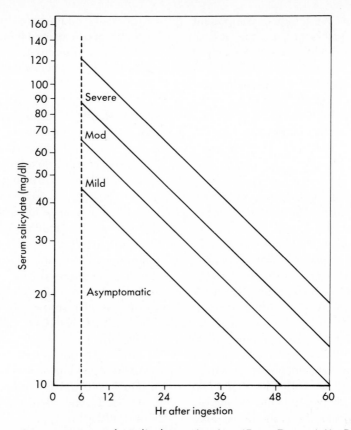

FIG. 55-2. Done nomogram for salicylate poisoning. (From Done, A.K.: Pediatrics **26:**805, 1960. Copyright American Academy of Pediatrics, 1960.)

Patients may develop slurred speech, hallucinations, vertigo, pulmonary edema, and cardiovascular collapse.

Chronic salicylism is associated with accentuated CNS findings and less prominent acid-base abnormalities. Thus levels do not indicate the seriousness of ingestion.

Complications

1. Metabolic
   a. Hypoglycemia, sometimes preceded by an initial hyperglycemia
   b. Metabolic acidosis and respiratory alkalosis. Children under 4 yr develop metabolic acidosis more rapidly, without the concurrent respiratory alkalosis, and this is often the predominant presentation.
   c. Electrolyte abnormalities
      (1) Potassium deficit secondary to acidosis with urinary losses
      (2) Hyponatremia because of inappropriate ADH
2. Noncardiogenic pulmonary edema (Chapter 19)
3. CNS findings in moderate to severe ingestions
   a. Seizures from hypoglycemia, hyponatremia, cerebral edema, or decreased ionized calcium caused by alkali therapy
   b. Coma. May occur in acute ingestions

when the level is very high or the patient has ingested more than one agent. Coma is more common with chronic salicylism (Chapter 15).

4. Bleeding from hypothrombinemia and platelet dysfunction
5. Chemical hepatitis
6. Allergic manifestations, particularly wheezing

Ancillary data

A qualitative test for the presence of aspirin in urine may be performed by adding 5 ml of urine to a few drops of 10% ferric chloride. The urine will turn purple and remain stable if salicylates are present, purple-brown with phenothiazines, purple-red (fades in minutes) with ketosis, and yellowish-green with isoniazid. Normal urine turns brownish, whitish, or yellowish.

To provide a semiquantitative measure of salicylate level one drop of serum may be applied to a Phenistix. A tan color is consistent with a level of <40 mg/dl, brown with a level of 40-90 mg/dl, and purple indicates a level >90 mg/dl.

1. A quantitative salicylate level should be done and interpreted by the Done nomogram (Fig. 55-2). It is not useful in chronic ingestions. Therapeutic: 15-30 mg/dl
2. Electrolytes, glucose, and ABG as indicated
3. Coagulation studies if indicated. Prolonged PT and bleeding time
4. ECG if electrolyte problems are suspected

DIFFERENTIAL DIAGNOSIS

1. Metabolic acidosis ("MUDPIES")
   a. Ingestions: methanol, paraldehyde, iron, isoniazid, ethanol, ethylene glycol
   b. Metabolic: uremia, diabetes mellitus, starvation
   NOTE: In general, metabolic acidosis results from ingestions of the specific drugs listed above, as well as cellular poisons (e.g., iron, cyanide) and drugs that cause seizures. Ad-

ditionally, poor perfusion ischemia or cellular death produces metabolic acidosis.
2. Infection: meningitis, encephalitis, pneumonia, Reye's syndrome

MANAGEMENT

After stabilization, oral absorption should be reduced by emesis (syrup of ipecac) or gastric lavage, activated charcoal, and catharsis. Mild ingestions require no additional therapy.

Moderate or severe ingestions require parenteral therapy with forced alkaline diuresis. Salicylates are weak acids (pKa = 3), and elimination may be facilitated by alkalinization of the urine to pH of 7-8 and correction of potassium and acid-base abnormalities. Ancillary data should be monitored.

1. If the patient is initially dehydrated, expand the vascular volume by D5W.45NS, adding 60 mEq/L $NaHCO_3$. Infuse at 10-20 ml/kg over 1-2 hr.
2. Following the resuscitation and establishment of good urine flow (>2 ml/kg/hr), infuse D5W with 88-132 mEq (2-3 ampules) $NaHCO_3$/L, and 30-40 mEq KCl/L at a rate of 4-8 ml/kg/hr.
   • If a severe metabolic acidosis is present, give an additional 1-2 mEq/kg $NaHCO_3$ IV slowly.
3. Treat hyperpyrexia with cooling blanket.
4. For seizures give diazepam (Valium) 0.2-0.3 mg/kg/dose IV q 10 min prn. Treat metabolic problems, if any.
5. For bleeding diathesis: vitamin K (infants—1-2 mg/dose IV; children and adults—5-10 mg/dose IV)

Dialysis is indicated for the following conditions:
1. Renal failure
2. CNS deterioration or poor response, particularly with chronic salicylism
3. Unchanging high salicylate level or level >130 mg/dl at 6 hr
4. Severe, unresolving metabolic acidosis
5. Pulmonary edema

Hemodialysis is more effective than peritoneal dialysis.

DISPOSITION

Patients with mild ingestions may be discharged with appropriate poison-prevention counseling. Patients who are significantly symptomatic, have serum levels ≥60 mg/dl at 6 hr, have ingested methyl salicylates, or have chronic or sustained release ingestions that are potentially toxic should be hospitalized.

REFERENCES

Burton, R.T., Bayer, M.J., Barron, L., et al.: Comparison of activated charcoal and gastric lavage in the prevention of aspirin absorption, J. Emerg. Med. **1**:411, 1984

Hill, J.B.: Salicylate intoxication, N. Engl. J. Med. **288**:1110, 1973.

Temple, A.R.: Acute and chronic effects of aspirin toxicity and their treatment, Arch. Intern. Med. **141**:364, 1981.

Carbon monoxide

ALERT: Several members of the same household with headache, nausea, or shortness of breath should be evaluated for exposure.

Carbon monoxide is an odorless, colorless gas produced by internal combustion engines and by combustion of natural gas, charcoal, and coal gas. Fire victims often have high levels after exposure. Methylene chloride (a solvent used in paint stripper) is metabolized to carbon monoxide. Carbon monoxide binds to hemoglobin 210 times more avidly than does oxygen.

DIAGNOSTIC FINDINGS

A high index of suspicion is essential, and evaluation is indicated if several members of the same household are experiencing similar symptoms.

Signs and symptoms progress with increased exposure, reflecting the levels of carboxyhemoglobin in the blood:

Carboxyhemoglobin level in the blood (%)	Clinical findings
10-20	No apparent findings
	Dyspnea (vigorous exertion)
20-30	Dyspnea (moderate exertion)
	Intermittent throbbing headache
30-40	Throbbing headache, dyspnea, irritability, fatigue, dizziness, blurred vision
40-50	Headache, confusion, syncope, tachycardia, tachypnea
50-60	Stupor, seizures, coma
60-70	Unconsciousness, fibrillation, tachycardia, death
>80	Immediately fatal

The levels listed on p. 289 are from data about adults. Children may have an increased susceptibility to CO toxicity. Children with levels above 25% carboxyhemoglobin (HGCO) consistently have syncope and lethargy in a recent study. Symptoms in all patients may correlate more closely with the length of exposure than with the carboxyhemoglobin levels. Furthermore, levels may be influenced by significant delays between exposure and presentation, particularly if oxygen therapy has been administered en route.

Complications

1. Cardiac
   a. Dysrhythmias (Chapter 6)
   b. Myocardial ischemia with ST/T wave changes (usually only in adults)
2. Pulmonary edema and hemorrhage either immediately or as delayed finding (Chapter 19)
3. Renal failure secondary to myoglobinuria
4. CNS
   a. Encephalopathy with associated seizures and coma (Chapters 15 and 21)
   b. Cerebral edema
   c. Long-term neuropsychiatric changes and memory defects

Ancillary data

1. HGCO level. Normally this is <1%, although it has been reported to be as high as 5% after driving on busy freeways. Heavy smokers may have levels up to 15%.
2. ABG with a measured, not calculated, oxygen saturation
3. ECG with any evidence of myocardial ischemia, chest pain, or shortness of breath
4. Chest x-ray film, with smoke inhalation. Often normal in first 24 hr (Chapter 53)

MANAGEMENT

Although it is clear that hyperbaric oxygen is the treatment of choice for patients in coma from CO poisoning, it is not at all clear what levels of HGCO require such treatment if the patient has minimal symptoms. It is not known if hyperbaric oxygen will decrease the long-term neurologic sequelae in these patients. Some experts have suggested that patients with HGCO levels >20%-25%, neurologic findings, acidosis, or syncope should be treated in the hyperbaric chamber, but the data regarding an absolute level is not available. While arranging transportation to such a unit, administration of 100% oxygen should continue.

1. Remove patient from source of combustion, and immediately administer high-flow oxygen while continuing resuscitation. 100% oxygen can be delivered through a mask with a nonrebreathing apparatus or an endotracheal tube.
   NOTE: Half-life of HGCO at room air is approximately 4 hr, and with 100% oxygen it is approximately 40 min. With hyperbaric oxygen (2 atm), this is reduced to less than 20 min.
2. Monitor for evolving complications, and treat aggressively.

Patients who are pregnant at the time of exposure place the fetus at great risk. Treatment should be continued for at least three times as long as the time recommended for the mother alone. Consultation should be obtained.

DISPOSITION

Patients who require admission for prolonged observation and treatment include:
1. Those with HGCO >20%-25%. This decision must be individualized.
2. Those with abnormal neurologic examination, ECG, or acidosis
3. Pregnant women with HGCO >15%. They require more prolonged oxygen therapy (approximately three times the amount calculated).

Before the patient is discharged, the source of CO must be eliminated in the household or car. The clinician suspecting CO poisoning should evaluate all household residents.

REFERENCES

Crocker, P.J., and Walker, J.S.: Pediatric carbon monoxide toxicity, J. Emerg. Med. 3:443, 1985.

Zimmerman, S.S., and Truxel, B.: Carbon monoxide poisoning, Pediatrics 68:215, 1981.

Hallucinogens: phencyclidine, LSD, mescaline

ALERT: Differentiate from other entities causing hallucinations.

A wide variety of agents produce hallucinogenic states. Phencyclidine (PCP, angel dust), lysergic acid diethylamine (LSD, acid), and mescaline (buttons, peyote, cactus) produce similar behavioral changes, although the systemic effects are markedly different. Of the three, phencyclidine is most widely used at present. Hallucinogens may be ingested along with other drugs, altering the presentation markedly.

DIAGNOSTIC FINDINGS
Phencyclidine

Children under 5 yr have symptoms different from those of older patients:
1. Bizarre behavior, including lethargy, staring spells, intermittent unresponsiveness, irritability, and poor feeding
2. CNS findings that may progress to coma—commonly ataxia, nystagmus, opisthotonos, and hyperreflexia
3. Tachypnea, tachycardia, and hypertension
Older patients have a progression of symptoms with increasing dosage.
1. Low doses (<5 mg). Induce associated agitation, excitement, disorganized thought process, incoordination, nystagmus, blank-stare appearance, and intoxication with drowsiness and apathy
2. Moderate doses (5-10 mg or 0.1-0.2 mg/kg). Often induce stupor or coma, decreased peripheral sensation, muscular rigidity, myoc-lonus, nystagmus, flushing, hypersalivation, and vomiting
3. High doses (>10 mg). Cause coma with seizures, decerebrate posturing, hypertension, nystagmus, opisthotonos, hypersalivation, and diaphoresis

LSD

Effect lasts for 4-12 hr with an accompanying hallucinogenic state. LSD may produce permanent psychosis in susceptible individuals and flashbacks months after the initial ingestion.

Ancillary data

1. Do urine toxicology, analysis for PCP, and other studies indicated for support.
2. Let the laboratory know if phencyclidine is suspected, as many urine screens do not specifically examine for it.

DIFFERENTIAL DIAGNOSIS

1. Intoxication
   a. Sedative. Hypnotics do not generally cause hypertension or hyperreflexia. Respirations are usually decreased.
   b. Anticholinergics: prominent peripheral and central findings. May cause hallucinations
2. Encephalitis, meningitis, Reye's syndrome, or high fever
3. Acute psychosis

MANAGEMENT

Supportive care is essential, and associated drug ingestion should be considered.
1. Administration of dextrose and naloxone as indicated
2. Gastric emptying
3. Diuresis. PCP is a weak base, and excretion may be increased 100-fold if the urine is acidified to a pH of ≤5.5, although the utility is controversial. Acidifying the urine, however, may increase the risk of precipitating myoglobin crystals in the urine if rhabdomyolysis has occurred.

- Maintain urine flow at 3-6 ml/kg, and give ammonium chloride 75 mg/kg/dose (maximum: 1.5 g) q 6 hr IV to a total maximum dose of 6-8 g/24 hr.

With agitated and hallucinating patients:

1. Avoid physical restraints if possible
2. With PCP, reduce stimuli
3. Try to maintain verbal contact and reassure patient
4. Consult psychiatrist for acute and long-term care

If sedation is necessary, use diazepam (Valium).

DISPOSITION

Most patients with significant findings require hospitalization for medical or psychiatric management.

REFERENCES

Aronow, R., and Done, A.K.: Phencyclidine overdose: an emerging concept of management, J.A.C.E.P. **7:**58, 1978.

Welch, M.J., and Correa, G.A.: PCP intoxication in young children and infants, Clin. Pediatr. **19:**510, 1980.

Hydrocarbons

ALERT: Pulmonary and CNS findings predominate, and specific guidelines for emesis or lavage should be followed.

The ingestion of hydrocarbons is a common occurrence in children, but management remains controversial. The toxicity of hydrocarbons varies with the relative viscosity (SSU: seconds for a quantity of liquid to pass through a standard aperture) and additives. The lower the viscosity, the higher the risk of pulmonary aspiration; certain additives have significant toxicity of their own.

ETIOLOGY

1. Viscosity (SSU)
   a. <60 SSU: gasoline, turpentine, benzene, kerosene, mineral seal oil (furniture polish)
   b. <100 SSU: lubricating grease, diesel oil, mothballs, paraffin
2. Toxic additives: "CHAMP"
   a. *C*amphor causes CNS excitement or depression.
   b. *H*alogenated hydrocarbons (i.e., carbon tetrachloride) produce hepatitis, nephritis, diarrhea, and CNS excitement or depression.
   c. *A*romatic (benzene) results in aplastic anemia, dysrhythmias, and CNS and respiratory depression.
   d. *M*etals (heavy metals such as mercury) result in GI bleeding, renal failure, and neurologic sequelae.
   e. *P*esticides, primarily organophosphates, also cause cholinergic signs and symptoms (p 297).

DIAGNOSTIC FINDINGS

These depend on the history of the amount ingested (one swallow in a child is about 4 ml), the material (container should be examined), and the time elapsed. Findings include the following:

1. Coughing, dyspnea, and choking accompanying the initial ingestion
2. Pulmonary symptoms. May be delayed up to 6 hr and include tachypnea, wheezing, and respiratory distress. The pneumonitis produces a fever that does not necessarily reflect a bacterial infection.
3. CNS depression or excitement
4. Nausea, vomiting, and abdominal pain
5. Pulmonary edema and dysrhythmias (Chapters 6 and 19)
6. Cyanosis developing shortly after ingestion. May be associated with a toxin that causes methemoglobinemia
7. Toluene (glue or paint sniffing). Produces psychiatric disturbances, CNS depression, abdominal pain, dysrhythmias, or renal tubular acidosis with associated hypokalemia and acidosis

Ancillary data

1. CBC. May demonstrate leukocytosis. Electrolytes are indicated if toluene ingestion is suspected.
2. ABG
3. X-ray studies. Chest films are abnormal in 90% of symptomatic patients, usually with a multilobar fluffy infiltrate. These findings may be delayed. Pulmonary edema may be present.
4. Other studies as indicated, including red cell cholinesterase and ECG.

MANAGEMENT

Initial management should include stabilization, with administration of oxygen, and decontamination of the patient by removal of clothing and washing the skin. Associated findings require treatment.

Indications for gastric emptying are controversial. At present they include the following: severe gastrointestinal or CNS symptoms, or hydrocarbon that contains one of the "CHAMP" additives (Fig. 55-3). Lavage should be done only after intubation and protection of the airway.

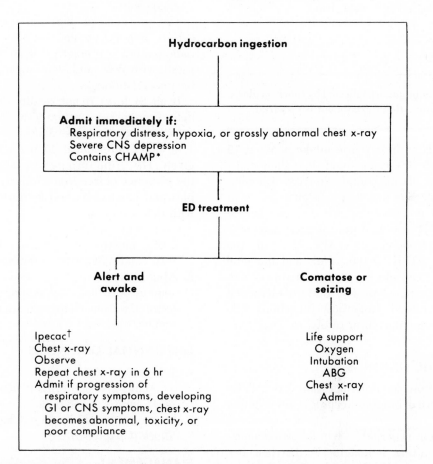

FIG. 55-3. Management of hydrocarbon ingestion. *Camphor, halogenated, aromatic (Benzene), metals (heavy), pesticides (organophosphates). †Although the use of syrup of ipecac is not contraindicated after hydrocarbon ingestion, the volume of hydrocarbon ingested is not always the best guide to using it. Most of the common hydrocarbons ingested (e.g., gasoline, kerosene, oil) need not be removed regardless of the volume swallowed.

Steroids and antibiotics are not indicated prophylactically.

DISPOSITION

Patients require admission in accordance with the protocol outlined in Fig. 55-3. Before the patient is discharged, poison-prevention counseling is required, and long-term follow-up of pulmonary status should be arranged.

REFERENCES

Eade, N.R., Taussig, L.M., and Marks, M.I.: Hydrocarbon pneumonitis, Pediatrics 54:351, 1974.

Kulig, K., and Rumack, B.H.: Hydrocarbon ingestions, Curr. Top. Emerg. Med. 3(4):1, 1981.

Iron

ALERT: GI symptoms are followed by shock, acidosis, and liver failure. Rapid treatment is required.

Normal daily dietary iron intake is about 15 mg, of which 10% is absorbed. It is then transported in the plasma bound to ferritin. Elemental iron content of ingested substance is a good measure of potential toxicity. Ferrous sulfate contains 20% elemental iron, ferrous gluconate 12%, and ferrous fumarate 33%. Normally the serum iron (SI) is 50-100 μg/dl, and the total iron-binding capacity (TIBC) of ferritin is 300-400 μg/dl. An ingestion of 60 mg/kg of elemental iron is considered dangerous. Ingestions <20 mg/kg of elementary iron rarely are symptomatic.

DIAGNOSTIC FINDINGS

Toxicity from an iron ingestion has a fairly classic pattern of progression unless intervention is timely.

1. Stage 1: initial period (½-6 hr following ingestion). Vomiting, hematemesis, diarrhea, hematochezia, and abdominal pain occur.
2. Stage 2: latent period (2-12 hr). The patient improves.
3. Stage 3: systemic toxicity 4-24 hr after ingestion. Shock, metabolic acidosis, fever, hyperglycemia, bleeding, and death may occur.
4. Stage 4: hepatic failure beginning at 48-96 hr. This is associated with seizures and coma, and the patient has poor prognosis.
5. Stage 5. Late sequelae of pyloric stenosis may develop at 2-5 wk.

Ancillary data

Levels of SI and TIBC should be ascertained.
1. Peak SI <350 μg/dl is rarely symptomatic.
2. Peak levels >500 μg/dl are considered very dangerous.

The presence of diarrhea, vomiting, leukocytosis, hyperglycemia, or a positive abdominal radiograph are predictive of an SI level >300 μg/dl, with WBC and blood sugar producing the best correlation.

If an SI level is not readily obtainable, the deferoxamine provocation test may be useful for asymptomatic patients. A dose of 90 mg/kg (or 1 hr of IV infusion at 15 mg/kg/hr IV) IM is given. The urine turning rose colored indicates the presence of free iron and ferrioxamine complex and is an indication for further treatment with deferoxamine.

Other data include:
1. CBC, electrolytes, glucose, liver function tests, and ABG with significant ingestion
2. Abdominal flat plate. Should be obtained as soon as possible. The presence of intact tablets in the stomach mandates aggressive therapy for removal.

DIFFERENTIAL DIAGNOSIS

1. Infection
   a. Acute gastroenteritis (Chapter 76)
   b. Hepatitis (p. 487)
2. Gastrointestinal bleeding (Chapter 35)
3. Shock (Chapter 5)

MANAGEMENT

Management should reflect the amount of iron ingested; the clinical status of the child in terms of GI, CNS, and vital signs problems; and laboratory data.

Initial fluid and acid-base resuscitation is imperative when it is indicated. Shock, GI hemorrhage, and significant metabolic acidosis may be present. After initial measures are taken, the patient should be lavaged. Emesis or lavage to reduce or eliminate absorption is important. Radiographs should be taken as soon as possible to detect undissolved tablets. Rarely, surgical removal is required.

1. Patients with peak levels <350 μg/dl require no further treatment if TIBC >350 μg/dl.
2. Patients with SI >TIBC or SI > 350 μg/dl and TIBC unavailable should be treated with IV or IM deforoxamine.

Patients with levels of ≥500 μg/dl must be treated immediately, with monitoring of electrolytes, hematocrit, and ABG.

1. For patient in shock or coma, give deferoxamine at 15 mg/kg/hr for 8 hr IV or as long as the urine remains colored. Start slowly and work up to this infusion rate over the first 15-30 min.
2. If patient is less seriously ill, give 90 mg/kg/dose IM q 8 hr.

Deferoxamine 100 mg can chelate 8.5 mg of elemental iron. It is contraindicated in renal failure and in patients shown to be sensitive to it.

1. Rapid IV administration of deferoxamine may cause hypotension, facial flushing, rash, urticaria, tachycardia, and shock.
2. If an SI level is unavailable or delayed and the patient is symptomatic, give deferoxamine 90 mg/kg/dose IM and repeat q 8 hr.
3. Exchange transfusion may be indicated in cases of life-threatening iron toxicity.

DISPOSITION

Patients with peak levels <350 μg/ml may be discharged after poison-prevention counseling.

All patients treated with deferoxamine should be admitted for observation and treatment. Such patients require follow-up after discharge in order to monitor long-term sequelae.

REFERENCE

Lacouture, P.G., Wason, S., Temple, A.R., et al.: Emergency assessment of severity in iron overdose by clinical and laboratory methods. J. Pediatr. **99**:89, 1981.

Narcotics and sedative-hypnotics

ALERT: CNS and respiratory depression and hypotension are prominent.

Narcotics and sedative-hypnotics in overdoses consistently produce CNS and respiratory depression, along with hypotension. Aggressive supportive care is the key to treatment.

ETIOLOGY

1. Narcotics
   a. Heroin (skag, dope, horse)
   b. Morphine
   c. Codeine
   d. Meperidine (Demerol)
   e. Methadone
   f. Propoxyphene (Darvon)
   g. Diphenoxylate (Lomotil)
2. Barbiturates
   a. Long acting (onset: 1 hr; peak: 6 hr: duration: days)—phenobarbital
   b. Intermediate acting (onset: 1 hr; peak: 3-6 hr; duration: 6-8 hr)—amobarbital, butabarbital
   c. Short acting (onset: minutes; peak: 3 hr; duration: 4-8 hr)—pentobarbital, secobarbital
   d. Ultra-short acting (onset: seconds; peak: seconds; duration: minutes)—thiopental
3. Sedative-hypnotics
   a. Benzodiazepines: chlordiazepoxide (Librium), diazepam (Valium)
   b. Cyclic ether: paraldehyde (Paral)
   c. Alcohols: chloral hydrate, ethchlorvynol (Placidyl)
   d. Propanediol carbamates: meprobamate (Miltown, Equanil)

   e. Piperidinediones: glutethimide (Doriden), methyprylon (Noludar)
   f. Quinazolines: methaqualone (Quāālude)

DIAGNOSTIC FINDINGS (Table 55-3)

Patients with overdoses of these drugs demonstrate variable levels of CNS depression with associated respiratory impairment. Other findings are outlined in Table 55-3. Associated ingestions may change the presentation.

Ancillary data

1. Toxicologic levels. Urine and blood should be sent for analysis for all patients whose diagnosis is uncertain.

2. Electrolytes, glucose, CBC, and ABG as indicated.
3. X-ray film: abdominal flat plate if chloral hydrate is suspected (radiopaque)
4. Other studies to exclude differential diagnostic considerations

DIFFERENTIAL DIAGNOSIS

See Chapter 15.

MANAGEMENT

1. Good supportive care is of primary importance, with particular attention to the airway, ventilation, and circulation.
   a. All patients with impaired mental status

TABLE 55-3. Narcotics and sedative-hypnotic overdose: clinical findings and treatment

	Narcotics	Sedative-hypnotics	Barbiturates
FINDINGS			
CNS			
Depressed/coma	Yes	Yes	Yes
Seizures	Meperidine, propoxyphene	Methaqualone, meprobamate	Butabarbital, pentobarbital, secobarbital
Cardiovascular			
Hypotension/shock	Yes	Yes	Yes
Dysrhythmias	No	Chloral hydrate, haloperidol, meprobamate	No
Miosis	Yes (not meperidine)	Variable	Variable
Respiratory			
Depression	Yes	Yes	Yes
Pulmonary edema	Yes	Meprobamate, ethchlorvynol, paraldehyde	Yes
Anticholinergic	Lomotil (early)	Glutethimide, OTC sleep medications	No
Other	Analgesia (GI, GU motility; bronchoconstriction)	Paraldehyde—acute renal failure	Cutaneous bullae
MANAGEMENT			
Support	Yes	Yes	Yes
Gastric emptying	Yes	Yes	Yes
Antidote	Naloxone	No	No
Diuresis	No	No	Phenobarbital (alkaline)
Dialysis	No	No	Phenobarbital

or respiratory function should have oxygen, cardiac monitor, and IV in place.

    b. D50W 0.5-1.0 g dextrose (1-2 ml)/kg/dose IV; and naloxone 0.8 mg (2 adult vials) IV. If no response, 2 mg (5 vials) IV should be given to all patients with altered mental status.

2. Gastric emptying, usually by lavage, is indicated with impaired mental status after oral overdose.

3. For narcotic overdoses, naloxone (Narcan 0.8 mg or two adult ampules) IV should be administered. If this is ineffective, an additional 2 mg (5 ampules) should be given, regardless of the patient's size. Propoxyphene (Darvon) and pentazocine (Talwin) overdoses may require larger than usual amounts of naloxone for adequate reversal. If there is a response to naloxone, a continuous infusion may be indicated. After the initial bolus, begin an infusion (2 ml in 500 ml D5W or 0.9%NS equaling 4 μg/ml). Start at 1-4 μg/kg/min (adult: 0.4 mg/hr) IV and titrate. Naloxone infusion should never replace careful observation and support. Use with caution after oral overdose. Naloxone is also available in multidose vials and 1 mg/1 ml ampules.

4. Alkaline diuresis may enhance excretion of phenobarbital. Urine flow should be established at 3-6 ml/kg/hr by giving an initial flush of 0.9%NS or LR at 20 ml/kg and then $NaHCO_3$ 1-2 mEq/kg/dose over 60 min with K supplements as necessary. Fluids should be infused at twice the maintenance level. Urine pH should be >7.5. Dialysis or hemoperfusion is rarely required.

5. Serial doses of activated charcoal (adults: 20-50 g q 2-4 h PO) in 70% sorbitol increases the elimination of oral or intravenous phenobarbitol, but the effect on clinical course is unclear. Mixing every other dose with a cathartic may be beneficial.

6. Dialysis may be useful in severe phenobarbital ingestions.

7. Associated ingestions should be treated as necessary.

DISPOSITION

All patients with significant overdoses should be hospitalized, and following their clearance, psychiatric consultation should be sought.

REFERENCES

Goldberg, M.J., and Berlinger, N.G.: Treatment of phenobarbital overdose with activated charcoal, JAMA **247**: 2400, 1982.

Lewis, J.M., Klein-Schwartz, W., Benson, B.E., et al.: Continuous naloxone infusion in pediatric narcotic overdose, Am. J. Dis. Child **138**:944, 1984.

Moore, R.A., Rumack, B.H., Conner, C.S., et al.: Naloxone: underdosage after narcotic poisoning, Am. J. Dis. Child. **134**:156, 1980.

Pond, S.M., Olson, I.C.R., Osterloah, J.D., et al.: Randomized study of the treatment of phenobarbital overdose with repeated doses of activated charcoal, JAMA **251**: 3104, 1984.

Organophosphates and carbamates

ALERT: The classic cholinergic syndrome is recognized by the mnemonic SLUDGE (*s*alivation, *l*acrimation, *u*rination, *d*efecation, GI cramping, and *e*mesis).

Organophosphate pesticides are widely used and produce the classic cholinergic syndrome by the inhibition of acetylcholinesterase. There are many different organophosphates with widely varying toxicities, including chlorthion, parathion, diazinon, malathion, TEPP, OMPA, and systox. Parathion is 600 times more toxic than malathion, the latter being used for household purposes. Carbamates have similar uses as insecticides but are less toxic, and the symptoms they produce are of shorter duraton. Absorption is primarily through the skin and gastrointestinal tract.

DIAGNOSTIC FINDINGS

The symptoms of cholinergic syndrome are usually evident within hours of exposure.

Specific findings reflect excessive acetylcholine.

1. *Muscarinic* (parasympathomimetic) findings
   a. Sweat glands: increased sweating
   b. Lacrimal glands: increased lacrimation
   c. Genitourinary: urinary incontinence
   d. Gastrointestinal: anorexia, nausea, emesis, diarrhea, fecal incontinence
   e. Eye: miosis, blurred vision
   f. Bronchial: bronchoconstriction, pulmonary edema
   g. Cardiovascular: bradycardia, hypotension
2. *Nicotinic* (motor) findings
   a. Striated muscle: fasciculations, weakness, hyperflexia
   b. Long-term peripheral neuropathy may be seen after serious exposure.
3. CNS: restlessness, ataxia, seizures, depression of respiratory and cardiovascular centers, emotional lability, confusion, coma

Ancillary data

1. Blood CBC, electrolytes, BUN, glucose, liver function tests, PT, and ABG
2. Chest x-ray film with evidence of pulmonary edema and ECG for dysrhythmias
3. Cholinesterase levels (either serum or red cell). They do not correlate well with clinical status of the patient and are only rarely available to the physician soon enough to make a difference in treatment. They are primarily useful in cases of chronic exposure where it is desirable to know if further protection from the organophosphate is needed. Usually expressed as a percentage of normal (>50%: no manifestations; 20%-50%: mild; 10%-20%: moderate; <10%: severe)

DIFFERENTIAL DIAGNOSIS

1. Intoxication: physostigmine, neostigmine, pyridostigmine, edrophonium (Tensilon)
2. Noncardiogenic pulmonary edema

MANAGEMENT

Stabilization of the airway and resuscitation are imperative. Additional measures include decontamination by removal of clothing and washing of skin for contact exposure and emesis or lavage and administration of charcoal and cathartic for ingestion.

Organophosphate and carbamate insecticides are rapidly adsorbed through the clothes and skin. Contaminated clothes must be removed, and skin must be decontaminated. This is optimally done outside a medical facility by personnel wearing gloves, rubber apron, and so on. Two separate water/detergent washes remove a total of 91%-94% of organophosphates, even when performed up to 6 hr after exposure. Hospital personnel must be protected during and after decontamination.

Specific treatment involves administration of anticholinergic medications to the symptomatic patient.

1. Atropine is given first: 0.05 mg/kg/dose (maximum: 2-5 mg/dose) IV. Test dose (child: 0.01 mg/kg IV; adult: 2 mg IV) is usually given. This may be repeated q 5 min until atropinization is achieved, with drying of pulmonary secretions. Mydriasis is not an adequate endpoint.
   a. Should be given for the first 24 hr as needed to maintain atropinization. Adults may need several 100 mg in the first 24 hr of therapy.
   b. Pralidoxime (2-PAM) reactivates acetylcholinesterase and is useful if given within 36 hr of exposure. It should be administered after adequate atropinization.
   (1) Dosage: pralidoxime 20-50 mg/kg/dose (maximum: 2 g/dose) IV slowly. In the adult, 1 g is mixed in 250 ml 0.9%NS and given over 30 min. If symptoms of weakness and fasciculations persist, it may be repeated in 1 hr and then q 8 h for additional doses.
   (2) No serious side effects noted from pralidoxime.

Carbamates have lower toxicity of shorter duration.

DISPOSITION

All symptomatic patients with exposure or ingestion require admission and usually consultation with a poison control center for guidance in drug therapy.

REFERENCE

Namba, R., Note, C.T., Jackrel, J., and Grob, D.: Poisoning due to organophosphate insecticides. Am. J. Med. **50**:475, 1971.

Phenothiazines

ALERT: Symptoms include sedation and anticholinergic findings; occasionally there may be prominent dystonic reactions.

Phenothiazines are widely used antipsychotics as well as antinauseants. They have anticholinergic, antidopaminergic, and alpha-blocking actions.

ETIOLOGY

See Table 55-4.

DIAGNOSTIC FINDINGS

The major finding in overdoses reflects anticholinergic and antidopaminergic effects. There is an inverse relationship between the anticholinergic potency and extrapyramidal side effects (p. 284).

Extrapyramidal dystonic reactions may be divided into several categories, although clinically different patterns may appear simultaneously. Dystonia is not necessarily dose related.

1. Oculogyric: upward-gaze paralysis, bizarre tics
2. Torticollis: may involve one side, often with arm involvement
3. Buccolingual: facial grimacing with dysphagia, mutism, trismus
4. Optisthotonic
5. Tortipelvic: abdominal wall spasms, bizarre gait, lordosis, kyphosis

Other side effects include the following.

1. Seizure threshold is reduced.
2. Anticholinergic findings (p. 284).

TABLE 55-4. Related side effects

	Sedation	Extrapyramidal	Hypotension
PHENOTHIAZINES			
Chlorpromazine (Thorazine)	+ + +	+ +	IM + + + PO + +
Triflupromazine (Vesprin)	+ +	+ + +	+ +
Thioridazine	+ + +	+	+ +
Trifluoperazine (Stalazine)	+	+ + +	+
Prochlorperazine (Compazine)	+ +	+ + +	
THIOXANTHENE			
Thiothixene (Navane)	+ or + +	+ +	+ +
BUTYROPHENONES			
Haloperidol (Haldol)	+	+ + +	+

Modified from Gilman, A.G., Goodman, L.S., and Gilman, A.: The pharmacological basis of therapeutics, ed. 6, New York, 1980, Macmillan, Inc. Copyright ©1980, Macmillan, Inc.
+, + +, + + +, Relative prominence.

3. Hypothermia may occur early, but the patient with sufficient thermal exposure may have hyperthermia.
4. Tachycardia and orthostatic hypotension are common.
5. Non-life-threatening side effects include hepatitis, photosensitivity, visual blurring, hirsutism, and gynecomastia. Thioridazine has been associated with retinal pigment degeneration.

Ancillary data

1. Granulocytopenia, hyperglycemia, and acetonemia are reported.
2. Other studies should include toxicology screen (in seriously ill patients), ECG, and x-ray film.
3. A few drops of 10% ferric chloride added to 5 ml of urine will turn urine purple-brown. Urine turns purple in presence of salicylates.

MANAGEMENT

Initial attention must be given to stabilization, with particular attention to airway, ventilation, and circulation. Obtunded patients should receive oxygen, dextrose, and naloxone. Hypotension should be treated initially with IV fluids. Rhythm should be monitored and dysrhythmias treated as appropriate.

Emesis should be induced. Lavage may be necessary, followed by charcoal and catharsis.

Extrapyramidal dystonic reactions should be treated with diphenhydramine (Benadryl) 1-2 mg/kg/dose IV or with benztropine (Cogentin) 1-4 mg/dose (adult) IV. Patients are maintained with one of these drugs for 1-2 days.

DISPOSITION

Disposition must reflect the severity of symptoms. Those with only extrapyramidal findings can usually be discharged with follow-up. Others often require hospitalization. Depending on the nature of the ingestion, psychiatric counseling or poison prevention should be stressed.

REFERENCE

Lee, A.: Drug-induced dystonic reactions. J.A.C.E.P. **6**:351, 1977.

Sympathomimetics

ALERT: CNS and cardiovascular stimulants may produce ventricular dysrhythmias or sudden death.

The sympathomimetics are a diverse group of stimulant drugs with primarily CNS and cardiovascular toxicity.

TYPES

1. Amphetamines: methamphetamine, phenmetrazine (Preludin) (much greater toxicity intravenously than orally)
2. Cocaine (street names: snow, gold dust, coke, speed ball—when combined with heroin)
3. Ephedrine: available alone or in combination with theophylline

DIAGNOSTIC FINDINGS (Table 55-5)

Ancillary data should include CBC, electrolytes, glucose, BUN, ABG, ECG, and toxicology screens as indicated.

DIFFERENTIAL DIAGNOSIS

The diagnosis must be differentiated from intoxication caused by phencyclidine, hallucinogens, anticholinergics, sedative-hypnotics, alcohol, theophylline, caffeine, and camphor.

MANAGEMENT

1. Supportive care is important, focusing particularly on potential cardiovascular instability and altered mental status.
   a. Patients should receive oxygen, dextrose, and naloxone if mental status is altered.
   b. Hyperthermia must be aggressively treated with cooling blankets.
2. Gastric emptying should be achieved either by emesis or lavage, as well as by charcoal and catharsis as outlined earlier.

TABLE 55-5. Sympathomimetic syndrome: common clinical findings

Clinical findings	Amphetamines	Cocaine	Ephedrine
CNS			
Stimulation	Yes	Yes	Yes
Hallucinations	Yes	Yes	Yes
Seizures	Yes	Yes	
Coma	Yes	Yes	
Cardiovascular			
Tachycardia	Yes	Yes	
Dysrhythmias	Yes	Yes	Yes
Hypertension	Yes	Yes	Yes
Nausea, vomiting, abdominal pain	Yes		Yes
Mydriasis	Yes	Yes	Yes
Hyperthermia	Yes	Yes	
Other	Intracranial hemorrhage, self-destructive behavior		Short duration

3. A calming, reassuring approach to the patient with an acute psychosis or hallucinations is important, as is an attempt to reduce stimuli.
4. The hypermetabolic state marked by tachycardia, dysrhythmias, and hypertension can be treated with propranolol 0.01-0.1 mg/kg/dose (maximum: 1 mg/dose) IV.
5. Sedation, if necessary, may be achieved with diazepam (Valium) 0.2-0.8 mg/kg/24 hr q 6-8 hr PO (adult: 5-10 mg/dose). Titrate response.
6. For behavioral changes caused by amphetamines, a dopamine-blocking antipsychotic such as chlorpromazine (Thorazine) 0.5 mg/kg/dose q 30 min prn IV or IM may be given but not in cases of street drug overdoses because of synergistic hypotension.

REFERENCE

Pentel, P.: Toxicity of over-the-counter stimulants, JAMA 252:1898, 1984.

Theophylline (p. 584)

ALERT: Seizures and cardiac dysrhythmias may occur with toxicity.

Because of its widespread use in the control of reactive airway disease, theophylline overdoses are common in children.

DIAGNOSTIC FINDINGS

Effects are primarily sympathomimetic in action, resulting in irritability and seizures as well as tachycardia, dysrhythmias (atrial fibrillation and ventricular tachycardia), and hypertension. Patients may be restless and agitated. Nausea, vomiting, diarrhea, and abdominal pain are seen frequently, even at nontoxic levels.

Overdoses with sustained release preparations can produce severe and prolonged CNS and cardiovascular toxicity.

Ancillary data

Theophylline levels are commonly available and should be obtained for all patients who are considered to have potentially toxic levels. Rapid office assays also are available for measuring levels. An ECG should usually be obtained.

MANAGEMENT

1. Supportive care is essential with ongoing cardiac monitoring. Gastric emptying either by emesis or lavage (reflecting level of consciousness, seizures, or absence of gag reflex) followed by charcoal and catharsis is done as outlined earlier.
2. In the asymptomatic patient with minimal overdoses, withholding drug and monitoring are usually adequate.
3. Significant theophylline overdoses may initially be treated with serial doses of activated charcoal (adult: 20-50 g q 2-4 hr PO; children: relatively less). This approach markedly decreases the half-life of elimination. If the level is >50 mg/dl, dialysis (and rarely, hemoperfusion) should be considered.
4. Seizures are treated initially with diazepam (Valium) 0.2-0.3 mg/kg/dose IV q 2-5 min prn (Chapter 21) and dysrhythmias treated with specific drugs (Chapter 6).

DISPOSITION

Patients who are symptomatic or have levels >30 mg/dl should generally be admitted for observation and treatment.

REFERENCES

Gal, P., Miller, A., and McCue, J.D.: Oral activated charcoal to enhance theophylline elimination in an acute overdose, JAMA **251**:3130, 1984.

Park, G.D., Spector, R., Roberts, R.J., et al.: Use of hemoperfusion for treatment of theophylline intoxication, Am. J. Med. **74**:961, 1983.

Tricyclic antidepressants

ALERT: Anticholinergic effects and cardiotoxicity are prominent. Immediate intervention is necessary.

Tricyclic antidepressants are a widely used class of medications. Beyond their use as antidepressants they are popular in the treatment of enuresis (e.g., imipramine). Their major toxicity is from their anticholinergic and quinidine-like effects. Plasma levels do not correlate with toxicity.

ETIOLOGY

Imipramine (Tofranil), amitriptyline (Elavil), desipramine (Norpramine), doxepin (Sinequan), and nortriptyline (Pamelor) are commonly used.

DIAGNOSTIC FINDINGS

Anticholinergic, both peripheral and central, effects may be prominent and usually develop within 6 hr (p. 285).

1. Peripherally, patients have dry, flushed skin and dry mucous membranes, dilated pupils, and urinary retention, with decreased bowel sounds. Tachycardia, dysrhythmias, hyperpyrexia, and hypertension may be present.
2. Centrally, patients have delirium with disorientation, agitation, hallucinations, and movement disorders. Seizures and coma are common.

Dysrhythmias result from the anticholinergic effects of tricyclics and from direct cardiotoxicity, blockage of norepinephrine uptake, and a quinidine-like action (myocardial depression and AV conduction delay). Superventricular tachyrhythmias, conduction blocks, and ventricular dysrhythmias are common, although their onset may be delayed. The best correlate with risk of seizures is a QRS ≥0.10 sec, whereas ventricular dysrhythmia occurs when the QRS is ≥0.16 sec.

Hypotension is common, secondary to myocardial depression and alpha blockade. Patients with fatal ingestion may present with trivial signs and symptoms that may have rapidly progressed to coma, conduction defects, dysrhythmias, hypotension, or seizures.

Ancillary data

1. Tricyclic antidepressant level. Although unreliable, documentation of the drug's presence by toxicology screens may be important.

Toxicology screens are not of predictive value regarding complications.

2. ECG on all patients; ABG and glucose as indicated.

DIFFERENTIAL DIAGNOSIS

Intoxications must be differentiated from anticholinergic and quinidine reactions.

MANAGEMENT

1. Life support is crucial because of the potential findings of respiratory depression and hemodynamic compromise. Patients should receive oxygen, IVs, and cardiac monitoring on arrival. Dextrose and naloxone should be administered as indicated by mental status.

2. Gastric emptying, charcoal, and cathartics should be administered.

3. Physostigmine is effective as a treatment for the anticholinergic effects, but because of significant side effects (seizures, dysrhythmias, and cholinergic crisis), its use should be reserved for situations where other modalities have failed (p. 285).

   a. Dosage—children: 0.5 mg IV slowly over 3 min q 10 min up to 2 mg; adult: 1-2 mg IV slowly over 3 min q 10 min until cessation of life-threatening condition or ineffective. Maximum dose: 4 mg in 30 min.

   b. Indicated with hemodynamically unstable supraventricular dysrhythmias, seizures, and dysrhythmias unresponsive to other measures and also behavior that is potentially harmful. It is best to reserve physostigmine for life-threatening situations because there are safer agents for treatment of seizures (phenytoin, phenobarbital, diazepam) and dysrhythmias (phenytoin, alkalinization, lidocaine).

4. Seizures should initially be treated with diazepam (Valium) 0.25 mg/kg/dose IV q 10 min prn (Chapter 21).

5. Patients with prolongation of the QRS or ventricular dysrhythmias should be alkalinized with $NaHCO_3$ 1-2 mEq/kg/dose IV q 10-20 min prn to maintain plasma pH of 7.5 or above. This appears to be prophylactic in preventing progression of dysrhythmias.

   • Ventricular dysrhythmias or conduction delays (QRS >0.16 sec) should be treated with phenytoin (Dilantin), 5 mg/kg loading dose IV and then with maintenance dose. Administer at <40 mg/min. Lidocaine also may be used (Chapter 6).

6. Coma usually requires supportive care but is self-limited and not an immediate indication for physostigmine.

7. Hypotension may respond to fluid challenge. If unsuccessful, use norepinephrine as the pressor agent (Chapter 5).

DISPOSITION

All patients require monitoring for at least 6 hr following ingestion. Significant ingestions or symptomatic patients with tricyclic overdose require admission to an ICU for treatment and cardiac monitoring. Those with minimal ingestions who after 6 hr have only minor signs or are asymptomatic may be discharged if there are bowel sounds and cathartics and charcoal have been administered. Appropriate psychiatric evaluation should also be completed. Follow-up is necessary.

REFERENCES

Boehnert, M.T., and Lovejoy, R.H.: Value of the QRS duration versus serum drug level in predicting seizures and ventricular arrhythmia after an acute overdose of tricyclic anti-depressants, N. Engl. J. Med. **313**:474, 1985.

Callaham, M.: Tricyclic antidepressant overdose, J.A.C.E.P. **8**:413, 1979.

Callaham, M., and Kassel, D.: Epidemiology of fatal tricyclic antidepressant ingestion: implications for management, Ann. Emerg. Med. **14**:1, 1985.

Hagerman, G.A., and Hanashiro, P.K.: Reversal of tricyclic-antidepressant induced cardiac conduction abnormalities by phenytoin, Ann. Emerg. Med. **10**:82, 1981.

IX TRAUMA

56 Evaluation and stabilization of the multiply traumatized patient

ROBERT C. JORDEN

ALERT: An aggressive, highly prioritized approach must be immediately implemented, employing a team approach to the stabilization of airway, ventilation, the spine, shock, and external hemorrhage. A multiply injured patient may be able to respond only to one major painful stimulus at a time. Thus a careful identification of all sites of injury is important.

The traumatized pediatric patient presents unique challenges to the physician but the principles of establishing treatment priorities are identical to those for older patients. However, beyond the principles of immediate stabilization, the psychologic impact on a child and family are immense and must be addressed with appropriate urgency through communication, support, and understanding. Furthermore, the pediatric patient presents logistic problems in respect to ensuring intravenous access, adjusting to limitations of equipment, monitoring and determining vital signs, and assessing fluid requirements.

PRINCIPLES OF MANAGEMENT
Organization

For optimal treatment, trauma care requires organizational structure and coordination at several levels: the region, the ED, the hospital, and the treating physicians. Although this text focuses on the physician-centered organization, to be effective, that physician must understand the other levels and be able to communicate effectively with the prehospital system.

Team approach

Effective trauma resuscitation requires a trauma team led by a senior member designated as the trauma captain. Although the exact composition of the team varies with the institution and availability of personnel, the need for some type of organized team approach is essential. Trauma injuries are complex, requiring multiple procedures and frequent reassessment in a timely fashion. Only through a team effort, orchestrated by a team captain, can optimal care be provided.

Aggressive management

Because the multiply injured child has a high potential for rapid deterioration, an aggressive approach must be the foundation for determining treatment priorities.

Treatment based on clinical findings

Diagnosis need not always be confirmed by x-ray study or laboratory work before treatment is initiated. Such delays in treatment may prove detrimental to patient survival. For example, the treatment urgency of tension pneumothorax, diagnosed by clinical findings of diminished breath sounds or subcutaneous emphysema, necessitates immediate placement of a chest tube without x-ray confirmation.

Assuming the most serious diagnosis

When a number of diagnostic possibilities exist to explain a physical finding, the most serious of these possibilities should be assumed and appropriate treatment instituted until that diagnosis can be excluded.

Consideration of the nature of the accident

Patients who are victims of potentially serious accidents should be considered seriously injured until proved stable. For example, the victim of a fall or auto-pedestrian accident should have IV lines started and be carefully monitored despite an initial stable appearance and absence of complaints.

Assessment of priorities

Evaluation of the trauma victim must be conducted in a prioritized fashion to guarantee that life-sustaining functions are addressed and maintained first.

Thorough examination

The trauma team rapidly ensures that the airway, ventilation, and circulation are adequate; obtains a history; and then does a more complete examination.

1. Remove all clothing to prevent overlooking an injury.
2. Perform concise and systematic, yet thorough, examination to ensure detection of all injuries.
3. Do not stop looking for injuries after one serious injury has been detected.
4. Examine the patient's back. If there is potential cervical spine injury, obtain an x-ray film before examining the back if the patient's condition permits. Otherwise, the patient may be logrolled.

Frequent reassessments

Trauma victims are dynamic in their clinical presentation and thus subject to sudden deterioration. Frequent assessment of vital signs and indicators of vital function (e.g., level of consciousness, pupils, ventilation) is essential. Vigilance in monitoring intake and output and correlation with vital signs is imperative in determining additional fluid or blood requirements.

Technical steps

These should be accomplished early to facilitate monitoring and intervention in seriously ill patients. *IV lines* should be placed, *oxygen* administered, *urinary catheter* (6 mo: 8 Fr; 1-2 yr: 10 Fr; 5 yr: 10-12 Fr; 8-10 yr: 12 Fr) inserted and urine examined for blood. *NG tube* (6 mo: 8 Fr; 1-2 yr: 10 Fr; 5 yr: 10-12 Fr; 8-10 yr: 14-18 Fr) inserted (after cervical spine is cleared), and *cardiac monitor* applied. *Laboratory* and *x-ray studies* are ordered as discussed later. Five tubes are virtually always required in situations where major trauma is suspected, that is, two IV tubes, an NG tube, a bladder tube, and type and cross-match.

ASSESSMENT BY PRIORITIES
Preliminaries

1. Assemble the trauma team, which will vary depending on the number and type of people available in the ED. A team captain must be identified who can orchestrate the resuscitation and task assignments, based on ambulance reports.
2. Take updated report from ambulance personnel while the patient is being transferred from the ambulance stretcher. Attempt to acquire additional history, including the details of the accident, significant past history, medications, and allergies.
3. Maintain any splinting and head and neck immobilization that have been instituted in the field.
4. Remove all clothing. Use overhead heating and lights to maintain body temperature, especially in smaller children.
5. Attach the patient to a cardiac monitor and administer oxygen. Initiate IV lines.

Approach

Initial management can be divided into stabilization of immediate life-threatening conditions and a brief but systematic head-to-toe evaluation. Life-threatening conditions include five high-priority areas: *airway, ventilation, spine, shock,* and *external hemorrhage.* These five areas require rapid assessment and intervention to permit survival (Chapter 4).

The second phase of management is a complete evaluation of other potentially injured systems. A reassessment of the high-priority areas and evaluation of neurologic status, abdomen, heart, musculoskeletal system, and soft tissue injuries is essential. Although of lower priority, these areas do have the potential for causing serious morbidity and mortality and must be addressed expeditiously.

Airway

1. Check for patency. If there is any question, open the airway, suction secretions, remove foreign debris, and insert an oral or nasal airway. Oxygen at 3-6 L/min must be administered.
2. Check for adequacy of air exchange; if insufficient, active intervention is necessary.
   a. If urgent airway management is needed before the cervical spine can be cleared:
      (1) Attempt nasotracheal intubation unless there is severe facial injury, which may cause the tube to pass into the cranium. Nasotracheal intubation is generally easier if there is some ventilatory effort by the patient.
      (2) In the presence of severe facial injury or if nasotracheal intubation is unsuccessful in the patient with a very high risk of cervical spine injury, perform a cricothyroidotomy on the child over 3 yr of age. In the younger child, the cricothyroid space is too small to accommodate a tube of sufficient size for adequate ventilation. A tracheostomy may therefore be necessary. As a temporizing measure, a noncuffed ET tube may be used through the surgically created airway. Unfortunately, this is a very difficult and time-con-

suming procedure, and it may be more practical to orally intubate the patient while maintaining axial traction, knowing that there is a risk of inducing further spinal cord injury.

   b. If there is no evidence of cervical spine injury, the likelihood of unstable injury is small, or the cervical spine has been cleared, oral intubation may be performed.

Ventilation

1. Inspection. Look for signs of respiratory distress, including dyspnea, tachycardia, tachypnea, cyanosis, diaphoresis, retractions, flail segments, external evidence of trauma, tracheal deviation, and subcutaneous emphysema.
2. Palpation. Feel for bony crepitus, subcutaneous emphysema, chest wall tenderness, and tracheal deviation.
3. Auscultation. Determine presence, character, and symmetry of breath sounds.
4. **Management**
   a. Evidence of inadequate ventilation indicates the need for active airway management or tube thoracostomy.
   b. Airway management may be achieved as outlined previously. If necessary, the child may be paralyzed with succinylcholine (1 mg/kg/dose IV) after establishing availability of skilled personnel and ancillary equipment, including suction. Ambu bag and appropriate mask, oral and nasal airways, and equipment for a cricothyroidotomy. Cricoid pressure should be maintained during fasciculations to prevent aspiration. Pretreatment with atropine 0.01 mg/kg/dose IV (minimum: 0.1 mg/dose) is indicated for children under 8 yr of age to prevent the reflex bradycardia commonly seen with succinylcholine.
   c. Chest tube insertion should be performed if there are any signs of pneumothorax or hemothorax (Chapter 62). If the patient is

relatively stable, tube thoracostomy may obviate the need for active airway management.

Cervical spine (Chapter 61)

1. The cervical spine of every multiply traumatized patient should be considered fractured until proved otherwise. This has direct bearing on airway management. Fracture or dislocation is unusual in the patient under 2 yr without neurologic defect.

2. In the awake, alert, and cooperative older child, palpation to detect misalignment or tenderness may be all that is necessary to rule out injury. If there is any doubt, particularly in the younger, uncooperative child or in those with an impaired sensorium, x-ray films should be taken, i.e., a portable, cross-table lateral view of the neck. This study, to be adequate, must include all seven cervical vertebrae. One person should maintain axial traction while a second person pulls the patient's arms caudad from the foot of the bed, thus lowering the shoulders enough to expose the lower cervical vertebrae.

3. **Management**
   a. Immobilize the head and neck with sandbags and tape until the entire cervical spine series is completed.
   b. If fractures or dislocation are detected or suspected, immobilize with Philadelphia or 4-poster collar with tape and sandbags; consider dexamethasone (Decadron) 0.25 mg/kg/dose IV or IM. Request immediate neurosurgical consultation.

Thoracic and lumbar spine (Chapter 61)

1. Thoracic or lumbar fractures are easily overlooked in the confused or obtunded child or in one with other painful injuries.

2. Palpation of the spinal column will frequently localize tenderness and step offs or, on logrolling, one may see ecchymoses.

3. Cross-table lateral views may not be easily obtainable anywhere but in the x-ray suite, but anteroposterior views often show thoracic or lumbar fractures. Moreover, it is the view from which to assess stability if there is a dislocation and also to obtain important information about other structures in the chest, abdomen, and pelvis.

4. Management
   a. The patient should be maintained in a supine position on a hard stetcher.
   b. An NG tube and urinary catheter should be inserted if the cervical spine is clear and there is no meatal bleeding.

Shock (Chapter 5)

1. Up to 25%-30% of blood volume can be lost before a child exhibits hypotension in the supine position. More subtle findings of tachycardia, a narrowed pulse pressure, or poor perfusion should be sought and treated aggressively.

2. Normal age-specific values of pulse and blood pressure must be considered in the evaluation of the patient. Normal systolic blood pressure in individuals 1-18 yr of age can be estimated by adding twice the age (yr) plus 80. Diastolic pressure is usually two thirds of systolic (Appendix C-2).

3. The initial hematocrit done in the ED is usually normal in acute hemorrhages and is therefore a poor indicator of volume status. If it is low, it may indicate that there was a preexisting anemia, chronic hemorrhage, or a massive acute hemorrhage.

4. The presence of shock demands a thorough, rapid evaluation to determine the source of bleeding. In the absence of external musculoskeletal hemorrhage, three cavity spaces must be evaluated: chest, abdomen, and retroperitoneum. Except in the small infant, isolated head trauma does not cause shock. Therefore another source of shock must be aggressively investigated in the presence of head trauma.

5. Management
   a. Estabish IV lines. In massive trauma, one line should be a CVP line.
   b. Initially administer a bolus of LR or 0.9% NS 20 ml/kg IV as rapidly as possible.

Subsequent crystalloid and blood administration should reflect response to the initial infusion and ongoing hemorrhage. Once 40-50 ml/kg of crystalloid has been infused during the initial resuscitation, blood should be administered if evidence of hypovolemia persists.

c. If completely cross-matched blood is not available, administer type-specific blood. It is usually available 10-15 min after delivery of a clot to the blood bank. O negative blood should be reserved for those patients who are in profound shock or cardiac arrest. Warm, fresh blood is optimal when available.

d. If massive transfusions are necessary (equivalent to one total blood volume), use blood warmers and micropore filters and also consider administration of fresh frozen plasma and platelets.

e. *MAST* suits are available for pediatric patients but are not presently widely used. If an appropriately sized suit is available, it may be used in conjunction with fluid resuscitation for the patient in shock secondary to hemorrhage once the lower extremities, back, and abdomen have been examined for injury. It also is useful in stabilization of fractures and in hemostasis following aortic aneurysm rupture or pelvic fractures. The use of MAST suits is contraindicated in patients with pulmonary edema, cardiogenic shock, pregnancy, an object impaled in the abdomen, or with eviscerated abdominal contents. Use with caution in patients with a tension pneumothorax or cardiac tamponade. Complications include compartment syndromes and acidosis.

The suit should be inflated in a stepwise fashion while monitoring the blood pressure response. Once inflated, it should normally only be deflated when the patient is hemodynamically stable. At that time, the compartments should be deflated one at a time starting with the abdominal component. Deflation should occur slowly, with close monitoring of vital signs and observation for acidosis that may result.

f. *Thoracotomy* is indicated for trauma arrests and persistent post-trauma shock that is unresponsive to fluid resuscitation. The thoracotomy permits cross clamping of the aorta and shunting of available blood to the cerebral and coronary circulations. It also permits immediate relief of pericardial tamponade and temporary control of certain cardiothoracic injuries. Obviously, it is only appropriate in rare patients and must be performed by persons with experience in the procedure while an operating room is being readied for definitive repair.

External hemorrhage

Significant external hemorrhage should be controlled by direct pressure. If an isolated bleeding vessel can be identified, it may be clamped, but blind clamping in the depths of a wound is never indicated.

Reassessment

Once the high-priority areas listed on pp. 307-310 have been evaluated and appropriate treatment administered, reassessment of vital signs and overall status should be done. If no further actions are necessary beyond those already initiated, a complete secondary survey, including a thorough examination and a more detailed history, should be initiated.

Neurologic considerations (Chapter 57)

Level of consciousness is the most important indicator of prognosis. The Glasgow Coma Scale (Table 57-1) provides an objective, reproducible means of assessing level of consciousness. A numerical score is assigned based on motor and verbal responses and eye movement.

1. Eyes. Evaluate size, shape, symmetry and reactivity of pupils, fundus, fullness of extra-

ocular movements, and evidence of obvious trauma.

2. Nose and ears. Hemotympanum, otorrhea, and rhinorrhea are indicative of a basilar skull fracture and often represent the only means of making that diagnosis.

3. Movement of extremities. Spontaneous movement or movement of all extremities in response to pain should be noted. Is movement symmetric? Any evidence of posturing?

4. Rectal tone. The presence of rectal tone in a patient paralyzed from spinal cord injury may indicate a central cord syndrome, which has a good prognosis. Absence of rectal tone in a comatose patient may be the only discernible clue to spinal cord injury.

5. Reflexes. Absent deep tendon reflexes are consistent with a cord injury; upward flexion of the toes (positive Babinski's reflex) is consistent with upper motor neuron damage.

Management

Any alteration of consciousness or abnormal neurologic findings warrants close and repeated observation, neurosurgical consultation, and consideration of a CT scan.

Persistent loss of consciousness requires intubation and hyperventilation, dexamethasone (Decadron) 0.25 mg/kg/dose IV or IM and furosemide (Lasix) 1 mg/kg/dose IV if the patient is hemodynamically stable. Mannitol 0.5-1.0 g/kg/dose IV should be added if there is evidence of cerebral herniation. A neurosurgeon should be consulted.

Cardiac considerations (Chapter 62)

Although usually not very enlightening in trauma cases, a cardiac examination should be performed, and cardiac monitoring is imperative. A full 12-lead ECG should be obtained for all patients with chest wall trauma.

1. Inspect for signs of anterior chest wall trauma, which may be the only evidence of cardiac contusion and the only means of assessing the jugular veins and locating the point of maximal impulse (PMI). Tachycardia may

be the only sign of myocardial contusion.

2. Auscultate to determine the character of the heart sounds and the presence of rubs or murmurs.

3. In penetrating chest trauma, exclude cardiac tamponade. Inspect for evidence of hypotension, tachycardia, dilated (full) jugular veins (elevated CVP), and muffled heart sounds. A pericardiocentesis may be indicated.

Management

1. Cardiac tamponade requires immediate pericardiocentesis or thoracotomy, depending on the status of the vital signs.

2. Myocardial contusion requires ICU monitoring of enzymes and dysrhythmias. Hemodynamic compromise may occur in cases of severe contusion.

The abdomen (Chapter 63)

The abdomen is difficult to examine. Older cooperative children without evidence of injury or unexplained hemodynamic instability may require no further evaluation. Younger children and those with any alteration in mental status with unexplained vital sign abnormalities should undergo diagnostic peritoneal lavage in consultation with a surgeon. Lavage should always be preceded by placement of an NG tube and urinary catheter to prevent accidental injury to the stomach and bladder.

Lavage may not be necessary in patients with unequivocal signs of a surgical abdominal condition following trauma or for those with persistent, unexplained shock. Instead, surgical intervention is required.

Examination of the abdomen

1. Inspect for signs of trauma, distention, or surgical scars.

2. Auscultate to determine the presence or absence of bowel sounds.

3. Palpate to elicit tenderness and rebound and to define any masses.

4. Do a rectal examination to evaluate tone, status of prostate, and presence of blood in stool.

5. Palpate, compress, and rock the pelvis over

the iliac crest and pubis to detect movement, tenderness, or crepitus suggestive of pelvic fracture.

6. Examine the genitalia for obvious trauma. Blood at the urethral meatus precludes the insertion of a urinary catheter and requires investigation.

7. Do a dipstick examination of urine for blood and, if present, a microscopic analysis. If >5-10 RBC/HPF, an IVP should generally be performed, although the indications are somewhat controversial (p. 375). With a pelvic fracture, a cystogram should be done. Blood at the urethra indicates the need to do a urethrogram after urologic consultation.

Management

A positive lavage or signs of peritoneal irritation or persistent unexplained shock are indications for laparotomy. Initial volume resuscitation, delineation of associated injuries, and type and crossmatching of blood should be done in the ED.

Musculoskeletal injuries (Chapters 66-70)

These are relatively low-priority injuries. Obvious extremity injuries require splinting and referral for a more detailed examination. Nevertheless, major bone fractures can contribute significantly to hypovolemic shock.

Examinations

1. Inspect and palpate all extremities for deformity, tenderness, bony crepitus, and joint laxity.

2. Assess distal pulses and neurovascular integrity distal to the injury.

3. Inspect and palpate the spine for deformity and tenderness.

Management

This involves appropriate x-rays, temporary splinting, and orthopedic consultation.

Facial and soft tissue injuries (Chapters 58, 60, and 65)

Facial injuries, unless massive, are not life threatening and require little initial treatment although they do affect airway management. Severe hemorrhage and distortion are indications for active intervention.

1. Contusions and lacerations of the soft tissues should be defined and pressure applied to control hemorrhage. Distal neurovascular function should be assessed. When time permits, sutures should be placed after defining structures, to avoid further injury.

2. Penetrating or significant soft tissue injuries to the neck require careful exploration of the depth and severity of the damage. A surgeon should be involved in evaluation and management if there is penetration of the platysma or extensive blunt soft-tissue involvement.

X-RAY AND LABORATORY EVALUATION
X-ray studies

1. Essential roentgenograms during the initial evaluation on any victim of multiple trauma include a chest, pelvis, and cross-table, lateral view of the cervical spine. The spine film is essential in diagnosing fractures and dislocations, and the chest and pelvic films may identify serious pathology requiring further assessment and treatment, as well as defining a source of blood loss.

2. Portable films should be obtained. Unstable patients should not be transported to the radiology department. Following stabilization, additional films can be obtained while the patient is being appropriately monitored.

3. CT scans and angiography may be necessary. Great care and judgment must be exercised in obtaining these studies in the unstable patient. Other priorities of care such as a laparotomy must be carefully weighed before obtaining diagnostic x-ray studies. Careful monitoring must be maintained throughout the examination.

Laboratory

1. Studies that should be done in the ED include a spun hematocrit, urinalysis, and ABG.

2. Type and cross-match is essential in all significant trauma cases.
3. Routine studies include a CBC, platelet count, electrolytes. BUN, glucose, amylase (with abdominal pathology), and coagulation studies (PT and PTT).

CONSULTATION

1. A trauma surgeon should be notified as soon as the facility is alerted that a patient with serious trauma is en route to the hospital. Depending on the reliability of the prehospital care assessment, this initial surgical contact may await arrival and primary assessment if the surgeon is not in the hospital.
2. A neurosurgeon should be notified if significant head injury is present.
3. Orthopedic, plastic surgery, and urology personnel may be notified after stabilization. Premature consultation may add chaos and confusion to the initial resuscitation.

DISPOSITION

Patients with multiple serious injuries should be admitted to the trauma service with coordination of the appropriate consulting services.

Transfer to another institution is indicated only if definitive care cannot be provided at the initial facility. Lines of referral for specific types of injury should be established in advance to facilitate communication and transfer.

- Before transfer, the patients must be stabilized. During transfer, the same levels of monitoring and treatment in the ED should be maintained. All records, x-ray films, and laboratory data should accompany the patient (Chapter 3).

PSYCHOLOGIC CONCERNS

For many reasons, the child who is the victim of trauma may be terrified and crying hysterically on arrival in the ED. Pain is present from either the injuries or their treatment. The child is separated from parents and is in a strange environment and surrounded by unfamiliar doctors and nurses.

Support is essential for the conscious child. Time must be taken to explain in a reassuring way that the youngster has been injured, is in the hospital, and is going to be all right. Touching the child in a soothing manner as well as speaking in a calm, controlled tone may be helpful in winning confidence and establishing rapport. Procedures should be explained if possible and the child warned that there may be accompanying pain. The patient should not be surprised.

Parents should be allowed to stay with the child whenever possible. This may not be feasible when the youngster is critically ill, requiring major resuscitative efforts, or when the parents are so upset that they are actually contributing to the patient's hysteria. If parents are not available, a member of the resuscitation team

1. Should be designated to support the child as a surrogate parent in these circumstances
2. Should make sure that there is adequate communication and support for the family when contact is made

SIZE CONSIDERATIONS

1. *Vital signs*, including respiratory rates, vary by age (Appendix C-2). Systolic blood pressure may be estimated by adding twice the patient's age to 80. The heart rate varies with age (infant: 100-160, child: 60-150, adult: 50-90).
2. *Fluid replacement* should be based on the patient's blood volume (70-80 ml/kg), the vital signs, the nature of the injury, and the presence of ongoing hemorrhage. Unless the patient is in profound shock, the initial approach is to give a fourth of the patient's blood volume (20 ml/kg) as crystalloid (0.9%NS or LR). Further treatment should be geared to the initial response and the other factors mentioned.
3. *Venous access* is somewhat more difficult in children, particularly if the youngsters are hypovolemic. If establishing a percutaneous line is impossible, a venous cutdown in the distal saphenous or external jugular should

be established. Central venous lines are infrequently used in children because of the increased risk of pneumothorax and vascular injury. If a central line is desired, the subclavian or internal jugular veins may be cannulated, employing the customary approaches but using somewhat smaller (16-18 gauge) needles. Increasing evidence substantiates the usefulness of interosseous infusions during initial fluid resuscitation in patients without readily available venous access (Appendix A-3, p. 629).

4. *Tube placement*, including thoracostomy and ET, NG, and urinary catheters, should be effected with the largest tube that the child can accommodate.

REFERENCES

Agran, P.F., Dunkle, D.E., and Winn, D.G.: Motor vehicle childhood injuries caused by non-crash falls and ejections, JAMA 253:2530, 1985.

American College of Surgeons Committee on Trauma: Advanced trauma life support course, Chicago, 1981, American College of Surgeons.

German, J.C.: Multiple-system injured children, Top. Emerg. Med. 6:46, 1984.

Gratz, J.R.: Accidental injury in childhood: a literature review on pediatric trauma, J. Trauma 19:551, 1979.

Harris, B.H.: Management of multiple trauma, Pediatr. Clin. North Am. 32:175, 1985.

Holmes, M.J., and Reyes, H.M.: A critical review of urban pediatric trauma, J. Trauma 24:253, 1984.

Jorden, R.C.: Multiple trauma. In Rosen, P., editor: Emergency medicine: concepts and clinical practice, St. Louis, 1983, The C.V. Mosby Co.

Kaback, K.R., Sanders, A.B., and Meislin, H.W.: MAST suit update, JAMA 252:2598, 1984.

Kanter, R.K., Zimmerman, J.J., Strauss, R.H., et al.: Pediatric emergency intravenous access, Am. J. Dis. Child. 140:132, 1986.

Moore, E.E., Eiseman, B., Van Way, C.W., III: Critical decisions in trauma, St. Louis, 1984, The C.V. Mosby Co.

Ordog, G.J., and Wasserberger, J.: Coagulation abnormalities in shock, Ann. Emerg. Med. 14:650, 1985.

Rivara, F.P.: Traumatic deaths of children in the United States: current available prevention strategies, Pediatrics 75:456, 1985.

Seidel, J.S., Hornbein, M., Yoshigama, K., et al.: Emergency medical services and the pediatric patient: are the needs being met? Pediatrics 73:769, 1984.

Thompson, J.D., Fish, S., and Ruiz, E.: Succinylcholine for endotracheal intubation, Ann. Emerg. Med. 11:526, 1982.

57 Head trauma

PETER T. PONS

ALERT: Any patient with head trauma must be considered to have spinal trauma and other associated injuries. Initial evaluation must focus on airway, ventilation, circulation, and immobilization of the cervical spine. Head injury as an isolated finding very rarely causes shock.

Automobile accidents account for the vast majority of head trauma. Although the primary mechanical injury to the brain from direct compression or acceleration/deceleration produces immediate findings, secondary complications of hypoxia, increased intracranial pressure, hypotension, and hypercapnia cause most morbidity and mortality. Intracranial injuries or skull fractures in children under 1 yr, in the absence of a history of significant accidental trauma, such as a motor vehicle accident, may constitute grounds for consideration of child abuse.

Aggressive early resuscitation with establishment of the integrity of the airway, ventilation, and circulation and the immobilization of the spine largely determines the outcome. This is then followed by systematic, definitive care of neurologic and associated injuries.

DIAGNOSTIC FINDINGS
History

The mechanism of trauma and associated signs and symptoms must be determined following initial resuscitation:
1. Mechanism of injury: direct blow (define implement) or acceleration/deceleration
2. Circumstances of accident: motor vehicle accident, diving accident, fall, or blow
3. Chronology
   a. Loss of consciousness immediately following accident or shortly thereafter
   b. Period of lucidity
   c. Progression of deficits
4. Associated findings
   a. Amnesia
   b. Disorientation
   c. Sensorimotor abnormalities
   d. Visual disturbances
   e. Dizziness
   f. Vomiting of nausea
   g. Seizures
5. Medications at the time of the incident including alcohol, drugs, and prescribed treatments
6. Past medical history and allergies
   Associated injuries, especially facial and neck, are often present.

Neurologic examination (Table 15-3)

Frequent repetition of the neurologic examination is essential to detect any signs of deterioration, as well as to monitor improvement. Specific consideration must be given to determining the extent of neurologic injury, the presence of a mass lesion effect, and the course of the injury.

315

Vital signs

1. Cushing's reflex. Produces elevated blood pressure, slowed pulse, and irregular respirations. Usually a late finding of increased intracranial pressure
2. Hypotension. Acute head trauma does not produce hypotension except in infants with open sutures and massive intracranial bleeding or in individuals with large scalp lacerations. If shock is present, look for other associated injuries
3. Dysrhythmias: ventricular and atrial. Prolonged QT interval and large T and prominent U waves have been noted without cardiac pathology
4. Airway. Often occluded by blood, mucus, fractures, or foreign bodies, leading to respiratory distress
5. Cheyne-Stokes respiration. Characterized by crescendo-decrescendo patterns of hyperventilation, followed by periods of apnea. Often accompanies decorticate posturing caused by cerebral hemispheric lesions and incipient temporal lobe herniation
6. Central neurogenic hyperventilation with deep, rapid ventilation. May accompany decerebrate posturing and is indicative of brainstem dysfunction, either as a primary injury or secondary to supratentorial herniation

Level of consciousness

1. Maximal depression in the level of consciousness occurs at the time of impact and should subsequently improve. Failure to improve indicates that additional or massive injury has occurred.

2. The level of consciousness may be recorded in a descriptive narrative indicating the patient's response to stimuli or characterized as follows:
   a. Alert: awake and responds verbally to questions
   b. Lethargic: sleeps when undisturbed but is incoherent when awakened
   c. Stupor: sleeps when undisturbed but is incoherent when awakened
   d. Semicoma: responds to painful stimuli in a purposeful, decorticate, or decerebrate posture
   e. Coma: does not respond to stimuli
3. The Glasgow Coma Scale for responsiveness (Table 57-1) standardizes assessment, predicts outcome, and is useful in monitoring patient.

Posturing

Decerebrate posturing and flaccidity are associated with the worst prognosis.

Pupils: size, equality, and reactivity

1. Unilateral pupillary dilation strongly suggests a mass lesion with actual or incipient herniation requiring immediate intervention. A dilated and fixed pupil is the most reliable sign of the side of the lesion. It results from pressure on the third cranial nerve (oculomotor).
2. Examination must exclude previous eye trauma, topical medications, or congenital anisocoria.
   NOTE: Retinal hemorrhage in children under 1 yr is usually associated with shaking injuries.

TABLE 57-1. Glasgow Coma Scale

Best motor response		Best verbal response		Eyes open	
Obeys commands	6	Oriented	5	Spontaneously	4
Localizes pain	5	Confused	4	To speech	3
Withdrawal	4	Inappropriate	3	To pain	2
Abnormal flexion	3	Garbled	2	None	1
Extension	2	None	1		
None	1				

Eye movements

1. Destructive lesions in the occipital or frontal lobes cause deviation of the eyes toward the lesion. Injury to the brainstem causes deviation away from the lesion.
2. Oculocephalic reflex (doll's eye) demonstrates intactness of the brainstem as does the oculovestibular reflex. These should be tested only after the cervical spine has been cleared.
   a. *Oculocephalic reflex* (doll's eyes) is performed with the eyes held open and the head turned quickly from side to side. A comatose patient with an intact brainstem will respond by the eyes moving in the direction opposite to that which the head is turned as if still gazing ahead in the initial position. Comatose patients with midbrain or pons lesions will have random eye movements.
   b. *Oculovestibular reflex* with caloric stimulation is done with the head elevated 30 degrees in the patient with an intact eardrum. Ice water is then injected through a small catheter lying in the ear canal (up to 200 ml is used in an adult). Comatose patients with an intact brainstem will respond by conjugate deviation of the eyes toward the irrigated ear, whereas those with a brainstem lesion will demonstrate no response.
   c. *Corneal reflex* is elicited by gently stroking the cornea with sterile cotton. A response demonstrates an intact brainstem and nucleus of cranial nerves V, VI, and VII.

Sensory and motor response

1. Motor responses may be determined by response to verbal commands, painful stimuli, and spontaneous movements. Tone and symmetry should be evaluated.
2. Sensory examination should include light touch and pain.

Reflexes

1. Presence, absence, and equality of reflexes should be ascertained.

2. The presence of an abnormal Babinski's reflex (dorsiflexive plantar response) is indicative of an upper motor neuron lesion.

Rectal examination

This must be performed to check for spinal cord integrity, indicated by the presence of sphincter tone.

Other findings

For a careful assessment the following signs are important:

1. Bulging fontanel
2. Palpable depression or crepitus of skull; unusual hematoma, particularly longitudinal ones
3. Battle's signs (ecchymosis posterior to ear) or raccoon (bilateral black eyes) eye sign
4. Evidence of basilar skull fracture:
   a. Battle's or raccoon-eye sign
   b. CSF rhinorrhea or otorrhea
   c. Hemotympanum or bleeding from middle ear
5. Diabetes insipidus; polyuria, nocturia, and polydipsia

Increased intracranial pressure

As the intracranial pressure rises, a relatively well-defined series of events will occur, ultimately leading to the patient's death unless appropriate actions are performed to slow or reverse the process. As the pressure rises in the supratentorial compartment, the brain (usually the uncus or medial temporal lobe) will be pushed against and through the opening of the tentorium. This produces compression of the ipsilateral third cranial nerve, leading to a fixed, dilated pupil.

Progression of the herniation leads to compression of the pyramidal tract, usually resulting in contralateral weakness or paralysis. Simultaneously, pressure on the reticular activating system results in impaired consciousness, which may be the first sign of deterioration.

In the infant with an open fontanel, initial findings may include a bulging fontanel, irritability, and listlessness, eventually progressing to focal findings. Those with closed fontanels present a more classic picture.

In patients with cerebellar tonsillar herniation, the midline force causes the low brainstem and cerebellar tonsils to herniate through the foramen magnum, leading to Cushing's reflex (bradycardia, hypertension, and apnea).

Prognostic factors

Prognostic factors in severe head trauma may be useful in the management of children's injuries. Severe head trauma is defined as unconsciousness over 6 hr and inability to obey commands, utter recognizable words, or open the eyes.

Children under 10 yr of age generally have the best prognosis. Those with a Glasgow Coma Score of 5-8 usually do not die, and only 20% have permanent focal deficits. Higher scores are associated with even fewer sequelae. The recovery to consciousness and function is usually complete within 3 wk, and 77% of the children in one study returned to a regular school setting.

The worst prognosis is for those children with flaccidity or decerebrate posturing. Although children with prolonged coma tend to have a poor outcome, in one study 9 of 14 children in coma for more than 2 wk had little or no handicapping neurologic sequelae.

Complications

The following are caused primarily by secondary complications of initial mechanical injury, including hypoxia, increased intracranial pressure, hypotension, and hypercapnia:
1. Altered neurologic examination
2. Seizures
3. Pulmonary edema
4. Transient cortical blindness

Death results from complications of the primary process or secondary complications.

Ancillary data

X-ray film of the cervical spine (Chapter 61)

This should be obtained on all patients with a posttraumatic altered mental status, neurologic deficit, and neck or back pain or for those who are poor historians, such as younger children and drug abusers.

A cross-table lateral cervical spine view should be the first radiograph obtained.

Skull x-ray film

This is usually not needed in the initial management since bone fracture is not the critical injury.

Patients for whom there is a high risk of fracture include those with:
1. Documented loss of consciousness over 5 min or lack of consciousness at the time of the evaluation
2. The possibility of a depressed skull fracture (palpable defect, crepitus) or a suggestive history (blunt injury with head of hammer or heel of high-heeled shoe). Tangential views may be required.
3. Focal neurologic signs
4. Penetrating trauma
5. Evidence of basilar skull fracture (Battle's or raccoon-eye sign, CSF from nose or ear, hemotympanum)
6. Head trauma where child abuse is suspected, particularly in children under 1 yr

Important findings are:
1. Fracture that crosses the middle meningeal artery groove associated with increased incidence of epidural hematoma
2. Depressed skull fracture
3. Open fracture

The absence of a fracture does not exclude significant pathology.

CT scan

This is the diagnostic procedure of choice. A noncontrast study of the acutely traumatized patient is usually sufficient, but a contrast study (3 ml/kg) may be useful for chronic subdural hematoma. Generalized cerebral swelling is common. If a CT scan is immediately available, a skull roentgenogram may be selectively omitted.

Indications for obtaining a CT scan are:
1. Unconsciousness at the time of evaluation

2. Focal neurologic deficits
3. Depressed skull fracture or fracture crossing middle meningeal artery groove
4. Deterioration of mental status or neurologic function
5. Children under 1 yr of with bradycardia, diastasis of sutures on skull x-ray study, or full fontanel

Magnetic resonance imaging (MRI) may offer detection of more subtle changes. More planes of visualization are available without patient manipulation, and evaluation of extracerebral fluid collections is improved.

Other data

1. ABG is important to ensure that the patient is being adequately ventilated and that hyperventilation is maintaining $PaCO_2$ at about 25 mm Hg.
2. Lumbar puncture (LP) is not indicated. If infection is considered, LP should be done only after a negative CT scan.
3. EEG rarely provides any information that is useful either therapeutically or prognostically.
4. Electrolytes should be checked if there is evidence of diabetes insipidus.

MANAGEMENT
Initial management

The initial management of severe head trauma is directed not at therapy of the head trauma but rather at immediate or potential life threats. Minimal head trauma requires a careful examination, appropriate laboratory studies, a short period of observation, and good follow-up and instructions.

Airway

1. Oxygenate.
2. Suction blood and secretions, and remove foreign material from airway.
3. If the patient is unable to maintain a patent airway, active management is essential while attempting to maintain cervical spine precautions, if necessary.
   a. Nasotracheal intubation may be attempt-

ed if major facial trauma has not obscured landmarks.
   b. If the cervical spine (cross-table lateral view) is negative, orotracheal intubation may be attempted. If unsuccessful, immediate cricothyroidotomy should be performed.
4. Acutely unconscious patients secondary to trauma, particularly those requiring prolonged diagnostic evaluation or transport, should generally be considered for intubation on a prophylactic basis, as well as to initiate hyperventilation.
5. Some clinicians recommend administration of lidocaine (1.5 mg/kg IV) 1 min before intubation to prevent an acute rise in intracranial pressure. Some also suggest administration of atropine to reduce potential bradycardia.

Respirations

Supplemental oxygen and assisted ventilation should be administered as necessary.

Circulatory status (Chapter 5)

Shock must be managed aggressively with crystalloid infused into large-bore IV lines. If shock is present, associated injuries should be determined after resuscitation has been achieved. Fluids are generally administered at a rate of two thirds of maintenance. Intake and output must be closely monitored. Cerebral perfusion pressure depends on an adequate blood pressure.

Immobilization of cervical spine

See Chapter 61.

Reduction of intracranial pressure (ICP)

1. Hyperventilation is the most rapid method of decreasing ICP.
   a. Hyperventilate the patient to maintain a $PaCO_2$ (ABG) of 20-25 mm Hg. Values ≤ 20 mm Hg provide no further benefit. Decreasing the $PaCO_2$ from 40 to 20 mm Hg reduces cerebral blood flow by nearly 60% of normal.
   b. Maintain PaO_2 of at least 90 mm Hg. Supplemented oxygen and PEEP may be required.

2. Elevate head to approximately 30 degrees if patient is not in shock.
3. Administer one or more:
   a. Furosemide (Lasix) 1 mg/kg/dose IV q 4-6 hr IV
   b. Dexamethasone (Decadron) 0.25 mg/kg/dose q 6 hr IV **or** methylprednisolone (Solu-Medrol) 1-2 mg/kg/dose q 6 hr IV. Steroids are controversial, with no documented efficacy.
   c. Mannitol
      (1) Dose: 0.25 g/kg/dose IV over 10-15 min q 3-4 hr prn
      (2) Not used in routine management but useful if there are signs of increased ICP
      (3) Risks: fluid and electrolyte imbalance and rebound cerebral edema. Should not be used for patients with hypovolemia shock or renal failure.
4. Monitor ICP in consultation with a neurosurgeon in cases of severe head trauma. Optimally, maintain ICP ≤20 mm Hg and CPP ≥50 mm Hg. An ICP >40 mm Hg is associated with a poor outcome.
5. Barbiturates are useful for significant cerebral edema associated with elevated and poorly responsive intracranial pressure. They decrease ICP and cerebral metabolism and stabilize cell membranes. Since the ability to evaluate neurologic status is lost, they should be given only in consultation with a neurosurgeon.
   • Pentobarbital (Nembutal) dosage is 3-20 mg/kg IV slow push while monitoring BP. Infusion is maintained at 1-2 mg/kg/hr to maintain level between 25-40 μg/ml. Levels above 30 μg/ml may be associated with hypotension in as many as 60% of patients.
6. The use of anticonvulsants prophylactically is controversial and is not generally done but should be discussed with the consultant neurosurgeon. Anticonvulsants should be initi-

ated if there is seizure activity and should be considered in patients with significant neurologic deficit, penetrating brain injuries, and depressed fractures with true penetration.
7. Induce hypothermia (Chapter 51) only as a last resort in patients whose ICP remains elevated despite other measures.
   a. It reduces cerebral metabolism and vulnerability to hypoxemia.
   b. In consultation with a neurosurgeon, temperature should be gradually reduced to 32°-33° C.
8. The potential role of calcium blockers is under investigation.

SPECIFIC CLINICAL ENTITIES
Contusion of scalp, forehead, or face

An x-ray film usually is not required since it would be normal.
Diagnostic findings
1. Localized swelling and tenderness. Variable hematoma or ecchymosis
2. No neurologic deficit
Management
1. Discharge patient.
2. Prescribe ice packs for swelling and analgesia (aspirin or acetaminophen) for pain.
3. Discuss head injury precautions.
4. Do not aspirate (commonly liquefies in children).

Concussion
Diagnostic findings
1. Transient neurologic dysfunction, which disappears within minutes to days, leaving a neurologically normal patient
2. May include transient loss of consciousness as well as isolated findings of dizziness, nausea, vomiting, amnesia, or confusion
3. X-ray study indicated with dysfunction >5 min
Management
1. Observation. In cases where there has been

>5 min of unconsciousness, persistent symptoms, or inadequate home environment, hospitalization is recommended.
2. Aspirin or acetaminophen analgesia. Narcotics should be avoided.

Skull fracture

Diagnostic findings
1. Pain, tenderness, and swelling over fracture site
2. Significance related not to bony defect but to intensity of injury and possible damage to underlying structures
3. Basilar skull fracture suggested by findings of hemotympanum, Battle's sign (bilateral postauricular ecchymoses), raccoon-eye sign (bilateral periorbital ecchymoses), or CSF rhinorrhea or otorrhea. Anosmia may indicate involvement of cranial nerves VII or VIII.
4. X-ray study (p. 318)
   a. Linear fractures may be noted involving the flat bones of the skull (frontal, temporal, parietal, or occipital)
      (1) Fractures crossing the middle meningeal artery have the potential of causing epidural hematoma.
      (2) Fractures of the occiput, particularly if stellate or comminuted, are associated with child being repeatedly struck against object (child abuse).
   b. Depressed fractures are recognized by areas of lucency adjacent to an area of increased density. This represents a double density of bone caused by depressed segment overlapping a nondepressed segment. Tangential views or CT scan may be helpful.
   c. Basilar skull fracture is commonly not detectable by roentgenogram. Rarely, a blood-air level may be noted on sphenoid sinus (with patient supine as film is taken). CT scan is the most sensitive diagnostic tool.

Management
1. All patients with skull fractures should be hospitalized for observation, with neurosurgical consultation.
2. Early CT scan should be considered for patients with fractures that either cross the middle meningeal artery or are depressed or if there is any degree of neurologic dysfunction, especially if progressive.
3. Aspirin or acetaminophen analgesia is prescribed (no narcotics).
4. Use of antibiotics for patients with basilar skull fractures is controversial, and the ultimate decision should rest with the neurosurgeon. Intracranial contamination by foreign bodies is often treated with ampicillin and chloramphenicol.

Cerebral contusion

Diagnostic findings
1. Decreased level of consciousness is usually present.
2. Associated neurologic deficits, if any, will reflect the contused area of brain. Pathologically, this represents an injury to the brain and is marked by hemorrhage and swelling.
3. CT scan will demonstrate an area of cortex with both increased and decreased density.

Management
1. Hospitalization and close observation are required.
2. Principles of head trauma management, including stabilization of airway, ventilation, circulation, and cervical spine, should be used, depending on the degree of injury and neurologic impairment. Other measures outlined previously should be implemented when appropriate.

Intracranial hemorrhage

Diagnostic findings
1. Epidural hematoma is usually associated with a skull fracture and associated meningeal artery bleeding. The classic history of loss of

consciousness followed by a lucid period and then deepening coma is rare (10%).

2. Subdural hematomas are more frequent than epidural hematomas and usually result from laceration of bridging veins.
3. Intracerebral hemorrhage is usually associated with a brain laceration. The anterior frontotemporal region is most common. Progression of findings may be gradual.

Since the clinical presentation of these entities is similar, it is impossible to differentiate them clinically. They show signs of a space-occupying lesion, with progressive increase in intracranial pressure.

Ancillary data

An x-ray film may demonstrate a fracture, particularly with epidural hematomas, whereas a CT scan will differentiate the cause of hemorrhage.

1. Epidural hematoma appears as a lens-shaped (biconvex) area of increased density. The size of the hematoma is limited by the dural attachments at the sutures.
2. Subdural hematomas appear as an increased density spread over the entire cerebral cortex. There is often cerebral edema on the side of the injury, with a midline shift.
3. Intracerebral hemorrhage has increased density within the cortex and is surrounded by small areas of decreased density, representing edema.

Management

1. Resuscitation and head trauma management are urgently required. Emergent intervention is mandatory. Suspicion and recognition determine the ultimate outcome.
2. Neurosurgical consultation is required with an immediate CT scan to define the lesion and then to evacuate the hematoma.
3. Rarely is emergent trephination without CT scan required. Probably the only circumstance would be the individual who arrived without evidence of herniation but who begins to show signs while in ED.

DISPOSITION

The criteria for hospitalization must be individualized, but indications may include coma, significant loss or altered level of consciousness, prolonged memory loss, seizure, persistent vomiting, skull fracture, severe and persistent headache, focal neurologic deficit, altered vital signs, suspicion of child abuse, and unreliable caretakers.

Parental education

All children discharged from the hospital following head trauma must be released to the care of a responsible adult who has been carefully and explicitly instructed in head precautions.

1. Limit activities and restrict patient to light diet. If trauma is recent, apply ice pack to reduce swelling.
2. Waken patient every 2 hr and observe.
3. Call physician immediately with any of the following:
   a. Increasing sleepiness, drowsiness, or inability to awaken patient from sleep
   b. Change in equality of pupils (black center of eye) or if blurred vision, peculiar movements of the eyes, or difficulty focusing develops
   c. Stumbling, unusual weakness, or problem using arms or legs or change in normal gait or crawl
   d. Seizures
   e. Change in personality or behavior, such as increasing irritability, confusion, unusual restlessness, or inability to concentrate
   f. Persistent vomiting (more than three times)
   g. Drainage of blood or fluid from nose or ears
   h. Severe headache
4. Aspirin or acetaminophen may be given for pain. Do not use narcotics.

REFERENCES

Berger, M.S., Pitts, L.H., Lovely, M., et al.: Outcome from severe head injury in children and adolescents, J. Neurosurg. **62**:194, 1985.

Billmire, M.E., and Myers, P.A.: Serious head injury in infants: accident or abuse, Pediatrics **75**:340, 1985.

Bruce, D.A., and Schut, L.: The value of CAT scan following pediatric head injury, Clin. Pediatr. **19**:719, 1980.

Bruce, D.A., Schut, L., and Bruno, L.A.: Outcome following severe head injury in children, J. Neurosurg. **48**:679, 1978.

Cooper, P.R., Moody, S., Clark, W.K., et al.: Dexamethasone and severe head injury: a prospective double-blind study, J. Neurosurg. **51**:307, 1979.

Dearden, N.M., Gibson, J.S., McDowall, D.G., et al.: Effect of high-dose dexamethasone on outcome from severe head injury, J. Neurosurg. **64**:81-88, 1986.

Dershewitz, R.A., Kaye, B.A., and Swisher, C.N.: Treatment of children with post-traumatic loss of consciousness, Pediatrics **72**:602, 1983.

Hamill, J.F., Bedford, R.F., Weaver, D.C., et al.: Lidocaine before endotracheal intubation: intravenous or laryngotracheal? Anesthesiology **55**:578, 1981.

Jacobson, M.S., Rubenstein, E.M., Bohannon, W.E., et al.: Follow-up of adolescent trauma victims: a new model of care, Pediatrics **77**:236, 1986.

Lillehei, K.O., and Hoff, J.T.: Advances in the management of closed head injury, Ann. Emerg. Med. **14**:789, 1985.

Mahoney, W.J., D'Souza, B.J., Haller, J.A., et al.: Long-term outcome of children with severe head trauma and prolonged coma, Pediatrics **71**:756, 1983.

Mayer, T.A., and Walker, M.L.: Pediatric head injury: The critical role of the emergency physician, Ann. Emerg. Med. **14**:1178, 1985.

Pons, P.: Head trauma. In Rosen, P., editor: Emergency medicine: concepts and clinical practice, St. Louis, 1983, The C.V. Mosby Co.

Raphaely, R.C., Swedlow, D.B., Downes, J.J., et al.: Management of severe pediatric head trauma, Pediatr. Clin. North Am. **27**:715, 1980.

Sainsbury, C.P.Q., and Sibert, J.R.: How long do we need to observe head injuries in the hospital? Arch. Dis. Child **59**:856, 1984.

58 Facial trauma

STEPHEN V. CANTRILL

ALERT: Protection of the airway is essential following facial trauma and often requires active intervention. Cervical spine and other associated injuries must be excluded.

Facial trauma in children is most commonly associated with vehicular accidents, usually because of failure to use restraints, as well as falls and child abuse. Home accidents, athletic injuries, bites (animal and human), child abuse, and interpersonal altercations are also sources of facial trauma.

The period of maximal enlargement of the face occurs during the sixth and seventh years. Facial proportions at that time are primarily influenced by the development of the midface and eruption of teeth. Therefore the development and treatment of the preadolescent must reflect the stage of facial development.

DIAGNOSTIC FINDINGS

Patients with facial trauma often have trauma to other organ systems, especially those involving the head, chest, and abdomen. Facial trauma rarely represents a life threat, and therefore its evaluation and treatment should be deferred until the other, more serious injuries are evaluated and treated.

1. A complete appraisal of facial trauma includes careful evaluation of soft tissue, bony structures, innervation, eyes, ears, and mouth. Specific attention to the eye is required as outlined in Chapter 59.
2. Inspection of the face must include assessment for deformity, asymmetry, dental malocclusion or displacement, CSF rhinorrhea, nasal septal hematoma, and examination of any obvious wounds.
3. Palpation of the face should include the infraorbital and supraorbital ridges, zygomas and zygomatic arches, nasal bones, maxilla (grasp the upper central incisors and attempt to move), and mandible. Examine for tenderness, bony defects, crepitus, and false motion.
4. Neuromuscular evaluation consists of evaluation of the facial nerves, trigeminal nerves, extraocular movements, visual acuity, and hearing. The facial nerves may be tested by having the patient wrinkle the forehead, smile, bare the teeth, and tightly close the eyes. All three branches of the trigeminal nerve (sensory) should be tested on each side of the face. Anesthesia in any area implies a disruption of that branch until proved otherwise. Extraocular movements are tested to uncover diplopia or entrapment, both signs of a blow-out fracture.

Complications

1. Disfigurement
2. Loss of function
3. Infection
4. Airway obstruction
5. Hemorrhage

6. Ocular injuries occur in as many as 67% of facial fractures, especially those that are mid-facial.

Ancillary data

X-ray study

The selection of radiographic studies should be based on physical findings, the clinician's suspicions, and the patient's overall status. If there is any possibility of cervical spine trauma, cervical spine x-ray films must be ordered and cleared before any other radiographic investigations.

Waters' view is the single most helpful x-ray film for the evaluation of facial trauma, especially maxillary fractures. This is usually accompanied by AP and lateral views of the facial bones. Zygomatic, Towne projection (especially for fracture of the condyle), mandibular, lateral obliques (especially for fracture of body or ramus of mandible), and nasal views should be ordered as indicated. A mandibular Panorex view may be helpful in detecting otherwise occult mandibular fractures. Findings may include fractures, air-fluid levels in the sphenoid sinus (implies basilar skull fracture), opacification or air-fluid level in the maxillary sinus (implies blowout fracture), and subcutaneous air (implies occult fracture until proved otherwise).

Computerized axial tomography (CT scan) is useful in defining fractures in selected patients following stabilization. It is usually more sensitive than routine tomography.

MANAGEMENT

Management procedures for specific soft tissue and bony injuries follow. However, several general principles must be carefully considered, as partially outlined in Chapter 65.

1. Provide for adequate airway and ventilation. Oxygen must be administered at 3-6 L/min while determining the necessity to actively intervene. Intubation may be required on either an emergent or prophylactic basis. Rarely is cricothyroidotomy appropriate.

2. Evaluate cervical spine (Chapter 61).
3. Begin stabilization of cardiovascular system. Control hemorrhage.
4. Administer tetanus prophylaxis, as indicated.
5. Arrange for specific management of the fracture in consultation with otolaryngologists, oral surgeons, or plastic surgeons.
6. Initiate antibiotics in patients with open facial fractures. Penicillin and cephalosporins are often used unless there is CNS involvement (orbital floor or maxillary or frontal sinuses), in which case nafcillin (or equivalent) and chloramphenical are used.
7. Stimulate prevention programs that encourage use of seat belts and motorcycle full-face helmets.

SPECIAL CONCERNS IN THE MANAGEMENT OF FACIAL SOFT TISSUE INJURIES

The general principles of management of soft tissue injuries are summarized in Chapter 65. Bony injuries usually require attention first, followed by management of soft tissue damage. All involved structures must be identified and bleeding controlled. The injury should be repaired within 24 hr. Anesthesia (local or regional), cleansing with copious irrigation, debridement, and removal of all imbedded particles are imperative.

Lip lacerations

Lacerations of the lips require extra attention since a displacement of 1-2 mm in the vermilion border (the mucocutaneous junction) is quite noticeable. Little, if any, wound revision should be done in this area.

1. The vermilion border, if violated, should be marked on both sides of the laceration before injection of anesthetic since injection causes distortion of landmarks. This may be done with a needle scratch or a needle dipped in methylene blue. Unless the laceration is very superficial, a layered closure should be employed to avoid tissue defects.

2. The first skin stitch placed to repair a facial laceration extending beyond the vermilion border should be at the vermilion border. The cutaneous component is then closed with nonabsorbable synthetic suture. The vermilion section is closed with 5-0 or 6-0 silk for patient comfort.

3. Lower lip anesthesia may be achieved by injecting 1-2 ml of 2% lidocaine with epinephrine in close proximity to the neurovascular bundle of the mental nerve intraorally at the point just posterior to the first premolar.

Lip burn, electrical

Burns to the lips from biting power cords deserve special consideration. They may initially appear quite localized but may spread over the subsequent 3-5 days.

Lip burns should not be debrided. Hemorrhage may occur in the subsequent 5-10 days and close observation is essential, often in the hospital. Bleeding is controlled by pressure with the area kept clean. Special feeding devices and arm splints may be necessary.

Mouth and tongue

1. Through-and-through lacerations of the mouth require a careful, layered closure. The inner mucosa should first be closed with 4-0 or 5-0 absorbable suture to give a watertight seal. The wound is then irrigated from the exterior and closed in layers. Many recommend that these lacerations be covered with antibiotics because of the degree of contamination. Penicillin VK 40,000 units (25 mg)/kg/24 hr q 6 hr PO for 10 days is adequate for these wounds.

2. Lacerations in the area of the submandibular or parotid salivary ducts require the physician to demonstrate patency of these structures before closure. If there is any doubt, a consultant should be used.

3. Superficial lacerations of the tongue need not be closed. However, larger lacerations should be repaired in a layered fashion with the mucosal layer closed with a synthetic absorbable suture so it need not be removed later. Exposure of a tongue laceration may be improved by having an assistant grasp the tongue with a piece of gauze and apply gentle traction.

4. Local care for mouth wounds should include rinsing the mouth three to four times a day with a mild antiseptic, such as half-strength hydrogen peroxide.

Nose

Any nasal injury requires an examination for a septal hematoma, a large, purple, grape-like swelling over the septum, which should be drained through a vertical incision to avoid eventual septal necrosis. An anterior nasal pack should then be placed to avoid reaccumulation of blood. The patient should be treated with penicillin and referred to a consultant for follow-up.

Through-and-through lacerations of the nose require a careful layered closure and antibiotic treatment.

Ear

1. Adequate anesthesia of the ear may be achieved by raising a wheal with lidocaine (Xylocaine) 1% without epinephrine about the entire base of the ear. Injuries to the ear require approximation of the cartilaginous structures with fine absorbable suture. The lateral skin should be closed with fine nonabsorbable suture; the medial skin may be closed with absorbable suture to avoid bending the ear back for suture removal. Ear canal injuries require alternative anesthesia.

2. All significant injuries to the cartilage of the ear should be splinted with moist cotton balls medially and laterally and then dressed with a circumferential bandage about the head. These injuries, if at all contaminated, should be treated with antibiotics to avoid the complication of a smoldering chondritis.

3. Subperichondrial hematomas of the ear, usu-

ally caused by direct blunt trauma, often require aspiration and a compression dressing applied to avoid the development of a "cauliflower" ear. Careful follow-up and possible reaspiration are indicated.

Eyelid (Chapter 59)

1. Lacerations involving the lid margin should be referred to an ophthalmologist. If the injury prevents the cornea from being bathed by tears, artificial tears should be instilled on a regular basis until repair is achieved.
2. Lacerations not involving the lid margin should be carefully closed in layers, with the skin sutured with fine silk for comfort.
3. Wounds near the medial canthus may violate the lacrimal apparatus and require probing of the tear duct by an opthalmologist to demonstrate its integrity.

Eyebrow

1. Debridement of lacerations to the eyebrow should be kept to an absolute minimum and should be done parallel to the hair follicles, not perpendicular to the skin, to minimize the scar.
2. The eyebrow should not be shaved, because the margins are important landmarks to observe in the closure.

Scalp

It is imperative to explore all scalp lacerations with the finger to exclude fractures and debris. There may be a great deal of blood loss. Lacerations may involve the skin, subcutaneous tissue, galea, subgalea, and periosteum or pericranium. Anesthetic agents should be deposited above the galea where most of the nerves and vessels rest. When involved, the galea is closed separately.

Neck

Penetrating injuries of the neck involving the platysma or deeper structures or extensive blunt soft tissue damage require surgical consultation and in-hospital observation for a minimum of 24-48 hr. Three zones of the anterior neck are commonly identified:

I. Below the level of the top of the sternal notch
II. Between the angle of the mandible and the sternal notch
III. The region cephalad to the angle of the mandible

Airway stabilization and ventilation must be considered along with fluid resuscitation and direct pressure (not clamping) for control of hemorrhage. Chest x-ray films, arteriography, endoscopy, and water-soluble contrast studies may assist in defining the extent of the injury. In the stable patient, cervical spine films and soft tissue films of the neck may be useful. Angiography often is indicated in asymptomatic level I injuries to identify damage to thoracic outlet vessels, whereas it may be done in level III wounds to exclude a high internal carotid injury at the base of the skull.

The necessity for mandatory versus selective surgical exploration is controversial. Findings requiring surgery include shock; active bleeding; moderate, large, or expanding hematomas; pulse deficits; bruits; neurologic deficits; dyspnea; hoarseness; stridor; dysphonia; hemoptysis; difficulty or pain on swallowing; subcutaneous crepitations or air; or hematemesis. If these do not exist, the edges of the wound can be spread apart gently to avoid dislodging a clot. If the platysma has been penetrated, the patient should be admitted for observation. The need for surgical exploration and repair must reflect individual experience and preference and the ability of the facility to provide close monitoring for the patient.

FACIAL FRACTURES AND DISLOCATIONS

Facial fractures are relatively rare in the pediatric age-group because of the elasticity of the child's facial bones and the protection offered by the relatively large skull in children. Any facial fractures in children should increase the physician's suspicion of child abuse (Chapter 25).

Facial fractures are frequently associated with other, more severe injuries that require emergent attention of a higher priority (e.g., closed head and cervical spine injuries, etc.) (Chapter 56).

The emphasis here is on diagnosis. Manual palpation of the facial skeleton is particularly helpful, especially the orbital rim, zygomatic arch, nasal bridge, and inferior border of the mandible. Ocular injuries are often associated with facial fractures, and it is imperative to exclude injuries to the eye, as well as associated injuries to the head, cervical spine, etc.

Facial fractures cannot be definitively treated in the ED but require referral to a consultant. However, if the fracture is not initially diagnosed, the child may suffer permanent impaired function, disability, and disfigurement. Delay in treatment may be required because of the patient's general condition and associated injuries. The outcome still can be excellent without extensive complications. Appropriate antibiotic therapy should be considered. Uncomplicated mandibular and maxillary fractures can be managed by routine methods with good outcome even after a delay of weeks. Cosmetic complications, however, are more likely to occur with prolonged delay in treatment of zygoma fractures.

Nasal fractures

Nasal fractures may be difficult to diagnose in children because of the relative immaturity of the nasal pyramid, which makes an adequate physical examination difficult. X-ray films may be of help in making the diagnosis, especially if there is a displaced fracture. Intranasal inspection should be done, searching for a septal hematoma or a fracture dislocation of the septal cartilage. A septal hematoma should be treated as outlined on p. 326.

1. Any continuing epistaxis should be controlled by an anterior nasal pack.

2. Because of the growth potential of a child's nose, any fracture should be reduced accurately to avoid future disfigurement. For this reason, any child with significant posttraumatic epistaxis, tenderness, and swelling is assumed to have a nasal fracture until proved otherwise.

3. Any child with a documented or suspected nasal fracture should be referred to a consultant for reevaluation in 4-6 days (after the swelling has subsided).

4. Trauma to the bridge of the nose may result in an ethmoidal fracture with possible violation of the cribriform plate followed by CSF rhinorrhea. This may be disguised by epistaxis. Patients with ethmoidal fractures with suspected CSF rhinorrhea should be admitted for observation and placed in a headup position. If a CSF leak is proved, prophylactic antibiotics may be used according to the recommendation of the neurosurgical consultant.

Mandibular fractures

The pediatric mandible is more susceptible to fracture than the adult mandible because of its inherent weakness from multiple tooth buds. The subcondylar area is the most common site of fracture, especially in children under 10 yr.

1. Patients with mandibular fractures have mandibular pain and tenderness, often exacerbated by movement of the mandible. Malocclusion, a step-off in dentition, or a sublingual hematoma may be present and is highly suggestive of a mandibular fracture. Ecchymosis on the floor of the mouth is pathognomonic. Laceration of the chin associated with hyperextension also may be noted. Crepitus felt by the fingers placed in the auditory meatus during mandibular movement may indicate a condylar fracture.

2. Because the mandible is a ring structure, multiple fractures are very common, with the fracture sites possibly distant from the point of trauma. Mandibular fractures involving

the teeth are considered open fractures.

3. Mandibular x-ray films, especially a Panorex view, will assist in the diagnosis. Almost all of these patients require admission for fixation by a consultant. Usually, closed immobilization for 3-4 wk is adequate

Zygomatic fractures

In children the frontozygomatic suture is weak and may be a common site of fracture. Severe trauma may result in a tripod or trimalar fracture with fracture lines at the frontozygomatic suture and the temporozygomatic suture and through the infraorbital foramen. Patients with this complex fracture often have flatness of the cheek, anesthesia over the infraorbital nerve (cheek and ala of nose and upper lip), a palpable step defect, or change in consensual gaze.

A zygomatic arch fracture may be sustained by lateral force over the area of the arch. These patients may have a palpable defect over the arch or difficulty with mandibular movement caused by impingement of the defect on movement of the coronoid process of the mandible.

• X-ray studies, specifically the Waters' (occipitomental) and the submental-vertex views, are helpful in diagnosing these fractures.

These patients usually do not require immediate hospitalization, but the case should be discussed with a consultant, as open reduction and fixation are frequently required.

Orbital floor fractures (blow-out fractures)
(Chapter 59)

Isolated fractures of the orbital floor are most often caused by the direct application of pressure to the globe of the eye with subsequent fracture at the weakest area of the orbit, the floor. This often results in herniation of orbital contents and flow of blood into the maxillary sinus.

These patients have impaired ocular motility with diplopia, secondary to entrapment of the interior rectus muscle, infraorbital hypesthesia, and enophthalmos. The impaired motility may

be difficult to see in a child and may require a forced-traction examination under anesthesia by a consultant. Periorbital crepitus is highly suggestive of a fracture.

• The Waters' view and tomograms are most helpful in radiographically diagnosing this injury. Presence of orbital contents or opacification of the maxillary sinus is presumptive evidence of an orbital-floor fracture until proved otherwise.

Although the question of hospitalization is controversial, these patients do not usually require admission but should be referred to a consultant for follow-up in 3-5 days. Definitive therapy remains controversial. Many delay the decision on selective repair for 10-14 days.

Maxillary fractures

Maxillary fractures are most often the result of massive facial trauma, such as that caused by a deceleration injury. These patients have midface mobility as demonstrated by movement of the hard palate and upper incisors during examination. They also have massive facial soft tissue injury and malocclusion. In addition, CSF rhinorrhea may be present.

An idealized classification scheme of maxillary fractures follows (however, fractures rarely appear in pure form).

1. LeFort I: fracture at the level of the nasal fossa
2. LeFort II: pyramidal disjunction involving fractures of the maxilla, nasal bones, and medial aspects of the orbits
3. LeFort III: craniofacial disjunction involving fractures to the maxilla, zygomas, nasal bones, ethmoids, and vomer

Because of the configuration of the child's head, LeFort II and III fractures are very rare in children, and when present, they are usually accompanied by other head trauma inconsistent with survival. LeFort I fractures may often be seen in conjunction with dentoalveolar injuries.

• Radiographically, these fractures are diagnosed by the lateral facial bones and Waters' views.

Immediate care of these injuries requires aggressive airway maintenance and intensive care monitoring. Patients with these injuries must also be suspected of having cervical spine injuries, especially those with an altered sensorium. In these cases, a CT scan is indicated, and a consultant should be immediately used, e.g., a neurosurgeon if the patient is comatose.

Temporomandibular joint dislocations

Dislocation of the temporomandibular joint may be the result of trauma or may be caused merely be the patient's opening the mouth widely. In these cases, the mandible dislocates forward and superiorly. The dislocation may be unilateral or bilateral.

These patients have moderate discomfort and inability to close the mouth. X-ray films are indicated before reduction in order to rule out fracture if the dislocation is posttraumatic.

1. Reduction is performed by placing the thumbs (wrapped in gauze for protection) on the third molars of the mandible with the fingers curled under the mandibular symphysis. The condyles are levered downward and posteriorly by applying downward pressure on the molars and slight upward pressure on the symphysis. In cases of severe spasm, IV diazepam may facilitate reduction.
2. Postreduction x-ray studies are indicated for the first occurrence of this dislocation if it is not trauma related.

Admission for occlusal fixation is indicated if severe pain, tenderness, or spasm is present after reduction. Otherwise the patient may be discharged and placed on a soft diet with instructions to avoid yawning or otherwise stressing the temporomandibular joints for several days.

REFERENCES

Cantrill, S.V.: Facial trauma. In Rosen, P., editor: Emergency medicine: concepts and clinical practice, St. Louis, 1983, The C.V. Mosby Co.

Carducci, B., Springs, C., Lower, R.A., et al.: Penetrating neck trauma: consensus and controversies, Ann. Emerg. Med. 15:208, 1986.

Holt, G.R., and Holt, J.E.: Incidence of eye injuries in facial fractures: an analysis of 727 cases, Otolaryngol. Head Neck Surg. 91:276, 1983.

Maniglia, A.J., and Kline, S.N.: Maxillofacial trauma in the pediatric age group, Otolaryngol. Clin. North Am. 16:717, 1983.

Mulliken, J.B., Kaban, L.B., and Murray, J.E.: Management of facial fractures in children, Clin. Plast. Surg. 4:491, 1977.

Narrod, J.A., and Moore, E.E.: Initial management of penetrating neck wounds — a selective approach, J. Emerg. Med. 2:17, 1984.

Press, B.H.J., Boies, L.R., and Shons, A.R.: Facial fractures in trauma victims: the influence of treatment delay on ultimate outcome, Ann. Plast. Surg. 11:121, 1983.

Rao, P.M., Bhatti, F.K., Gaudino, J.; Penetrating injuries of the neck: criteria for exploration, J. Trauma 23:47, 1983.

Walton, R.L., Hagan, K.F., Parry, S.H., et al.: Maxillofacial trauma, Surg. Clin. North Am. 62:73, 1982.

Zook, E.G., editor: The primary care of facial injuries, Littleton, Mass., 1980, John Wright PSG, Inc.

59 Eye trauma

JAMES SPRAGUE

ALERT: Visual acuity must be screened and if abnormal indicates an acute need for referral to an ophthalmologist. Associated injuries, especially facial fractures, must be excluded.

The traumatized eye requires prompt attention because of potential damage and the high level of anxiety for the patient. Both can be reduced by a systematic approach emphasizing visual acuity and external examination. Visual acuity determination is frequently neglected or is done in a cursory fashion. It is helpful to remember that an injured eye with good acuity, regardless of its appearance, is unlikely to have sustained an injury requiring immediate referral or surgery. Ocular injuries commonly are associated with facial fractures.

The following equipment will facilitate the examination and treatment of the eye:

1. Visual acuity chart
2. Bright pen light
3. Ophthalmoscope
4. Irrigation setup
5. Fluorescein strips (and Wood's or cobalt blue light)
6. Topical anesthetics
7. Topical antibiotics
8. Lid retractor
9. Foreign body spud
10. Patch
11. Paper/plastic tape

GENERAL EXAMINATION TECHNIQUE
Visual acuity

Visual acuity should be assessed first. The only exception is an acute chemical injury to the eye, which requires immediate irrigation. If the patient is experiencing a great deal of pain, application of a topical anesthetic may facilitate the examination if there is no question of a penetrating injury.

1. For children under 3 yr of age, a picture-card test is easy to administer. Older preschool children can usually do the "E" test. By 7 yr most children can use the Snellen chart.
2. Each eye should be checked individually, with the patient wearing eyeglasses, if previously prescribed.
3. Many preschool children do not have 20/20 acuity, despite normal examinations. Some may have delayed myelination of the optic nerve. Useful age-specific acuity levels for screening are:

3 yr	20/50
4 yr	20/40
5 yr	20/30

A difference of more than two lines between the eyes is probably more significant than the absolute acuity and suggests unequal refractive error, amblyopia, or trauma.

In patients who are unable to cooperate in reading the eye chart, the following may be helpful: light perception by watching response (blinking, aversion, discomfort, identifying of two lights) or the ability to recognize movement of object, count fingers, distinguish faces, or recognize objects or pictures.

Patients with diminished acuity may obviously have preceding trauma. Nontraumatic conditions that should be considered include amblyopia (primary cause of monocular poor vision in early childhood), refractive errors (myopia—nearsightedness, hyperopia—forsightedness, astigmatism, or anisometropia—unequal refractive error in the two eyes), cataract, glaucoma, optic neuritis, retinal detachment, retinoblastoma, congenital problems, retinal dystrophy, and cortical blindness. Sudden loss of vision may be associated with optic neuritis, cerebral retinal artery occlusion, vitreous hemorrhage, or retinal detachment.

External examination

1. Orbital bones. Palpate the orbital rim for a step-off or marked local tenderness.
2. Infraorbital nerve. Compare sensation on both cheeks.
3. Lids. Retract lids with a lid retractor. If unavailable, use two paper clips shaped like a U. Instill topical anesthestic drops to anesthetize the cornea.
4. Position of the globe: exophthalmos or enophthalmos
5. Cornea: clarity and absence of fluorescein staining
6. Anterior chamber: clarity and depth
7. Pupil: size, reactivity, symmetry, regularity
8. Ocular motility. Test all six positions for limitation or diplopia.

Funduscopic examination

This examination is performed to evaluate for optic nerve pallor, papilledema, and retinal or vitreous hemorrhage.

Fluorescein stains

Fluorescein stains show corneal epithelial defects and should be used if there is a question of abrasion. A fluorescein strip is moistened (sterile saline or water) and applied to the conjunctiva. A staining area appears green with white light. A cobalt blue flashlight or Wood's light will cause the dye to fluoresce, which facilitates the examination.

X-ray studies

1. Waters' view to evaluate the orbital rim and maxillary sinus
2. CT scan for localization of a foreign body. Soft tissue films of the globe may be helpful.
3. To define an orbital floor blow-out fracture: tomography of the orbital floor if the plain film is abnormal.

TOPICAL MEDICATIONS

1. Topical antibiotics for bacterial conjunctivitis are normally given four times per day for 3 days (a patient who does not respond should be seen again):
   a. Sulfa: sulfisoxazole 4% (Gantrisin), sulfacetamide 10% (Sulamyd)
   b. Polymyxin B-bacitracin (Polysporin) if patient is allergic to sulfa
   c. Polymyxin B-bacitracin-neomycin (Neosporin) (may cause local sensitization with prolonged use)
2. Mydriatics/cycloplegics
   a. Tropicamide (Mydriacyl): onset, 15-20 min; duration, 2-6 hr (useful for ocular examination)
   b. Homatropine 2%-5%: onset, 30 min; duration, 24-48 hr (useful for more prolonged action, as with corneal abrasion)
3. Anesthetic: proparacaine 0.5% (Alcaine, Ophthaine, Ophthetic): 1-2 drops provides immediate corneal anesthesia. Not for home use.
4. Topical steroids: indicated for some allergic conditions, iritis, and phlyctenular disease. Should be prescribed only by an ophthalmologist if consultation is available. Complications include exacerbation of herpes, glaucoma, and impaired healing.

EYE PATCHES

These are applied by asking the patient to close both eyes, after which two pads are placed on the eyelids (an additional patch may be necessary depending on the depth of the orbital recess). Secure with a single piece of paper tape. Place strips (up to eight) of tape from the hairline to the angle of the jaw, creating pressure by pulling the skin. Patching is indicated in treatment of corneal epithelial defects of any cause. Do not patch eye infections.

Children lose CNS fusional mechanisms rapidly. After only 1-2 days, esotropia may develop; therefore children with an occlusive eye bandage should be seen by an ophthalmologist every 24 hr.

TYPES OF INJURIES
Corneal abrasion, burn, and foreign body

See Table 59-1.

Lid ecchymoses and lid and lacrimal lacerations

The eyelids provide protection and lubrication of the eye.

Ecchymosis of the eyelid ("black eye")

This requires examination to exclude more significant pathology such as an orbital fracture or hyphema. It is treated with cold compresses, analgesics, and head elevation.

Lacerations

Lid lacerations may be associated with ocular injuries and may lead to other complications if improperly treated.

1. Complications
   a. Full-thickness lacerations of the lid may be associated with penetrating injuries of the globe
   b. Improper repair of the eyelid may result in poor lacrimal function with secondary irritation and lacrimation
   c. Lacerations of the medial aspect of the lid may involve the lacrimal system, which, if not treated, may lead to poor lacrimal drainage and epiphora.
   d. Penetration. Rupture or perforation of the globe may occur and is associated with a soft globe, subconjunctival hemorrhage,

and impaired vision. Sharp lacerations or missiles are the most common causes. Immediate involvement of an ophthalmologist is imperative. The eye should initially be patched, and sedation may be required to minimize agitation that may increase venous and intraocular pressure.

2. Management (Chapter 65)
   a. Examine the eye. Be certain there is no penetration of the globe. If there is any suspicion, avoid direct pressure of excessive manipulation. Immediate ophthalmologic consultation is indicated. If there is any doubt, treat as a penetration. In general, start systemic antibiotics, keep patient NPO, and apply a loose patch and metal shield until patient can be seen. With question of foreign body penetration, obtain CT scan or soft tissue globe film.
   b. All wounds should be carefully irrigated. Debridement should be minimized.
   c. Careful apposition of the lid margins is essential in vertical lacerations, usually requiring general anesthesia in children and involvement of an ophthalmologist.
      (1) Lid avulsion requires reattachment of the eyelid to the canthal tendons.
      (2) Interruption of the lacrimal system will necessitate intubation of the lacrimal system and suturing of the canaliculus. Medial portion of the lid includes the lacrimal drainage canaliculi, whereas the lacrimal duct runs along the outer third of the upper lid.
   d. Horizontal lacerations may disrupt the levator palpebra, causing ptosis. Careful apposition is essential. A through-and-through laceration requires a three-layered closure (conjunctiva, levator aponeurosis, and skin). An ophthalmologist should be consulted.

Subconjunctival hemorrhage

The subconjunctival space is defined by the conjunctiva anteriorly, the sclera posteriorly, the

TABLE 59-1. Corneal abrasion, burn, and foreign body

	Corneal abrasion	Foreign body	Radiation burn	Chemical burn
Etiology	Direct trauma, contact lens, foreign body		Sun lamp, snow reflection	Alkali much worse than acid
Diagnostic findings	Pain, photophobia, lacrimation, fluorescein positive; small, vertical linear abrasion suggests foreign body beneath upper lid	Pain, photophobia, lacrimation, fluorescein positive; may see foreign body*	Pain, photophobia, lacrimation, fluorescein pos Punctate keratitis or diffuse abrasion; stain may be difficult to see without magnification	Pain, photophobia, lacrimation Cornea: hazy to opacified Conjunctiva/sclera: no ischemic change to blanched
Visual acuity Complications	WNL Infection	Usually WNL Penetration, infection	Decreased Infection	Markedly decreased Corneal opacification, necrosis
Treatment	Visual acuity check Topical anesthetic† Topical antibiotic Cycloplegic if >40% involved Eye patch Systemic analgesia Recheck in 24 hr‡ Avoid contact lens for 4-5 days	Visual acuity check Topical anesthetic† Remove with spud or 25-gauge needle if superficial; otherwise refer Topical antibiotics Topical cycloplegic Eye patch Recheck in 24 hr	Visual acuity check Topical anesthetic,† eye patch, analgesia Recheck in 24-48 hr	Irrigate with 1-2 L saline per eye *immediately* Evert eyelids Clear fornices Refer to ophthalmologist

*If there is any question of intraocular foreign body, particularly following hammering metal on metal, orbital x-ray studies and direct ophthalmoscopy should be performed. Penetrating injuries require immediate repair by an ophthalmologist.
†Topical anesthetics facilitate examination. They should not be dispensed for prn use.
‡On reevaluation in 24 hr, check to make certain that staining and edema have decreased. If not, refer.

cul-de-sac above and below, and the limbus centrally. The conjunctiva lines the inside of the eyelid and then is reflected in the cul-de-sac before it spreads over the globe and inserts at the corneal-scleral limbus. This space is therefore extraocular. Subconjunctival hemorrhage is associated with trauma, coughing, Valsalva's maneuver, or a coagulation disorder.

Diagnostic findings

1. The symptoms are usually those associated with the initial trauma.
2. Vision is normal if there is no damage to the intraocular contents. The hemorrhage spreads out as a thin sheet and appears bright red and homogeneous. It comes up to the limbus. There is usually no involvement of conjunctival vessels in areas where hemorrhage is not present.
3. The condition resolves in 1-2 wk without sequelae.
4. Cases of trauma to the eye followed by a 360-degree subconjunctival hemorrhage should be referred, especially if associated with anterior chamber or vitreous hemorrhage, because of the potential of posterior rupture of the globe.

Management

If there is conjunctival prolapse, sterile ointment prevents keratinization.

Hyphema

Hyphema occurs with bleeding into the anterior chamber of the eye. It usually is caused by blunt trauma although it may complicate a penetrating injury.

Diagnostic findings

There is usually a history of blunt trauma with an object small enough to fit within the ocular rim margins such as a fist, bottle, ball, etc. Vision may be decreased with marked bleeding, and pain may be present. Other symptoms are usually related to associated ocular injuries such as corneal abrasion, blow-out fracture, etc. There may be associated ecchymosis of the eyelid.

1. Initially, before the blood settles, vision is impaired, the anterior chamber shows a diffuse decrease in iris detail and less intense iris color compared to the normal eye. A complete hyphema may obscure the pupil.
2. As the blood begins to layer out, a meniscus will form and a blood-aqueous level can be seen in the inferior chamber angle.
3. **Complications**
   • Secondary hemorrhage, which occurs 3-5 days after the initial injury, is typically larger than the primary hemorrhage and may fill the anterior chamber. This can lead to acute glaucoma, corneal blood staining, and, ultimately, optic nerve damage.

Differential diagnosis

1. The usual problem is to diagnose the hyphema initially.
2. Conditions to be considered in posttraumatic loss of vision include:
   a. Corneal injury
   b. Vitreous hemorrhage
   c. Traumatic cataract or subluxation of the lens
   d. Retinal detachment
   e. Injury to the optic nerve
   f. Cortical blindness from hematoma, ischemia, or anoxia
   g. Hysteria or malingering

Management

Management is directed toward reducing the incidence of secondary hemorrhage. The following approach, although controversial, represents one plan:

1. Hospitalization and sedation with complete bed rest, with head of bed elevated
2. Bilateral eye patching to reduce saccadic eye movement, which might dislodge blood clot (also serves as a reminder that the child needs complete bed rest)
   • Bilateral patching may disorient some children. If it is not tolerated, switch to monocular patching.
3. Metal shield for injured eye
4. If dilation of the pupil was necessary to conduct the admission examination, continue dilation with scopolamine ophthalmic solution (0.25%) or 5% homatropine

- The use of topical and systemic medications, as well as the importance of pupillary dilation, is controversial.
5. Administer amino caproic acid (an initial dose of 200 mg/kg [maximum: 6 g] PO and then 100 mg/kg/dose q 6 hr PO) if the patient develops a secondary hemorrhage. Prophylactic use is presently controversial.

The anterior chamber drainage angle should be examined by gonioscopy 4-6 wk after the initial injury. If there is evidence of angle recession, annual examinations for secondary glaucoma are necessary. A dilated funduscopic examination for traumatic retinal detachment also should be performed.

Blow-out fracture (Chapter 58)

Blunt trauma from being hit with something small enough to enter between the orbital rims results in the eyeball absorbing the force of the blow and being compressed backward into the orbit. The marked increase in intraorbital pressure results in a blow-out fracture of the orbital floor, which is thin.

Diagnostic findings
1. Pain is related to the injury, periorbital swelling and ecchymosis, subcutaneous emphysema, and ipsilateral epistaxis.
2. Associated injuries include corneal abrasions, traumatic cataracts, hyphema, vitreous hemorrhage, and retinal damage in 15%-40% of patients.
- Complications
1. Hypesthesia in the distribution of the intraorbital nerve, which is best tested by evaluating sensation of the upper lip and cheek. Regeneration usually occurs.
2. Limitations of upward gaze with vertical diplopia, caused by entrapment of the inferior rectus muscle and orbital fat in the orbital floor break.
3. Enophthalmos of the injured eye, which becomes obvious as the swelling resolves.
- Ancillary data
1. X-ray film: Waters' view shows antral clouding.

2. Tomograms may be needed.
Differential diagnosis
1. Restriction of vertical motion may result from mechanical entrapment of the inferior rectus muscle or damage to the nerve of that muscle. This distinction can be made by a forced traction test, which may require general anesthesia to perform.
2. Posttraumatic diplopia occurring with entrapment must be considered in the differential of a number of entities, including:
   a. Orbital fracture
   b. Extraocular muscle avulsion, contusion, transection, or hematoma
   c. Palsy of the third, fourth, or sixth cranial nerves
Management
1. A careful examination to exclude intraocular damage and other entities in the differential diagnosis must be conducted.
2. An ophthalmologist should be involved in the acute and long-term care of the patient.
3. If the vision is normal and there are no associated facial or other major injuries, the patient can usually be followed as an outpatient. Analgesics, ice packs, elevation, and bed rest are indicated.
4. If the motility defect persists or there is frank enophthalmos initially, surgical exploration is usually necessary. The timing of surgery is controversial. Some of the restrictions in eye movement may result from hemorrhage and edema in the orbital fat, which typically resolves and may not require surgery. However, some consider it important to explore the orbital floor early and remove any orbital material in the defect.

REFERENCES

Brinkley, J.R.: Emergency management of ocular trauma, Top. Emerg. Med. **6**:35, 1984.
DeJaun, E., Sternberg, P., and Michels, R.G.: Penetrating ocular injuries: types of injuries and visual results, Ophthalmology **90**:1318, 1983.
Paton, D., and Goldberg, M.D.: Management of ocular injuries, Philadelphia, 1976, W.B. Saunders Co.
Sternberg, P.J., DeJaun, E., and Michels, R.G.: Penetrating ocular injuries in young patients: initial injuries and visual results, Retina **4**:5, 1984.

60 Dental injuries

GARY K. BELANGER

PAUL S. CASAMASSIMO

ALERT: After management of associated injuries, traumatic dental problems usually require referral.

The examination of the oral cavity requires a systematic approach to the soft tissues and teeth. The mechanism and time of traumatic injuries must be determined, as well as the onset and nature of other complaints and complicating medical problems (e.g., cardiac disease, which requires antibiotic prophylaxis, or bleeding diatheses). Status of tetanus immunizations should be assessed.

BASIC CONSIDERATIONS
Soft tissues

1. Lips: pink, moist, continuous vermilion border, possible glandular inclusions (Fordyce's granules)
   - Abnormal: tenderness, ulcers, swelling, lacerations, hemorrhage, hematoma, burn
2. Mucosa: pink, moist, possible glandular inclusions, major salivary duct openings, possible areas of hyperkeratosis associated with chewing
   - Abnormal: same as for lips; possible torn frenulum
3. Tongue: pink, papillated dorsum (possibly coated), smooth ventral surface, normal range of motion and strength
   - Abnormal same as for lips; weakness, loss of function
4. Palate: hard palate—pink, firm, rugae normal in anterior position. Soft palate—pink, mobile, functional
   - Abnormal: same as for lips: for soft palate, abnormal function or loss of function
5. Floor of the mouth: pink with areas of high vascularization (varices) appearing blue-gray; moist, major salivary duct openings, tissue tags
   - Abnormal: same as for lips; excessive firmness or elevation may indicate cellulitis or mucus-retention phenomenon

Teeth

See Fig. 60-1.
1. Color: white (permanent can appear sightly more yellow than primary)
   - Abnormal: caries, pulp degeneration; environmental and genetic defects can cause range-of-color changes
2. Integrity: complete crown without interruptions of surface morphology
   - Abnormal: caries, fractures, hypoplasias, anomalous crown forms
3. Mobility: lateral and AP movement slight to imperceptible; vertical movement nonexistent; exfoliating primary teeth may normally be very mobile
   - Abnormal: displacement by light finger pressure

337

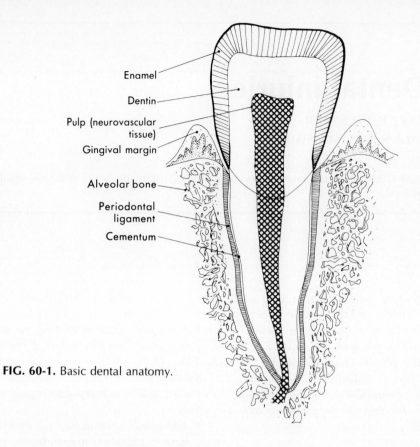

Enamel

Dentin

Pulp (neurovascular
tissue)

Gingival margin

Alveolar bone

Periodontal
ligament

Cementum

FIG. 60-1. Basic dental anatomy.

4. Position: upper teeth overlap lower teeth; mirror imaging of teeth left to right; teeth in each arch arranged in arch form
   • Abnormal: asymmetries and obvious displacements
5. Pain and sensitivity: ascertained by questioning patients about abnormal pain on percussion or sensitivity to air, cold, heat, or chewing in both involved and uninvolved areas
6. Development status (Fig. 60-2)
   • Abnormal: more than 1 yr deviation from chart

Mandible

See Chapter 58.
1. Observe opening and closing movements of mouth.

2. Check bite for malocclusion.
3. Palpate for tenderness, crepitus, deformity, asymmetry, and mental nerve anesthesia.

TRAUMATIC INJURIES TO THE TEETH

Tooth fractures are usually caused by a blow to the tooth from a fall, sports, fights, or abuse. It is important to define whether the injury is to a primary or permanent tooth.

Diagnostic findings

The signs and symptoms vary with the site of fracture. Cracks, loss of tooth structures, hemorrhage at the gingival margin or from an exposed pulp, pain, and sensitivity to stimuli can all result.
1. Crown cracks (crazing), which are incomplete

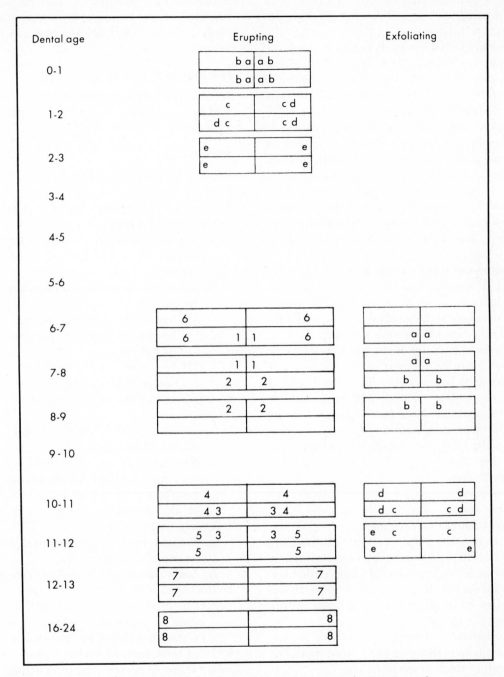

FIG. 60-2. Most common pattern of dental development. **a-e,** Primary teeth. **1-8,** Secondary (permanent) teeth.

fractures of the enamel without loss of tooth structure, may be associated with other injuries to the tooth.

2. Uncomplicated crown fractures involve the enamel or dentin. If the dentin is involved, a yellow area will appear at the center of fracture site and may demonstrate sensitivity to thermal or direct stimuli (air, heat, cold) because of proximity of the pulp.

3. Complicated crown fractures extending through the pulp almost uniformly produce sensitivity to thermal or direct stimuli (e.g., touch, air, ice). There is usually hemorrhage from the exposed dental pulp. Pulp injuries may lead to subsequent inflammation, necrosis, and abscess formation, with progressive pain.

4. Crown-root fractures appear as a "split tooth" and involve the enamel, dentin, cementum, and almost always the pulp. There is usually hemorrhage at the gingival margin, and if the fracture extends through the pulp, there is bleeding along the fracture line as well.

5. Root fractures are rare in the anterior primary teeth before 18 mo of age. They involve the cementum, dentin, and pulp and, on physical examination, may be associated with movement of the tooth.

6. Periodontal injuries are often found with dental fractures.

Complications
1. Imbedding of tooth fragments into the soft tissue (tongue, lips)
2. Aspiration of tooth fragment
3. Damage to the pulp, resulting in subsequent inflammation, necrosis, or abscess formation. May be secondary to initial injury to the neurovascular bundle at time of trauma or to secondary bacterial contamination and inflammatory response
4. Dentoalveolar abscess
5. Damage to underlying permanent tooth bud
6. Death of tooth or eventual loss

Ancillary data
Dental x-ray films, if available, are particularly important in evaluating all injuries involving fractures of the dentin, pulp, or roots. X-ray study is a required diagnostic modality for root fractures.

Differential diagnosis
1. Dental attrition (normal wear)
2. Loss or fracture of a previously placed restoration

Management
Life-threatening conditions must be stabilized.

1. Uncomplicated crown fractures or cracks not involving the pulp
   a. Primary tooth: nonurgent referral to a dentist for follow-up for definitive treatment
   b. Secondary tooth: dental referral within 24 hr for
      (1) Smoothing of sharp, jagged edges of remaining surface to prevent damage to soft tissues
      (2) Restoring tooth appearance, using composite resin material
2. Complicated crown fracture involving the pulp
   a. Primary tooth: urgent dental referral within 24 hr
   b. Secondary tooth: immediate referral to minimize bacterial contamination of the pulp and to provide subsequent endodontic therapy and crown
3. Crown-root fracture
   a. Primary tooth: urgent referral within 24 hr, usually for extraction
   b. Secondary tooth; immediate referral
4. Root fractures
   • Immediate referral to a dentist for stabilization or extraction of fracture segment. Primary teeth may be removed.
5. Long-term goals of dentist include:
   a. Maintenance of vitality of tooth, if possible
   b. Treatment of the pulp and its complica-

tions, often requiring root canal therapy and a crown

c. Restoration of clinical crown
d. Extraction and prosthesis if other goals not achieved

Disposition

Close dental follow-up is essential for all patients with dental trauma and any findings on physical examination—both for acute management and long-term monitoring of dental health.

TRAUMATIC PERIODONTAL INJURIES

Periodontal injuries involving the alveolar bone or socket and the periodontal ligament are almost always caused by a blow. Teeth are abnormally mobile or displaced.

Diagnostic findings

The extent of mobility or displacement reflects the severity of the injury. Pain and increased sensitivity are commonly present.

1. Concussion results in minimal damage to the periodontal ligament. The tooth is sensitive to percussion or pressure such as chewing, biting, or mobility testing but is not displaced or excessively mobile.
2. Subluxation produces abnormal looseness and mobility of the tooth from moderate damage to the periodontal ligament with slight displacement. The tooth is displaced out of the socket. Hemorrhage at the gingival margin may be noted.
3. Intrusive displacement is common in primary teeth and involves the tooth being driven into the socket. The tooth may appear avulsed. Compression fractures of the alveolar socket are common.
4. Extrusive displacement occurs with relocation of the tooth outside of the alveolar socket into an abnormal position and is often associated with a fracture of the alveolar socket and tear of the periodontal ligament.
5. Avulsion of a tooth is common, particularly in 7- to 10-year-olds

6. Periodontal injuries may be associated with dental fractures

Complications

1. Those involving traumatic injuries to the teeth
2. Root resorption
3. Ankylosis (fusion of tooth to bone)
4. Eruption problem for a permanent successor tooth (i.e., delays, space loss)

Ancillary data

Dental x-ray films, if available, are particularly important to identify associated root fractures.

Differential diagnosis

1. Root fracture
2. Normally exfoliating primary tooth (variably mobile, possibility of slight bleeding)
3. Newly erupting primary and secondary teeth (slightly mobile, possibility of being malpositioned)
4. Dentoalveolar infection
5. Systemic disease with bone loss (e.g., hypothyroidism, diabetes, leukemia)

Management

First priority must be given to stabilization of life threatening conditions.

1. Concussion. No immediate therapy indicated but requires long-term follow-up to ensure that complications of root resorption, pulp injury, and ankylosis do not occur
2. Subluxation. Usually requires immobilization with an acrylic splint and long-term follow-up
3. Intrusive displacement
   a. Primary tooth: urgent referral to dentist within 24 hr. Unaffected permanent tooth will be allowed to erupt with careful observation and close follow-up.
   b. Secondary tooth: initial care giver should attempt to reposition, particularly in adolescents. Younger patients' secondary teeth may be allowed to erupt. Immediate dental referral for stabilization.
4. Extrusive displacement

a. Primary tooth: urgent referral to dentist within 24 hr (usually extracted)
b. Secondary tooth: immediate dental referral for stabilization and positioning
   (1) Initial care giver should attempt to reposition, using gentle pressure.
   (2) Delays in repositioning the tooth increase the chance that the tooth will stabilize in an ectopic position.
5. Avulsion
   a. Primary tooth: nonurgent dental referral (usually left out)
   b. Secondary tooth: immediate dental referral and careful handling of the tooth and rapid reimplantation to maximize the success of replacement. Dentists will immobilize tooth with acrylic splint and arrange close follow-up.
      (1) Hold the tooth carefully by the crown. Do not touch the roots.
      (2) Wash the tooth with saline. Plug the drain to avoid losing tooth. Rinse off foreign material.
      (3) Insert the tooth into the socket as soon as possible (lacerations should be cared for after reimplantation if bleeding is controlled).
      (4) See a dentist immediately. In the interim, have the child hold the tooth in place with a finger or bite on a gauze to stabilize the tooth.
      (5) If immediate reimplantation is not possible, place the tooth under the child's or parent's tongue to bathe in saliva. Other options include soaking in milk or normal saline.
6. Long-term goals of dentist
   a. Maintaining the tooth in the dentition; stabilizing the tooth via interdental acrylic splinting immediately after the injury
   b. Monitoring and treating later pulp and root resorption problems
   c. Considering possible later orthodontic repositioning
   d. Extraction and prosthesis if other goals are not achieved

Disposition

Dental follow-up is essential.

REFERENCES

Berkowitz, R., Ludwig, S., and Johnson, R.: Dental trauma in children and adolescents, Clin. Pediatr. 19:166, 1980.

Courts, F.J., Mueller, W.A., and Tabeline, H.J.: Milk as an interim storage medium for avulsed teeth; Pediatr. Dentistry 5:183, 1983.

Josell, S.D., and Abrams, R.G.: Traumatic injuries to the dentition and its supporting structures, Pediatr. Clin. North Am. 29:717, 1982.

61 Spine and spinal cord trauma

RONALD D. LINDZON

ALERT: Exercise extreme caution when the type and mechanism of injury are sufficient to cause spinal or spinal cord trauma.

The majority of spinal cord injuries are partial or incomplete. With care from the onset of trauma, substantial recovery may ensue, thereby avoiding the catastrophic physical and psychologic morbidity associated with major neurologic involvement. Motor vehicle accidents remain the single most common cause of spinal and spinal cord trauma, followed by falls, diving accidents, electrical injuries, and in newborns, birth trauma.

Initial stabilization of the spine in all major trauma, particularly of the head and face, with collar, sandbags, and tape is imperative in the interval before the cervical spine can be evaluated. This stabilization is maintained until x-ray studies have excluded injury or appropriate intervention has been initiated if pathology is present.

ETIOLOGY
Mechanisms of injury

1. Flexion
   a. Stretching of the posterior ligamentous complex produces tears or spinous process avulsions.
   b. Wedge (tear-drop) fractures of vertebral bodies result from mechanical pressure of one vertebral body on the next.
   c. Ligamentous disruptions result in vari-able degree of subluxation and dislocation of bony spinal elements.
2. Rotation
   a. Simultaneous flexion and rotation about one of the facet joints may cause unilateral facet-joint dislocation.
   b. Rotational forces produce unstable articular process fractures in the lumbar region.
3. Extension
   a. With extension, compression of the posterior neural arch of C1 or the pedicles of C2 from the heavy occiput above can result in fractures of these elements. The latter is known as a hangman's fracture.
   b. Stretch of the anterior longitudinal ligament can produce ligamentous tears or avulsion (tear-drop) fractures of the vertebral body.
   c. Buckling of the ligamentum flavum into the posterior spinal canal can produce central or posterior cord syndromes.
4. Vertical compression/axial loading
   • The cervical and lumbar spines straighten at the time of impact from above or below, potentially compressing the nucleus pulposus (disk matter) into the vertebral body, with compromise of the anterior spinal canal, causing the anterior cord syndrome.

DIAGNOSTIC FINDINGS

A high index of suspicion must be maintained in all traumatic injuries with potential spinal injury. At high risk are those patients with the following:

1. Injury compatible with causing spinal injury as outlined on p. 343
2. Postraumatic neck or back pain
3. Postraumatic neurologic complaints or deficits, whether stable or progressive
4. Postraumatic impaired level of consciousness or an inability to give an accurate history (e.g., infants, alcohol or drug abusers, and those who have had a concussion or are postictal)
5. Breathing difficulty
6. Presence of severe associated injuries or shock

The ability to ambulate after an accident does not exclude spine or spinal-cord trauma since 15%-20% of patients may be able to walk initially. Severe head and facial injuries carry a 15%-20% risk of concomitant spine or spinal cord trauma. Other associated injuries must be defined. The neck and back should be palpated for tenderness, step deformity, crepitus, and paraspinous spasm.

Vital signs

1. Breathing pattern may indicate loss of diaphragmatic breathing and hypoventilation or apnea with injuries to C3, C4, and C5, which supply the phrenic nerve. Although lower cervical lesions preserve diaphragmatic function, there may be a loss of abdominal and intercostal breathing.
2. Hypotension may exist with spinal shock. Hypovolemic shock must be excluded.
3. Temperature regulation is impaired with associated hypothermia or hyperthermia.

Neurologic findings (Chapters 15 and 57)

1. Mental status and level of consciousness
2. Cranial nerves. Assess for associated intracranial injury.

3. Motor
   a. Tone
      (1) Flaccid: lower motor neuron (LMN) lesion or spinal shock (with areflexia)
      (2) Spastic: upper motor neuron (UMN) lesion (with hyperreflexia)
   b. Power (Table 61-1)
      (1) Comparison of strength of upper to lower extremities and right to left. Muscles that are essential for maintaining normal posture usually have bilateral innervation and are not useful in lateralizing weakness. Best muscle groups to use for rapid examination are:
         (a) Upper extremity: dorsiflexion of wrist and extension of forearm
         (b) Lower extremity: dorsiflexion of great toe and flexion of lower leg at knee
      (2) Mass flexion withdrawal movements in response to stimulation may occur in infants with paralyzed limbs and may be indistinguishable from normal movements.
4. Sensation. Upper level of sensory impairment is best guide to accurate localization (Table 61-1 and Fig. 61-1)
   a. Light-touch sense assesses ipsilateral posterior spinal column and contralateral anterior column.
   b. Pain sense (pinprick) assesses contralateral anterolateral spinal column.
   c. Position sense assesses ipsilateral posterior spinal column.
5. Reflexes
   a. Deep tendon, superficial (Table 61-1)
   b. Primitive: Babinski's reflex, Hoffmann's reflex, and others, if present beyond 4 wk of life, may be indicative of a UMN lesion.
   c. Rectal. Very important prognostically to assess rectal tone in children with quadriplegia or paraplegia. If rectal tone is present, sacral sparing is implied, with subsequent partial or complete neurologic

TABLE 61-1. Spinal cord injuries: motor, sensory, and reflex deficits

Level of lesion	Motor function lost	Sensation lost at and below	Reflex
C2	Breathing	Occiput	
C3	Spontaneous breathing and trapezius function	Thyroid cartilage	
C4		Suprasternal notch	
C5	Shoulder flexion and abduction	Infraclavicular +/− lateral arm sparing	Biceps brachialis*
C6		Infraclavicular +/− lateral arm, fore-arm sparing	Brachioradialis*
C7	Elbow and wrist extension	Infraclavicular with sparing as above to middle finger	Triceps*
C8	Small muscles of hand (lumbricales and interossei)	Infraclavicular with sparing as above to little finger	
T1		Infraclavicular with upper extremity sparing to axilla	
T4	Intercostal and abdominal musculature	Nipple line	Upper abdominal†
T7		Inferior costal margin	
T10		Umbilicus	Lower abdominal†
T12			
L1	Hip flexion	Groin	
L2		Anteromedial thigh	
L3	Hip adduction and knee extension	Medial knee	Knee/patellar*
L4	Hip abduction and knee extension	Anterior knee and medial calf	
L5	Foot and great toe dorsiflexion	Lateral dorsum foot and lateral sole foot	
S1	Foot and great toe plantar flexion	Lateral dorsum foot and lateral sole foot	Ankle/Achilles*
S2	Perianal and rectal sphincter tone	Perianal and rectal sensation	
S3			
S4			

*Deep tendon.
†Superficial.

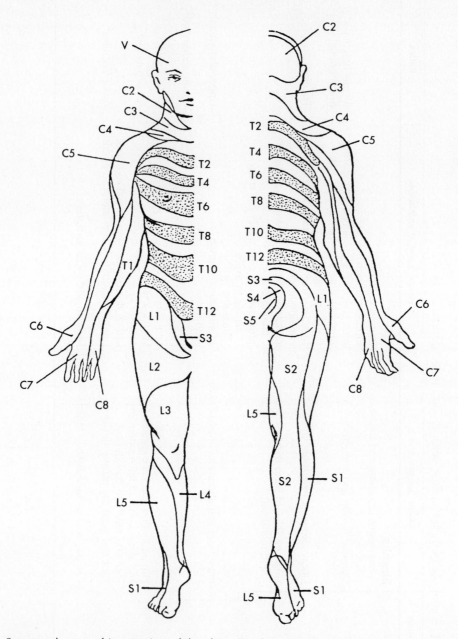

FIG. 61-1. Segmental areas of innervation of the skin. Overlapping of one segment occurs between adjacent dermatomes. (From Clark, R.G.: Essentials of clinical neuroanatomy and neurophysiology, Philadelphia, 1975, F.A. Davis Co.)

recovery in up to 30%-50%. Absence of rectal tone implies only a 2%-3% chance of partial or complete recovery.

   d. Bulbocavernous reflex is performed by pressing the glans penis or pulling on urinary catheter. An intact reflex results in distinct rectal sphincter contraction. The absence of an intact reflex indicates the presence of spinal shock. No accurate estimate of prognosis can be made until this reflex has returned.

   e. Autonomic reflex paralysis produces vasomotor paralysis with flushed, warm, dry skin, loss of temperature regulation (if lesion above T8), hypotension, and bradycardia.

6. Mental status changes, craniofacial injuries, range of motion abnormalities, and focal neurologic findings are not always present in acute cervical spine injuries.

Cervical spine injury stability

1. Intact anterior structures with disrupted posterior elements often are unstable.
2. Intact posterior elements with disrupted anterior elements are occasionally unstable.
3. Disruption of both anterior and posterior structures usually causes instability.
4. Mechanically stable fractures may still cause neurologic defects.

Complications

1. Quadriplegia or paraplegia; paralysis
2. Spinal shock. Flaccid paralysis, areflexia and sensory loss distal to lesion. Impaired temperature control. Hypotension with bradycardia. Skin is warm, flushed, and dry as a result of loss of sympathetic tone and decreased peripheral vascular resistance. Priapism
3. Acute urinary retention or incontinence
4. Paralytic ileus with potential for aspiration
5. Gastric stress ulcer
6. Incomplete spinal cord syndromes
   a. Anterior cord. Complete paralysis and hypalgesia with preservation of touch and proprioception. Flexion or vertical compression injury with anterior spinal cord compressed by bony fragments, disk material, or hematoma
   b. Central cord. Motor weakness in arms greater than in legs, with variable bladder and sensory involvement. Extension injury, with buckling of ligamentum flavum into posterior spinal canal
   c. Posterior cord. Loss of proprioception with variable paresis. Extension injury as in *b*. Rare
   d. Brown-Séquard's syndrome. Cord hemisection with ipsilateral motor, proprioception, and light-touch deficit, with contralateral pain and temperature impairment. Usually penetrating injury.
   e. Horner's syndrome. Unilateral ptosis, miosis, anhidrosis, facial flushing with apparent enophthalmos. Disruption of the cervical sympathetic chain arising at C7-T2.

7. Death secondary to respiratory failure, cardiovascular collapse, hypothermia or hyperthermia, or associated injuries
8. Long-term sequelae including psychiatric trauma, repeated pulmonary and genitourinary infections, muscle contractures, progressive spinal deformity, and decubitus ulcers.

Ancillary data

Cervical x-ray studies (Fig. 61-2)

All cervical vertebrae except C1 have a body. C1 moves in union with the occiput. C2 (axis) has the odontoid process (dens) protuding from its body to rest posterior to the anterior arch of C1 and anterior to the transverse atlantal ligament, allowing for rotation of the neck.

The most important initial x-ray film is the *cross-table lateral cervical spine*. This film will identify over 75% of cervical spine fractures, dislocations, and subluxations. It should be obtained early in the resuscitation and the cervical

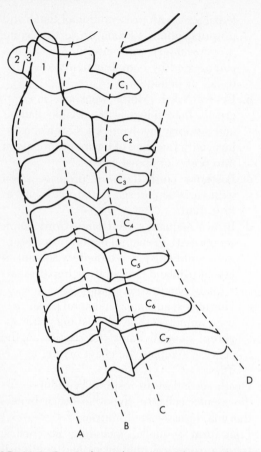

FIG. 61-2. Cervical vertebrae. Lateral cervical spine: **A,** anterior vertebral bodies; **B,** posterior vertebral bodies and anterior spinal canal; **C,** spinolaminal line and posterior spinal canal; **D,** spinous process tips C2-C7. *1,* Odontoid process or dens of C2; *2,* anterior arch of C1; *3,* predental space between posterior surface of anterior arch of C1 and anterior surface of odontoid process.

spine should be immobilized during this phase. All seven cervical vertebrae must be included.

In order to visualize C7-T1, it is usually necessary to have one person hold the patient's head, applying in-line axial traction, while another pulls gently down on the arms from the foot of the bed. Lead aprons should be worn by care providers.

Swimmer's (transaxillary) view should be obtained if C7-T1 is not visualized using the above technique.

Complete cervical spine trauma series must include, as a minimum, the cross-table lateral view, anteroposterior view, and the open-mouth odontoid radiograph.

- Assessment of the lateral cervical spine *(ABC)*
1. *Alignment:* four continuous curvilinear lines without step-offs. Loss of the normal lordotic curve is seen in 20% of normal patients with spasm, or it may be the only evidence of severe spinal injury.
2. *Bony integrity.* Compare uniformity, shape, mineralization, density. Look for fracture lines, displacements, subluxations, or dislocations in systematic manner by first assessing each vertebral body and then each pedicle, facet joint, lamina, and spinous process.
3. *Cartilaginous spaces*
   a. Assessment of disk-space uniformity. Isolated disk-space narrowing in a child with the appropriate type and mechanism of injury is suggestive of acute disk herniation. Lengthening of the disk space implies disruption of the anulus fibrosus and possibly the longitudinal ligaments.
   b. The inferior articular facets above and the superior facet below articulate and must line up in parallel. Widening, facet overriding, or vertebral body rotation over 11 degrees above the facet joint is pathologic.
   c. Interspinous widening is suggestive of ligamentous disruption of the interspinous and supraspinous ligaments.
4. Soft tissue spaces
   a. Predental space (space between the posterior aspect of the anterior arch of C1 and the anterior aspect of the odontoid process of C2 on lateral view) should ≤5 mm in children and ≤3 mm in adults. Greater distance may represent odontoid fractures with posterior displacement or transverse atlantal ligament tear.

b. Normal prevertebral spaces:
 (1) Anterior to C2; ≤7 mm in children and adults
 (2) Anterior to C3,C4: ≤5 mm in children and adults or < 40% of the AP diameter of the C3 and C4 vertebral bodies
 (3) Between C6 and trachea: ≤14 mm in children (under 15 yr) and ≤22 mm in adults
  NOTE: NG or ET tubes may invalidate these measurements. Soft tissue swelling may be secondary to hemorrhage, abscess, infection, foreign body, tumor, air, or bony injury.
c. Since the retropharyngeal space may be widened during expiration, inspiratory film should be attempted.
d. The body of the hyoid bone should normally lie entirely below a line that is parallel to the top of C3. The hyoid bone crosses the epiglottis and is helpful in identifying an inflamed epiglottis.
• Other considerations
1. The odontoid film (open-mouth view preferable) will ensure that the dens is centered between the lateral masses of the atlas, and the AP view is useful in assessing C3-C7. Both should be obtained after initial stabilization of the patient and after ensurance that the lateral view is normal.
2. Oblique, flexion, and extension views and tomograms are occasionally required.
3. Epiphyseal growth plates may resemble fractures. Other developmental changes must be considered in interpretation of films.
 a. Pseudosubluxation of C2 occurs anterior to C3 and, rarely, at C3-C4. Maximum normal: 2.7 mm
 b. Posterior arch of C1 fuses at 4 yr and anterior arch at 7-10 yr
 c. Epiphyseal plate at base of odontoid fuses with body of C2 at 3-7 yr
4. CT scan often is preferred in selected circumstances when routine films are negative

and a fracture is still suspected. The anatomy can be well documented without unnecessary movement of the patient.
5. Minimal wedge shape of body of C3 may be normal.
6. Up to 15%-50% of pediatric patients with major neurologic involvement have normal roentgenograms.
 Thoracic and lumbar spine x-ray studies
1. A cross-table lateral view of the thoracic or lumbar spine should be obtained first, with the patient immobilized on a firm backboard.
2. AP view is taken next (obliques periodically needed).
3. Interpedicular space must be assessed, as well as the *ABC's* delineated on p. 348.
• Other considerations
1. The distance between the medical aspects of the two pedicles overlying each vertebral body (on the AP view) gradually increases in a caudal (cervical-to-lumbar) direction. A marked increase in this distance is indicative of posterior disruption and probable instability.
2. Most fractures of the lower spine occur in the region of T10-L4 although in the multiply injured patient, injuries are common at T2-T7. In multiple level, noncontiguous fractures, the secondary lesions occur at L4-L5 and C1-C2.
3. Fractures of T1-T5 may produce mediastinal hematomas with widening of the mediastinum.
4. Thoracolumbar compression fractures in children may appear as beaklike projections on the anterior margin of the vertebral body, usually superior.

DIFFERENTIAL DIAGNOSIS

1. Hysterical paralysis
2. Trauma
 a. Bilateral brachial plexus injury
 b. Nerve root injury
 c. Cauda equina syndrome
3. Vascular: ischemia resulting from atheroscle-

rosis, thromboembolic disease, thoracic aorta dissection, epidural hematoma

4. Spinal tumor

MANAGEMENT

Initial attention must be paid to resuscitation and support while immobilizing the spine at the levels of suspected injury. Immediate consultation with a neurosurgeon is necessary.

1. Airway stabilization, with ventilatory support as necessary and administration of oxygen
   a. Bag-valve-mask ventilation, nasotracheal intubation, or cricothyroidotomy in patients with severe respiratory compromise
   b. Oral ET intubation—contraindicated because excessive C-spine motion may occur
   c. Forced vital capacity determination may be useful in the evaluation.
2. Circulation (Chapter 5)
   a. If shock is present, treat as hypovolemic. Look for source of internal hemorrhage. Excessive transfusion of crystalloid in the presence of spinal shock may precipitate pulmonary edema. Urinary output rather than blood pressure is the best monitor.
   b. Once hypovolemic shock has been excluded neurogenic shock should be considered. Patients are hypotensive with bradycardia and have warm, flushed, dry skin—in contrast to hypovolemic shock.
      (1) Use pneumatic antishock trousers (MAST) to increase peripheral vascular resistance. Trendelenburg position. Ensure adequate ventilation and oxygenation.
      (2) To treat decreased sympathetic tone: low-dose norepinephrine (Levophed) drip infusion at 0.1-1.0 µg/kg/min IV, with close attention to vital signs
      (3) To treat increased parasympathetic tone: atropine 0.01-0.02 mg/kg/dose IV repeated q 5-10 min as necessary, used alternatively or concurrently with norepinephrine

      (4) Insert NG tube and Foley catheter. Consider cimetidine 20-40 mg/kg/24 hr (maximum: 300 mg) q 6 hr IV
      (5) Steroids: dexamethasone (Decadron) 0.25 mg/kg/dose (maximum: 20mg/dose) q 4-6 hr IV for 72 hr. Controversial
3. Immobilization and stabilization of neck from the outset
   a. Place in neutral position with sandbags and 1 to 2-inch tape across the forehead and chin with the patient on a rigid backboard or scoop.
   b. Apply gentle in-line traction with neurologic abnormalities. Cervical spine stabilization can be achieved with a semi-hard Philadelphia collar or a four-poster collar. Tape and sandbags alone or in combination with the Philadelphia collar is most effective. Soft collars offer no demonstratable stability.
4. When there is cervical neurologic impairment, *skeletal traction* is indicated on an emergent basis. Traction can be applied using halo, Gardner-Wells, Crutchfield, or Vinke tongs. A neurosurgeon is best involved in these procedures.
   a. The patient is then transferred to a suitable frame and 1-5 lb of weight/interspace (adult) is applied. Lateral spine roentgenograms are repeated to assess alignment. If alignment is not achieved, muscle relaxants are often required.
   b. Thoracic and lumbar injuries are treated by immobilizing the patient to allow for postural reduction. Concurrent stabilization of other life-threatening injuries with appropriate consultations is essential.
5. *Surgical decompression*, when required, should be done in a timely fashion. When performed more than 8 hr after injury, it is significantly less successful. The indications include progressive neurologic deterioration, penetrating injuries of the spinal cord, and a

foreign body within the spinal canal. Surgical stabilization and realignment may be necessary for potentially unstable injuries or for relief of pain.

DISPOSITION

All patients with spine or spinal cord injury require hospitalization and immediate neurosurgical consultation. A team approach to the management of such patients is mandatory. After they are stabilized, patients often require transfer to neurosurgical spinal trauma centers.

Parental education

Prevention

1. Automobile restraints should always be used.
2. Swimming and diving in uncontrolled areas should be avoided.
3. Trampolines should be forbidden.

REFERENCES

Blahd, W.H., Iserson, K.V., and Bjelland, J.C.: Efficacy of the post-traumatic cross-table lateral view of the cervical spine, Ann. Emerg. Med. 2:243, 1983.

Gaufin, L.M., and Goodman, S.J.: Cervical spine injuries in infants: problems in management, J. Neurosurg, 42:179, 1975.

Gerlock, A.J., Krichner, S.G., Heller, R.M., et al.: The cervical spine in trauma, Philadelphia, 1978, W.B. Saunders Co.

Hockberger, R.S., and Doris, P.E.: Spinal injuries. In Rosen, P., editor: Emergency medicine: concepts and clinical practice, St. Louis, 1983, The C.V. Mosby Co.

Kelen, G.D., Noji, E.K., and Doris, P.E.: Guidelines for use of lumbar spine radiography, Ann. Emerg. Med. 15:245, 1986.

Podolsky, S.: Efficacy of cervical spine immobilization methods, J. Trauma 23:461, 1983.

Walter, J., Doris, P.E., Shaffer, M.A.: Clinical presentation of patients with acute cervical spine injury, Ann. Emerg. Med. 3:512, 1984.

62 Thoracic trauma

VINCENT J. MARKOVCHICK
BENJAMIN HONIGMAN

ALERT: Blunt or penetrating thoracic trauma requires a rapid assessment of pulmonary, cardiac, and mediastinal injuries. These may necessitate lifesaving procedures without a complete data base.

Traumatic injuries of the chest are common and require urgent attention to therapy and diagnosis. The physician must rapidly assess the status of the patient and may have to intervene without a full diagnosis more than with any other anatomic area. Delays in management are often life threatening, while life-saving procedures such as pericardiocentesis and the insertion of a chest tube are associated with minimal complications.

The initial evaluation of the patient must take into consideration the totality of the injuries (Chapter 56). The airway, ventilation, and circulation are of primary concern. Specific attention must be focused on the mechanism and severity of the injury and the progression of signs and symptoms since the trauma.

1. *Blunt trauma* is associated with chest-wall injuries (rib fractures or flail chest), hemothorax, pneumothorax, pulmonary contusion, myocardial contusion, aortic tears, diaphragmatic rupture, and esophageal rupture.
2. *Penetrating injuries* cause hemothorax, pneumothorax, penetrating cardiac injuries and tamponade, direct vessel damage, and diaphragmatic injuries.

The duration since injury and the current status provide some indication of the urgency of intervention.

Diagnostic findings by a quick physical examination must include blood pressure (including an evaluation for pulses paradoxus and orthostatic changes if appropriate), respiratory rate and pattern, and heart sounds. Evidence of upper-airway obstruction must be sought, including stridor and facial and neck injuries, with active intervention initiated when indicated. If the upper airway appears intact, lower-airway compromise must be excluded by evaluating chest wall stability, symmetry and adequacy of air movement, and presence of subcutaneous emphysema.

If the patient is in obvious respiratory distress, immediate therapy is required. Oxygen should be administered and, simultaneously, an airway ensured. Unilateral or bilateral chest tubes may be required, often solely on the basis of the physical examination.

Shock must be treated. With isolated thoracic injuries shock is most commonly caused by massive pulmonary hemorrhage, pericardial tamponade, or tension pneumothorax. With multiple trauma, other etiologies must be excluded.

Ancillary data that are mandatory in any thoracic injury include chest x-ray film (portable supine if the patient is unstable), ECG, ABG, and CBC (Hct done in ED). Patients with major injuries also should have a type and cross-match performed immediately. However, these studies should not delay intervention in the patient with respiratory distress following a traumatic injury.

RIB FRACTURE

ALERT: Rib fractures are rare in children because of their highly elastic chest wall; therefore, when a rib fracture is noted, significant underlying organ injury (e.g., liver, lung, spleen) must be suspected. Upper-rib fractures are associated with pulmonary and major vessel injuries; lower-rib injuries are associated with potential liver, spleen, lung, and kidney injury. Conversely, the absence of a rib fracture does not preclude serious injury to the underlying soft tissue structures.

Fractured ribs are caused by blunt trauma resulting from motor vehicle accidents, falls, blows with blunt objects, child abuse, and athletic injuries. With minor trauma, rib fracture is unlikely, whereas in major trauma a rib fracture may lacerate underlying structures.

Diagnostic findings

The mechanism of injury and estimate of the degree of impact may predict the type of injury.
1. Dyspnea and chest pain are common symptoms with isolated rib fractures.
2. Point tenderness over the rib is uniformly present. Anterior-posterior and lateral-lateral compression is painful. Referred pain is present on proximal compression of the fractured rib.
3. Tachypnea, tachycardia, and shock are associated with underlying organ damage and respiratory failure.
   #### Complications
1. Pneumothorax
2. Hemothorax
3. Pulmonary laceration or contusion
4. Myocardial contusion
5. Solid visceral damage (liver, spleen, kidney), particularly with fractures of ribs 9-12
6. Neurovascular tears (e.g., subclavian, brachial plexus, aorta) with fractures of ribs 1 and 2

Ancillary data
1. Chest x-ray studies. Most useful in evaluating status of pulmonary parenchyma and mediastinum. Over 50% of single-rib fractures are missed on the initial chest x-ray film.
2. Hct (to be done in ED) and urinalysis
3. ABG with any respiratory distress or complications
4. ECG for major blunt chest injury
5. Angiogram for widened mediastinum (aortic tear) or fractures of the first or second rib, particularly if displaced

Differential diagnosis
1. Infectious/inflammatory: pleurisy, pneumonia, perichondritis
2. Trauma: rib contusion, costochondral separation (snapping sound with breathing)

Management
1. Treatment of any complications
2. Simple rib fractures without complications
   a. Analgesia
   b. Intercostal nerve block, using long-acting local anesthetic agent such as bupivacaine (Marcaine) with epinephrine. 1-2 ml is injected in the subcostal space at the posterior axillary line. The intercostal nerve above and below the fracture should be blocked.
3. Instructions to patients
   a. Patients should be taught deep-breathing exercises.
   b. Patients should not use binders or rib belts because they inhibit adequate ventilation.

Disposition
1. Hospitalization should be strongly considered for young children and infants with *any* rib fracture because of the extreme force necessary to break a rib in this age-group and, therefore, the high probability of complications and the high possibility of child abuse.
2. Hospitalization for observation should be

strongly considered for older children and adolescents who sustain multiple (>2) fractures.
3. All children with any complications require admission.

Parental education
1. Continue child's deep-breathing exercises.
2. Call if child develops cough, fever, dyspnea, or increased pain.

FLAIL CHEST

ALERT: Flail chest is invariably associated with pulmonary contusion and abnormal respiratory physiology.

Flail chest results from blunt trauma when three or more adjacent ribs are fractured at two points resulting in a freely movable chest-wall segment. This results in paradoxic movement on respiration (inward with inspiration and outward with expiration), which may compress lung tissue, decrease ventilation on the ipsilateral side, and cause mediastinal shift to the opposite side. Venous return is decreased secondary to lung compression. More importantly, the underlying pulmonary contusion contributes to hypoxia and increasing respiratory distress.

Diagnostic findings
1. Usually associated with multiple trauma
2. Tenderness over ribs with crepitus and ecchymoses
3. Common occurrence of increased heart and respiratory rates. Shock may occur secondary to complications or related injuries.
4. Visible or palpable paradoxic movement, which may require a tangential light to see. Up to 30% is missed on the initial examination in the first 6 hr.

Complications
Complications are commonly associated with rib fracture. Respiratory insufficiency is caused by pulmonary contusion, atelectasis, and decreased tidal volume and vital capacity, with resultant hypoxia, AV shunting, and, ultimately, shock.

The respiratory embarrassment results primarily not from the paradoxic movement of the chest but from the underlying injury to lung parenchyma.

Ancillary data
Chest x-ray studies and ABG are required.

Management
1. For multiple trauma management, treat and diagnose complications and associated life-threatening injuries: oxygen, IV, chest x-ray film, ABG, and Hct.
2. Stabilize flail chest with sandbags and pressure over unstable segment, or position patient on side of injury, if possible.
3. Correct associated respiratory complications, e.g., thoracostomy for pneumothorax or hemothorax. If respiratory distress continues, intubate and internally stabilize with positive-pressure ventilation.
4. Intubate if flail chest is associated with:
   a. Shock
   b. Three or more related injuries
   c. Five or more rib fractures
   d. Underlying pulmonary disease
   e. Respiratory failure, with PaO_2 <50 mm Hg and $PaCO_2$ >50 mm Hg
      (1) Relative indications include increasing respiratory rate, restlessness, anxiety, or A-a gradient, or a decreasing PaO_2.
      (2) Some clinicians recommend intubation only when flail chest is associated with respiratory failure.
5. Strongly consider thoracostomy if the patient is to have general anesthesia or if the patient requires ventilator support (especially if PEEP is to be used). In addition, thoracostomy is required for hemothorax or pneumothorax (Appendix A-9).
6. Do not give antibiotics prophylactically. Steroids are not indicated.

Disposition
All patients require admission to an ICU.

STERNAL FRACTURE

ALERT: Sternal fractures and dislocations in children are unusual but when present suggest underlying myocardial contusion, cardiac rupture, pericardial tamponade, or pulmonary contusion. Mortality rate is 25%-45%.

Diagnostic findings

Simple sternal fractures, which are unusual, are accompanied by anterior chest pain with point tenderness and ecchymoses over the sternum. More commonly, there are associated complications.

Complications
1. Flail chest
2. Myocardial contusion or rupture, pericardial tamponade
3. Pulmonary contusion

Ancillary data
1. Chest x-ray study. Reveals fractures on lateral view, although special sternal views may be necessary. Differentiate from nonossified cartilage of sternum. Will not be seen on PA or rib films.
2. ECG reveals nonspecific ST-T wave changes and a persistent tachycardia. Dysrhythmias may be seen.

Management
1. Treatment of life-threatening injuries and complications with oxygen, IV, cardiac monitor, specific intervention
2. Analgesia
3. Surgery may be required if fracture is displaced

Disposition

All patients require admission to an ICU.

TRAUMATIC PNEUMOTHORAX

ALERT: A simple pneumothorax may cause respiratory distress. Bilateral or tension pneumothoraxes are life threatening and require immediate intervention.

A *simple* pneumothorax occurs when air accumulates in the pleural space without mediastinal shift. It is invariably present with penetrating chest injuries and in 15%-50% of blunt chest trauma cases. A *tension* pneumothorax is produced when there is progressive accumulation of air in the pleural space with shift of mediastinal structures to the opposite hemithorax and compression of the mediastinum and contralateral lung. Tension pneumothorax can progressively decrease cardiac output. Massive shunting of blood occurs from perfused but nonventilated areas, resulting from lung compression, atelectasis, and collapse.

Etiology
1. Blunt trauma: complication of fractured ribs, cardiopulmonary resuscitation, or violent chest impact with closed glottis.
2. Penetrating trauma: complication of stab, gunshot, or other penetrating wounds or complication of insertion of a central venous catheter

Diagnostic findings
1. Patients have dyspnea, chest pain, and a history of trauma.
2. With a small, uncomplicated pneumothorax, patients have normal vital signs, although respiratory and heart rates may be increased. Large defects are associated with respiratory distress and sometimes cyanosis.
3. Tension pneumothorax is accompanied by hypotension, pulsus paradoxus, increased jugular venous pressure (JVP), tachycardia, and respiratory distress, as well as restlessness, agitation, altered mental status, tracheal shift, and, at times, cyanosis. Air hunger is marked.
   a. If the patient is being ventilated with bag-valve-mask, an early indication of tension pneumothorax is an increasing resistance to bag ventilation. If the patient is being mechanically ventilated, increasing airway pressure may be needed to deliver the same volume of air.

b. Other clues are increased CVP, decreased BP, electromechanical dissociation, and marked intercostal and supraclavicular retractions.

4. Decreased breath sounds and hyperresonance to percussion are present. Subcutaneous emphysema with crepitus is common, increasing rapidly if positive-pressure ventilation is being used.

   NOTE: Soon after penetrating injuries, and in children with small chests, transmission of breath sounds from the unaffected lung may simulate normal breath sounds, making clinical diagnosis more difficult.

5. Pneumomediastinum may accompany pneumothorax.

   ### Complications

   Complications include respiratory distress, hypotension, and cardiac arrest.

   ### Ancillary data

1. Chest x-ray film for simple pneumothorax
   a. Definitive diagnostic procedure
   b. On occasion, may only be found in an expiratory view, which increases intrapleural pressure, pushing the lung and visceral pleura away from the chest wall
   c. Classification: small (<10%), moderate (10%-50%), large (>50%)

   NOTE: Tension pneumothorax should be a clinical diagnosis and not await x-ray confirmation. X-ray film shows marked lung compression with mediastinal shift away from the affected side.

2. ABG when patient is stabilized

Differential diagnosis

Many other entities besides trauma cause pneumothorax:

1. Asthma and other reactive airway diseases with hyperexpansion
2. Spontaneous pneumothorax secondary to apical blebs in adolescents
3. Meconium aspiration and hyaline membrane disease in the newborn (Chapter 11)

Management

Life-threatening injuries must be treated immediately.

1. Tube thoracostomy is the treatment of choice for pneumothorax, sometimes before making a definitive diagnosis (Appendix A-9)
   a. Indications for insertion of a chest tube include:
      (1) Tension pneumothorax
      (2) Traumatic etiology, especially penetrating injuries
      (3) Any pneumothorax with respiratory symptoms
      (4) Increasing pneumothorax after initial conservative therapy
      (5) Pneumothorax with need for mechanical ventilation or general anesthesia
      (6) Associated hemothorax
      (7) Bilateral pneumothorax

      NOTE: Small (<10%), simple pneumothorax—one that shows no increase on repeat x-ray—in a symptom-free patient who does not require general anesthesia or mechanical ventilation may be observed in the hospital without a chest tube.
   b. Position for chest tube
      (1) Insert in fourth or fifth intercostal space in midaxillary line directed posteriorly and apically.
      (2) Insert superior to rib since neurovascular bundle runs inferior to rib in the lateral interspaces.
   c. Size. As large a tube as possible should be inserted, particularly if a hemothorax is present.
      • Newborn (8-12 Fr), infants (14-20 Fr), children (20-28 Fr), adolescents (28-42 Fr)
   d. Use tube with radiopaque line (for placement verification by roentgenogram.)
   e. Drainage. All chest tubes should be connected in an underwater seal drainage. Patients with continuous air leaks or associated hemothorax may require suction (15-25 cm H_2O).

2. Chest venting may be required as an initial therapeutic maneuver when tension is suspected and when there is some delay in placement of a chest tube.

  a. Venting can be done with a needle, Angiocath, or one-way flutter valve.

  b. Venting necessitates the eventual use of a chest tube.

  c. Venting should be done in the second or third intercostal space at the midclavicular line in the anterior chest wall. Care must be taken to prevent the vent from being dislodged before the chest tube is placed.

Disposition

All patients with pneumothorax require hospitalization. The level of monitoring is dependent on the degree of respiratory distress and associated injuries.

PULMONARY CONTUSION

ALERT: Pulmonary contusion is a significant cause of respiratory failure following major blunt injury in children, particularly rapid deceleration injuries.

Pulmonary contusion occurs when there is lung parenchymal damage with intraalveolar hemorrhage and edema. This is secondary to increased capillary membrane permeability, which impairs gas exchange.

Diagnostic findings

Patients have experienced a rapid-deceleration injury and arrive with dyspnea and cyanosis. Hemoptysis is rare in children. Tachycardia, tachypnea, anxiety, restlessness, labored respiration, and hypotension may be present. Localized rales or wheezing, with decreased breath sounds, are common. Significant hypoxia may be delayed 4-6 hr from the time of injury.

Obvious evidence of external trauma may not be present. Approximately 80%-90% of patients have associated injuries.

Complications

Pneumonia is a complication.

Ancillary data

1. Chest x-ray film. For all patients with increased respiratory or heart rate following trauma even if there is no external evidence of injury

  a. Findings vary from patchy areas of alveolar infiltrates to frank consolidation. They may be delayed 4-6 hr or they may be rapid in onset.

  b. Usually clear in 48-60 hr

2. ABG

  a. Hypoxemia is invariable but may be delayed in onset for 4-6 hr (deteriorates over the ensuing 24 hr).

  b. The A-aO$_2$ difference (gradient) at room air (A-aO$_2$ = 150 − PaO$_2$ − 1.2 PaCO$_2$)—normally ≤15—is the first to increase.

  c. Respiratory rate will increase and is a noninvasive clue to onset of insufficiency when followed serially.

Differential diagnosis

1. Trauma: multiple causes of acute respiratory distress syndrome (ARDS) in children include smoke inhalation and fat emboli (fracture, penetrating chest wound). ARDS is usually delayed in onset, beginning 24-48 hr after the injury, and it has diffuse involvement.

2. Medical causes of infiltrates and hypoxia: CHF, embolism, pneumonia

Management

1. Treat associated life-threatening injuries.

2. Maintain oxygenation and ventilation.

  a. Intubation and ventilation are indicated if PaO$_2$ <50 mm Hg at 100% O$_2$ (sea level).

  b. Positive end-expiratory pressure (PEEP) or continuous positive airway pressure (CPAP) may shorten the length of ventilatory assistance. Begin at 5 cm H$_2$O and increase slowly, monitoring oxygenation and cardiac output.

3. Intravenous fluids

  a. Patients with pulmonary contusion benefit from low levels of fluid administration. However, associated injuries may require high volumes of crystalloid. This infusion may increase pulmonary interstitial fluid, worsening the respiratory status.

    b. Ideally, the goal is to combine blood products and crystalloid to maintain adequate perfusion, CVP, and urinary output.

4. Steroids should not be used.
5. Analgesics may be required but must be used sparingly in view of the potential respiratory compromise.
6. Antibiotics are reserved for demonstrated infections.

Disposition

All patients require admission to an ICU.

HEMOTHORAX

ALERT: Hemothorax can cause hypovolemic shock and respiratory failure from compression of the lung.

As a result of blunt or penetrating trauma, large amounts of blood can accumulate in the pleural space, secondary to injury to intercostal and internal mammary arteries, the heart, great vessels, or the hilar vessels. Lung lacerations usually have self-limited bleeding. Hemostasis, eventually occurs in hemothorax as a result of low pulmonary arterial pressures, large concentrations of thromboplastin in lung tissue, and the compressive effects of the pleural blood volume.

Diagnostic findings

1. With small amounts of blood loss (<10% of blood volume), diagnosis may be difficult in an isolated injury; however, over 75% are associated with extrathoracic injuries. The physical examination will usually demonstrate evidence of trauma.
2. Larger accumulations of blood (>25% of blood volume) will produce pallor, restlessness, anxiety, tachycardia, vasoconstriction, and eventually, orthostatic and resting hypotension.

3. Chest examination will demonstrate evidence of external trauma and decreased breath sounds. Pneumothorax is often an associated finding.

Complications

1. Respiratory failure, hypotension, and shock
2. Infection with empyema

Ancillary data

1. Chest x-ray study will demonstrate blunting of the costophrenic angle on an upright film when over 175 ml of blood accumulates in the adolescent
    a. Supine chest film will demonstrate haziness of the affected side.
    b. Pneumothorax may be present.
    c. Lateral decubitus film may be helpful if upright cannot be obtained or interpreted.
2. ABG will reflect degree of respiratory compromise.

Differential diagnosis

1. Pleural effusion of any etiology, for example, congestive heart failure, pneumonia, empyema, chylothorax, or hydrothorax (from improperly placed CVP catheter)
2. Trauma: pulmonary contusion (upright or decubitus chest x-ray film should differentiate)

Management

1. Priorities should be established with respect to concurrent life-threatening injuries, that is, maintenance of oxygenation and ventilation. Fluid resuscitation is commonly needed.
2. Tube thoracostomy is the treatment required immediately, sometimes solely on the basis of respiratory distress and physical examination (Appendix A-9).
    a. Indications
       (1) Penetrating injury with obvious or suspected hemothorax, respiratory distress, or shock. Required immediately, before chest x-ray film
       (2) Blunt injuries with suspected hemothorax (decreased breath sounds, mul-

tiple rib fractures, etc.), respiratory failure or shock. Required immediately

(3) Unsuspected thoracic injuries in a child with multiple trauma. A chest x-ray film is indicated before intervention.

(4) The child in hemorrhagic shock with no evidence of internal blood loss from the abdomen, retroperitoneal space, pelvis, or external blood loss associated with an extremity fracture. In these patients, bilateral chest tubes may be required as a diagnostic and therapeutic modality if hemothorax is present on chest x-ray film or instability prevents chest x-ray film.

b. Size. Large-bore Silastic tubes should be used for blood drainage: newborn (8-12 Fr), infants (16-20 Fr), children (20-28 Fr), adolescents (28-42 Fr)

c. Position: fourth or fifth intercostal space in midaxillary line directed superiorly and posteriorly. If large amounts of blood return or if the tube becomes clotted, a second chest tube one or two interspaces below the first may be required.

NOTE: The chest tube should be connected to an underwater seal drain and 15-25 cm H_2O suction.

3. Autotransfusions are useful if appropriate equipment is available.

4. Thoracotomy is only rarely needed but may be life-saving in rare circumstances.

a. When the blood drainage from the initial thoracostomy tube is $>\frac{1}{3}$ of patient's blood volume (blood volume in child: 80 ml/kg; in adult: 70 ml/kg).

b. With persistent bleeding >10% blood volume/hr

c. With increasing hemothorax on chest x-ray film, despite therapy

d. With persistent hypotension despite adequate crystalloid and blood replacement and when other areas of blood loss have been excluded.

Disposition

All patients require admission to an ICU.

SUBCUTANEOUS EMPHYSEMA AND PNEUMOMEDIASTINUM

ALERT: The presence of subcutaneous emphysema or pneumomediastinum in a trauma patient requires a careful search for laryngeal fracture, esophageal tear, or tracheobronchial injury, as well as pneumothorax.

Air in the subcutaneous tissue or mediastinum following trauma may be caused by an underlying intrapleural leak from a pneumothorax or bronchial tear, or it may be secondary to a penetrating injury with spread through the fascial planes.

Etiology

1. Trauma: blunt or penetrating (usually secondary to laryngeal tear). May involve pulmonary or mediastinal structures. May be secondary to foreign body

2. Infection: respiratory

3. Allergy: asthma

4. Intoxication: marijuana inhalation or heroin injection—may cause increased intrathoracic pressure from Valsalva's maneuver and bronchial tear

5. Valsalva's maneuver for any reason, including yelling, coughing, emesis, marijuana smoking

6. Iatrogenic: following intubation of trachea or esophagus

Diagnostic findings

1. History of trauma or excessive Valsalva's maneuver

2. Pain and crepitus overlying the upper thorax and neck

3. "Hammond's crunch" on auscultation

Complications

Complications are directly related to the etiology (e.g., mediastinitis from perforation of esophagus secondary to contamination with gastrointestinal contents)—in contrast to the benign course of only a pneumomediastinum caused by a simple Valsalva's maneuver.

Ancillary data

1. Chest x-ray film reveals air in the tissue planes of the thorax, neck, or mediastinum.
2. Laryngoscopy, bronchoscopy, or an esophagram may be indicated to determine the etiology.

Differential diagnosis

There may be infection by gas gangrene.

Management

1. Treat underlying etiology. May need surgical intervention with certain entities (e.g., with esophageal perforation or laryngeal fracture).
2. Administer 100% oxygen to facilitate resorption secondary to nitrogen washout.
3. Administer antibiotics (penicillin or cephalosporin) if esophageal tear is present.

Disposition

1. Hospitalize patient to evaluate etiologies and facilitate nitrogen washout.
2. Follow those with benign etiologies as outpatients (marijuana, simple Valsalva's maneuver, etc.) if there are no complications.

DIAPHRAGMATIC RUPTURE

ALERT: **Frequently overlooked, diaphragmatic rupture may be an asymptomatic lesion or a large herniation presenting with severe respiratory distress. Presentation may be acute or delayed in onset.**

Diaphragmatic tears may result from blunt or penetrating forces and most often (>90%) are on the left side. Blunt abdominal compression generates increased intraabdominal pressure, which can tear the diaphragm with herniation of stomach, colon, small bowel, spleen, or liver. The negative intrathoracic pressures create a gradient that keeps the diaphragmatic rupture open and facilitates herniation of abdominal contents into the thorax.

Diagnostic findings

1. Presentation varies considerably, depending on whether the signs and symptoms are acute or delayed in onset, on the side of the defect, and on the degree of herniation of abdominal organs.
2. In acute cases patients complain of abdominal and chest pain with dyspnea, nausea, and vomiting. Delayed presentation may be accompanied by nausea, vomiting, abdominal pain, and intermittent episodes of abdominal cramping and colic, with radiation to the associated shoulder.
3. Vital signs may be normal, or there may be tachycardia, hypotension, and tachypnea.
4. A large herniation produces cardiac dullness, with displacement of the point of maximal impulse (PMI) to the right, decreased breath sounds and tympany in the left chest, and bowel sounds or borborygmi in the chest. The abdomen may be distended with obstruction or scaphoid if large amounts of abdominal contents are in the thoracic cavity.

Complication

The complication is bowel obstruction with strangulation of herniated bowel.

Ancillary data

1. Chest x-ray film demonstrates an elevated diaphragm (usually on the left), pleural effusion, silhouetting of the diaphragm, and bowel or viscus in the chest. There may be a mediastinal shift to the right, atelectasis, and an air-fluid bubble, or the NG tube may be above the diaphragm.

   NOTE: 20%-40% of films are read as normal because of misinterpretation of the findings. A common error is to misread the herniated bowel and other abdominal organs as a hemopneumothorax.
2. Laparotomy for associated injuries may reveal an unsuspected diaphragmatic tear.
3. Contrast studies (diluted upper GI or barium enema) may reveal intrathoracic abdominal contents. Usually performed in stable cases with delayed presentation

4. Peritoneal lavage. A low RBC count (>5,000 RBC/ml) in the peritoneal fluid is indicative of diaphragmatic injury associated with a penetrating wound of the lower thorax; and is considered positive (Chapter 63).

Differential diagnosis

See Chapters 14, 20, and 63.

Management

1. Stabilization of the patient, with particular attention to airway management, oxygen, IV lines, and cardiac monitor. Treat life-threatening conditions and hypovolemic shock.
2. NG tube for decompression of the stomach. An NG tube may be a useful aid in diagnosis if it is visualized within the chest on x-ray film.
3. Surgery as the definitive treatment. Acute herniated bowel must be reduced and vascular compromise avoided. With delayed presentation, resection for strangulated bowel is commonly needed.

Disposition

Patients must be hospitalized for fluid resuscitation and surgery.

MYOCARDIAL CONTUSION

ALERT: Children with major blunt chest trauma and persistent tachycardia or other ECG changes require monitoring and admission for cardiac evaluation.

Myocardial contusion results from blunt trauma to the anterior midchest from auto accidents, falls, or blunt objects. The injury may cause a cardiac concussion with sudden disruption of cardiac activity, ventricular fibrillation, or dysrhythmias and cellular injury from edema leading to necrosis, ischemia, valvular or ventricular rupture, or pericardial tamponade.

In the multiply traumatized patient, the diagnosis can be difficult or impossible because of the more obvious presentation of associated problems such as hypovolemic shock, pneu-mothorax, head trauma, etc. The condition must be suspected in any young patient without previous heart disease who has sustained chest trauma and has a persistent unexplained tachycardia or dysrhythmia.

Diagnostic findings

1. Chest pain is often present with associated chest wall trauma. Unfortunately, the pain may be delayed until several days postinjury when cellular swelling and ischemia ensue. Chest pain is unrelieved by nitrates.
2. Patients have a persistent tachycardia and may have tachypnea caused by associated pulmonary injuries or hypotension from ventricular dysfunction.
3. Contusions or tenderness over the precordium may be present, but associated rib and sternal fractures are unusual in children because of the compliance of their chest wall.
4. A new murmur may be present secondary to disruption of the septum, cardiac valve, or papillary muscle. Rales may be a later finding associated with left ventricular failure or pulmonary contusion.

Complications
1. Low cardiac output state secondary to ventricular dysfunction
2. Increased sensitivity to fluid overload
3. Cardiac tamponade (muffled sounds, hypotension, and paradoxic pulse)
4. Dysrhythmias

Ancillary data
1. ECG
   a. Any new finding including persistent, unexplained sinus tachycardia and nonspecific ST/T wave changes
   b. Acute ST-segment elevation or T-wave inversion
   c. Any dysrhythmia (e.g., premature atrial or ventricular contractions, atrial fibrillation, or atrial flutter)
2. Chest x-ray film. May demonstrate rib or sternal fracture and associated pulmonary injury. A lateral film must be obtained.

3. Isozymes. CPK-MB band peaks within 24 hr but may not rise until days after injury at the point at which edema and ischemia occur; therefore it is not very useful.
4. Radionuclide studies (ventricular angiography) have been demonstrated to be useful in detecting myocardial dysfunction following blunt chest trauma.
5. Echocardiography (2-D) may be useful.

Management

1. Stabilization of life-threatening conditions. Administer oxygen, fluids, initiate cardiac monitoring. Avoid overzealous fluid administration, which may precipitate left ventricular failure.
2. Analgesics as required.
3. Treatment of dysrhythmias (Chapter 6)
4. Treatment of cardiogenic shock, if present (Chapter 5)

Disposition

1. Patients with myocardial contusion should be hospitalized for at least 24-72 hr for monitoring in the following situations:
   a. Anterior chest wall injury secondary to violent blunt trauma
   b. Persistent tachycardia when other causes have been ruled out
   c. Any new changes on ECG or signs of dysrhythmia
   d. As required by associated injuries
2. If tachycardia has subsided and if the home environment is adequate, the patient with no signs of cardiac dysfunction need not be hospitalized.

PERICARDIAL TAMPONADE

ALERT: With an overlying penetrating wound, hypotension, distended neck veins (increased CVP), tachycardia, and muffled or faint heart sounds require immediate pericardiocentesis after tension pneumothorax has been ruled out. If vital signs are unstable, consider thoracotomy.

Penetrating wounds of the chest may injure the pericardium or myocardium, resulting in pericardial pressure and volume with resultant impaired diastolic filling, increased CVP, hypotension, and tachycardia.

Diagnostic findings

Patients are agitated and hypoxic and have poor peripheral circulation, elevated CVP, tachycardia, and hypotension. A penetrating wound to any area of the thorax, epigastrium, or supraclavicular area may result in tamponade.
1. A paradoxical pulse of >10 mm Hg is usually present.
2. If hypovolemic shock is present, the neck veins may not be distended until the patient is resuscitated with fluid.
3. Beck's triad (hypotension, increased venous pressure with distended neck veins, and muffled, distant heart sounds) is not usually present in the acutely traumatized patient.
4. If bradycardia occurs, the patient is about to arrest. Tamponade must be relieved immediately.

Complications are hypovolemic and cardiogenic shock and death.

Ancillary data
1. Chest x-ray film is usually nondiagnostic.
2. ECG may have nonspecific ST/T waves changes and low voltage. ECG has no pathognomonic changes. Pulsus alternans may rarely be seen with chronic effusion.
3. Echocardiography will demonstrate pericardial fluid but is contraindicated in unstable patients.

Differential diagnosis

1. Constrictive pericarditis (p. 425)
2. Tension pneumothorax

Management

1. Initiate resuscitation, including oxygen, fluids, cardiac monitoring, and MAST trousers.
2. Insert CVP catheter.

3. An initial fluid push of 0.9%NS 10-20 ml/kg over 20 min may provide support of blood pressure while preparing for a pericardiocentesis.

4. Pericardiocentesis may be a lifesaving procedure that permits temporary improvement in cardiac output. Rarely is a patient stable enough to permit a diagnostic evaluation such as an echocardiogram before pericardiocentesis (Appendix A-5).

   a. An 18-gauge metal spinal needle is attached to a syringe by a 3-way stopcock. If a rhythm is present, one end of an alligator clip is fastened to the needle's base and the other end to chest lead V of the ECG with the limb leads attached normally.

   b. The needle is introduced into the left subxiphoid region and aimed cephalad and backward, toward the tip of the left scapula, exerting constant negative pressure on the attached syringe. Others recommended aiming the needle toward the right scapula.

   c. On contact with the epicardium, the ECG will demonstrate an injury current, and the needle should be withdrawn slightly. This should be the pericardial space.

   d. Aspiration of only a few milliliters of blood may provide temporary decompression.

   e. A negative pericardiocentesis does not exclude the possibility of a pericardial tamponade.

5. Thoracotomy is indicated in the arrested patient, particularly in the presence of electromechanical dissociation, or if the patient has become bradycardiac or has lost vital signs. The pericardial sac may be very tense if it is filled with blood and requires a pericardiotomy to relieve the tamponade.

   NOTE: Do not mistake a tense tamponade for adhesive pericarditis.

6. Definitive surgical care is the ultimate treatment. The patient should be moved expeditiously to the operating room once the di-

agnosis is made and the patient is temporarily stabilized.

7. If pericardiocentesis is positive, it may help to leave a catheter in the pericardial space. Even if the catheter does not drain, it may relieve the pressure in the pericardial space. If the patient's condition deteriorates again, the pericardiocentesis should be immediately repeated, and, if it is successful, a thoracotomy should be immediately performed.

Disposition

1. The patient should be immediately transported to the operating room.

2. If a thoracic surgeon or trauma surgeon is not available, repeated pericardiocentesis may be needed to enable transfer to an appropriate facility.

AORTIC INJURY

ALERT: Violent acceleration-deceleration injuries with associated chest trauma, upper rib fractures, or widened mediastinum require emergent evaluation.

Injury to the aorta may occur from acceleration-deceleration injuries occurring in automobile accidents (usually front seat occupants), falls from heights, or from sudden massive compressing injuries, resulting in a shearing force on the mobile aorta at points of fixation, most commonly at the isthmus distal to the left subclavian artery. Injury may also occur from pressure waves generated in the aorta by the compression and decompression.

High-risk injuries include those occurring at high speed (>45 mph accident), where there is chest trauma, fractured first or second ribs, or damage caused by the steering wheel.

Diagnostic findings

1. Patients complain initially of retrosternal or interscapular pain, although the location may change with progression of the dissection. Dyspnea, stridor, and dysphagia occur

secondary to pressure of hematoma on left recurrent laryngeal nerve, trachea, and esophagus. Ischemic extremity pain may be present.

2. Patients develop harsh systolic murmur of precordium and interscapular area.
   a. A pseudocoarctation syndrome with upper extremity hypertension and decreased femoral pulses may be noted. Carotid bruits may be present with decreased carotid pulse and a pulsatile mass at the base of the neck.
   b. Generalized hypertension may occur.

Complications

Hypovolemic shock and death are common (80%-90%) secondary to rupture.

Ancillary data

1. Standard upright chest x-ray film if patient is stable enough (supine chest film may be falsely positive and normalize when repeated as upright)
   a. Widened mediastinum (in adult >8 cm at superior margin of anterior fourth rib) present in 50%-85% of patients (exclude upper thoracic spinal fracture)
   b. Blurring of the aortic knob with loss of sharp aortic outline
   c. Depression of left mainstem bronchus
   d. Left pleural effusion
   e. Deviation of NG tube to the right at T4 level
   f. Left apical pleural cap
2. Aortography
   a. Definitive study for establishing diagnosis
   b. Indicated if patient is stable enough to tolerate. If peritoneal lavage is grossly positive, aortogram is usually not done and patient is taken directly to surgery.
3. CT scan may be obtained to ascertain presence of periaortic hematoma.

Management

1. Supportive resuscitation measures, including oxygen, fluids, blood
2. Immediate thoracic surgical consultation
   a. Obtain thoracic aortogram.
   b. If the patient is unstable, immediate surgery is indicated, sometimes without aortography.
3. Exclusion of concomitant intraabdominal injuries. If peritoneal lavage is positive, abdomen should be explored before aortography.
4. Problem of concomitant head injury. CT scan should be delayed until abdomen and chest are evaluated.

REFERENCES

Bickford, B.J.: Chest injuries in childhood and adolescence, Thorax **17**:240, 1962.

Kilman, J.W., and Charnock, E.: Thoracic trauma in infancy and childhood, J. Trauma **9**:863, 1969.

Marcovchick, V.J.: Thoracic trauma. In Rosen, P., editor: Emergency medicine: concepts and clinical practice, St. Louis, 1983, The C.V. Mosby Co.

Marnocha, K.E., Maglinte, D.D.T., Woods, J., et al.: Blunt chest trauma and suspected aortic rupture: reliability of chest radiograph findings, Ann. Emerg. Med. **14**:644, 1985.

Mellner, J.L., Little, A.G., and Shermata, D.W.: Thoracic trauma in children, Pediatrics **74**:813, 1984.

Smythe, B.T.: Chest trauma in children, J. Pediatr. Surg. **14**:41, 1979.

63 Abdominal trauma

JOHN A. MARX

ALERT: Intraabdominal trauma poses an immediate life threat. Aggressive volume resuscitation and timely peritoneal lavage, surgical consultation, and laparotomy are the foundations of therapy. Multisystem involvement is common.

In 80%-90% of cases intraabdominal injuries are the result of blunt trauma. Hypovolemia in the presence of significant blunt trauma requires that intraperitoneal hemorrhage be excluded.

MECHANISM OF INJURY
Blunt trauma

This is caused primarily by vehicular accidents, falls, contact sports, and child abuse. With infants and small children, pedestrian accidents predominate because of the child's limited ability to avoid or respond to potentially dangerous traffic situations. Passenger accidents are more common among the adolescent population. More recently the use of motor bikes poses an increasing hazard.

The spleen and then the liver are the most likely organs to be injured, whereas small-bowel contusions and perforations cause the most frequent damage to the hollow viscus. The rib cage in the child, although resilient and less prone to fracture, affords only partial protection for the liver and spleen. Intraabdominal injuries are often part of multisystem pathology resulting from vehicular accidents. Injury to two or more intraabdominal organs occurs in up to 30% of blunt-trauma victims.

Type of injury
1. Crush injuries occur with compression of organs between external forces and the posterior thoracic cage or spine, resulting in contusions, lacerations, or disruption.
2. Shear injuries occur when acceleration and deceleration forces cause tearing of viscera and vascular pedicles, particularly at relatively fixed points of attachment.
3. Burst injury of hollow viscera follows the generation of sudden and pronounced increases in intraabdominal pressure (e.g., by seat belts)

Penetrating injuries

In children under 13 yr these are likely to be caused by accidental impalement on objects like scissors or picket fences or by misfiring of a weapon. In patients over 13 yr of age, 75% of penetrating trauma episodes are caused by knife or handgun wounds inflicted by an assailant.
1. Stab wounds to the abdomen cause intraperitoneal organ damage in 30% of cases. Penetration of the peritoneum occurs 70% of the time.
2. Gunshot wounds enter the peritoneal cavity in 80% of cases, causing visceral injury in 95%-99% of patients.
3. Penetrating trauma to the lower chest (below the fourth intercostal space anteriorly and sixth to seventh laterally and posteriorly)

places the abdomen and diaphragm at risk. Coincident injury to the lower chest and abdomen occurs in 25%-40% of patients. The peritoneal cavity may also be entered via back or flank wounds.

DIAGNOSTIC FINDINGS
History

The ability to obtain an accurate history may be compromised by the urgency of the situation, communication skills of the child, concomitant intracranial injuries, reluctance of parents, and interfering toxic agents (e.g., drugs or alcohol). Information about underlying cardiorespiratory disease, coagulopathies, and medication usage will help guide volume resuscitation.

With vehicular trauma it is helpful to know the amount of damage to the automobile and what, if any, restraint systems were used for the child. With penetrating injuries the type of weapon, number of shots or stabs inflicted, and blood loss at the scene should be ascertained.

Child abuse should be suspected when the child has difficulty or fear relating the circumstances of the injury or the history is inconsistent with the injuries.

Symptomatology

1. Volume loss secondary to acute hemorrhage (solid viscera or vascular) or later development of bacterial or chemical peritonitis (hollow viscus or pancreas) leads to inadequate perfusion, causing dizziness and confusion, which may be orthostatically induced.
2. Pain is usually caused by hematic, infectious, or enzymatic irritation of the peritoneum. It may be localized or diffuse. Diminished ability to sense pain (e.g., because of alcohol, concussion, or spinal injury), ineffectual communication, or significant injury elsewhere may impair the recognition of abdominal pain.
   - Splenic and liver injury can cause diaphragmatic irritation and radiation of pain to the ipsilateral shoulder, especially when the patient is in Trendelenburg's position.
3. Nausea and vomiting are nonspecific. They may result from peritoneal irritation or obstruction caused by a duodenal hematoma.

Physical findings

These are unreliable in 30%-40% of cases, particularly those in which CNS trauma coexists. Serial examinations by a single observer are invaluable, especially with the patient whose sensorium is clearing.

1. All clothing must be removed to allow careful inspection of axilla, skin folds, and scalp for entrance and exit wounds.
2. Inspection may reveal superficial abrasions or contusions, which are often deceptively unremarkable in the majority of cases of intraabdominal injury.
3. Acute hypotension is caused by hemorrhage from a solid organ or major vessel injury. Hypotension may be delayed when there is third spacing or significant vomiting with pancreatitis or hollow-viscus damage. Delayed findings occur hours to days following trauma. Splenic injuries are usually obvious immediately but may, rarely, also have delayed presentations.
4. Tenderness is found in up to 90% of patients with intraabdominal pathology and alert mental status. It may be localized to the quadrant of injury (e.g., spleen, liver), or it may be diffuse. Abdominal wall rebound tenderness and rigidity are more specific but less common.
5. Bowel sounds may be decreased or absent and can be helpful in predicting injury. However, they may be present with significant injury or absent because of vertebral fractures, electrolyte disturbances, or other pathology.
6. Gastrointestinal hemorrhage may occur following blunt or penetrating trauma and is identified with NG tube placement and rectal examination.
7. Distension secondary to hemorrhage requires extreme intravascular volume loss and

is accompanied by profound shock. It may occur gradually secondary to third spacing and peritonitis.

Ancillary data

Peritoneal lavage

This is a relatively safe and extremely accurate (98%) method of detecting intraperitoneal hemorrhage. It is particularly useful in those circumstances where the physical examination is equivocal or unreliable. Its use has greatly reduced the frequency of unnecessary laparotomies and has aided in the early discovery of injuries not suspected by abdominal examination.

1. Relative indications
   a. Blunt trauma
      (1) Unreliable examination because of CNS or spinal cord injury, alcohol or drug intoxication, or communication barriers
      (2) Unexplained history of hypotension in the field or ED but now corrected in an environment where intensive observation and immediate surgical availability are not possible
      (3) Multiple trauma patient requiring general anesthesia for repair of extraabdominal injury
      NOTE: Unstable patients whose source of bleeding is unidentified require immediate laparotomy. Stable patients with no history of hypotension and with significant blunt abdominal trauma who are to be observed may be alternatively considered for a liver-spleen scan in lieu of immediate lavage.
   b. Penetrating injury
      (1) Local stab wound exploration that is
         (a) Positive or equivocal
         (b) Contraindicated or technically difficult because of low chest penetration or multiple stab wounds
      (2) Gunshot wound with questionable peritoneal cavity penetration
2. Contraindications

a. Absolute: indications for laparotomy already exist
b. Relative: technically difficult because of previous abdominal surgery or intraperitoneal infection and adhesions, pregnancy, or massive obesity

3. Procedures
   a. A decompressive NG tube and urinary catheter should be placed.
   b. Open technique is preferred. Following sterile preparation and injection of epinephrine-containing local anesthetic, the peritoneal cavity is entered infraumbilically under direct vision. The catheter tip is directed toward the pelvis. Aspiration of 10 ml of free blood is immediately positive. If this does not occur, instill 15 ml/kg (adult 1 L) of normal saline and recover by gravity drainage. Usually done after surgical consultation

4. Results of studies on the recovered peritoneal fluid that are indicative of a positive tap and intraperitoneal hemorrhage in adults:
   a. Red blood cell (RBC) criterion is the most accurate.

Type of trauma	RBC (/mm³) on peritoneal fluid
Blunt	>100,000
	(20,000-100,000: equivocal)
Penetrating	
Stab wound	
Anterior abdomen	>100,000
	(50,000-100,000: equivocal)
Lower chest	>5,000
Gunshot wound	>5,000

Lavage in patients with possible diaphragmatic injury is considered positive with >5,000 RBC/mm³. Lower chest penetrating injuries are those in the area between the fourth intercostal space anteriorly, the seventh intercostal space posteriorly, and the costal margins. This incorporates the area of possible diaphragmatic excursions.
   b. Elevated peritoneal lavage alkaline phosphatase (>3 IU/L) is seen in small bowel injury.

c. Other relative criteria include a WBC $>500/mm^3$ or an amylase >175 μg/dl (usually elevated 4-6 hr following hollow visceral injury). Bile and Gram's stains are of relatively little use in acute trauma.

d. If the initial results are equivocal, a repeat lavage in 4-6 hr may be diagnostic.

NOTE: No comparable data exist for children. These guidelines attempt to minimize missed significant injury, accepting a low rate of negative laparotomy.

5. **Complications**

a. Open technique greatly helps to avoid misplacement of the catheter and consequent inaccurate results and iatrogenic injury.

b. Hollow viscera or vascular punctures may occur.

Other laboratory tests

1. Hematocrits must be obtained early and followed throughout the period of observation. They reflect sustained blood loss, endogenous plasma refilling, and parenteral fluid administration. WBC elevation lasting 48 hr is a nonspecific response to injury. A prolonged leukocytosis may be seen with visceral injury or bacterial peritonitis.

2. Elevated serum amylase is an insensitive and nonspecific marker of pancreatic or proximal small-bowel injury. Persistently high or increasing values may be suggestive.

3. X-ray studies should be performed following initial stabilization and when additional diagnostic data are necessary for management. Patients suspected of having serious injuries must be monitored by experienced personnel in the radiology suite.

a. Plain films are useful to detect small quantities of free intraperitoneal air, but normal studies do not exclude a perforation. Patients should be maintained in the upright or left-lateral decubitus position, if possible, for 10-15 min before x-ray film to mobilize air. Peritoneal lavage causes iatrogenic pneumoperitoneum. Retroperitoneal rupture of a hollow viscus reveals a stippling pattern, outlining the duodenum, kidney, or psoas margins. Foreign bodies, hemoperitoneum, and skeletal fractures may be visualized or localized.

NOTE: These should be obtained before peritoneal lavage, if possible. However, peritoneal lavage must often take first priority.

b. Contrast studies are useful in defining non-life-threatening conditions. Intramural duodenal hematomas are best diagnosed with barium. Water-soluble contrast should be used for suspected gastric, duodenal, and rectal perforations. IVP is indicated in the patient with posttraumatic hematuria where there is a risk of urogenital trauma (Chapter 64). Limited studies may be indicated before laparotomy in the compensated but unstable patient.

c. Scintigraphic liver-spleen scans are accurate in detecting subcapsular hematomas, parenchymal damage, lacerations, and intrahepatic hematomas and may be particularly useful in the stable patient with suspected injuries for whom a peritoneal lavage is not definitely indicated.

d. A CT scan offers simultaneous visualization of all organs in the peritoneal cavity and the retroperitoneum. It defines intraabdominal hemorrhage and the extent of damage to solid viscera. It shows promise, but its sensitivity and specificity have been controversial.

e. Angiography is the most accurate method to visualize vascular injury and active bleeding, but it has limited application for acute trauma.

MANAGEMENT
General principles

Resuscitation of the injured child must be tailored to the specific requirements of the case and the nature of the trauma. Aggressive and systematic treatment as outlined in Chapter 56 becomes crucial in view of the frequency of associated injuries in abdominal trauma. Delivery of adequate replacement fluid volume is critical. Immediate thoracotomy or laparotomy may be indicated. In the stable patient, extensive evaluation and diagnostic studies may be appropriately performed to establish the nature of the injuries and the patient's status.

Certain general principles apply. The emergency physician must do the initial assessment and stabilization while organizing resources within the ED. Assignment of specific tasks to members of the team should be done rapidly, preferably before the patient's arrival. Surgical staff should be contacted as early as possible to assist in the assessment, stabilization, and definitive care of the patient.

Primary assessment

This must ensure an adequate airway and ventilation and initiate treatment of shock, when appropriate. The spine requires immobilization in multiply traumatized patients with suspected spinal injury and in those with altered mental status from blunt trauma injuries (pending spine films) (Chapter 61).

1. All patients require oxygen and cardiac monitoring on arrival. Airway intervention, as appropriate, should be initiated.
2. Clothing should be removed while vital signs are being obtained.
3. Hemorrhage is the immediate life threat. Large-bore catheters should be placed as dictated by the clinical situation. A central line may be required for monitoring if there is intercurrent cardiothoracic pathology or if it is necessary to gain rapid venous access.
   a. Initially, a bolus of LR 20 ml/kg IV is given rapidly. Additional administration of crystalloid must reflect the response to the initial infusion and the presence of ongoing hemorrhage. In general, once 40-50 ml/kg of crystalloid has been infused during the initial resuscitation, blood

should be administered if continuing evidence of hypovolemia exists.
   b. MAST suits may appropriately be used for hypovolemic shock.
   c. Fluid given below the diaphragm following abdominal injury may not reach the right atrium if there is vascular disruption.
4. Initial laboratory studies are required. Hematocrit should be done in the ED and a clot of blood sent for type and cross-match. An ABG may be helpful.
5. Other considerations
   a. An NG tube, when appropriate, will decompress the stomach, permitting improved ventilation and a more reliable examination. It will assist in determining if there is upper GI hemorrhage. The cervical spine must be cleared first.
   b. A urinary catheter may be required for sampling blood in the genitourinary tract and helping monitor fluid management. The urethral meatus should be examined for blood. If blood is present, this precludes insertion.
   c. Reassessment is constantly required, with ongoing measures of vital signs and serial examinations by the same examiner. Once the primary assessment has been completed, a more complete physical should be done and history obtained.
6. Early rectal examination should be performed to assess the integrity of spinal cord function.
7. It is easy to overlook trauma to the thoracic or lumbar spine and the bony pelvis. These should be cleared with chest, abdomen, and pelvic x-ray studies.

Blunt trauma (Fig. 63-1)

Certain victims of blunt trauma are candidates for immediate laparotomy following the initial resuscitation. In hemodynamically stable patients, further diagnostic evaluations and expectant management may be suitable.

1. Urgent laparotomy following stabilization

MANAGEMENT PROTOCOL*

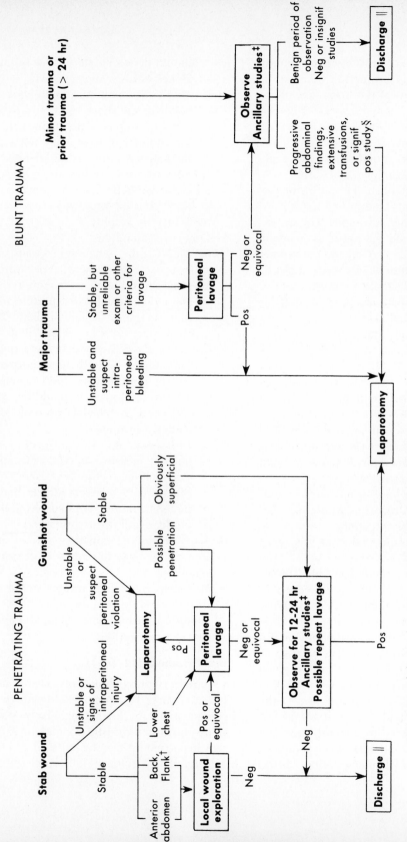

FIG. 63-1. Abdominal trauma. *Assumes optimal resuscitation (Chapters 4 and 56). Associated injuries may modify protocol. †Flank and back do not include areas overlying the thoracic cage. ‡Ancillary studies include plain abdominal film (upright), liver-spleen scan, serial Hct, etc. §Degree of significance will reflect the actual pathology as well as the ability of the facility to monitor patient and intervene emergently, if necessary. Peritoneal lavage before surgery may be indicated. ‖On discharge, all patients require close follow-up.

NOTE: Patients with major blunt trauma and positive peritoneal lavages should have a laparotomy if unstable but may be considered for observation and ancillary studies if stable and adequate support services are available.

should be performed in the following circumstances:

a. Unstable vital signs and suspected or documented intraperitoneal hemorrhage
b. Positive peritoneal lavage
c. Evidence of pneumoperitoneum, diaphragmatic injury, or significant GI hemorrhage

2. Conservative management is appropriate when physicians experienced in pediatric abdominal trauma are present and the facilities and personnel necessary for intensive observation of the child are available. Onset of instability, progressive abdominal findings, or the need for extensive blood transfusions (over 20-30 ml/kg) to supplement crystalloid mandate operative intervention. Criteria for observation in a nontrauma center should be more stringent, favoring earlier peritoneal lavage and surgical intervention or transfer with trained personnel to a better equipped facility.

Splenic injury

This is variably associated with moderate intraabdominal bleeding, which may stop secondary to tamponade. Some patients may have massive bleeding. Left upper quadrant pain, guarding, and rigidity, as well as left shoulder pain, may be present.

1. Splenectomy increases a patient's risk of overwhelming infection 50-60–fold. Therefore maximal splenic preservation is attempted whenever possible, utilizing splenoplasty, partial splenectomy, hemostatic agents, and, more recently, autotransplantation. Patients with penetrating abdominal trauma probably are not candidates for nonoperative management because of the high incidence of associated injuries. Total splenectomy rarely is required and is reserved for the pulverized, nonsalvageable organ.
2. Laparotomy is indicated for the unstable patient with suspected splenic trauma.
3. A liver-spleen or CT scan should be obtained in stable patients with suspected splenic trauma. The need for laparotomy (major lacera-

tion or hematoma), for close intensive observation with serial Hct (minor laceration), or for minimal observation (normal study) is dictated by the clinical status and results of the scan.

NOTE: Children with positive scans who do not require surgery should be maintained at bed rest with daily Hct for 1 wk. During this period, the rate of bleeding and the results of physical examination and monitoring parameters are the main determinants of the need for laparotomy. More than 4 units of blood in adults (or relative equivalent in children) over 48 hr or progressive peritoneal irritation usually necessitates laparotomy. Patients may return to full activity after 2-6 mo of convalescence and a normal study on repeat liver-spleen scan.

Liver injury

The liver follows the spleen in frequency of injury from blunt trauma but tends to result in more massive hemorrhage, one third of patients dying before transport. It is the major cause of immediate mortality related to abdominal trauma. With significant injury, patients may be in shock or have protuberant abdomens and right upper quadrant or diffuse abdominal pain.

The same basic principles of splenic management apply to injuries to the liver although there is rarely time for diagnostic studies beyond peritoneal lavage.

Pancreatic and duodenal injuries

Because these structures have a retroperitoneal location, signs and symptoms may be obscure and delayed.

Pancreatic contusions, the most common type of injury to the pancreas, cause variable degrees of midepigastric, diffuse abdominal, or back pain. Lacerations cause focal hemorrhage and release of enzymatic contents toxic to the surrounding tissues. If this contamination is contained within the lesser sac, severe localized abdominal and back pain may be present. With leakage, there is diffuse chemical peritonitis. Elevated or rising serum or peritoneal lavage amylase levels may be seen. Conservative therapy with NG suction and parenteral nutrition is helpful. Worsening clinical signs may prompt surgical exploration.

Trauma is the leading cause of pancreatic pseudocysts in children and may occur days to months following injury. Capsulized collections of pancreatic secretions and debris form in the lesser sac causing chronic, intermittent attacks of abdominal pain, nausea, vomiting, and weight loss. Ultrasound and CT are valuable in securing the diagnosis. Resolution may spontaneously occur. Otherwise, surgery is required.

Duodenal intramural hematoma causes signs and symptoms of proximal intestinal obstruction. The diagnosis is confirmed by barium contrast studies. Transection of the duodenum should be specifically considered if the barium does not at least partially pass, if extravasation has occurred, or if there is unexplained diffuse abdominal tenderness. The hematoma frequently resolves following 8-10 days of conservative management including an NG tube and parenteral nutrition. Surgery is necessary if this approach fails. Duodenal perforations cause a range of abdominal pain and tenderness, often developing hours after injury. Intraabdominal or retroperitoneal free air may be demonstrated radiographically. Surgery is necessary.

Bowel injuries

Injury to the remainder of the small bowel or colon may also lead to subtle or delayed findings. Perforation usually results in signs of peritonitis 4-12 hr after injury and radiologic evidence of free air. Peritoneal lavage is not diagnostic immediately following injury. Elevated WBC count may occur 4-6 hr after perforation in the peritoneal lavage effluent.

Penetrating wounds (Fig. 63-1)

Stab wounds

1. Immediate exploration is required for hemodynamically unstable patients or for those with clear physical or radiographic evidence of intraperitoneal injury.
2. In the stable, cooperative child, local wound exploration with meticulous hemostasis and possible extension of the wound to facilitate inspection are employed to assess the extent of the penetration. An equivocal examination must be considered positive.
   a. If the end of the wound tract is clearly demonstrated superficial to the posterior rectus fascia, wound care is provided and the patient may be safely discharged if the stab wound was an isolated injury.
   b. If the end cannot be clearly seen or if the peritoneum is violated, peritoneal lavage should be performed. If results are negative or equivocal, observation for 12-24 hr with additional studies and possible repeat lavage are indicated. Positive lavage is an indication for laparotomy.
3. The care of flank and back wounds (excluding areas overlying the thoracic cage) should be individualized. Since retroperitoneal structures are at greater risk, peritoneal lavage may not be diagnostic, and other ancillary diagnostic techniques such as ultrasound and CT scan may be helpful. Local wound exploration is useful for superficial entry.
4. Penetrating injury from lower chest (below the fourth intercostal space anteriorly or sixth to seventh posteriorly) wounds places the abdomen at risk. However, local wound exploration over the rib cage is hazardous and contraindicated because of the risk of causing a pneumothorax. Peritoneal lavage should be performed unless there is other clinical evidence that already dictates the need for laparotomy.

Gunshot wounds

The incidence of intraabdominal injury exceeds 95% when the missile has entered the peritoneal cavity. Therefore the criteria for selective management are greatly restricted as compared with stab wounds.

1. Unstable patients are immediately explored. When peritoneal violation is suspected on the basis of entrance and exit wounds or radiographic findings or if other evidence of in-

traabdominal injury exists, laparotomy is undertaken.

2. Local wound exploration is technically more difficult and less reliable. It is not generally used. Patients with obviously superficial injuries should be observed. Those in whom an intraabdominal penetration is unclear should undergo peritoneal lavage.

3. If the situation permits, patients with lower-chest gunshot wounds should have peritoneal lavage to ascertain existence of concomitant diaphragmatic or intraabdominal injury. Many times these patients require immediate thoracic surgery, which precludes peritoneal lavage.

REFERENCES

Bresler, M.J.: Computed tomography of the abdomen, Ann. Emerg. Med. **15**:280, 1986.

Giacomantonio, M., Filler, R.M., and Rich, R.H.: Blunt hepatic trauma in children: experience with operative and nonoperative management, J. Pediatr. Surg. **19**:519, 1984.

Karp, M.P., Cooney, D.R., Pros, G.A., et al.: The nonoperative management of pediatric hepatic trauma, J. Pediatr. Surg. **18**:512, 1983.

Kuhn, J.P.: Diagnostic imaging for the evaluation of abdominal trauma in children, Pediatr. Clin. N. Am. **32**:1427, 1985.

Marx, J.A.: Abdominal injuries. In Rosen, P., editor: Emergency medicine: concepts and clinical practice, St. Louis, 1983, The C.V. Mosby Co.

Moore, E.E., and Marx, J.A.: Penetrating abdominal wounds: rationale for exploratory laparotomy, JAMA **253**:2705, 1985.

Moore, J.B., Moore, E.E., Markovchick, V.J., et al.: Diagnostic peritoneal lavage for abdominal trauma: superiority of the open technique at the infraumbilical ring, J. Trauma **21**:570, 1981.

Thompson, J.S., Moore, E.E., Van Duzer-Moore, S., et al.: The evolution of abdominal stab wound management, J. Trauma **20**:478, 1980.

Zucker, R., Browns, K., Rossman, D., et al.: Non-operative management of splenic trauma: conservative or radical treatment, Arch. Surg. **119**:400, 1984.

64 Genitourinary trauma

GREGORY W. ZOLLER

ALERT: Anyone with trauma to the perineum, back, abdomen, flank, or genitalia should be suspected of having genitourinary (GU) trauma. Hematuria, oliguria, tenderness, pain, masses, or lower rib fractures must be carefully evaluated for associated pathology.

Automobile accidents, sports injuries, or falls cause 75% of GU trauma. After the brain the kidney is the most frequently injured internal organ in children. The kidney, primarily an intraabdominal organ in younger children, is more mobile and not protected by perinephric fat. Urologic injuries are noted in 13.5% of pelvic fractures.

The diagnosis of GU trauma must be entertained anytime a patient has hematuria (>5 RBC/HPF), decreased urinary output, an unexplained abdominal mass or pain and tenderness, penetrating trauma, a fractured pelvis, blood at the urethral meatus, or scrotal swelling and hematoma.

Preexisting congenital anomalies such as hydronephrosis and polycystic disease are present in 10% of children evaluated for renal trauma. Other causes of hematuria (Chapter 37) and infection (p. 620) must also be considered in the initial evaluation. Epididymitis, testicular torsion, and penile disorders are discussed in Chapter 77.

EVALUATION

Evaluation must include a careful urinalysis and radiographic studies when indicated.
1. Urinalysis
   a. Dipstik may show false positive values when urine is contaminated with povi-done-iodine (Betadine) or hexachlorophene. It is positive if there is hemoglobin or myoglobin in the urine. Drugs and chemicals may turn the urine dark or red (p. 277).
   b. Microscopic examination for red cells is mandatory if the dipstik is positive.
   c. The absence of hematuria does not exclude significant renal injury. Renal vascular thrombosis, renal pedicle injury, and complete transection of the ureter are common causes of false negative values.
2. Abdominal flat plate and chest x-ray film. May have a variety of findings associated with GU injuries requiring further evaluation:
   a. Fracture of lower rib
   b. Fractured vertebrae or transverse process in lower thoracic or lumbar vertebrae
   c. Pelvic fracture
   d. Other findings, including ileus, scoliosis of vertebral column toward injured side, unilateral enlarged kidney shadow, loss of psoas muscle margin, displaced bowel secondary to hemorrhage or urine extravasation, or an elevated ipsilateral hemidiaphragm
3. Retrograde urethrogram. Done before urethral instrumentation or catheterization, if indicated
   a. Indications include:

(1) Blood at meatus
(2) Significant scrotal or perineal hematoma
(3) Obvious urethral trauma (Penetrating or foreign body)

b. Procedure: 10-30 ml of standard water-soluble renograffin is drawn into a catheter-tipped syringe, the tip of which is inserted into the urethral meatus. Anterior, posterior, and oblique x-ray films are obtained as the dye is injected. Patient sedation may be required.

4. Cystogram. Indicated when the injury and findings are consistent with bladder injury, pelvic fracture, inadequate urine production, or gross hematuria.

a. If indicated performed after urethrogram

b. Procedures: 150-300 ml (depending on size of child) of 10% solution water-soluble renograffin is placed in bladder through urethral catheter by gravity. Smaller volumes may be required in infants to fill bladder. AP and oblique views are required with filled and postevacuation films.

5. Excretory urogram (IVP)

a. Indications after trauma
(1) Hematuria
(2) Penetrating injury to flank, back, or abdomen, possibly involving GU tract
(3) Flank mass or costovertebral angle (CVA) tenderness
(4) Unexplained ileus or abdominal pain
NOTE: The indications for IVP are controversial at present. Patients with gross hematuria or microscopic hematuria and shock after blunt trauma require study, as do those with penetrating trauma and concern over renal involvement. Although at present most clinicians consider microscopic hematuria following blunt trauma without shock to be an indication, increasing data would suggest that this approach may not be justified because of the low incidence of injuries requiring surgical intervention (i.e., IVP's either demonstrate contusion or normal kidneys).

b. Procedure: sodium diatrizoate (Conray) 60% IV at 2 ml/kg (<4.5 kg: 4ml/kg). Films at 1, 5, 10, and 20 min if possible. Rarely, a rapid, high-dose infusion study may be indicated with films at 1 and 15 min.

6. Renal arteriogram. Indicated when the kidney is not visualized (total or partial) on IVP or with major extravasation

7. Renal scans. May be used to monitor patients with known renal injury and to detect recovery or loss of function of renal parenchyma

8. Renal sonography. Useful in monitoring the expansion or resolution of a urinoma or hematoma over a period of time.

RENAL TRAUMA

Over 90% of direct renal trauma is caused by blunt injuries from automobile accidents or significant falls. Males, particularly under age 30, are at greatest risk. The kidney can move on the pedicle and can therefore be contused or lacerated by ribs or spinal transverse process. Gerota's fascia surrounding the kidney may restrict bleeding.

Diagnostic findings

There is abrasion, ecchymosis, pain, or tenderness over the back, flank, or abdomen following trauma, often accompanied by an unexplained ileus and diffuse abdominal tenderness.

Associated injuries are present in 44% of patients—up to 25% of whom have intraabdominal pathology. Fractures of lower ribs, thoracic or lumbar vertebrae, or the transverse processes are common.

Classification of degree of renal trauma

1. Class I: renal contusion, which accounts for 80% of injuries. Hematuria with no evidence of decreased renal function, extravasation, or pelvicaliceal injury on IVP

2. Class II: renal cortical laceration with or with-

out hematoma. Hematoma with extravasation of dye from cortical laceration seen on IVP
3. Class III: caliceal laceration. Hematuria with intrarenal extravasation of dye on IVP demonstrating disruption of pelvicaliceal system. Intact capsule. Flank pain present on physical examination
4. Class IV: complete renal tear or fracture (shattered kidney). Separation of parenchyma from the pelvicaliceal system to the capsule with intrarenal and extrarenal dye extravasation (combination of Class II and III). Shock often present
5. Class V: vascular pedicle injury. Nonvisualization of kidney on IVP with damage seen by selective renal arteriogram. Hematuria variably present. Shock

Complications
1. Extravasation of urine variably associated with infection or obstruction
2. Vascular compromise of the kidney
3. Acute tubular necrosis (ATN) with renal failure
4. Hemorrhage with hypovolemic shock
5. Delayed complications, including hypertension, chronic infection, hydronephrosis, calculus formation, chronic renal failure, arteriovenous fistula, pseudocyst formation, and nonfunction

Ancillary data
These include CBC, urinalysis, abdominal flat plate, and IVP. If the IVP does not show the renal unit, selective arteriogram is performed and then, for follow-up, renal scan and sonography.

Urinalysis may be normal, especially with pedicle injury or renal vascular thrombosis.

Management (Fig. 64-1)

1. Class I injuries. These patients may be discharged if there are no other significant injuries.
   a. They may ambulate but must avoid physical contact sports for 2-6 wk.

   b. Urinalysis and examination should be repeated in 1-2 wk.
2. Class II injuries. These patients should be admitted for bed rest and observation after urologic consultation.
   a. Renal scan and sonography may be helpful to monitor kidney changes while patient is hospitalized. IVP should be done in follow-up.
   b. Physical contact sports should be avoided for at least 6 wk.
   c. Blood pressure and renal follow-up are required for at least 1 yr.
3. Class III injuries. These patients require admission and immediate urologic consultation.
   a. The necessity to repair is controversial. Many prefer a nonsurgical approach with frequent monitoring of vital signs, bed rest, and serial Hct.
   b. Renal scan and sonography can assist in monitoring the patient's course.
4. Class IV injuries. These patients require hospitalization, replacement of fluid deficits, and nephrectomy. On arrival patients are usually hypovolemic with multiple injuries.
5. Class V injuries. These patients usually have multiple injuries and require immediate vascular repair after the renal arteriogram, concomitant with stabilization of other pathology.
   a. Low renal salvage rate. If the kidney is preserved, long-range blood pressure and renal function monitoring are necessary.
   b. The ischemic lifetime of a warm kidney is estimated at 40-60 min.

URETERAL TRAUMA

Blunt injuries result from a hyperextension, with bowstringing of the ureter, causing complete or partial laceration. They are common in children after automobile-pedestrian accidents because of the flexibility of the torso and limited retroperitoneal fat for protection. The tear almost always occurs at the ureteropelvic junction (UPJ). Penetrating ureteral injuries as well as surgical damage are more frequent in adults.

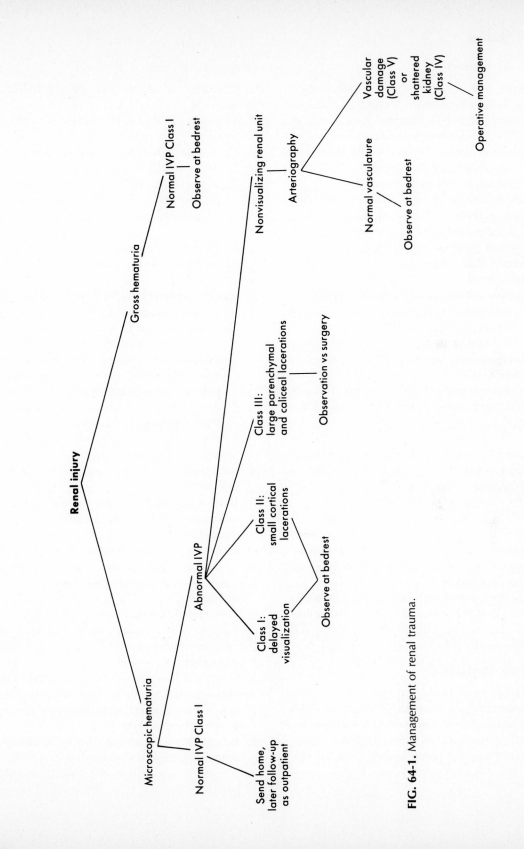

FIG. 64-1. Management of renal trauma.

Diagnostic findings

Patients may have lumboiliac pain from a blow, a flank mass from extravasated urine or blood, frequency of urination, hematuria, or pyuria. The diagnosis is often missed because of the severity of other associated multiple injuries and the subtleness of the findings. There is a better prognosis with early repair.

Delayed retroperitoneal mass, back pain, unexplained fever, or urine drainage from a wound or operative incision site may be noted. Over 50% of patients with delayed repair lose ureter and kidney function.

Complications

1. Extravasated urine may cause peritonitis if the peritoneum is ruptured or empyema if the diaphragm is involved.
2. Ureteral strictures secondary to obstruction or infection may occur.

Ancillary data

1. Hematuria is present in 66% of cases but may not be noted with complete transection of the ureter.
2. IVP demonstrates extravasation of dye. If the injury is near the UPJ, the dye may travel up and around the kidney, simulating a lacerated renal cortex or pelvis.

Management

1. A urologist should be consulted for primary repair and cutaneous ureterostomy as indicated. A nephroureterectomy may be done if the diagnosis is delayed.
2. Long-term follow-up must include monitoring of blood pressure and ensuring that a ureteral stricture or obstruction does not develop.

BLADDER TRAUMA

The majority of bladder ruptures occur from blunt trauma to patients with full bladders, often during automobile or auto-pedestrian accidents. Penetrating injuries may occur from guns, knives, or fractured pelvic bones.

Diagnostic findings

1. Bladder contusion results in bruise to bladder wall.
2. Intraperitoneal bladder rupture is more common in younger children than adults because the pediatric bladder is an abdominal organ. Break is usually at bladder dome.
   a. Suprapubic tenderness, abdominal pain, ileus, extreme desire but inability to void, hematuria, pallor, tachycardia, hypotension
   b. Delayed symptoms 24-72 hr after rupture, including fever, abdominal tenderness, vomiting
3. Extraperitoneal bladder rupture is less common, occurring more frequently in the older child and adolescent with pelvic injury.
   a. Symptoms are similar to intraperitoneal except that patient can pass a small amount of urine, and a hematoma may be palpated in suprapubic region. Urine can dissect up to the kidney or down into the legs, scrotum, and buttock.
   b. Red, indurated suprapubic area may develop if diagnosis is delayed.
4. Intraperitoneal and extraperitoneal rupture may occur.
5. Urethral injuries and associated abdominal or pelvic pathology are common.

Complications of misdiagnosis

These include peritonitis, abscess, sepsis, ileus, osteomyelitis, bladder neck contractures, and poor bladder muscle function.

Ancillary data

Hematuria is present in over 95% of patients. The degree of hematuria does not correlate with the severity of injury.

• Cystogram

1. Contused bladder will show normal vesicle outline and a teardrop shape if there are bilateral hematomas or a half-moon shape with unilateral hematoma.
2. Intraperitoneal rupture may have intraperitoneal organs outlined by dye.

3. Extraperitoneal rupture demonstrates dye in contact areas after dye is drained from bladder on postevacuation film.

Management

1. Bladder contusion is treated by hospitalizing patient and placing indwelling catheter for 7-10 days. Minor contusions can be observed at home without catheter placement. Close follow-up is essential. Contact sports should be avoided for 2-6 wk. Prognosis is good.
2. Bladder ruptures may be evaluated by cystoscopy and, if small, treated with indwelling catheter for 7-14 days. Larger deficits require operative repair and suprapubic cystoscopy.
3. A urologist should be consulted when the diagnosis is first suspected.

URETHRAL INJURIES

These commonly follow blunt trauma and are associated with pelvic fractures. They may be a complication of urethral catheterization.

Diagnostic findings

Posterior urethral injuries are those above the urogenital diaphragm, and they involve the prostatic and membranous urethra. They usually follow crush pelvic injuries or surgical complications.
- Blood at the urethral meatus and inability to void are the most common complaints. Pelvic fracture is usually present. Prostate is boggy and high riding in older individuals.

An anterior urethral tear involves the bulbous and pendulous or penile urethra; it results from a straddle fall or from foreign bodies.
- Perineal pain is prominent. There is blood at the meatus and a good urinary stream when voiding. If patient is seen late after injury, penile and perineal edema, necrosis, and ecchymosis may be present.

Complications
These include stricture, impotence, or urinary incontinence.

Ancillary data
These include urinalysis and retrograde urethrogram before urinary catheter is placed.

Management

1. A urologist must be consulted immediately on identifying blood at the meatus or on defining the pathology.
2. Anterior injuries, if small, may be treated with a urethral catheter; otherwise operative repair is needed.
3. Posterior injuries are controversial. There is question as to whether immediate or delayed intervention provides the best repair.
4. Since urethral injuries may be iatrogenic, careful technique in catheterization is advisable. The catheter should not be forced.

EXTERNAL GENITALIA TRAUMA (p. 505)

Penile, scrotal, and testicular injuries may occur from missiles (bullet or knife); from strangulation secondary to a condom, string, hair, or constricting metal band; from blunt injury to an erect penis during intercourse or fall; from being caught in a zipper; or from amputation. Vulvar lesions usually follow blunt trauma.

Diagnostic findings

Penile swelling, ecchymosis, and other direct injury can be present. With constricting band, close inspection is necessary since edema can hide a small constricting band such as hair.

Ancillary data
These include urinalysis to evaluate for blood, which indicates urethral injury requiring a retrograde urethrogram. Ultrasonography may be useful in the assessment of significant blunt scrotal and testicular trauma.

Management

Urology consultation is necessary.
Lacerations of the penile skin
These can be sutured with absorbable suture.
1. If the wound is not deep beyond the Colles'

fascia, it can be closed in the ED with two layers of Vicryl or Dexon sutures. If deeper, it should be explored in the OR.

2. If the corpus cavernosum penis is violated, it should be explored in the operating room.

3. Constricting devices should be removed as soon as possible. The distal penis that appears necrotic should be treated conservatively. Often, an apparently nonviable penis will survive.

Zipper injuries

These are best treated by breaking or cutting the small bridge (U-shaped bar) between the anterior and posterior faceplates of the zipper fastener with a bone cutter. Others recommend local anesthetic of the involved skin and then unzipping by moving one tooth at a time, alternating sides.

Amputation of penis

This requires immediate consultation.

Lacerations of the scrotum

1. Laceration of scrotal skin alone: debridement and closure with absorbable suture

2. Scrotal skin and dartos layer only: debridement and two-layered closure with absorbable suture to reduce chance of hematoma formation

3. Penetrating wound or major blunt trauma: exploration in the OR. Conservative treatment leads to high incidence of atrophied testes and loss of viability.

Injury to vulva

This requires examination (often under anesthesia) to exclude extension of injury to the vagina, rectum, bladder, and urethra. Lacerations in the perineal area in prepubertal girls are more likely to involve the vagina.

Vulvar hematomas are usually treated conservatively and commonly result from handlebar or crossbar injuries. Patients may be placed on strict bed rest, ice packs, analgesia, stool softener and close monitoring of urinary output. Rarely is a urinary catheter needed.

REFERENCES

Levitt, M.A., Criss, E., Kobernick, M.: Should the emergency IVP be used more selectively in blunt trauma? Ann. Emerg. Med. 14:959, 1985.

Morse, T.: Symposium on childhood trauma: renal injuries, Pediatr. Clin. North Am. 22:379, 1975.

Nicolaisein, G.S., McAninch, J.W., Marshall, G.A., et al.: Renal trauma: reevaluation of the indication for radiographic assessment, J. Urol. 133:183, 1985.

Palmer, J.K., Benson, G.S., and Corriere, J.N.: Diagnosis and initial management of urologic injuries associated with 200 consecutive pelvic fractures, J. Urol. 130:712, 1983.

Reichard, S.A., Helikson, M.A., et al.: Pelvic fractures in children—review of 120 patients with a new look at general management, J. Pediatr. Surg. 15:727, 1980.

Uehara, D.T., and Eisner, R.F.: Indications for intravenous pyelography in trauma, Ann. Emerg. Med. 15:266, 1986.

Zoller, G.W.: Genitourinary trauma. In Rosen, P., editor: Emergency medicine: concepts and clinical practice, St. Louis, 1983, The C.V. Mosby Co.

65 Soft tissue injuries

VINCENT J. MARKOVCHICK
STEPHEN V. CANTRILL

Soft tissue injuries are common in children. They often are caused by falls, contact with sharp objects, or motor vehicle accidents. Since many involved areas are visible, such as the face (Chapter 58), it is imperative that the principles of meticulous wound care and repair be practiced to maximize cosmetic and functional results.

DIAGNOSTIC FINDINGS

The following should be ascertained: the mechanism (cut, fall, crush, bite, or electrical injury) and the time of injury, whether the wound was clean or dirty, the amount of blood loss, the history of foreign body sensation, and the degree of paresthesia or impaired motor function distal to the wound. Child abuse must be considered in cases where the history and injury are inconsistent.

The status of tetanus immunization as well as allergies to antibiotics, local anesthetic agents, and other medications, in addition to underlying medical problems, should be noted. True allergies to local anesthetics are extremely rare.

Local pain and swelling are common with all soft tissue trauma. Furthermore, children tend to be fearful and anxious.

All wounds must be carefully inspected to determine the depth of injury and involvement of underlying tissues, including vessels, nerves, muscles, tendons, ligaments, bone, joints, and ducts.

1. Attention must be given to the physical examination and to documentation of an accurate description of the wound for the record. The wound should be described with respect to location, length, depth, nature of the edges, cleanliness, and involvement of any underlying structures.
2. The integrity of arterial circulation is determined by palpation of peripheral pulses, skin color, temperature, and capillary filling. Contusions over the forearm and leg may lead to delayed onset of compartment syndromes.
3. Sensory deficits are tested by determination of distal sensation, often requiring two-point discrimination distal to the lesion. This can easily be done by using a paper clip and separating the ends by 8 mm.
   - Nerve injuries are classified as neuropraxia (nerve continuity maintained and no axonal degeneration secondary to compression or contusion), axonotmesis (preservation of anatomic continuity of nerve with axonal degeneration) or neurotmesis (complete division of nerve).
4. After a careful sensory examination, infiltration of local anesthesia may be provided for a painless yet accurate examination, cleansing, debridement, and definitive treatment.
5. Tendons, ligaments, and muscles should be tested distal to the injury individually and by muscle group.
6. Foreign bodies should be identified and removed.

381

7. Injuries of the hand or foot require very careful assessment. The examination of the hand, which is commonly injured in children, is outlined in Chapter 68. Open wounds require direct visualization since motor function may remain normal with incomplete laceration of tendons or ligaments.

Complications

Infections can be minimized by meticulous wound preparation, irrigation and debridement, careful closure of the wound, and application of appropriate dressings and splints.

Other complications include:

1. Failure to recognize deep structure injury to nerve, tendon, bone, or joint capsule with sensory or motor deficits (fractures underlying lacerations must be considered open fractures)
2. Delayed recognition of a foreign body
3. Cosmetic deformity

Ancillary data

X-ray studies should be obtained before testing motor function or range of motion:

1. For injuries secondary to blunt trauma or crush injury
2. To exclude a radiopaque foreign body
3. Glass fragments usually can be seen on a standard x-ray film. Small (0.5-1.0 mm) or thin glass fragments are more difficult to see but can be detected if there is no overlying bone.

MANAGEMENT (Chapter 58 on facial injuries)

Although unusual, massive hypovolemia from a vascular injury or extensive laceration of the scalp or face may cause hypotension, which is usually responsive to crystalloid administration (0.9%NS or LR at 20 ml/kg over 20-30 min). Stabilization of life-threatening conditions is of greatest priority.

1. If hypotension is present, an injury, in addition to the soft tissue damage, should be sought.
2. Hemorrhage can usually be controlled by direct pressure alone. If placement of hemostats is required for control of hemorrhage, this must always be done under direct vision (never blindly) to avoid iatrogenic injury to nerves, vessels, or tendons.
3. Tetanus immunizations must be updated (p. 546).

Immediate consultation should be requested if the injury is very complex or if extensive follow-up will be required.

Anesthesia

Lidocaine

Lidocaine (Xylocaine) 1%-2% is adequate for most infiltration and regional anesthesia. Infiltration is done with a small needle (25-gauge) directly through the wound margins.

1. Lidocaine containing epinephrine (1:100,000) may assist with hemostasis but should *never* be used on the digits, hands, feet, ear, tarsal plate of the eye, bridge of the nose, nipple, or penis.
2. Regional anesthesia may be achieved using proper anatomic landmarks, but it often requires additional local infiltration. It minimizes distortion.
3. The ear may be adequately anesthetized by raising a wheal with lidocaine 1% without epinephrine about the entire base of the ear. This will not anesthetize the external canal.
4. Before injection a small amount of 4% lidocaine may be applied topically to the wound to decrease the pain of injection. Pain also may be minimized by using a small needle, injecting the smallest volume possible, and performing the injection slowly while the needle is being withdrawn.
5. Toxic levels may be achieved with local administration of >4 mg/kg plain lidocaine or >7 mg/kg of lidocaine with epinephrine. Toxicity includes sinus arrest, bradycardia, hypotension, AV block, irritability, respiratory depression, seizures, and coma.

Topical mixtures

Topical mixtures may be useful for superficial injuries, particularly in young children. Do not use on mucosal lesions or where epinephrine is contraindicated.

1. *TAC:* Topical *t*etracaine 2% (2.2 ml), topical *A*drenaline (epinephrine) (1:1,000) (4.25 ml), *c*ocaine 1 g, and bacteriostatic saline (1.2 ml) to make up 8.5 ml
2. Also transient anesthesia can be obtained by topical application for 5-15 min of gauze saturated with 2%-4% lidocaine.
3. Ethyl chloride spray may also be used.

Sedation

Sedation is not required for most injuries and is usually not worth the risk of iatrogenic problems. However, there are occasions when it may be used *cautiously* to expedite a repair:

1. Meperidine (Demerol) 1 mg/kg/dose IM (hydroxyzine [Atarax, Vistaril] 0.5-1 mg/kg IM will potentiate); **or**
2. Meperidine (Demerol) 1-2 mg/kg/dose (maximum: 50 mg/dose) **and** promethazine (Phenergan) 0.25-0.5 mg/kg/dose (maximum: 12.5 mg/dose) **and** chlorpromazine (Thorazine) 0.25-0.5 mg/kg/dose (maximum: 12.5 mg/dose) give IM. Usually mixed in ratio of 1:0.25:0.25 (DPT cocktail)
   NOTE: Sedation may be partially reversed with naloxone (Narcan) 0.8-2.0 mg/dose IV.
3. Fentanyl (Sublimaze) 2-3 µg/kg IV *slowly* over 3-5 min recently has been used with great success. It has a half-life of 20 min and can easily be reversed. Older children often require less than the calculated dose.
4. Nitrous oxide (50%-70% mixture) is a useful supplement to local anesthetics.

Wound cleansing

This is best done (after local anesthesic is injected) with a high-velocity jet stream accomplished by attaching a 16- or 18-gauge IV catheter to a large syringe. Normal saline is adequate as an irrigating solution. Volume is important: 500 ml should be used for a normal-sized wound. Foreign material in an abrasion must be removed within 24 hr to avoid the creation of a permanent traumatic tattoo, particularly in such cosmetically important areas as the face. Anesthesia of the abrasion may be achieved by direct application of gauze to the wound that has been saturated with 4% lidocaine or *TAC* (above). The abrasion should then be scrubbed with a scrub brush or toothbrush. An 11-blade or 18-gauge needle may be used to remove material not removed by the scrubbing process.

Position and draping

Wounds in small children are most easily repaired if the child is restrained, e.g., on a papoose board.* This necessitates careful attention to the child's respiratory status and the potential for aspiration of vomitus. A sterile field should be created by the use of drapes. However, the face should not be draped.

If extensive bleeding is associated with a finger laceration, an excellent field and tourniquet can be achieved by cleansing the patient's finger and then slipping the hand into a sterile glove, snipping the end of the glove on the involved finger, and then rolling the finger of the glove back to provide exposure and tourniquet. Careful scrubbing is then done.

Wound exploration

This should be performed on all injuries so that the extent of the damage may be fully appreciated, violation of underlying structures realized, undetected fractures and tendon lacerations discovered, and removal of all foreign bodies ensured. Optimally the wound is explored after injection of local anesthesia and sensory examination.

Embedded, inert foreign bodies such as glass or metal should be removed if possible. X-ray films are often helpful in localization. The precise location of an embedded object can be identified by taping paper clips or a flexible radiopaque marker such as wire to the skin overlying the suspected location and getting an AP and a lateral view at 90 degrees to each other. However, if foreign bodies are small and if they are

---

*Available from Olympic Surgical Co., Seattle, Wash.

embedded deeply into muscle and cannot be easily removed, they may be left in place. The patient should be informed of the presence of the foreign body and follow-up arranged.

NOTE: Organic foreign bodies such as wood should be removed whenever possible to prevent local inflammatory reactions. Xeroradiography may be necessary to localize some foreign bodies not seen on standard soft tissue radiographs. Surgical consultation should usually be obtained unless the material is superficial.

Hemostasis

Direct pressure and tourniquets occasionally are needed for hemostasis. Vessels should not be sutured or clamped blindly because of the risk of injury to other underlying tissues.

Wound revision and debridement

This may require very conservative debridement, after anesthesia, of devitalized or severely contaminated tissue. Ragged and uneven edges may need to be incised. Most wounds do well with little or no revision. It should be explained to the parents that the wound may leave a noticeable scar, which may be further revised by a consultant after 9-18 mo of healing.

Associated abrasions can lead to permanent tattooing if foreign particulate material is not removed. Scrubbing and selective debridement are important.

Wound closure

Wounds should be closed as soon as possible. In general, wounds over 8-12 hr old should not be closed. Clean wounds on the face may be closed, if necessary, up to 24 hr after the injury.
1. Contaminated or dirty wounds are optimally treated with vigorous cleansing, appropriate dressings, and a delayed closure at 48-72 hr.
2. Puncture wounds should not be closed. Bites are rarely closed, except on the face.
3. Subcutaneous sutures should be placed equal in depth and distance from the wound edges.
4. Cutaneous tape closure may occasionally be used for superficial wounds in areas without motion. The area should be dried, tincture of benzoin applied, and the edges approximated without tension or underlying dead space.
5. Undermining of the subcutaneous layer may be necessary if there has been extensive loss of tissue secondary to trauma or revision. Undermining should be at least equal to the gap at its widest point to diminish tension.

Wound-closure techniques

These vary with the location of the injury. If the primary goal is a good cosmetic closure, it often requires at least two layers. The top sutures should be removed within 5 days to minimize the possibility of suture marks being part of the scar. If a good functional result is the goal, as on the hand or foot, then a single-layered closure is desirable. Guidelines are provided in Table 65-1. A sterile scalpel blade or stitch cutter* facilitates removal.

Primary repair of nerve injuries

Repair is more effective in children than in adults. Neuropraxia or axonotmesis should be observed for 3-6 mo along with electrodiagnostic studies before surgical repair is performed. Neurotmesis requires an early epineural repair by a surgeon.

Dressing and splints of the hands and feet

1. A large bulky dressing of the hand or foot is optimal for most children, particularly when immobilization will only be necessary for several days.
2. Injuries of the hand requiring immobilization usually involve wounds over the joints and are best dressed in the "hooded cobra" position. The wrist is in neutral position, the metacarpophalangeal (MCP) joints are flexed at about 60-70 degrees, the interphalangeal

---

*An excellent cutter is available from Medeira, P.O. Box 43068, Cincinnati, OH 45243, (513) 489-6654.

TABLE 65-1. Suture repair of soft tissue injuries

Location	Anesthetic	Suture material	Type of closure	Suture removal	Special considerations
Scalp	Lidocaine 1% with epinephrine	3-0 or 4-0 nylon	Interrupted in galea; single tight layer in scalp	7-12 days	Control initial hemorrhage with lidocaine (Xylocaine) with epinephrine and with pressure; digital exploration for foreign body or fracture; pressure dressing if early hematoma noted (p. 327)
Pinna (ear)	Lidocaine 1% (field block)	6-0 nylon 5-0 Vicryl in perichondrium	Close perichondrium with 5-0 Vicryl interrupted; close skin with 6-0 nylon interrupted	4-6 days	Stent dressing is necessary for 24-48 hr to prevent hematoma formation with resultant pain and risk of cartilaginous pressure necrosis (p. 326)
Eyelid	Lidocaine 1%	6-0 nylon or silk	Single layer interrupted	3-5 days	If through tarsal plate, should be referred to consultant; check for ptosis (Chapter 59)
Lip	Lidocaine 1% with epinephrine or use field block	4-0 silk (mucosa) 5-0 Vicryl (SQ, muscle) 6-0 nylon (skin)	Three layers (mucosa, muscle, and skin) if through and through, otherwise two layers	3-5 days	Exact approximation of vermilion border is necessary; water-tight closure of through-and-through laceration (p. 325)
Face	Lidocaine 1% with epinephrine	4-0 or 5-0 Vicryl (SQ) 6-0 nylon (skin)	If full-thickness laceration, layered closure is desirable	3-5 days	Careful attention to evaluation of underlying surface anatomy such as nerve VII and parotid duct (p. 325)
Neck	Lidocaine 1% with epinephrine	4-0 Vicryl (SQ) 5-0 nylon (skin)	Two-layered closure for best cosmetic results	4-6 days	Control hemorrhage by direct pressure; avoid blind clamping; if puncture wound violates platysma, involve consultant
Trunk	Lidocaine 1% with epinephrine	4-0 Vicryl (SQ, fat); 4-0 or 5-0 nylon	Single or layered closure	7-12 days	Exclude abdominal pathology
Extremity	Lidocaine 1% with epinephrine	3-0 or 4-0 Vicryl (SQ, fat, muscle) 4-0 or 5-0 nylon (skin)	Single-layered closure is adequate although layered closure may give better cosmetic result	7-14 days	Evaluation of distal circulation and neurologic and motor function must be performed
Hand and feet	Lidocaine 1% (if field block, 2%)	4-0 or 5-0 nylon	Single-layered closure only with interrupted suture, at least 5 mm from cut wound edges; vertical mattress sutures should be used if much tension on wound edges	7-12 days	Control hemorrhage with direct pressure only; evaluate for underlying surface anatomy; usually explore all wounds; dress and splint in position of function (p. 390)

NOTE: Dexon is equivalent to Vicryl. Plain or chromic catgut should not be used because both are rejected rather than hydrolyzed. Nylon is available as Prolene, Ethilon, Surgilon, etc.

(IP) joints are flexed at 10-20 degrees, and the thumb abducted. A volar plaster splint may be incorporated over the dressing for additional immobilization.

3. The foot may require temporary immobilization if extensive injuries are present, particularly those involving tendons. This may be achieved by maintaining the ankle at 90 degrees with a posterior plaster splint.

Antibiotics

Antibiotics are not required for clean lacerations. Grossly contaminated wounds are best left open and treated with delayed closure. Antibiotics may be used in special circumstances, such as animal bites, but are certainly not totally effective (Chapter 45).

Fishhooks

Fishhooks commonly become embedded in fingers and other areas. Techniques for removal include:

1. Introducing an 18-gauge needle along the barbed side of the hook, with the bevel toward the inside of the hook curve. Apply a slight pressure upward on the hook shank to disengage it from the soft tissues. Push the needle upward and rotate until the lumen locks firmly over the barb. Keep the needle locked on the barb with gentle upward pressure. Then, with a slight rotation of the hook shank upward, the hook and needle can be removed through the original wound with a slight downward movement.

2. Hook a thread around the curve of the hook. Push downward on the hook's eye and shank to disengage the barb, and align the string with the long axis of the shank. Pull gently.

Splinters, subungual/hematomas and paronychia

See discussion on these problems in Chapter 68, p. 407.

PARENTAL EDUCATION

Parental education and follow-up should be specifically delineated on printed instruction sheet.

1. Mild bleeding and some discomfort may occur after suturing as anesthesia wears off.
2. Keep wound clean and dry for 2 days. Then begin gentle cleaning of wound with soap and water. Peroxide may be useful if there is significant scab formation to facilitate suture removal.
3. Call if the wound becomes red, painful, swollen, drains pus, or if red streaks appear.
4. Change dressing as directed.
5. Return for suture removal as instructed.

REFERENCES

Stewart, R.D.: Nitrous oxide sedation and analgesia in emergency medicine, Ann. Emerg. Med. **14**:139, 1985.

Tandberg, D.: Glass in the hand and foot: will an x-ray film show it? JAMA **248**:1872, 1982.

X ORTHOPEDIC INJURIES

DOUGLAS MAYEDA

66 Management principles

ALERT: Management of orthopedic injuries must follow stabilization of the patient. The unique growth characteristics of the child affect the nature of potential injuries.

Most orthopedic injuries seen in the ED are not life threatening. However, those involving multiple trauma must be appropriately prioritized, and when the pelvis or femur is broken, vascular support may be required (spinal injuries are discussed in Chapter 61). For all patients the diagnosis and management must be precise to maximize permanent function.

Children's bones are more easily injured than adults'. Less force is often required to produce an injury than might be expected. Anatomic considerations of growing bones and ligaments with abundant vascular supply make pediatric orthopedics unique in its approach to management.

The elasticity of children's bones allows the bone to deform before breaking and may result in a greenstick or torus fracture. A *greenstick* fracture involves the diaphysis of one side of a long bone, thus resulting in a fracture of one side of the cortex with an intact opposite side. A *torus* fracture is a buckling of one side of the cortex without an actual fracture line. This is usually seen in the metaphysis. The cortex in the developing skeleton and the microstructure and macrostructure dictate that the pattern of failure will be torus deformation rather than a complete transverse fracture. Torus fractures comprise one of the most common fracture patterns affecting the developing skeleton.

An accurate history of the time of the event,

mechanism of injury, and direction of forces and any history of previous injury and aggravating disease processes or bleeding diatheses should be obtained. The mechanism of injury is particularly important in defining the potential and type of injury and may assist in developing treatment plans by reducing a fracture or dislocation using a force that is opposite to that which led to the injury. Frequently, the injury was not witnessed and the child may be either unable (because of age) or too frightened to give a reliable history. Pseudoparalysis secondary to pain is common in the younger child. Children rarely complain persistently unless there is pathology. It is particularly important to recognize that pain may be referred, the classic example being hip injuries presenting as knee pain. Histories that are vague or inconsistent with injuries or delay in seeking medical care suggest child abuse. Approximatley 25% of fractures in children under 3 yr of age are caused by nonaccidental trauma (NAT) (Chapter 25).

Observation and examination for obvious deformities, swelling, ecchymoses, and point tenderness should be performed. In addition, evaluation of skin integrity, neurovascular status, muscle and tendon function, and pretreatment x-ray films are required.

Because of difficulty with physical evaluation and the lack of history in many cases, if there is any suspicion of an underlying fracture, x-ray films should be obtained. Routine AP and lateral views, with inclusion of the joints above and below the suspected fracture site, will help ensure that all potentially involved areas are studied. If there is any doubt because of the growth plates, comparison views should be obtained on a selective basis. Gonadal shields should be used. Those fractures missed most commonly by x-ray study include fractures of the ribs, elbow, and periarticular regions of the phalanges. Other problem areas include fractures of the navicular and calcaneous.

Fracture modeling and growth are rapid with particular stimulation of longitudinal growth and therefore may lead to overgrowth of an extremity when they occur between 2-10 yr. However, angulation should be reduced as much as possible. It is tolerated better in children under 2 yr with fractures near the ends of bones, where there is bayonet opposition, or if the deformity is in the plane of motion of the joint. Displaced intraarticular fractures; fractures that are grossly shortened, angulated, or rotated; fractures at marked angles to the plane of motion of a joint; or fractures that cross the growth plate need accurate reduction. It is unusual for children to need open reductions, but early orthopedic consultation is usually desirable.

Dislocations are rare, and when they do occur, they most commonly involve the radial head or patella. *Fractures often accompany dislocations because the ligamentous structures are more resistant to trauma than the epiphyseal plates*. In general the dislocation should be reduced before treatment of the fracture. An orthopedist should be involved. Neurologic function should be evaluated and in most instances x-rays obtained before and after reduction. Open dislocation or those with neurovascular compromise are true emergencies. A deformity is best corrected by an orthopedic consultant with gentle, steady, in-line traction, if such traction does not further impede circulation, increase pain significantly, or result in increased resistance with correction.

Patients with any fracture or dislocation in-

volving a potential for vascular compromise (e.g., supracondylar, humerus, posterior knee dislocation) should be admitted to the hospital following immediate ED orthopedic consultation and management. Should there be any suggestion of vascular compromise, it is also wise to have immediate vascular consultation to assist in making a decision about angiography or surgery. The absence of a pulse does not always indicate that the vascular status is compromised nor does the presence of a pulse assure adequate circulation. Severe pain in the forearm or calf, pain with passive stretching of the fingers or toes, or a sensory deficit in the distal extremity are more sensitive indicators of ischemia, which may be caused by arterial injury or a compartment syndrome.

Analgesia (meperidine [Demerol] 1-2 mg/kg/dose IM or IV [maximum: 50 mg/dose]) and muscle relaxation (diazepam [Valium] 0.1-0.2 mg/kg/dose PO or IV) usually are required before reduction in treating dislocations or poorly aligned fractures. Some prefer the lytic *(DPT)* cocktail consisting of meperidine (Demerol) 1-2 mg/kg/dose (maximum: 50 mg/dose); promethazine (Phenergan) 0.25-0.5 mg/kg/dose (maximum: 12.5 mg/dose); and chlorpromazine (Thorazine) 0.25-0.5 mg/kg/dose (maximum: 12.5 mg/dose) IM. Fentanyl 2-3 μg/kg IV, slowly over 3-5 min, may be another alternative. Half-life is 20 min. Older children may require less than the calculated dose. Nitrous oxide (50%) is also a useful adjunct as are Bier's blocks for some fractures. Judicious use of tape, sandbags, and foam blocks, as well as gentle handling, are usually adequate to obtain x-ray films.

Although stiffness is unusual, long-term care is essential for children in order to monitor growth and development. Communication with parents regarding treatment, home care, and possible complications is essential in initiating the management plan. In general, sprains and strains should be elevated, with use of ice packs for 12-24 hr. Ice packs are best prepared by crushing ice and placing it with some water in a plastic bag and applying for 15-20 min every 3-4 hr with continuing use of an elastic bandage in between. The elastic ACE bandage, if used, should be rewrapped as necessary if too loose or too tight. The cast should be kept dry. Parents should call immediately if there is severe pressure or pain within the cast, increasing blueness, coldness, swelling, or decreased motion of the toes or fingers.

SPLINTS

All suspected fractures should be splinted when the patient arrives at the ED. Splinting can be performed with firm materials, slings, and tape and is used primarily as an initial treatment to rest an injured area. Casts are usually not applied for at least 48 hr after acute injuries, which should be splinted over adequate padding (webril, stockinette, etc.) with plaster of paris (10 layers for upper extremities and 20 layers for lower extremities). The splint is then affixed with cotton or elastic bandages. An alternative is to place a circular cast and immediately bivalve it. Commercial splints are also available.

Swelling during this period can cause neurovascular compromise if confined to a compartment. One joint above and one below should be incorporated. Delayed casting is particularly important in children who are often unable to follow after-care instructions of elevation, rest, and cool packs. They can then be immobilized and followed by an orthopedist.

Those with obvious deformities should be stabilized on arrival and before complete evaluation unless there is compromised sensation or circulation distal to the injury, indicated by pain, pallor, pulselessness, paralysis, paresthesias, and pain with passive movement. If neurovascular deficits exist, gentle longitudinal traction in line with the extremity should be performed.

Fractures of the femur are usually immobilized using a Thomas' splint or Hare's or Buck's traction.

Commonly used splints include the following.

Sling and swathe

This is used for injuries between the sternoclavicular joint and elbow. It is made by placing the arm at 90 degrees of flexion with a sling and immobilizing it against the chest using a swathe wrapped around the body.

Long-arm splint

This is employed for injuries between the elbow and wrist, most commonly involving fractures of the forearm and distal radius. A posterior plaster slab extends from the axilla to the midpalmar region of the hand.

Hand splints

These are used for injuries between the wrist and tip of the fingers and are made by applying a posterior plaster splint from the back of the forearm, extending over the back of the fingers to the tips of the fingers. The hand is splinted in the position of function.

The best position for splinting is the "hooded cobra." The wrist is in neutral position (long axis of forearm roughly lines up with long axis of thumb), the MCP joints are flexed to about 60-70 degrees, the IP joints are flexed 10-20 degrees, and the thumb is widely abducted (p. 405). The tips of the fingers must be visible for neurovascular examination.

Long-leg posterior splint

This is used for injuries between the knee and ankle and is applied from the groin to the toes.

Short-leg posterior splint

This is used for injuries between the ankle and tips of the toes and is applied from just below the knee over the back of the leg to the toes, with the ankle at a 90-degree angle. Toes must remain visible.

SPRAINS AND STRAINS

The diagnosis of sprain or ligamentous tears, as an isolated injury, is unusual in children. A *sprain* is a tear of a ligament joining bone to bone around the joint and is caused most commonly by outside forces, especially contact sports. *Strains* are tears of the muscle or of fascia joining muscle to bone (musculotendinous unit), often resulting from a dynamic injury and usually not a contact sport.

Buckle fractures or epiphyseal injuries, rather than sprains and ligamentous injuries, often occur in young children because of the ease of injury to the epiphysis. However, adolescents do suffer ligamentous injuries.

First-degree sprain

This consists of minimal tearing of a ligament. There is point tenderness with neither abnormal motion nor joint instability and little or no swelling. The patient can bear weight.

Second-degree sprain

This consists of appreciable tearing of a ligament (5%-99% of fibers disrupted). There is point tenderness with moderate loss of function and variable presence of abnormal motion and joint instability. Weight-bearing is painful, there is localized soft tissue hemorrhage and hemarthrosis, testing of stability of joint causes pain, and there is possible persistent instability.

Third-degree sprain

This consists of complete disruption of the ligament surrounding a joint. There is extreme pain, loss of function, abnormal motion with absolute joint instability, deformity with tenderness and swelling, and diffuse hemorrhage. The patient is unable to bear weight, and there is persistent instability without surgical repair.

The patient may complain of little discomfort after the initial insult, and testing of the stability of the joint may cause little pain. Dislocations may have reduced spontaneously (common in fracture dislocation of knee). The only clue may be the unwillingness or inability of the patient to bear weight across the joint.

Strains

Strains are classified like sprains. First-degree strains involve minimal tearing of a musculotendinous unit, whereas second-degree strains involve more significant tears. Third-degree strains are marked by complete tears and may be painless initially. Injuries are marked by tenderness and pain, usually accompanied by no evidence of joint instability.

Management

Elevation, ice, and analgesia may reduce symptoms. Splint immobilization may be used prior to consultation for second- and third-degree injuries.

EPIPHYSEAL FRACTURES (Fig. 66-1)

A long bone can be divided into four parts. The first part is the shaft of the bone and is known as the diaphysis. The metaphysis is adjacent to the growth plate. The third part is the growth or epiphyseal plate and is a radiolucent horizontal line near the end of the bone where longitudinal growth occurs. The epiphysis is the end of the bone near a joint and is separated from the metaphysis by the epiphyseal plate.

Five types of epiphyseal fractures are identified by Salter and Harris, with the risk of growth disturbance increasing from a Type I to a Type V fracture.

Type I

This consists of separation of the epiphysis from the metaphysis without displacement or injury to the growth plate. There is tenderness and pain at the point of the growth plate without other findings. The x-ray film is initially normal but when repeated 7-10 days later may show calcification and new bone formation at site of injury. The fracture should be immobilized for 3 wk. Growth disturbance rare.

Type II

This consists of an epiphyseal plate slip with fracture through the metaphysis, producing a

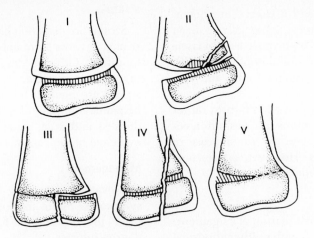

FIG. 66-1. Epiphyseal fractures: Salter classification.

triangular metaphyseal fragment. This is the most common type of fracture. Treatment is achieved with a closed reduction with immobilization for 3 (upper extremity) to 6 (lower extremity) wk. Growth disturbances are rare.

Type III

This consists of an epiphyseal plate slip with intraarticular fracture involving the epiphysis. The most common site is distal tibial epiphysis. Accurate reduction (often surgical) with maintenance of blood supply is essential to reducing risk of growth disturbance.

Type IV

This consists of an intraarticular fracture extending through the epiphysis, epiphyseal plate, and metaphysis. The lateral condyle of humerus is the most common site. It requires surgical open reduction and internal fixation, and the prognosis regarding growth is guarded.

Type V

This consists of a crush injury to the epiphyseal plate, producing growth arrest. This usually occurs in joints that move in one plane (flexion-extension), such as a knee, when a force in another plane is applied (abduction or adduction), such as smashing a dashboard or direct-crush

injury. The x-ray film may initially be normal. Despite treatment (no weight bearing for 3 wk) the prognosis for normal growth is poor. Therefore this type of injury must be treated with immobilization and early follow-up. It is important to advise parents of growth problems. Early orthopedic consultation is vital.

OPEN FRACTURES

Open fractures require immediate treatment unless life-threatening injuries supersede. It is important to note how much bone is exposed and if it is comminuted, the degree of soft tissue damage, and the extent of contamination and bleeding. The only clue to an open fracture may be the collection of blood with fat globules from what is thought to be a small puncture wound. Regardless of the exposure of bone, the injury should be considered an open fracture and cleaned, debrided, cultured, covered, and immobilized. A sterile dressing soaked in antiseptic solution is applied to the wound. Tetanus toxoid or antitoxin should be given, when appropriate (p. 546). Cephalothin (Keflin) 75-125 mg/kg/24 hr q 4 hr IV should be initiated, with an initial dose of 25-50 mg/kg IV.

The goal is to convert an open wound to a clean, closed wound as much as possible before definitive surgery.

67 Upper extremity injuries

CLAVICULAR FRACTURE

This fracture may be associated with chest trauma. In preschool children it is usually a greenstick fracture, with middle-third fracture most common.

Mechanism of injury

A fall or blow onto the shoulder or extended arm is the common cause.

Diagnostic findings

1. Pain on movement of affected arm or shoulder
2. Tenderness and possibly deformity at point of fracture
3. Possible injury to the subclavian vessels. It is important to examine for this possibility. Clues include the presence of an unusual degree of swelling or ecchymosis, pulse changes, and occasionally a bruit over the involved vessel, which may radiate down the arm or to the heart.

   #### X-ray film
   A clavicular view is indicated.

Management

1. Fractures should be immobilized for 3 wk in figure of 8 splint to maintain abduction of shoulder. A commercial clavicular strap or one made of tubular stockinette filled with felt or cotton padding may be used.
   a. Prevent skin maceration with a powdered pad in the axilla.
   b. Tighten to maintain abduction of shoulder (may have to be adjusted occasionally).
   c. Observe continually for axillary artery or brachial plexus compression.

2. Fractures of the distal (outer) tip of the clavicle should be treated as acromioclavicular separations.
3. Fractures of the proximal (inner) third may be treated with a simple sling if the figure of 8 splint distracts the pieces.

ACROMIOCLAVICULAR SEPARATION

This is partial to complete disruption of the acromioclavicular (AC) ligaments.

Mechanism of injury

Falling or a blow to the point of the acromion of the shoulder produces the injury.

Diagnostic findings

1. Tenderness over the AC articulation
2. Limited abduction of the arm
3. If third degree, step-off with upward displacement of the clavicle, representing complete rupture of the sternoclavicular and costoclavicular ligaments

   #### X-ray film
   An AC joint view is indicated. This is done initially without weights but, if normal, weight-bearing (0.03 kg weight/body weight up to 2 kg) films are obtained. Comparison views of opposite shoulder are necessary in all but third-degree separations.
   1. First degree: no evidence of displacement or joint subluxation
   2. Second degree: with weight bearing, <1 cm of upward displacement of the distal clavicle, indicating partial subluxation
   3. Third degree: with weight bearing, >1 cm of upward displacement

Management

1. First- and second-degree separations require immobilization with sling and swathe or shoulder immobilizer and follow-up with an orthopedist.
2. Third-degree separation requires ED consultation for consideration of surgical repair.

SHOULDER DISLOCATION: ANTERIOR

Anterior dislocation accounts for 95% of cases of shoulder dislocations.

Mechanism of injury

A blow to or fall on the abducted arm while it is in external rotation, abduction, and extension produces this dislocation.

Diagnostic findings

1. Prominent acromion process with flattening of deltoid muscle
2. Head of the humerus palpable anterior, inferior, and medial to the glenoid fossa
3. Limitation of abduction and absence of external rotation

Complications

1. Greater tuberosity fractures or others secondary to manipulation
2. Associated pathology of glenoid (labrum detachment, tear of anterior capsule and subscapularis muscle, or Hill-Sachs lesion, the latter representing a compression fracture of the posterior humeral head
3. Axillary nerve (lack of sensation over the lateral portion of shoulder and upper arm with deltoid muscle palsy) and distal vascular compromise

X-ray films

AP and axillary views are indicated. The humeral head lies inferior to the coracoid process. Fractures should be excluded. Postreduction x-ray films may reveal a fracture not seen initially or one that is secondary to reduction.

Management

1. Relaxation of subscapularis and pectoralis major with intravenous analgesia (meperi-

dine [Demerol]) and muscle relaxation (diazepam [Valium])
2. Reduction of dislocation
   a. With the patient prone and the involved arm and shoulder hanging in a dependent position over the table, have the patient hold a weight (about 1 lb weight/7 kg body weight). Reduction is usually achieved in 20-30 min. With younger children weight may have to be taped.
   b. In older children, especially where it is desirable to avoid large doses of opiates (e.g., long trip from point of injury to definitive medical care), an alternative reduction technique is to help child to reach behind the head (as if to scratch head). Then with an assistant supporting the trunk, outward traction is applied in the line of the long axis of humerus while the head of the humerus is pushed up into the fossa using pressure applied in the axilla.
   c. An alternative is to place the child in a prone position and push the scapula toward the midline (spine). Simultaneously, apply upward pressure on the head of the humerus in the axilla as above.
      NOTE: The methods described in *b* and *c* (especially useful for recalcitrant dislocations) require little if any analgesia, although nitrous oxide is a useful adjunct.
3. Other considerations
   a. Arm should be examined by physical assessment and x-ray film before and after reduction.
   b. After reduction, any fractures should be treated. These often require surgery.
   c. Sling and swathe or shoulder immobilizer (splinted in internal rotation) for 4 wk allows the capsule to heal.
   d. There is a 70% recurrence rate for those under 20 yr of age. Surgery may be required.

SHOULDER DISLOCATION: POSTERIOR

Posterior dislocations are uncommon.

Mechanism of injury

Violent internal-rotation motion of shoulder such as a seizure or electrial shock or direct trauma to the shoulder joint when the arm is outstretched can produce a posterior dislocation.

Diagnostic findings

1. There is an inability to abduct or externally rotate arm.
2. The affected shoulder is flat anteriorly or full posteriorly. There is a defect in the position of the humeral head, which is felt as a vague prominence behind and below the acromion. The injury may be bilateral.
3. There may be associated fracture.

X-ray films

The AP view may be normal, but the dislocation will be apparent on an axillary or transthoracic view. The humeral head may overlie the glenoid rim. Prereduction and postreduction x-ray studies should be obtained.

Management

1. Muscle relaxation and analgesia usually are required, sometimes necessitating general anesthesia.
2. Reduction of dislocation
   a. Consultation is usually advisable.
   b. Pressure is exerted on the posterior aspect of the shoulder joint with the arm in external rotation.
   c. Two-person approach involves application of traction along the long axis of the humerus while it is in 45 degrees of adduction with the elbow flexed to 90 degrees. A second person then pushes on the humeral head from behind.
   d. Anterior shoulder dislocation techniques also may be used.
3. Other considerations
   a. Treatment of any associated fractures after reduction
   b. Reexamination by physical assessment and x-ray film after reduction
   c. Immobilization with sling and swathe for 4-6 wk

ROTATOR CUFF INJURY
Mechanism of injury

Strenuous shoulder motion, such as in throwing, heavy lifting, or a fall on the shoulder, causes injury to the rotator cuff.

NOTE: The rotator cuff (*SIT: s*upraspinatus, *i*nfraspinatus, and *t*eres minor) stabilizes the shoulder in the glenoid fossa in abduction and allows the shoulder to abduct and externally rotate.

Diagnostic findings

1. Severe pain worsening with attempts at abduction or external rotation. Abduction of the shoulder may not be possible. Passive range of motion of the shoulder joint may be normal.
2. Tenderness is located over the insertion of the rotator cuff into the tuberosities.
3. May be only partial tear with abduction being weak, painful, and lacking endurance.

X-ray films

AP and lateral views of the shoulder may be normal or show a fracture of tuberosity. If significant with persistent weakness, arthrogram demonstrates leakage of contrast material from the shoulder joint capsule into the subacromial bursa.

Management

1. Minimal tears are treated with initial immobilization while maintaining good passive range of motion. Analgesia is administered.
2. Large tears require surgical intervention after confirmation. Early repair also is required in cases of an avulsion fracture of the tuberosity.

BRACHIAL PLEXUS
Mechanism of injury

There is traction on the brachial plexus during delivery, particularly in nulliparous mothers with large babies.

Diagnostic findings

1. Arm held loosely at side of thorax in internal

rotation with extension of the elbow, pronation of the forearm, and flexion at the wrist
2. Swelling in the region of the shoulder
   X-ray films
   Upper extremity and clavicle are indicated to exclude fractured clavicle, humerus, dislocated shoulder, or cervical spine injury.

Management

1. Prescribe physical therapy to avoid contractures.
2. Consider neurosurgical consultation.
   The majority of children have at least partial recovery by 18 mo of age.

SCAPULAR FRACTURE
Mechanism of injury

Severe blunt trauma produces scapular injuries.

Diagnostic findings

1. Swelling and localized tenderness
2. Possible associated injuries
   X-ray films
   Scapular views are indicated. A chest x-ray film, as well as other indicated studies, are important in cases of severe trauma (Chapter 56).

Management

Sling and swathe are indicated after caring for other injuries.

PROXIMAL HUMERAL EPIPHYSEAL FRACTURE
Mechanism of injury

Blunt trauma to the arm or shoulder may cause the fracture.

Diagnostic findings

1. Shoulder deformed by pain and tenderness
2. Possible associated neurovascular injury
   X-ray films
   A Salter type II epiphyseal slip is most commonly seen. Rarely, a Salter type I is found.

Management

1. Separation (<1 cm) with angulation of <40 degrees and absence of malrotation can be treated with a shoulder immobilizer or sling and swathe. Greater angulation requires closed reduction.
2. Fractures involving three pieces must be surgically corrected and four-piece fractures often involve replacement with a prosthesis.

HUMERAL SHAFT FRACTURE

A middle-third fracture is the most common.

Mechanism of injury

1. Spiral fractures result from twisting motion.
2. Transverse fractures result from direct blow.

Diagnostic findings

Tenderness with or without deformity is noted.
   Complications
   Complications are associated with arterial and radial nerve injury, particularly mid- or distal–humeral shaft injuries. Test sensation (first dorsal web space) and motor (extension of wrist and MCP joint) function should be assessed.
   X-ray films
   AP and lateral views of humerus, including shoulder and elbow, are indicated.

Management

1. Immobilization in long-arm splint (sugar tong) from the axilla to the wrist with flexion of the elbow at 90 degrees. Place in sling and swathe.
2. Specific therapy for radial nerve involvement
3. May require surgical repair to release entrapped radial nerve

CONDYLAR AND SUPRACONDYLAR FRACTURES OF DISTAL HUMERUS

These are the most common fractures of the elbow.

Mechanism of injury

1. Fall on outstretched hand with the elbow extended or fall on the flexed elbow
2. May also occur from snapping force as in throwing a baseball too hard

Diagnostic findings

1. Tenderness and deformity of the distal humerus. Distal fragment displaced upward, posterior and medial
2. Pain with flexion of elbow
3. May have associated dislocation of elbow (see next topic)
4. Lateral condyle fracture more common than medial, which is commonly associated with ulnar nerve injury

Complications

1. Nerve injury is associated with 20% of supracondylar fractures.
2. Pain with extension of fingers is an early sign of Volkmann's ischemia, which results from a volar-compartment syndrome of the forearm, leading to permanent hand disability.

X-ray films

AP and lateral views and, possibly, oblique views are indicated. Posterior displacement is recognized by extending a line down the anterior of the cortex of the distal humerus on the lateral x-ray film. Normally, this line intersects the middle third of the capitellum. With posterior displacement accompanying a supracondylar fracture, the line intersects anterior to the capitellum or the anterior third.

A subtle sign of a nondisplaced fracture is the "fat-pad sign." The sign is nonspecific and reflects hemorrhage into the elbow joint. This may be related to injury of the radial head, capitellum, trochlear, olecranon, or coronoid process. The "fat-pad sign" is an area of radiolucency seen on the lateral x-ray view of the elbow just above the olecranon process posteriorly or above the radial head anteriorly. The posterior "fat-pad sign" is of greatest importance since the anterior sign may be seen normally (see discussion following on elbow dislocation: posterior).

Management

1. Orthopedic consultation in ED
   a. Early reduction and immobilization with elbow held at 90-degree flexion. Test radial pulse before and after flexion.
   b. If there is any question of neurovascular compromise, immediate reduction is mandatory (traction, supination of the forearm, and flexion with direct pressure to align the displaced segment).
   c. Open reduction often required with condylar fracture
2. Hospitalization. Neurovascular compromise must be closely monitored, for at least 24 hr.

ELBOW DISLOCATION: POSTERIOR

This is the second most common dislocation in children.

Mechanism of injury

Fall on hyperextended arm causes the dislocation.

Diagnostic findings

There is obvious deformity, swelling, and effusion. The two epicondyles and the tip of the olecranon normally form an isosceles triangle. In a dislocation the sides of the triangle are unequal, while in a nondisplaced supracondylar fracture they remain equal.

There may be associated fracture, often supracondylar (see preceding topic).

Complications

Neurovascular compromise is common. There is nerve injury (median) in as many as 5%-10% of patients.

X-ray films

AP, lateral, and oblique views of elbow are indicated. There may be associated fracture. Posterior "fat-pad sign" is pathognomonic for elbow injury (dislocation, fracture, or possibly a sign of spontaneous reduction of elbow). Anterior "fat-pad sign" may be normal or pathologic (see condylar and supracondylar fractures of distal humerus).

Management

1. Administer analgesia (meperidine [Demerol]) or muscle relaxation (diazepam [Valium]) (p. 389)
2. With patient prone and arm in dependent position over edge of bed, apply gentle traction, with guidance of olecranon process into normal position.
   NOTE: Ensure that there is no trapped medial epicondyle fracture, which requires open surgery.
3. Order postreduction x-ray films and perform physical examination to check neurovascular and motor function and exclude fractures
4. Immobilize in splint with elbow flexed 90 degrees for 14-16 days. Test radial pulse before and after flexion.
5. Arrange close follow-up to monitor range of motion and exclude compartment syndrome or myositis ossificans.
6. Arrange ED orthopedic consultation.

RADIAL HEAD DISLOCATION OR SUBLUXATION (NURSEMAID'S ELBOW)

It occurs more commonly in younger children than in older ones.

Mechanism of injury

1. Sudden longitudinal pull on the forearm while patient's arm is pronated
2. Reported in children under 6 mo following rolling over

Diagnostic findings

1. Arm in passive pronation. Child will usually not move arm.
2. Resistance to and pain with full supination
3. Pain over the head of the radius
4. Rarely associated with a fracture of the proximal ulna (**Monteggia's fracture**)
   X-ray films
   Radiographs are usually normal. X-ray diagnosis is usually not required unless the mechanism of injury is unusual or the patient does not

become rapidly asymptomatic. In fact, if pre-reduction films are obtained, reduction is usually achieved by the radiology technician in process of supinating forearm for x-ray films.

1. A line drawn along the proximal shaft of the radius should pass through the capitellum. If it does not, there is a dislocation.
2. If x-ray films are obtained, the forearm should be evaluated to rule out Monteggia's fracture.

Management

Orthopedic consultation is usually not necessary.

1. Reduction by supination of the forearm while feeling the head of the radius (anulus) and, in a continuous motion, flexing the elbow. There is usually a palpable click over the radial head.
   a. The patient should be asymptomatic after 5-10 min, although in those that have been subluxed for several hours, return of function may take 6-12 hr.
   b. Those patients not rapidly asymptomatic should have x-ray studies.
2. Sling usually not required except for comfort
3. With Monteggia's fracture, following reduction, casting of the forearm in neutral position, with flexion of >90 degrees at the elbow for at least 6 wk. Orthopedic consultation should be obtained for this fracture.

RADIAL HEAD FRACTURE
Mechanism of injury

Falls on an outstretched hand produce fractures of the radial head.

Diagnostic findings

1. Tenderness over the radial head
2. May be associated with supracondylar, olecranon, or epicondyle fracture
   X-ray films
   AP and lateral views are indicated.

Management

1. **Nondisplaced fracture:** long-arm splint, including immobilization of wrist and sling
2. If more than one third of the articular surface is displaced, excision required. Angulation does not require reduction with displacement <20 degrees.

DISTAL ONE-THIRD RADIUS AND ULNAR FRACTURES

This is common in late school- and adolescent-age groups.

Mechanism of injury

A fall on the palm of the hand or blow to forearm causes forearm fractures.

Diagnostic findings

There is swelling and tenderness over the fracture site.
1. If a single bone is fractured and there is overriding, there must be a radial head dislocation (**Monteggia's fracture**) or a distal radioulnar dislocation (**Galeazzi's fracture**)
2. **Torus fracture:** common in children—a buckling or angulation of the cortex with no actual fracture line. A torus fracture usually is seen in the metaphyseal area.
3. **Greenstick fracture:** involves the diaphysis of a long bone—a fracture of one side of the cortex
4. **Colles' fracture:** transverse fracture of the distal radius with dorsal angulation and loss or reversal of volar tilt of distal radial articular surface; patient may have an accompanying fracture of the ulnar styloid. Usually Salter II epiphyseal injury
5. **Smith's fracture:** fracture of distal radius with increase in the volar tilt of the distal radial articular surface; reverse of Colles' fracture. Caused by blow on dorsum of wrist or distal radius with forearm in pronation.
6. **Barton's fracture:** marginal fracture of the dorsal or volar surface of the radius with dor-

sal or volar (corresponding to involved surface) dislocation of the carpal bones and hand
7. **Hutchinson's or chauffeur's fracture:** fracture of radial styloid process secondary to direct trauma or from impact of the styloid process against the navicular bone. Typically nondisplaced

Occasionally, median or ulnar nerve injury occurs, with self-limited neuropraxia.

Management

Rotational deformities must be eliminated. Angulation >15 degrees (especially proximal) in children leads to decreased function. Potential for longitudinal bone growth depends on distance from growth plates, especially the distal one where 80% of forearm growth occurs. The fracture should be immobilized for 4-6 wk. If both the radius and ulna are broken or dislocated, alignment is more difficult to attain and hold and open reduction and internal fixation may be required.

Torus fracture

It is immobilized for 4-6 wk in a long-arm splint.

Colles' fracture

1. Reduce by traction in the line of the deformity to disimpact the fragments, followed by pressure on the dorsal aspect of the distal fragment and volar aspect of the proximal fragment. Pressure should also be placed on the radial aspect of the distal fragment to correct radial deviation.
2. Test for reduction by palpation, lack of recurrence of deformity, and x-ray film.
3. Immobilize the hand in maximum ulnar deviation, the wrist neutral, and the forearm in full pronation. (If markedly displaced, immobilization in supination may be helpful.) Use anterior and posterior splints wrapped in place or an immediately bivalved cast. Cast should extend from knuckles to midhumerus. Some orthopedists prefer a short-arm cast. Once swelling resolves, a circular cast may be applied.

4. Ensure that there is no neurovascular compromise.
5. Consult with ED orthopedist.
   Smith's fracture
1. Reduce by longitudinal traction until fragments are distracted. Supinate and apply dorsal pressure on distal fragment.

2. Immobilize with anterior and posterior splint, with forearm in supination and wrist in extension.
3. Consult with ED orthopedist.
   Barton's fracture
   This usually requires open reduction.

68 Hand and wrist injuries

Hand and wrist injuries are common in children, and it is imperative to recognize their extent. A seemingly benign injury, if inappropriately managed, can lead to significant functional deficit. Historical data must include the time and mechanism of injury, defining whether it was a crush or puncture wound, whether it is dirty or clean, if there is tissue loss, the location of the injury, whether it is the dominant hand of the patient, immunization status, allergies, history of previous hand injuries, and, if possible, subjective motor and sensory deficits.

The physical examination is often more difficult because of decreased cooperation of the frightened child as well as the size of the structures. Skin, nerves, vessels, tendons, bone, joints, and ligaments must be evaluated. The nomenclature of the fingers is thumb, index, long, ring, and little fingers.

BASIC HAND EXAMINATION

This must be systematically and rapidly performed.

Observation

The hand should be observed at rest, looking for tendon injuries and obvious deformities. Fingers on flexion should normally point toward the scaphoid tubercle. If they deviate, there is a rotational injury. Digital cyanosis and capillary filling should be assessed.

Sensation

The hand should be observed for sweating, which should be present if digital nerve (sympathetics) is intact.

1. Radial nerve: dorsal thumb—web space
2. Median nerve: tip of the index finger
3. Ulnar nerve: tip of the little finger

Sensation distal to the injury should be examined. Two-point discrimination is particularly useful to determine abnormality. It can be performed by determining discrimination at 8 mm separation, using a paper clip.

Motor function

Each individual tendon should be checked for function in the fingers and as part of the group in the hand and wrist:

1. Flexor digitorum profundus. Stabilize the proximal interphalangeal (PIP) and metacarpophalangeal (MCP) joints while asking the patient to flex the distal interphalangeal (DIP) joint.
2. Flexor digitorum sublimis. Hold the fingers extended and ask the patient to flex only the PIP joint.
3. Extensor tendons. Extend each joint individually.
4. Flexor tendons. Flex each joint individually.

The following nerves should be checked:

1. Radial nerve: extension of the wrist and digits at the metaphalangeal (MP) joint
2. Median nerve: pointing the thumb upward or pinching the thumb and little finger tips together
3. Ulnar nerve: interossei muscles tested by having patient abduct and adduct the long finger from midline

Other considerations

1. Where there is injury around a joint, it

401

should be checked for stability.

2. X-ray films are useful in showing fractures, foreign bodies, and air in the joint. A true AP and lateral view of involved digits must be obtained, using the fingernail as a landmark.

3. Fractures are less common than in adults. They usually heal rapidly because of the thick periosteum. Surgical repair is rarely needed, and early functional use is essential.

PERILUNATE DISLOCATION

Mechanism of injury

Fall on an outstretched hand produces the dislocation.

Diagnostic findings

There are pain and tenderness in the wrist, which may be accompanied by minimal swelling or deformity.

X-ray films

Normally, on lateral roentgenogram, the long finger metacarpal, capitate, lunate, and radius line up in a straight line, and the lunate and navicular form an angle no greater than 50 degrees. This normal alignment is disrupted with a dislocation. A true lateral x-ray film is necessary since dislocation is easily missed on AP view.

If the dislocation is missed, the patient will have long-term disability. Thus the injury must not be passed off as a sprain.

Management

1. Immediate orthopedic consultation
2. Open reduction often required

NAVICULAR (SCAPHOID) BONE FRACTURE

This is the most common. Other fractures of the carpal bones are rare in children.

Mechanism of injury

Falling on an outstretched (dorsiflexed) hand results in navicular fractures.

Diagnostic findings

1. Tenderness over the anatomic snuffbox. Largely based on clinical suspicion.
2. Decrease in grip strength.

X-ray films

A view of the wrist, including the navicular view, is indicated. The x-ray film may be normal, but if the patient has clinical snuffbox tenderness, it should be treated as a fracture.

Management

Nondisplaced fractures should have a long-arm cast, which includes the thumb, MCP joint, and the elbow. Immobilization is for 7-8 wk unless no fracture was seen on the initial x-ray film, in which case the wrist should be reevaluated by x-ray examination in 10 days.

Even though nonunion and avascular necrosis of the navicular bone is rare in children, it is wise to have an orthopedist follow the child. If the fracture is displaced, an ED consultation should be obtained.

METACARPAL BONE FRACTURE

Mechanism of injury

A direct blow to the hand produces the fracture.

Diagnostic findings

1. Swelling and point tenderness
2. Deformity with displacement (need to assess the degree of rotation and angulation)
3. Types of fracture:
   a. **Boxer's fracture:** fracture of the little-finger metacarpal head. Usually has good functional result with up to 35-40 degrees of volar angulation
   b. **Bennett's fracture:** fracture of the thumb-metacarpal base into the joint. Unusual in children

X-ray films

AP and lateral views of the hand are indicated.

Management

1. Immobilization for 3-4 wk with splinting (of-

ten casting) from the mid forearm to the distal phalanges. The MCP joint should be splinted at 45-90 degrees of flexion (to prevent MCP contracture) and the wrist in extension.

2. Once reduced and immobilized, the fracture should be rechecked with x-ray examination to ensure that rotation and alignment have been corrected.

3. Bennett's fractures, even if reduced, usually require internal fixation to hold reduction because of the opposing forces of the abductor pollicis longus and adductor pollicis.

In general, more deformity is tolerated in the ring and little fingers than in the thumb, index, or long-finger metacarpals.

PHALANGEAL FRACTURE

This is the most frequently fractured bone in children.

Mechanism of injury

There is a direct blow to the tip of the finger, such as being caught in car door.

Diagnostic findings

1. Swelling and point tenderness of the phalanx
2. Deformity with displacement. On flexion, the fingernails normally point toward the scaphoid tubercle. If they do not, there is a rotational injury.
   #### X-ray film
   AP and lateral views are indicated. A true lateral view of the individual digits must be obtained, using the fingernail as a landmark.

Management

1. With the middle or distal phalanx fracture of the involved digit and the neighboring one should be immobilized in a finger splint. If involved, the long and ring fingers should always be splinted together since their lumbricales are mutually dependent.
2. If the proximal phalanx is fractured, a dorsal splint should incorporate the wrist at 30 degrees of extension, the MCP joint flexed at

30-50 degrees, and the IP joint flexed at 10-15 degrees.

3. Open fractures and intraarticular fractures, with or without displacement, that involve a large portion of the joint space should be referred to a hand or orthopedic surgeon.

4. Rotational or angulation deformities are difficult to correct and require consultation. A fracture of the phalangeal neck is a transverse fracture through the neck of either the proximal or middle phalanx. Maintaining reduction is difficult, and loss of reduction may be functionally significant.

5. Epiphyseal fractures usually occur in the proximal phalangeal base of the little fingers—usually Salter type II. They require reduction and splinting to a neighboring phalanx, with flexion at the joint. Complete separation of the plate requires open reduction.

FINGER DISLOCATION

Ligaments and capsular structures in children are stronger than an epiphyseal plate. Trauma that might dislocate a finger in an adult may instead produce a fracture in a child. Dislocations are rare.

Mechanism of injury

There is a blow to the tip of finger.

Diagnostic findings

1. Obvious deformity and tenderness at the joint
2. Swelling and inability to flex the finger
3. Complex dislocation if the MCP joint is involved
   a. Phalanx displaced on metacarpal—not at 90 degrees as in a simple dislocation but more parallel, with slight displacement and less angulation
   b. Dimpling of palmar skin
   #### X-ray films
   These should be done before attempting reduction since there may be an underlying frac-

ture. Dislocated bones are usually at 90 degrees to each other.

A complex fracture has widened joint space and parallel position. The sesamoid bone may be in the joint space, which often signifies the need for an operation.

Management

1. Refer to orthopedist.
2. Reduce by hyperextension of joint while pushing the distal bone over into position from above. Do not pull. Immobilize for 1-2 wk.
3. After reduction, check for ligamentous instability and immobilize with splinting for 1-2 wk.

BOUTONNIÈRRE DEFORMITY

This is a rupture of central slip of extensor tendon at PIP joint, with volar subluxation of the lateral bands.

Mechanism of injury

A direct blow or laceration produces the deformity.

Diagnostic findings

1. Tenderness and swelling over dorsal PIP joint may make diagnosis clinically difficult.
2. Distal IP joint is held in extension while proximal IP joint is held in flexion.
   X-ray film
   Fracture should be excluded.

Management

If fracture is not present, splint in extension and arrange follow-up with a hand surgeon. Patients seen days after injury without treatment will probably need operative repair.

MALLET FINGER

This is a fracture of the lip of the base of the distal phalanx with disruption of the extensor tendons at the DIP joint. It is common in ado-

lescents and may be a Salter type III epiphyseal injury. Younger children typically have a Salter type I or II injury.

Mechanism of injury

There is blunt trauma, with a blow to the tip of the finger by a softball or football striking finger ("jammed finger").

Diagnostic findings

1. Patient is unable to extend distal phalanx because of terminal slip rupture, laceration of terminal slip, or avulsion fracture.
2. Tenderness and swelling of the DIP joint
3. Finger held with distal phalanx flexed
   X-ray films
   AP and lateral views of digit are indicated. These views may show a chip fracture of the phalanx at the DIP joint.

Management

1. Fracture <25% of joint surface (without subluxation) is splinted in hyperextension and the patient referred. Finger may be splinted on either dorsal or volar surface, but tape must be changed daily while fingers are held in extension. Use foam and aluminum splints.
2. With fracture >25% of the joint surface or subluxed joint, operative reduction and fixation are required.
3. In older adolescents injury may occur without fracture, and the involved finger may be splinted with the DIP joints in hyperextension. Strict immobilization for 6 wk is necessary.

GAMEKEEPER'S THUMB (SKIER'S THUMB)

This is injury to the ulnar collateral ligament of the thumb.

Mechanism of injury

There is hyperextension of the MCP joint of the thumb (a common ski-pole injury with fall on outstretched hand while clasping pole).

Diagnostic findings

1. Swelling and tenderness over the ulnar aspect of the MCP joint of the thumb with increased pain on radial deviation of MCP joint
2. Laxity of the joint with stressing
   ### X-ray films
   AP and lateral views are indicated to exclude avulsion fracture of proximal phalynx.

Management

1. Apply thumb spica splint with the thumb in extension for 6 wk and follow-up with a hand surgeon.
2. With stress instability >30%-45%, initial surgical repair is needed.

LACERATION

See Chapter 65: Soft tissue injuries.

Diagnostic findings

1. Evaluate the wound to determine the depth of injury and involvement of underlying tissues including vessels, nerves, muscles, tendons, ligaments, bone, and joints.
2. Sensation and motor function must be specifically tested focusing on the three major nerves (radial, median, and ulnar) as well as sensation distal to the injury. Two-point discrimination is particularly useful. Each individual tendon must be evaluated. Consider the stance of fingers when the tendon was lacerated (p. 401).

Management

1. Use direct pressure and elevation to obtain hemostasis. Never use a clamp, hemostat, or deep suture. If extensive bleeding is associated with a finger laceration, an excellent field and tourniquet can be achieved by cleansing the patient's finger and then slipping the hand into a sterile glove, snipping the end of the glove on the involved finger, and then rolling back the finger of the glove to provide exposure and tourniquet. Careful scrubbing is then done.
2. Following sensory examination, infiltrate with lidocaine (Xylocaine) without epinephrine to facilitate cleansing and laceration repair. Epinephrine-containing medications should *not* be used.
3. Partial tendon tears may or may not cause functional deficits and these, as well as complete lacerations, require referral. Extensor tendon repairs have an excellent prognosis, whereas flexor injuries, even with meticulous surgical technique, have a poorer prognosis.
4. Repair lacerations using either 4-0 or 5-0 nylon (Prolene, Ethilon, Surgilon, etc.) suture material on a P3 needle. Never use deep sutures. Do not suture if over 8 hr since injury.
5. Children require extensive dressing and splints to maintain position and thereby minimize further injury and facilitate repair.

In children with extensive injuries, particularly when there is associated tendon damage, the best position for splinting is the "hooded cobra." The wrist is in neutral position (long axis of forearm roughly lines up with the long axis of thumb), the MCP joints are flexed to about 60-70 degrees, the IP joints are flexed 10-20 degrees, and the thumb is widely abducted. The first layer of dressing, when required, is a nonadherent material. The second layer maintains the position of the hand and is a noncircumferential, noncompressible material (such as fluffs or sponges), mostly occupying the palm and the dorsum of the hand, wrist, and forearm. The final layer should have decreasing tension and compression from the distal end, proximally. A plaster of paris splint of 10-15 layers may be incorporated into the volar (palmar) side of the dressing.

FINGERTIP INJURIES

Crush injuries are common in children and may be associated with tuft fracture.

Mechanism of injury

There is a blow to the distal phalanx between two firm objects.

Diagnostic findings

1. Discoloration, swelling, local tenderness
2. Frequently associated with subungual hematoma
3. Possibility of associated nail-bed injury
   X-ray films
   Views should be taken to exclude underlying fracture.

Management

1. **Subungual hematoma:** drain with electric cautery or red-hot paper clip.
2. If there is a laceration, it should be cleansed thoroughly and sutures used sparingly, with only loose approximation of the skin. Antibiotics often recommended.
3. If the nail bed is injured with partial avulsion or if it is lacerated, the nail should be left on to act as a splint and to protect the nail bed. If it is avulsed at the base and there is a transverse fracture of the distal phalanx, there is usually a laceration of the nail bed. Under these circumstances the nail should be removed and the nail bed repaired to prevent distortion with 5-0 fine absorbable (Vicryl, Dexon) sutures.
4. Distal tuft injuries usually heal without treatment other than good wound cleansing, dressing, and splinting.

AMPUTATION OF FINGERTIPS

This is common in children.

Management

1. If the subcutaneous tissue is intact, initial cleaning and debridement with a bulky dressing are adequate. It will heal well by secondary intention.
2. If there is partial or not quite total laceration of the fingertip, it should be loosely approximated. Children heal remarkably well, and little is lost if the tissue becomes necrotic and demarcates and subsequently must be removed.
3. X-ray examination is necessary to ensure that there is no bony involvement. A hand surgeon should be consulted.
4. Amputation at or distal to the distal half of the fingernail may be treated with careful cleansing and debridement and covered with ointment and gauze and immobilized in a nonoperative fashion. Antibiotics are indicated if there is significant contamination. Such conservative treatment also may be useful in very distal (distal to insertion of extensor and flexor tendons of distal phalynx) amputations. Consultation should be obtained.
5. For the completely amputated digit, treatment depends on the availability of microsurgery. The amputated part should be wrapped in sterile gauze, soaked in lactated Ringer's solution, placed and sealed in a plastic bag, and then placed in ice water. This prevents immersion and water logging. Rapid transport is essential.

WRINGER INJURY
Mechanism of injury

The involved limb is caught in roller, producing a crushing friction burn. A shearing force component is added if the individual attempts to pull away.

Diagnostic findings

1. There is swelling of the involved soft tissue area.
2. Fractures are uncommon. Dislocations may occur.
   Complications
1. There is extensive hematoma and compartmental swelling with neurovascular compromise.
2. Skin slough is common.

Management

1. Control of swelling by application of sterile occlusive dressing after cleansing of extremity

2. Elevation of extremity and hospitalization for observation for 24 hr
   - In rare circumstances, with mild injury and assurance of good follow-up, the patient may be discharged with q 12 hr reexaminations. In such cases, the arm should be splinted.
3. Possible need for fasciotomy of the forearm or carpal tunnel decompression because of neurovascular compromise
4. Possible need for skin graft

AMPUTATION OF THE HAND OR PARTS
Management

1. Examine hand completely. Preserve any viable tissue.
2. Clean the hand, wrap in sterile gauze, soak in lactated Ringer's solution, place in a plastic bag, and then put on ice.
3. X-ray hand to determine integrity.
4. Immediately refer to center capable of reimplantation.

RING ON A SWOLLEN FINGER
Management

Several alternatives exist:
1. Place a piece of string under the ring and from the distal end of the finger wrap it in close loops. Exert a slow pull on the proximal end, gently pulling the ring distally as the string unwinds.
2. Alternate at 5 min intervals between soaking the finger in cold water and elevating the fingers. This is repeated for 30 min and oil (mineral or cooking) applied while the hand is elevated. With a steady motion, the ring is pushed off.
3. Cut the ring with a ring cutter.

SUBUNGUAL SPLINTER
Management

A splinter under the nail can be removed by gently shaving over the distal end of the splinter until the splinter can be exposed. A single-edge razor or scalpel can be used.

INFECTIONS
Felon

Mechanism of injury
Improper trimming of nails or puncture wound to the volar aspect of the distal phalanx causes felons.

Diagnostic findings
Swelling, erythema, and tenderness of the volar aspect of the distal phalanx are present.

Management
1. Drainage. Incision can be made at site of maximum tenderness or laterally, taking care to avoid the neurovascular bundle. Penrose drain promotes drainage. Incision and drainage should be carried out before the wound becomes fluctuant, since intercompartmental pressure will produce ischemic necrosis.
2. Elevation, soaks

Paronychia

Mechanism of injury
Hangnail or any bacterial inoculum causes irritation leading to infection.

Diagnostic findings
There is swelling, erythema, and tenderness alongside the nail, which may extend under the nail.

Management
1. Digital block is essential. Do not use epinephrine-containing anesthetics.
2. If relatively acute, lift the cuticle up around the entire nail to relieve pus and insert cotton wick. Continue treatment with soaks.
3. If chronic, excise medial or lateral edge of nail to permit drainage.

Acute suppurative tenosynovitis

Mechanism of injury
Extension of local infection can involve the synovium.

Diagnostic findings
1. Erythema and tenderness along the tendon sheath, often with maximal pain over metacarpal head
2. Finger held in flexed position. Passive extension of DIP joint causes severe pain.

Management

1. Hospitalize.
2. Immobilize entire length of tendon.
3. Consider incision and drainage by orthopedist.
4. Give high-dose antibiotics: nafcillin (or equivalent, 100 mg/kg/24 hr q 4 hr IV in absence of penicillin allergy.

Palmar (thenar and midpalmar) space infection

Mechanism of injury

Extension of a localized puncture wound, laceration, or an animal bite leads to infection.

Diagnostic findings

Swelling, tenderness, and erythema are present.

Management

1. Hospitalize.
2. Arrange incision and drainage by hand surgeon.
3. Administer antibiotics: nafcillin (or equivalent) 100 mg/kg/24 hr q 4 hr IV in absence of penicillin allergy, unless Gram's stain or culture indicate other choices.

Herpetic whitlow

Etiology

Herpes simplex 1 virus is usually acquired from oral lesions.

Diagnostic findings

1. In contrast to bacterial paronychia, the lesions are more blistered, the exudate is serous, and the pain is described as burning. The lesions may be subungual and difficult to see.
2. Gram's straining of the exudate may show giant cells but no bacteria. If recurrent, viral cultures are useful.
3. **Complications**
   a. Superimposed bacterial infection
   b. Recurrence and long, indolent course

Management

1. The involved digit should be splinted.
2. Oral analgesics may be useful.
3. In general, surgery is avoided because it spreads the infection. However, if the lesions are subungual, incision and drainage with decompression may increase the patient's comfort.
4. Topical acyclovir (Zovirax) 5% ointment may shorten the course and diminish recurrences.

69 Lower extremity injury

PELVIC FRACTURE

The injury is usually incurred while the patient is a pedestrian or a passenger in an automobile collision. There are often major associated injuries, and the mortality rate is high (5%).

Mechanism of injury

Fracture results from blunt trauma to the pelvic area.

Diagnostic findings

1. Local tenderness. Excessive movement or crepitus on pelvic rocking or pressure on symphysis
2. Since the pelvis is a bony ring, fractures of one part are usually associated with fractures elsewhere in the ring, particularly if the fracture is displaced. The ischiopubic ring follows this ring concept independently.
3. Blood loss. May be significant, with up to 2,500 ml of hemorrhage common in adults. Massive retroperitoneal hematoma can occur with shock and vascular collapse.
4. Injuries to the bladder or urethra (Chapter 64)
   a. If there is blood at the meatus or inability to void with a distended bladder, a retrograde urethrogram should be obtained before passage of a catheter.
   b. If the urethra is intact, a cystogram followed by an IVP should be done.
   c. Hematuria is present in 50%-60% cases, but only 10% will have significant injuries.
5. Rectal and vaginal examination. Direct vaginal and perineal injuries may occur, or the examination may demonstrate communication with an open fracture.
6. High association with head trauma
7. Infrequent injuries to the obturator, femoral, or sciatic nerves

X-ray films

These consist of AP and frog-leg projections. Multiple ossification sites are present and must not be confused with a fracture.

Management

1. Life-threatening injuries should be managed first (Chapter 56).
2. IV fluids should be initiated with normal saline or lactated Ringer's and, shortly thereafter, blood. Massive hemorrhage is less common in pediatric pelvic fractures but ultimately determines mortality.
3. Orthopedic and urology consultants should be involved as needed.
4. Pneumatic antishock trousers (MAST) may be helpful in both the initial immobilization of the patient and subsequent therapy. Pediatric MAST suits are available.
5. If profuse bleeding is present, angiography may be required to localize site.
6. Pelvic fractures with a gravid uterus present a major risk of fetal injury and death. Obstetrics consultation is necessary. Fetal distress must be assessed by monitoring scalp pH and heart tones. If there is evidence of distress, an emergency cesarean section is indicated. Mother must be cared for at an appropriate institution.

409

HIP FRACTURE

This is rare in children.

Mechanism of injury

A fall onto the hip region with transmission of a large energy force causes the injury.

Diagnostic findings

1. Externally rotated and shortened
2. Localized swelling and tenderness, with pain on movement of leg
3. Large blood-loss potential

Management

1. Immobilization
2. Orthopedic consultation in ED

HIP DISLOCATION: POSTERIOR

This is rare in children, and there is usually an associated fracture. Anterior and obturator dislocations are less common.

Mechanism of injury

Longitudinal forces applied to the knee with the hip and knee in 90-degree flexion and slight abduction (knee hits dashboard in car) produce a posterior dislocation.

Diagnostic findings

1. Leg is shortened, internally rotated, and slightly adducted
2. Associated fractures, especially posterior wall of acetabulum, and sciatic nerve injury (10%)
   Complication
   Avascular necrosis of femoral head may follow, particularly if reduction is delayed.
   X-ray films
   AP and lateral views of the hip are indicated.

Management

1. Reduction without delay, preferably by orthopedist, using spinal or general anesthesia. If transfer of patient is necessary with a long transit time, the dislocation should be reduced to prevent aseptic necrosis. Traction in the line of deformity should be followed by gentle flexion of the hip to 90 degrees and then internal-to-external rotation.
2. Bed rest and long-term follow-up is essential.

HIP DISLOCATION: CONGENITAL

This should be diagnosed in infancy when prognosis for recovery is excellent. The child may limp or be unable to walk and should be referred to an orthopedist for care.

TOXIC SYNOVITIS OF THE HIP

This occurs in 1½ to 7-year-olds, with a peak at 2 yr of age. It often follows respiratory infection.

Diagnostic findings

1. Inability to bear full weight. Child may limp and complain of knee pain (Chapter 40).
2. Minimal (or no) pain on abduction and external rotation, with variably limited range of motion
   X-ray films
   These are usually normal or show small effusion.

Management

1. Self-limited. Symptomatic treatment with aspirin and follow-up
2. Must be certain to exclude septic arthritis by arthrocentesis or incision and drainage if necessary. If any question, admit and evaluate.

LEGG-CALVÉ-PERTHES DISEASE (AVASCULAR NECROSIS OF THE FEMORAL HEAD)

This is a common cause of limp in 4 to 10-year-olds.

Diagnostic findings

1. Limited hip movement, particularly internal rotation and abduction. Limp is common (Chapter 40).
2. Tenderness over anterior capsule
   X-ray films
   There is widened joint space between ossified head and acetabulum, progressing to collapse of

head, increased neck width, and head demineralization.

Management

1. Bracing and protection of hip
2. Orthopedic monitoring

EPIPHYSEAL SEPARATION OF THE HEAD OF THE FEMUR (SLIPPED CAPITAL FEMORAL EPIPHYSIS)

This is usually seen in obese or rapidly growing adolescent males (12-15 yr). It may be bilateral.

Mechanism of injury

1. Upward blow transmitted through shaft of femur
2. May be no history of trauma

Diagnostic findings

1. Leg may be shortened, externally rotated, and adducted. Pain with movement. Limitation of internal rotation and abduction.
2. Impaired weight bearing. Limp is present (Chapter 40).
3. Pain on palpation. Pain may be referred to knee, groin, or hip.
   #### X-ray films
   AP and frog-leg views are indicated. Widening and irregularity of epiphyseal plate is noted. If displaced, it usually is downward and posterior.

Management

1. Often requires surgical reduction and immobilization for 12 wk
2. Follow-up important—to watch for avascular necrosis of the femoral head

FEMORAL SHAFT FRACTURE
Mechanism of injury

A direct blow to the thigh (bumper injury) produces the fracture.

Diagnostic findings

1. Swelling, deformity, tenderness, and pain on movement

2. Impaired weight bearing
3. Possible significant blood loss
4. Possible neurovascular compromise
5. Rare fat embolus, especially with associated injuries of hip, knee, or pelvis
   #### X-ray films
   AP and lateral views to include entire femur, including hip, are indicated.

Management

1. Immediate reduction of fracture with Hare's or Thomas' traction splinting
2. Orthopedic consultation for long-term therapy, using traction or internal rod depending on age of child

COLLATERAL LIGAMENT INJURY TO KNEE

The medial collateral ligament is most commonly affected.

Mechanism of injury

A twisting injury or blow to the outer aspect of knee causes ligamentous injury.

Diagnostic findings

1. Pain on flexion and palpation
2. Knee effusion
3. Pain and instability with varus and valgus stress testing. With the knee extended, stress is applied to one side of the knee joint while applying counterpressure against the opposite side.
   #### X-ray films
   AP and lateral views of knee are indicated. There may be a need for arthroscopy and arthrogram.

Management

1. Immobilize with knee immobilizer.
2. Avoid weight bearing.
3. Refer to orthopedist.

MENISCUS INJURY TO KNEE

Medial meniscus is most commonly affected. It is uncommon in children but does occur in adolescents.

Mechanism of injury

This is a squatting or twisting injury. While the knee is weight bearing and slightly flexed, a twisting motion is applied. Internal rotation injures medial meniscus, whereas external rotation damages lateral meniscus.

Diagnostic findings

1. Pain on flexion. May lock in flexion or prevent full extension
2. Knee effusion, with tenderness over involved meniscus
3. McMurray's maneuver. In a supine patient, hold foot under arch with one hand and cup the knee with the other. Flex the knee. The knee is then extended with the leg in internal or external rotation. A clicking or rattling on extension in internal rotation indicates a tear of the lateral meniscus and, on external rotation involvement of the medial meniscus.
   ### X-ray films
AP and lateral views of knee are indicated. There may be a need for arthroscopy and arthrogram.

Management

1. Orthopedic consultation for immobilization, arthroscopy, and possible removal of meniscus
2. Definitive care needed within 1-2 days

CRUCIATE LIGAMENT INJURY TO KNEE

The anterior cruciate ligament is most commonly affected, occurring in children over 8 yr of age.

Mechanism of injury

Forcible hyperextension or abduction and external rotation of leg damages the ligament.

Diagnostic findings

1. Patient may feel or hear pop of knee if anterior cruciate ligament is ruptured.
2. Effusion

3. AP drawer sign. With patient supine, hip 45 degrees, knee flexed 90 degrees, and foot resting on table in external rotation: pushing or pulling produces sliding motion indicative of ligamentous injury. If there is increased anterior mobility, anterior cruciate ligament instability is present; if there is increased posterior mobility, posterior cruciate ligament damage has occurred.
4. Lachman's test: anterior drawer sign with knee in 15-20 degree flexion and then anterior stability test
   ### X-ray films
AP and lateral views of the knee are indicated. Small avulsion fragment of tibial spine should be excluded. Patient may need arthroscopy and arthrogram.

Management

1. Immobilization and orthopedic referral for evaluation for surgical repair
2. With associated tibial spine fracture, hospitalization and orthopedic consultation

PATELLAR DISLOCATON

This is most common in adolescent females.

Mechanism of injury

1. Internal rotation of leg or direct blow to outer aspect of the knee
2. Rare occurrence with forcible contraction of the quadriceps muscle

Diagnostic findings

1. Displaced patella palpated lateral to normal position
2. Effusion and tenderness over medial collateral ligament and along articular surface of patella
3. Subluxation of patella usually reduced spontaneously. Sense of knee "giving out" or buckling
4. Pain reproduced by pushing the patella laterally with knee flexed at 30 degrees and foot

supported (patellar apprehension)

5. Possibility of associated fracture of medial border of patella or osteochondral fracture of the lateral condyle

X-ray films

AP and lateral views of knee and tangential (sunrise) view of patella are indicated

Management

1. Reduction by extending the knee and flexing the hip (relaxing quadriceps). Slight medial pressure should be applied to the patella. Often happens spontaneously
2. Immobilization of knee in extension for 6 wk and avoidance of weight bearing
3. If recurrent, surgical reimplantation of patellar tendon

PATELLAR FRACTURE
Mechanism of injury

Blunt force over the anterior aspect of knee can fracture the patella.

Diagnostic findings

1. Effusion and tenderness. Fracture may be palpable.
2. Extension of knee is limited if fracture is transverse with complete transection of the extensor tendon. May also lose extensor function from rupture of patellar or quadriceps tendons or fracture of tibial tubercle
3. If caused by pressure applied through the femur, such as the knee hitting the dashboard, must also exclude posterior dislocation of the hip

X-ray films

AP and lateral views of knee and tangential (sunrise) view of patella are indicated.

Management

1. Immobilization of knee in extension and referral
2. Possibility of hospitalization and surgery with complete fracture

DISTAL FEMUR OR TIBIAL PLATEAU FRACTURE
Mechanism of injury

A direct blow or indirect valgus or varus stress is the cause of injury.

Diagnostic findings

A knee effusion is commonly present.

X-ray films

AP and lateral views are indicated. The patient may need stress films after consultation with orthopedist.

Management

Temporary immobilization and referral to orthopedist are required.

KNEE DISLOCATION

This is usually associated with a fracture and is rare in childhood.

Mechanism of injury

Severe trauma disrupting all ligaments permits the dislocation.

Diagnostic findings

An obvious deformity of the knee is present.

Complications

Neurovascular compromise is common. With absence of peripheral pulse, immediate reduction (without x-ray studies) is required.

X-ray films

AP and lateral views are required before and after reduction.

Management

1. Immediate orthopedic referral and reduction, usually with internal fixation
2. Possibility of immediate vascular consultation

OSGOOD-SCHLATTER DISEASE

This is usually seen in active children, 11-15 yr of age.

Mechanism of injury

Constant pulling of the patellar tendon on its insertion causes this partial separation of the tibial tubercle.

Diagnostic findings

1. Localized swelling, pain, and tenderness over the tibial tuberosity
2. Possibility of a partial avulsion of the tubercle
   X-ray films
   AP and lateral knee views are required. Tibial tuberosity is normally irregular in adolescents.

Management

1. Immobilization of knee in extension for 2-4 wk
2. Restricted activity in mild cases or immobilization of knee in extension for 2-4 wk if severe
3. With avulsed fracture, possibility of nonunion or avascular necrosis, requiring surgery at later date
4. Best followed by orthopedist

CHONDROMALACIA PATELLAE

This is softening of the patella.

Mechanism of injury

A fall on a flexed knee or chronic, strenuous exercise such as jogging causes the damage.

Diagnostic findings

1. Pain following exercise, with sensation of knee grating or "giving out"
2. Pain when sitting for long periods with the knee flexed or when walking up or down stairs
3. Pain and crepitus with palpation of the patella as it moves over its articular surface
   X-ray film of patella
   The film is normal.

Management

Restriction of activity with strengthening of quadriceps muscles is indicated.

TIBIAL OR FIBULA FRACTURE (BOOT-TOP FRACTURE)
Mechanism of injury

A direct blow or indirect stress to the bone produces the fracture.

Diagnostic findings

1. Tenderness, swelling, deformity, and impaired weight bearing
2. Spiral and oblique fractures usually are located at the junction of the middle and distal thirds, the weakest region of the tibia. Tibial shaft fractures associated with a fibular reciprocal fracture is considered eccentric if the fibular site is subcapital or malleolar in location. In children it is unusual to have an eccentric fibular fracture, which may reflect the greater flexibility of the ligamentous structures anchoring the proximal and distal fibula in children.
   Complications
1. Open fractures
2. Distal neurovascular injuries are common (e.g., compartment syndrome). If proximal third of the tibia is fractured, there may be injury at the bifurcation of anterior and posterior tibial arteries.
   X-ray films
   AP and lateral views are indicated. The patient may not have a fracture seen on radiograph, but epiphyseal separation may have occurred. Toward the end of adolescence, the medial aspect of the distal tibial epiphysis closes first.

Management

1. Isolated fibular fractures are managed with short-leg walking cast. Undisplaced tibial fractures can be immobilized in a long-leg posterior splint, with the patient non-weight bearing and followed at home for 4-6 wk. Early orthopedic consultation
2. Displaced closed tibial fractures require hospitalization for observation of circulatory status. Orthopedic consultation in ED
3. Open fractures require immediate consultation for surgical cleansing and stabilization.

70 Ankle and foot injuries

ANKLE SPRAIN

Ankle sprain is a ligamentous injury. The talus articulates primarily with the tibia. The medial and lateral malleoli provide horizontal stability. On the medial side of the ankle, the deltoid ligament binds the medial malleolous to the talus and calcaneus. On the lateral side, stability is achieved by three ligaments (anterior talofibular, posterior talofibular, and calcaneofibular ligaments).

Mechanism of injury

Twisting of the foot produces ankle sprains. Inversion (supination) and eversion (pronation) are more frequent than plantar and dorsiflexion injuries. Inversion is the most common.

Diagnostic findings

Local swelling, discoloration, and tenderness with impaired weight bearing are present.
1. Tenderness anterior and inferior to the lateral malleolus (attachment of talofibular and calcaneofibular ligaments) is common with inversion injuries.
2. Eversion injuries damage the deltoid ligament that is important for ankle stability. Separation >5 mm between the medial malleolus and talus is evidence of deltoid ligament injury. Deltoid ligaments, which almost never tear without associated fracture, have associated local tenderness.

X-ray

AP, lateral, and mortise views are indicated. With severe sprain, after routine films rule out fractures, ankle should be stressed to demonstrate stability of ankle mortise.

Management

1. First degree (mild sprain): ice and elevation; non-weight bearing for 3-4 days; once swelling resolved, passive exercises; once start walking, support with ankle wrap
2. Second degree (partial tear): immobilization in plaster splint or cast for 3-4 wk. Adolescents: non-weight bearing; preadolescents: limited activity and placed in short walking cast
3. Third degree (complete tear): often requires surgical repair. Refer to consultant.

ANKLE FRACTURE

Lateral malleolus is the most common type of ankle fracture.

Mechanism of injury

Usually an inversion or eversion injury is causative.

Diagnostic findings

1. Swelling, ecchymosis, and tenderness over the malleolus with impaired weight bearing
2. Pain when the foot is directed toward tibial surface
3. Inversion injury produces oblique fracture of medial malleolus and either horizontal fracture of lateral malleolus or tear of lateral ligament. Eversion injury causes opposite damage.

415

X-ray films
1. AP and lateral ankle views
2. Mortise if question of instability
3. Yield on x-ray film is greatest in the presence of localized bone pain

Management

1. Lateral malleolus: immobilization for 4 wk and non-weight bearing
2. Medial malleolus: immobilization and referral. Size of fragment determines therapy.

ANKLE FRACTURE-DISLOCATION

Mechanism of injury

Severe force applied to the area of the tibiotalar interface causes the fracture-dislocation.

Diagnostic findings

Obvious deformity and swelling are present.
X-ray films
1. AP, lateral, and mortise ankle views
2. Displaced talus (posterior and lateral to the tibia)
3. Prereduction and post reduction films

Management

1. Rapid reduction to reduce swelling and neurovascular compromise
2. Open reduction and internal fixation usually required for associated fractures

CALCANEAL FRACTURE

This is associated with a spinal compression injury and with fractures of the hip and knee in as many as 50% of cases.

Mechanism of injury

A fall from a height on extended legs can produce a fracture of the calcaneus.

Diagnostic findings

1. Local swelling, tenderness, impaired weight bearing, ecchymosis on posterior sole of foot

2. Frequent associated injuries, especially vertebral
X-ray films
AP, lateral, and calcaneal views are indicated. Bohler's angle is flattened. Angle described by anterior and posterior halves of the superior cortex of the bone.

Management

Compression dressing, immobilization, and orthopedic consultation are necessary.

METATARSAL FRACTURE
Mechanism of injury

The base of the fifth metatarsal is fractured as a result of inversion, with avulsion of the insertion of the peroneus brevis tendon. Fractures of the metatarsal midshaft are usually crush injuries.

Diagnostic findings

1. Local swelling with impaired weight bearing
2. **March fractures:** hairline stress fractures at the base of the metatarsal, often after hiking, jogging, or jumping. Pain is usually over the second, third, or fourth metatarsals. X-ray film may be initially negative.
X-ray films
AP, lateral, and oblique views are indicated.

Management

1. Immobilization in a posterior short-leg splint or short-leg walker cast for 5-6 wk
2. March fractures of the fifth metatarsal: hard-soled shoes or, with significant pain, a short-leg walking cast
3. For displaced fracture, possible surgery. Refer to consultant.

PHALANGEAL FRACTURES

Mechanism of injury

"Stubbing" on an immovable object produces the fracture.

Diagnostic findings

Local swelling and tenderness are present over the involved phalynx.

X-ray films

AP and lateral views of toe are indicated.

Management

The injury is managed by splinting the toe by taping to the adjacent one for 2-3 wk.

DISLOCATIONS OF BONES OF FOOT

These are uncommon but may occur at the phalangeal, metatarsophalangeal, talonavicular, subtalar, and tarsometatarsal joints.

Mechanism of injury

Twisting movement with associated force applied to foot

Diagnostic findings

Obvious deformity, tenderness, and decreased motion are characteristic.

X-ray films

AP, lateral, and oblique views are indicated.

Management

1. Phalangeal and metatarsophalangeal dislocations can usually be reduced by manual manipulation. After infiltration with local anesthetic, compression splint is useful for several days before mobilization.
2. Other dislocations require either closed reduction under general anesthesia or open reduction, and patient should be referred.

REFERENCES

Barber, F., and Marx, J.A.: Accuracy of emergency radiograph interpretation by emergency physicians, J. Emerg. Med. **1**:483, 1984.

Crawford, A.H., and Cionni, A.S.: Management of pediatric orthopedic injuries by emergency medicine specialists, Top. Emerg. Med **4**:61, 1982.

Farrell, R.G., Swanson, S.L., Walter, J.R., et al.: Safe and effective IV regional anesthesia for use in the emergency department, Ann. Emerg. Med. **14**:288, 1985.

Freed, H.A., and Shields, N.N.: Most frequently overlooked radiographically apparent fractures in a teaching hospital emergency department, Ann. Emerg. Med. **13**:900, 1984.

Green, D.P.: Hand injuries in children, Pediatr. Clin. North Am. **24**:903, 1977.

Lamon, R.P., Cicero, J.J., Frascone, R.J., et al.: Open treatment of fingertip amputations, Ann. Emerg. Med. **12**:358, 1983.

Rang, M.C., and Willis, R.B.: Symposium on common orthopedic problems: fractures and sprains, Pediatr. Clin. North Am. **24**:759, 1977.

Segal, D.: Pediatric orthopedics, Pediatr. Clin. North Am. **26**:793, 1979.

XI DIAGNOSTIC CATEGORIES

71 Cardiovascular disorders

Bacterial endocarditis

REGINALD L. WASHINGTON

ALERT: A high index of suspicion should lead to blood cultures and treatment for children with predisposing factors.

Bacterial endocarditis is a microbial infection of the endocardial surface of the heart, most frequently involving a heart valve. It is rare in children under 2 yr of age.

Approximately 90% of children developing endocarditis have underlying heart disease either congenitally or secondary to acute rheumatic fever. Patients at greatest risk include those with cardiac abnormalities associated with jet formation and vortex shedding rather than those with low-pressure, high-pressure conditions. Lesions include systemic-pulmonary arterial communications (tetralogy of Fallot and other cyanotic heart disease), ventricular septal defect, left side valvular disease including mitral stenosis and regurgitation, aortic stenosis, aortic insufficiency, bicuspid aortic valve, coarctation of the aorta, and pulmonary stenosis. High-velocity blood ejected into a chamber or vessel causes endocardial or intimal erosion and subsequent vegetations. Postoperative patients with artifical valves or conduits are at the highest continuous risk for endocarditis and represent an increasingly large percentage of patients with infectious endocarditis.

Bacteremia and infective carditis are associated with many predisposing events:

1. Dental cleaning, irrigation, or extractions, particularly with gingival bleeding
2. Tonsillectomy
3. Bronchoscopy
4. Cystoscopy or urethral catheterization
5. Sigmoidoscopy
6. Intravenous drug abuse

ETIOLOGY
Bacterial infection

1. *Streptococcus viridans* accounts for 46% of cases and is increasingly associated with post-surgical and catheterization-related cases.
2. *Staphylococcus aureus* is causative in 32% of cases.
3. Other: *Streptococcus faecalis*, *Streptococcus pneumoniae*, *Haemophilus influenzae*, enterococci, gram-negative organisms. Rarely are fungi involved.

DIAGNOSTIC FINDINGS

1. Fever is the most consistent finding. It is often prolonged without other systemic manifestations.
2. A heart murmur is commonly (98%) present. Chest pain may be noted.
3. Anorexia, malaise, weight loss, chills, weakness, and arthralgias are reported.
4. Splenomegaly and arthritis often are noted.
5. Peripheral manifestations: petechiae, Osler's nodes (small, tender, intradermal nodules in the pads of the fingers and toes), Janeway's lesions (painless erythematous hemorrhagic maculae on the palms or soles), and linear splinter hemorrhages under the nails are infrequent in children.
6. Neurologic manifestations, including confusion, seizures, stroke, or severe headache

7. A careful dental examinaton should be performed on all patients with endocarditis.

Complications

1. Congestive heart failure most commonly occurs with involvement of the aortic or mitral valves
2. Neurologic complications from mycotic, embolic, and cerebral abscesses. *S. aureus* endocarditis presents the greatest risk.
3. Diffuse glomerulonephritis and renal failure
4. Progressive cardiac destruction including mycotic aneurysm, pericarditis, rupture of the sinus of Valsalva, obstructive heart disease, acquired ventricular-septal defect, and conduction defects

Ancillary data

1. CBC demonstrates a leukocytosis and mild hemolytic anemia. ESR is elevated. Urinalysis shows microscopic hematuria. ECG and chest x-ray film may be important.
2. Echocardiogram often will demonstrate vegetative lesions and is useful in diagnosis and monitoring of treatment.
3. Blood cultures are 85%-95% positive when three separate cultures are obtained. This is crucial to the diagnosis and requries meticulous care to avoid contaminants.

MANAGEMENT

Initial stabilization of the cardiac and respiratory status must be achieved immediately, with oxygen and therapy for CHF (Chapter 16).

Antibiotics

1. Antibiotics must be compatible with organisms suspected or proved, and they may require alteration once sensitivity data are available.
2. Antibiotic levels must achieve at least a 1:8 serum-bactericidal level at all times. Antibiotic levels and potential toxicity must be constantly assessed.
3. Treatment course is 6-8 wk. *S. viridans* infections usually require 6 wk, whereas 8 wk is the usual course for *S. aureus*, gram-negative organisms, or unusual pathogens or if the etiology is unknown.
4. Therapy with a penicillin-type antibiotic and an aminoglycoside is recommended for their synergistic effect:

Etiologic agent	Drug	Dose
Unknown	Nafcillin (or equivalent) and	150 mg/kg/24 hr q 4 hr IV
	gentamicin	5.0-7.5 mg/kg/24 hr q 8 hr IV
S. viridans	Penicillin G and	300,000 units/kg/24 hr q 4 hr IV (maximum: 20 million units/24 hr IV)
	gentamicin	5.0-7.5 mg/kg/24 hr q 8 hr IV
S. aureus	Nafcillin and	150 mg/kg/24-hr q 4 hr IV
	gentamicin	5.0-7.5 mg/kg/24 hr q 8 hr IV

5. If the patient is allergic to penicillin, cephalothin (Keflin) 100 mg/kg/24 hr q 4 hr IV may be substituted for penicillin or nafcillin if indicated by sensitivity data.

Surgical intervention

This is indicated if there is increasing CHF, if the infection is uncontrolled by antibiotics, or if there are recurrent septic emboli or extensive cardiac destruction. If an artificial valve or conduit is present, surgical removal is often required.

Prevention

Prophylaxis of high-risk patients is mandatory in preventing bacterial endocarditis. Approximately 90% of children developing endocarditis have underlying heart disease either congenitally or secondary to acute rheumatic fever (p. 426). Conditions at greatest risk include:

1. Prosthetic cardiac valves (including biosynthetic valves.) These patients are at the highest continuous risk for endocarditis and represent an increasingly large percentage of patients.
2. Most congenital cardiac malformations
3. Surgically constructed systemic-pulmonary shunts
4. Rheumatic and other acquired valvular dysfunction
5. Idiopathic hypertrophic subaortic stenosis
6. History of bacterial endocarditis
7. Mitral valve prolapse with mitral insufficiency (low-risk)

At lower risk are patients with dilated secondum atrial septal defects, secondum atrial septum defects repaired without a patch over 6 months earlier, patent ductus ligation at least 8 months earlier, and postoperative coronary artery bypass surgery.

Bacteremia and infective endocarditis are associated with many predisposing events:

1. All dental procedures likely to induce gingival bleeding (not including simple adjustment of orthodontic appliance or shedding of deciduous teeth)
2. Tonsillectomy or adenoidectomy
3. Surgical procedures or biopsy involving the respiratory mucosa
4. Bronchoscopy, especially with rigid bronchoscopy
5. Incision and drainage of infected tissue
6. Genitourinary and gastrointestinal procedures including cystoscopy, urethral catheterization, prostatic, urinary tract, gallbladder, or colonic surgery, esophageal dilation, colonoscopy, endoscopy with biopsy, or proctosigmoidoscopy. In addition, if infection is suspected or the patient is at very high risk, prophylaxis is indicated for uterine dilation and curettage, cesarean section, therapeutic abortion, and sterilization. Many clinicians recommend that intrauterine devices should not be used in patients with a risk of endocarditis.

Specific regimens reflect the nature of the procedure, the relative risk to the patient, and the route of administration desired.

1. Antibiotic regimen for dental/respiratory tract procedures

  a. Standard regimen for *dental procedures* that cause gingival bleeding and oral/respiratory surgery

    (1) For children >60 lb and adults: penicillin V 2 g PO 1 hr before and then 1 g 6 hr later. For patients unable to take oral medications, 2 million units aqueous penicillin G given IV or IM 30-60 min before a procedure and 1 million units 6 hours later may be substituted.

    (2) For children <60 lb (<27 kg): penicillin V 1.0 g PO 1 hr before the procedure and then 500 mg 6 hr later. For children unable to take oral medications: 50,000 units/kg aqueous penicillin G IV or IM 30-60 min before and 25,000 units/kg 6 hr later.

  b. Parenteral regimen for use when maximal protection is required, such as in patients with prosthetic valves

    • Ampicillin 50 mg/kg (adults: 1.0-2.0 g),

plus gentamicin 1.5-2.5 mg/kg, both IM or IV ½ hour before the procedure, followed by penicillin V 25,000 units/kg (adult: 1.0 g) PO 6 hr later. Alternatively, the parenteral regimen may be repeated once 8 hr later.

  c. Oral regimen for penicillin allergic patients: erythromycin 20 mg/kg (adult: 1 g) PO 1 hr before and then 10 mg/kg (adult: 500 mg) 6 hr later

  d. Parenteral regimen for penicillin allergic patients: vancomycin 20 mg/kg/dose (adult: 1.0 g) IV slowly over 1 hr, starting 1 hr before procedure. No repeat dose is necessary.

2. Antibiotic regimen for *gastrointestinal/genitourinary* procedures

  a. Standard regimen: ampicillin 50 mg/kg (adult: 2.0 g) IM or IV **plus** gentamicin 1.5-2.0 mg/kg IM or IV given 30-60 min before procedure. One follow-up dose may be repeated 8 hr later.

  b. For patients allergic to penicillin: vancomycin 20 mg/kg/dose (adult: 1 g) IV slowly over 1 hr **plus** gentamicin 1.5-2.0 mg/kg IM or IV, both given 1 hr prior to the procedure. Dose may be repeated once 8-12 hr later.

  c. Oral regimen for minor or repetitive procedures in low-risk patients: amoxicillin 50 mg/kg (adult: 3.0 g) PO 1 hr before the procedure and 25 mg/kg (adult: 1.5 g) 6 hr later

3. Patients undergoing cardiac surgery should have maximal prophylaxis beginning before surgery and continuing for no more than 2 days postoperatively. Nafcillin (or equivalent) or a first-generation cephalosporin is recommended. Vancomycin is a good alternative.

4. Patients with indwelling transvenous cardiac pacemakers should receive prophylaxis during all procedures, as should renal dialysis patients with indwelling arterial-venous shunts and individuals with ventriculoatrial shunts for hydrocephalus.

DISPOSITION

All patients with bacterial endocarditis require hospitalization in an ICU for monitoring, immediate laboratory evaluation, and initiation of antibiotics. Mortality, especially with artificial valves or conduits, is as high as 50%.

REFERENCES

Gersony, W.M., and Hordof, A.J.: Infective endocarditis and disease of the pericardium, Pediatr. Clin. North Am. **25**:831, 1978.

Shulman, S.T., Amren, D.P., Bisno, A.L., et al.: Prevention of bacterial endocarditis: a statement for health professionals by the Committee on Rheumatic Fever and Bacterial Endocarditis of the Council on Cardiovascular Disease in the Young of the American Heart Association, Am. J. Dis. Child. **139**:232, 1985.

Stanton, B.F., Baltimore, R.S., and Clemens, J.D.: Changing spectrum of infective endocarditis in children, Am. J. Dis. Child. **138**:720, 1984.

Wolfson, J.S., and Swartz, M.N.: Serum bactericidal activity as a monitor of antibiotic therapy, N. Engl. J. Med. **312**:969, 1985.

Myocarditis

REGINALD L. WASHINGTON

ALERT: A high index of suspicion is necessary.

Myocarditis is an inflammatory lesion characterized by cellular infiltrate of the myocardium, usually predominantly mononuclear. Because of decreased myocardial contractility. Congestive heart failure (CHF) often results. Viral agents are most frequently causative.

ETIOLOGY

1. Rheumatic fever (p. 426)
2. Infection
  a. Viral
    (1) Enterovirus; coxsackievirus A and B, echovirus, and poliomyelitis
    (2) Influenza A and B
    (3) Other: mumps, variola, vaccinia, varicella-zoster, rubella, hepatitis
  b. Bacterial: diphtheria, beta-hemolytic

streptococci, meningococci, staphylococci, salmonellae, tuberculosis

c. *Mycoplasma pneumoniae*
d. Fungal
e. Congenital syphilis
f. Parasitic diseases: toxoplasmosis, trichinosis, Chagas' disease

DIAGNOSTIC FINDINGS

The onset is usually gradual and preceded by an upper respiratory infection (URI) or a "flu-like" syndrome. A high degree of suspicion is necessary because the early symptoms will mimic a severe URI, and only after cardiac decompensation will the diagnosis become obvious. Rarely, the myocarditis is isolated without preceding illness. The onset may be acute.

Cardiac examination may include tachycardia with a gallop rhythm, atypical systolic murmur, weak or distant heart sounds, and hepatomegaly. Evidence of CHF with pulmonary edema may be present with tachypnea, wheezing, rales, and respiratory distress.

There are associated signs and symptoms of the etiologic agent or condition.

Complications

1. Congestive cardiomyopathy and CHF
2. Constrictive pericarditis
3. Hemopericardium
4. Cardiac arrest and death

Ancillary data

1. Chest x-ray film: cardiomegaly. Pericardial effusion may be present.
2. ECG
   a. Tachycardia
   b. Lowered QRS-complex voltages
   c. Nonspecific elevation of ST segment and flattening or inversion of T waves
3. ABG, with cardiac decompensation
4. Echocardiogram: reveals dilated cardiac chambers with decreased function. Pericardial effusion may be present.
5. Other studies as indicated by etiologic considerations

DIFFERENTIAL DIAGNOSIS

1. Infection: pericarditis (p. 425)
2. Autoimmune: acute rheumatic fever (p. 426)
3. Vascular: congenital heart disease
4. Other: endocardial fibroelastosis, glycogen storage disease

MANAGEMENT

1. Initial stabilization of the cardiac and respiratory status must be achieved in symptomatic patients.
2. Oxygen at 3-6 L/min should be administered to all symptomatic patients. Airway patency should be assessed and intervention initiated if necessary. ABG should be monitored.
3. Cardiac contractility must be improved while reducing workloads in patients with CHF (Chapter 16).
   a. Digoxin may be helpful but must be used with *extreme caution* because the inflamed myocardium is sensitive, and signs of toxicity appear at low dose (Table 16-3). In acute situations pressor agents (Table 5-2) may be required.
   b. Vasodilators such as nitroprusside may be used if cardiac function is not improved by digoxin and the preload is adequate.
   c. Beta-blocking agents should not be used.
   d. Diuretic therapy: furosemide (Lasix) 1 mg/kg/dose q 2-6 hr prn IV (Table 16-3)
   e. Dysrhythmia and conduction disturbances are common and require treatment (Chapter 6).
4. Antibiotics should be used for defined bacterial etiologies.

DISPOSITION

The patient should be admitted to the hospital and monitored closely until the cardiovascular status has stabilized. The clinical course may be erratic. A cardiologist should be involved in initial care and follow-up.

REFERENCE

Greenwood, R.D., Nadas, A.S., and Fyler, D.C.: The clinical course of primary myocardial disease in infants and children, Am. Heart J. **92:**549, 1976.

Pericarditis

REGINALD L. WASHINGTON

ALERT: The possibility of cardiac tamponade must be ruled out.

There is a broad spectrum of inflammatory diseases that involve the pericardium and the pericardial space. Fluid accumulation may rapidly cause cardiac decompensation. Viral and autoimmune etiologies are most common, although pericarditis is often considered idiopathic.

ETIOLOGY

1. Infection
   a. Viral: coxsackievirus, influenza
   b. Bacterial: *S. aureus*, *S. pneumoniae*, beta-hemolytic streptococci, *H. influenzae*, *Escherichia coli*, *Pseudomonas*, and meningococci
   c. Other: fungal, tuberculosis, parasitic
2. Autoimmune: acute rheumatic fever, polyarteritis nodosa, systemic lupus erythematosus
3. Metabolic: uremia
4. Postpericardiotomy syndrome

DIAGNOSTIC FINDINGS

There is a pericardial friction rub associated with sharp, stabbing pain, located midchest with radiation to the shoulder and neck. The rub is best heard at any point between the apex and left sternal border. It is intensified with deep inspiration and decreased by sitting up and leaning forward. It is differentiated from pleural friction rubs when the patient holds the breath.

If there is a pericardial effusion, the heart may appear big to percussion, and ausculation reveals distant, muffled heart sounds. Friction rub may be present. The presence of pulsus paradoxus (decrease in amplitude of blood pressure on inspiration—significant if >15 mm Hg) indicates at least a moderate accumulation of pericardial fluid. This may be indicative of a cardiac tamponade, particularly if there is distension of the jugular veins, tachycardia, enlargement of the liver, peripheral edema, and, rarely, hypotension. Urgent intervention is required.

1. Dyspnea and fever may be present.
2. Associated signs and symptoms of the etiologic entity may be present.

Complication

Cardiac decompensation, often from cardiac tamponade, is a common complication.

Ancillary data

1. Chest x-ray film: varies with the amount of pericardial fluid. As accumulation increases, the cardiopericardial silhouette enlarges, and the contours become obscured, often in the shape of a water bottle. Fluoroscopy will demonstrate the absence of pulsations of the cardiac borders.
2. ECG
   a. ST-T wave elevation with inverted T waves
   b. Decreased QRS-complex and T-wave voltages
3. Echocardiogram: pericardial effusion is diagnostic
4. CBC, ESR, and cultures as indicated by potential etiologic agents

MANAGEMENT

Cardiac function must be rapidly assessed and decompression of the pericardium achieved if necessary. If there is a large volume of pericardial fluid, a pericardiocentesis should be performed for diagnostic and therapeutic objectives (Appendix A-5).

1. Fluid should be sent for cell count, glucose, protein, LDH, Gram's stain, and culture.
2. Rapid infusion of fluids may be necessary if the removal of pericardial fluid results in hypotension.
3. Resection of the pericardium through a surgical incision is often required following needle aspiration.

Treatment of the underlying disorder should be initiated:

1. Antibiotics as appropriate for bacterial, fun-

gal, tuberculosis, or parasitic disease. If bacterial etiology is likely and initial Gram's stain is nondiagnostic, initiate nafcillin (or equivalent) 150 mg/kg/24 hr q 4 hr IV **and** chloramphenicol 100 mg/kg/24 hr q 6 hr IV pending culture results. A surgical pericardial window is required.
2. Dialysis, if uremia is the etiology

Antiinflammatory agents are useful for autoimmune or idiopathic etiology. They improve long-term resolution but are not helpful in the immediate situation if there is evidence of cardiac decompensation.
1. Aspirin
   a. Load with 100 mg/kg/24 hr q 4 hr PO for 1-2 days and then reduce to 60 mg/kg/24 hr q 6 hr PO for 4-6 wk
   b. Ideal drug level: 15-25 mg/dl
2. Indomethacin 1.5-2.5 mg/kg/24 hr q 6-8 hr PO (maximum: 100 mg/24 hr) may be used instead of aspirin in older patients.
3. If no resolution with aspirin or indomethacin, initiate prednisone 1-2 mg/kg/24 hr q 6 hr PO for 5-7 days, and slowly taper.

DISPOSITION

The patient should be hospitalized for observation. If there is any evidence of cardiac decompensation, intensive care and evaluation for potential pericardiocentesis are necessary. Rarely, in early cases without evidence of cardiac decompensation, outpatient status may be tried after cardiology consultation.

REFERENCE

Benzing, G. III, and Kaplan, S.: Purulent pericarditis, Am. J. Dis. Child **106:**289, 1963.

Acute rheumatic fever

Acute rheumatic fever is a delayed, nonsuppurative, autoimmune disease occurring as a sequela of group A streptococcal infections. It peaks in 6 to 15 year olds and is more common in inner cities and black populations. The average annual incidence is declining. In the 1960s the rate was 10-15 cases/100,000 children 5-15 yr, whereas in 1978-1981 this rate had declined to 0.5 cases/100,000 children 5-15 yr.

DIAGNOSTIC FINDINGS

The Jones' criteria are the basis for making the diagnosis, based on either two major or one major and two minor criteria plus evidence of a preceding streptococcal infection.

Major criteria

1. Carditis. New murmur, tachycardia disproportionate to fever, and, rarely, pericarditis and CHF. Mitral and aortic valve are most commonly involved.
2. Polyarthritis. Two or more joints involved—most commonly the ankles, knees, wrist, and elbow. Exquisitely tender
3. Chorea. Marked emotional lability with involuntary motor movements. Usually self-limited but may last several months
4. Erythema marginatum. Rapidly spreading, ringed eruption, forming serpiginous or wavy lines primarily over the trunk and extremities
5. Subcutaneous nodules. Variably sized, hard, painless nodules that are freely mobile. Commonly found overlying joints, scalp, and spine. Also seen in rheumatoid arthritis and erythema nodosum

Minor criteria

1. Previous history of rheumatic fever or rheumatic heart disease
2. Polyarthralgia. Pain in two or more joints without swelling, warmth, or tenderness. Cannot be used as criterion for patients with arthritis
3. Fever (found in 90% of patients)
4. Elevated acute-phase reactions. ESR, C-reactive protein, leukocytosis
5. Prolonged PR interval: nonspecific

Streptococcal infection

All patients must have evidence of a preceding streptococcal infection.

1. Positive culture to rule out carrier
2. Scarlatiniform rash
3. Elevated streptococcal antibodies associated with evidence of rise or fall in titer (Streptozyme)

Complications

1. Cardiac
   a. Dysrhythmias (Chapter 6)
   b. Mitral or aortic valvular disease
   c. Pericarditis (p. 425)
   d. CHF (Chapter 16)
2. Rheumatic lung disease: pleurisy or pneumonia
3. Renal disease: glomerulonephritis or interstitial nephritis
4. Recurrence

Ancillary data

1. CBC, ESR, and C-reactive protein
2. Streptozyme measuring antistreptolysin (ASO), antihyaluronidase (AH), antistreptokinase (ASK), antideoxyribonuclease (ADNase), and antinicotinamide-adenine dinucleotidase (ANA-Dase)
3. Throat culture
4. ECG and chest x-ray film

DIFFERENTIAL DIAGNOSIS

See Chapters 16 and 27.

MANAGEMENT

1. Initial management must focus on cardiac stabilization, if necessary (Chapter 16).
   a. Digoxin is the drug of choice (Table 16-2).
   b. Furosemide (Lasix) 1 mg/kg/dose IV may be useful (Table 16-3).

2. Acute phase reactions should be monitored throughout the course of disease as an indication of resolution.
3. Antibiotics should be given to all patients:
   a. Penicillin V 25,000-50,000 units/kg/24 hr q 6 hr PO for 10 days **or**
   b. Benzathine penicillin G alone (or with procaine) in the dosages listed at the bottom of the page.
4. Antiinflammatory agents
   a. Aspirin for fever and joint pain
      (1) Initially give 100 mg/kg/24 hr q 4-6 hr PO for a maximum of 5,000 mg/24 hr.
      (2) Maintain levels at 20-25 mg/dl.
      (3) After 1 wk decrease to 50 mg/kg/24 hr q 6 hr PO for an additional 4-6 wk of therapy.
   b. Steroids with evidence of carditis or CHF
      (1) Begin prednisone 2 mg/kg/24 hr q 12-24 hr PO.
      (2) After 1 wk decrease to 1 mg/kg/24 hr for 1 wk, and begin aspirin at 50 mg/kg/24 hr.
      (3) Taper prednisone over the next 2 wk.
5. For chorea: haloperidol 0.01-0.03 mg/kg/24 hr q 6 hr PO (adult dose: 2-5 mg/24 hr q 8 hr PO). May be useful
6. Bed rest
7. Prevention: prophylactic antibiotics, using either oral (200-250,000 units q 12 hr PO) or every 4 wk, benzathine penicillin (1.2 million units IM) injections. Recent data indicate that injections are more effective when given every 3 wk. Prophylactic antibiotics are given indefinitely to those with cardiac involvement and those with chorea initially. Those

Weight (lb)	Benzathine penicillin G (Bicillin)	Benzathine with procaine penicillin G (Bicillin C-R) (900,000 benzathine : 300,000 procaine)
<30	300,000	300,000 : 100,000
31-60	600,000	600,000 : 200,000
61-90	900,000	900,000 : 300,000
>90	1,200,000	Not available

without cardiac involvement should receive antibiotics for at least 5 yr.

DISPOSITION

1. Patients should be admitted to the hospital for stabilization and initiation of treatment.
2. On discharge, the importance of prophylactic antibiotics must be emphasized, as well as the increased risk of endocarditis if abnormal valves are present.

REFERENCES

DiSciascio, G., and Taranta. A.: Rheumatic fever in children, Am. Heart J. 99:635, 1980.

Kaplan, E.L.: Acute rheumatic fever, Pediatr. Clin. North Am. 25:817, 1978.

Lue, H.C., Wu, M.H., Hsieh, K.H., et al.: Rheumatic fever recurrences: controlled study of 3-week versus 4-week benzathine penicillin prevention programs, J. Pediatr. 108:299, 1986.

Majeed, H.A., Shaltout: A., and Yousof, A.M.: Recurrences of acute rheumatic fever: a prospective study of 79 episodes, Am. J. Dis. Child. 138:341, 1984.

Deep vein thrombosis

Although uncommon in children and adolescents, deep vein thrombosis does occur in the presence of one of a number of predisposing factors.

ETIOLOGY
Predisposing factors

1. Trauma: injury to the endothelium
   a. Leg injury
   b. Pelvic injury
2. Vascular: stasis or reduction in venous return
   a. Extended bed rest or immobilization
   b. Cyanotic heart disease or CHF
3. Endocrine: hypercoagulability
   a. Pregnancy
   b. Birth control pills

DIAGNOSTIC FINDINGS

The clinical diagnosis of deep vein thrombosis is unreliable, but several findings should be sought:

1. Leg warmth, tenderness, or swelling
2. Homans' sign (unreliable) with the knee extended, dorsiflex the foot. Pain or soreness in the calf or increased muscular resistance to dorsiflexion is considered positive.
3. Pulmonary embolism in the absence of other sources

Complications
Pulmonary embolism

Clinically, pulmonary embolism (PE) is accompanied by dyspnea (80% of patients), pleuritic pain (75%), hemoptysis (20%), cough, and anxiety. Physical examination reveals tachypnea, tachycardia, rales, and increased secondary heart sound (pulmonary component).

There may be few symptoms. The classic triad (hemoptysis, pleuritic chest pain, and dyspnea) is seen in only 28% of patients.

Helpful laboratory tests include the following.

1. ABG may demonstrate hypoxia, although 10%-20% of patients with severe PE have normal ABG.
2. ECG may demonstrate nonspecific ST-T changes (S1Q3T3, RV1, S1, S2, S3).
3. Chest x-ray film may be normal or show elevated hemidiaphragm, infiltrate, effusion, and segmental or subsegmental atelectasis.
4. Ventilation-perfusion scan is diagnostic.
5. Definitive diagnosis may require pulmonary arteriography.

Ancillary data

1. CBC, platelet count, PT, and PTT
2. Venogram (usually only indicated in patients with uncertain diagnosis) to define the location, extent, and age of the thrombus. Doppler and plethysmography are useful techniques that may provide definitive diagnostic information, particularly in pregnant patients.

DIFFERENTIAL DIAGNOSIS

1. Infection: cellulitis (p. 423)
2. Trauma
   a. A sudden onset of leg tenderness, red-

ness, and swelling and a palpable venous cord with superficial thrombophlebitis. Pulmonary embolism can occur if the thrombus is in the proximal saphenous vein.
b. Muscle contusion
c. Compartment syndrome
d. Torn medial head of the gastrocnemius muscle. History of acute onset of pain while exercising, usually while up on toes (basketball, tennis, or skiing)

MANAGEMENT

1. Elevation of the leg
2. Heat packs applied to the leg
3. Bed rest
4. Anticoagulation (an important part of therapy)
   a. Heparin is given as a continuous intravenous infusion.
      (1) Initial dose is 50 units/kg IV
      (2) Continuous drip is 10-15 units/kg/hr IV
      (3) Goal is to maintain PTT at two times control
      (4) Heparin therapy should be given for 7-10 days, the last 4 concurrent with the administration of warfarin (Coumadin).
      (5) Antidote: protamine sulfate (1 mg IV for each 100 units of heparin given concurrently; 0.5 mg IV for each 100 units of heparin given in preceding 30 min and so on); maximum: 50 mg/dose NOTE: No heparin effect is present in normal patients 4 hr after cessation of therapy.
   b. Oral warfarin (Coumadin) should be initiated 4-5 days after beginning anticoagulation with heparin.
      (1) Adult dose ranges from 2-10 mg/24 hr PO.
      (2) Dosage should be titrated to maintain PT at two times control.
      (3) Duration of effect is 4-5 days.
      (4) Therapy should be continued for 4-6 wk.
      (5) Antidote: vitamin K (infants: 1-2 mg/dose IV; children and adults: 5-10 mg/dose). Fresh frozen plasma may be given for a more immediate effect.
   c. Contraindications to anticoagulation therapy are:
      (1) Active bleeding or blood dyscrasia
      (2) Cerebral vascular hemorrhage
      (4) Pregnancy
      (5) Poor compliance
   d. Drug interactions with warfarin include antibiotics, barbiturates, thyroid medications, prostaglandin inhibitors (aspirin), alcohol
5. Fibrinolytics. Their use should be initiated only after consultation with the admitting physician and consulting hematologist.

DISPOSITION

All patients should be hospitalized if the diagnosis is proved or suspected, the latter group until diagnostic studies have excluded the diagnosis.

72 Dermatologic disorders

Acne

Acne vulgaris occurs in as many as 85% of children with the onset between 8-10 yr of age in 40%. Neonates may develop a self-limited form of acne in the first 4-6 wk of life in response to maternal androgens. This form requires no treatment.

Acne results from outlet obstruction of the follicular canal with accumulation of sebum and keratinous debris. Sebaceous follicles are primarily located on the face, upper chest, and back. Acne is a multifactorial process involving anaerobic pathogens such as *Propionibacterium acnes*.

DIAGNOSTIC FINDINGS

Obstruction of the follicle leads to a wide, patulous opening filled with stratum corneum cells known as open comedones or "blackheads," which are commonly seen early in adolescent acne. Obstruction beneath the opening of the neck of the sebaceous follicle produces cystic lesions known as closed comedones or "whiteheads," which can progress to inflammatory acne with papules, pustules, cysts, and also draining sinus tracts that result in permanent scarring.

MANAGEMENT
Mild to moderate acne

Topical keratolytic agents are usually adequate in 80%-85% of adolescents. These agents

See Chapter 42: Rash.

inhibit bacterial growth and have a comedolytic and sebostatic effect. The two most commonly used are benzoyl peroxide gel in 5% concentration and retinoic acid 0.05% cream. Either agent may be used once a day, or if there is significant inflammation, retinoic acid cream may be applied to acne-bearing skin in the evening and the benzoyl peroxide gel may be applied in the morning.

Moderate to severe acne

In the presence of marked disease with tremendous inflammation, oral antibiotics should be initiated. Tetracycline 0.5-1.0 g/24 hr PO is given for 2-3 months until lesions are suppressed. This should not be done in children under 9 yr or if there is any potential of adolescent pregnancy.

Severe cystic acne

Severe cystic disease may additionally need oral retinoids. 13-cis-retinoic acid (isotretinoin [Accutane]) may be started at an initial dose of 40 mg once or twice daily PO. It should not be used in women of child-bearing age.

DISPOSITION

All patients may be followed on a regular basis to ensure compliance with the treatment regimen and to monitor progress. The management is directed at control and not eradication, with a response expected in 4-8 weeks.

Atopic dermatitis (eczema)

Atopic dermatitis is both an acute and a chronic dermatologic problem, often associated with asthma or allergic rhinitis. There is often a family history of allergic disorders.

DIAGNOSTIC FINDINGS

The severity of the disease varies tremendously. Exacerbations are associated with erythema and edema, as well as crusting and weeping. Lesions are often intensely red at the center, gradually tapering out at the periphery and fading into normal skin. Patients develop thickened, lichenified skin areas. Some have symmetrically distributed coin-shaped patches of dermatitis, primarily in the extremities. This is called nummular eczema.

Intense itching is commonly present, leading to excoriation and secondary bacterial infection. In the absence of acute dermatitis, children with eczema tend to have dry skin with a fine, gritty feel.

Most children have their initial episode in the first few months of life, with the condition resolving by 2 yr of age. Recurrences occur between 5 and 8 yr and again at puberty.

The pattern varies with the age of the child.
1. Infants typically have fine, scaly erythematous patches on the extensor surface and face, which are generally symmetric in location but not severity.
2. Children primarily have symmetric involvement of the flexor surfaces. The lesions may be papules with plaques.
3. Adolescents have dry, scaly lesions over the hands, feet, and genitalia.

Complications

1. Secondary bacterial infection from *Staphylococcus aureus*.
2. Secondary infection from herpes simplex virus (eczema herpeticum)

Ancillary data

Cultures of the infected sites are useful.

DIFFERENTIAL DIAGNOSIS

Eczema must be differentiated from superficial infections and inflammatory processes caused by:
1. Seborrheic dermatitis (p. 443)
2. Contact dermatitis (p. 435)
3. Tinea corporis (p. 436)

Other unusual conditions that may be considered in children include psoriasis (thick, reddened, well-defined plaques with silvery scales on exterior surface of arm, legs, and pressure areas), Wiskott-Aldrich syndrome (eczema, thrombocytopenia, purpura, and immunodeficiency), and acrodermatitis enteropathica (zinc deficiency).

MANAGEMENT
Acute exacerbation

Mild disease
1. If there is no significant weeping or crusting, hydration is required. This is best achieved by bathing the child and then applying Eucerin to the involved areas without drying off the youngster. Do not use soap since it is drying.
2. If there are well-circumscribed areas with marked erythema, hydrocortisone cream (1% four times a day) is useful for short periods and should be applied before the Eucerin.

Moderate to severe disease
1. For significant weeping and crusting, hydration is essential. The parent should use the following schedule for 2-3 days.
   a. During the day, apply wet compresses (gauze or soft dish towels) that are damp but not soaking with warm water. Keep them wet and remove them every 5 min, reapplying damp ones for a total of 15 min of treatment. Repeat 3-5 times/day.
   b. At night, bathe the child. Have the child wear cotton pajamas that are wet (not soaked) with warm water. Then put on a pair of dry pajamas over the wet ones.
   c. Do not use soap.
2. Topical steroids are usually necessary. They

should be applied after the wet-compress treatment, before putting on child's pajamas.

a. Fluorinated steroids are particularly effective but should not be used on the face:

(1) Fluocinolone acetonide cream 0.01% (Synalar)

(2) Triamcinolone cream, 0.01% (Kenalog)

b. Hydrocortisone cream (1%) may be used on facial areas.

3. Antipruritic (antihistamines) agents are useful to reduce scratching and may produce some sedation:

a. Diphenhydramine (Benadryl) 5 mg/kg/24 hr q 6 hr prn PO (over-the counter) or

b. Hydroxyzine (Atarax, Vistaril) 2 mg/kg/24 hr q 6 hr prn PO

4. Antibiotics are often indicated if there is evidence of secondary bacterial infection.

a. Dicloxacillin 50 mg/kg/24 hr q 6 hr PO for 10 days or

b. Cephalexin (Keflex) or cephradine (Velosef) 25-50 mg/kg/24 hr q 6 hr PO for 10 days

Ongoing management

This is crucial to minimizing acute problems.

1. Hydration should be maximized with daily baths and with application of Eucerin to the wet skin, without drying off the child. If the problem is mild, lubricating creams such as Nivea may be easier to use. This is particularly important in dry areas or those that are recurrent problems. Some recommend placing bath oils like Alpha Keri in the water.

2. Use of soap should be discouraged since it is a drying agent. Cetaphil lotion cleanser may be used as a soap substitute.

3. Occlusive ointments such as Vaseline should not be used.

4. The child's fingernails should be kept short to minimize scratching.

DISPOSITION

Most children can be sent home with appropriate management as described above. Hospi-

talization is indicated with severe disease, particularly if there is evidence of bacterial infection, eczema herpeticum, poor compliance, or if the child fails to respond to home management.

Parental education

1. Maintain skin hydration and reduce scratching. Patience and persistence are required.

2. Avoid skin-sensitizing agents that cause contact dermatitis: wool, soaps, chlorine, detergents, etc.

3. Call physician if

a. There is increasing redness, crusting, pustules, large blisters, or evidence of fever or toxicity

b. There does not seem to be response in 2-3 days

4. Follow-up is essential. Keep appointments.

Cellulitis and periorbital cellulitis

Cellulitis is an acute suppurative infection of the skin and the subcutaneous tissue.

ETIOLOGY

Cellulitis is caused by bacterial infection (Table 72-1).

DIAGNOSTIC FINDINGS

The lesions are generally erythematous, with swelling, tenderness, and edema. The edges are indefinite.

1. Common sites of involvement are the face and periorbital region, neck, and extremities.

2. There is often a preexisting break in the skin caused by animal or insect bites, lacerations, abrasions, or chickenpox.

3. The violaceous (purplish) swelling associated with facial cellulitis can be caused by most pathogens, not only *Haemophilus influenzae*.

4. Lymphangitis appears as red lines spreading rapidly from the focus of infection in the di-

TABLE 72-1. Cellulitis: etiologic characteristics and treatment

Etiology	Special clinical characteristics	Antibiotics
Haemophilus influenzae	Facial; periorbital; purplish swelling; under 9 yr	Ampicillin 100-200 mg/kg/24 hr q 4 hr IV **and** chloramphenicol 100 mg/kg/24 hr q 6 hr IV; **or** cefotaxime 50-150 mg/kg/24 hr q 6 hr **or** ceftriaxone 50-75 mg/kg/24 hr q 12 hr IV (**or** cefuroxime 50-100 mg/kg/24 hr q 6-8 hr IV)
Streptococcus pneumoniae	Facial	Penicillin G 25,000-50,000 units/kg/24 hr q 4 hr IV; **if PO:** penicillin V 25,000 units (40 mg)/kg/24 hr q 6 hr PO
Staphylococcus aureus	Often preexisting break in skin	Nafcillin 100-150 mg/kg/24 hr q 4 hr IV; **if PO:** dicloxacillin 50 mg/kg/24 hr q 6 hr PO
Group A streptococci	Often preexisting break in skin; rapidly spreading erythema, induration, pain, lymphadenitis	Penicillin G, as above
Anaerobes (*Clostridium perfringens*)	Possibly preexisting injury with necrotic tissue; dirty, foul-smelling, seropurulent discharge	Penicillin G, as above

rection of regional lymph nodes. It is most common with group A streptococci.

There is often concomitant fever, malaise, and regional lymphadenopathy. Periorbital cellulitis is often accompanied by otitis media and systemic bacterial infection at other sites. Sinusitis may be a predisposing condition.

Complications

1. Bacteremia with secondary focus
2. Infection of underlying joint or bone. Subcutaneous air implies myonecrosis secondary to clostridial infection.
3. Deeper involvement of the orbit (Table 72-2)

Ancillary data

Although empiric treatment is usually appropriate, when there is widespread cellulitis in-

volving the face or periorbital region or in cases of systemic toxicity, additional data are useful:
1. Needle aspiration of the edge of the lesion with a 23- to 25-gauge (face) or 18-gauge (extremity) needle, after thorough povidone-iodine preparation of the insertion site. The needle is inserted at an angle while maintaining negative pressure with a 10 ml syringe. If no material is obtained, 0.5 ml of nonbacteriostatic saline is injected and the material withdrawn. Aspirate is sent for Gram's stain and culture. Aspiration of periorbital cellulitis should be done only if the edge extends beyond the orbit.
2. Blood cultures in the toxic child. Over 80% are positive with facial cellulitis, whereas they usually are negative in patients with extremity cellulitis.
3. WBC: elevated with a shift to the left

TABLE 72-2. Periorbital cellulitis: differentiating clinical features

	Lid swelling and erythema	Ophthalmoplegia	Proptosis	Vision
Periorbital cellulitis	Positive	Negative	Negative	Negative
Orbital cellulitis	Positive	Positive	Positive	Variable
Subperiosteal abscess	Negative	Negative	Lateral	Negative
Orbital abscess	Positive	Positive	Positive	Positive
Cavernous sinus thrombosis*	Positive	Positive	Positive	Positive

From Barkin, R.M., Todd, J.K., and Amer, J.: Pediatrics **62**:390, 1978. Copyright American Academy of Pediatrics, 1978. Positive, Commonly present. Negative, Usually absent.
*Plus papilledema, meningismus, prostration, and cranial nerve involvement.

DIFFERENTIAL DIAGNOSIS
Infection

1. Erysipelas is an infection with acute lymphangitis of the skin secondary to group A streptococci. There is erythema with marked induration. The margins are raised and clearly demarcated. Fever, vomiting, and irritability may be present.
2. Osteomyelitis or septic arthritis is difficult to differentiate from simple cellulitis. Bone scans and aspirates are useful.
3. Lymphadenitis or abscess (particularly cervical) may have an overlying cellulitis. With appropriate treatment, the cellulitis will resolve rapidly, leaving a clearly defined lymph node. Abscesses should demonstrate fluctuance.
4. **Periorbital or preseptal cellulitis** must be distinguished from other infections of the orbit (Table 72-2). Spread to deeper structures is rare. Although the CT scan will give a definite answer about the extent of involvement, the physical examination should delineate the structures involved.

Allergy

Insect bites may cause a tense, warm, erythematous area. The history of insect exposure, presence of an entry point, and partial response to antihistamines are helpful in differentiation.

Trauma

Following known or unknown trauma, patients may develop contusions or hematomas. In addition, environmental stresses such as hypothermia (frostbite), sunburn, or chemical burns may produce tissue injury.

MANAGEMENT

Antibiotics are the major form of treatment. The choice of antibiotics must reflect the likely etiologic agents, the toxicity of the patient, and the involved site as well as information from Gram's stain and culture of the needle aspirate. A total course of 10 days is required, often with a combination of parenteral and oral medications.

1. Patients with only a localized cellulitis (not involving the face and with no evidence of systemic toxicity) can usually be treated as outpatients on an empirical basis:
   a. Dicloxacillin 50 mg/kg/24 hr q 6 hr PO; **or** cefazolin (Ancef) or cephradine (Velosef) 25-50 mg/kg/24 hr q 6 hr PO for 10 days
   b. With lymphangitis consistent with a group A streptococcal infection, penicillin alone: penicillin V 25,000 units (40 mg)/kg/24 hr q 6 hr PO for 10 days
2. Patients with systemic toxicity or facial involvement require parenteral therapy. If the

organism is unknown, the following guidelines are used.

a. For patients under 9 yr with toxicity or with large areas of involvement or facial location:

(1) Nafcillin (or equivalent) 100-150 mg/kg/24 hr q 4 hr IV **and** chloramphenicol 100 mg/kg/24 hr q 6 hr IV

(2) Alternatives: cefotaxime 50-150 mg/kg/24 hr q 6 hr IV **or** ceftriaxone 50-75 mg/kg/24 hr q 12 hr IV **or** cefuroxime 50-100 mg/kg/24 hr q 6 hr IV

(3) If there is a break in the skin, thereby increasing the likelihood of *Staphylococcus aureus*, nafcillin (as above) should be used in addition to one of the cephalosporins suggested.

b. For patients over 9 yr of age: nafcillin, as above

c. Following resolution of the cellulitis and defervescence: a change to oral medications for a total course of 10 days. These agents may include amoxicillin, Augmentin, or trimethoprim-sulfamethoxazole, depending on isolates and sensitivity.

DISPOSITION

Patients with only localized cellulitis and no involvement of the face or systemic toxicity may be followed closely as outpatients. Others require hospitalization.

Parental education

1. See that child takes all medications and keeps appointments for follow-up.
2. Call physician if
   a. Fever increases
   b. Area of cellulitis increases or becomes fluctuant
   c. Underlying joint or bone remains tender or painful once cellulitis has resolved

REFERENCE

Fleisher, G., Ludwig, S., and Campos, J.: Cellulitis: bacterial etiology, clinical features, and laboratory findings, J. Pediatr. **97**:591, 1980.

Contact dermatitis

Contact irritant dermatitis results from contact with an exogenous substance. It may be caused primarily by an irritant, such as an alkali or a detergent, or by prolonged contact of the skin with urine and feces as in diaper dermatitis (p. 437). It is usually mild in nature.

Allergic contact dermatitis is lymphocyte-mediated and caused by a variety of substances including plants (poison ivy or oak), topical medications, shoes, nickel, and cosmetics.

DIAGNOSTIC FINDINGS

1. The distribution and patterning of the lesions, as well as the history of contact, are diagnostic. The lesions often are limited to exposed contact surfaces, and they may be sharply delineated or have bizarre symmetric distribution.
2. The dermatitis is initially erythematous with edema but may progress to vesicle formation, weeping, and crusting.

MANAGEMENT

The offending allergen or irritant, if identifiable, should be removed.

Severe, generalized, allergic contact dermatitis

A short course of systemic steroids is indicated if there is extensive involvement over the body, face, or genitalia. Exacerbation may occur if therapy is not prolonged enough.

1. Prednisone is given 1-2 mg/kg/24 hr q 6-24 hr PO for 1 wk and then tapered over the next 2 wk for a total therapeutic period of 3 wk.

2. Therapy may be initiated parenterally: dexa-methasone (Decadron) 0.25 mg/kg/dose IV or IM.

Moderate allergic contact dermatitis

Topical steroids and compresses are adequate as described for atopic dermatitis (p. 431).

Mild allergic or irritant contact dermatitis

1. Topical steroids are usually adequate.
2. Hydration of the involved area may be useful and, after baths, application of Eucerin or Nivea. Others prefer applying compresses of tepid water, saline, or Burow's solution to weeping areas to dry up the involved region.

DISPOSITION

1. Patients may be discharged but followed until resolution occurs.

2. Patch testing may be useful in defining potential allergens that should be avoided.

Dermatophytosis

See Table 72-3.

Ancillary data

1. Wood's light. In dark room, shine Wood's light. Obtain fluorescence.
2. KOH prep. Place specimen taken from just inside the advancing border of the infection on slide. Add 1-2 drops of 10%-20% KOH; place coverglass on slide and heat gently (do not boil); do microscopic examination. Ideally, the hyphae are seen branching.

TABLE 72-3. Dermatophytoses: clinical characteristics

	Location	Diagnostic findings	Differential diagnosis	Management
Tinea capitis	Scalp, hair	Initially, noninflammatory—bald, scaly patch; 2-8 wk; inflammatory phase—edematous nodule with pustule (kerion)	Alopecia areata (scalp WNL); trichotillo-mania; pyoderma	Griseofulvin
Tinea corporis	Nonhairy parts of body	Dry, scaly, annular lesion with clear center	Pityriasis rosea, atopic dermatitis	Topical
Tinea pedis	Feet	Vesicle, erosion of fourth and fifth toes, extending to other toe and arch of foot; adolescent	Atopic or contact dermatitis	Topical
Tinea fachei	Face	Erythematous, scaly lesion; butterfly distribution	Systemic lupus erythematosus	Topical
Tinea cruris	Groin	Sharply demarcated erythematous, scaly lesion; scrotum not involved; adolescent		Topical
Tinea un-guium	Nails	Nail is thickened, friable, subungual debris; nail discoloration; adolescents	Psoriasis	Griseofulvin and topical; possibly surgery (if poor response)

3. Culture. Sabouraud's agar or dermatophyte test medium (DTM). Latter turns red if dermatophyte is present. Incubate up to 4 wk.

MANAGEMENT (Table 72-3)

1. Topical. Apply cream or solution 2-3 times/day for at least 1 wk after eruption has cleared. May take 2-4 wk.
   a. Tolnaftate (Tinactin)
   b. Clotrimazole (Lotrimin)
   c. Miconazole (MicaTin)
   d. Haloprogin (Halotex)
2. Tinea capitis and ungulum. Oral griseofulvin (microsize: 10 mg/kg/24 hr; or ultramicrosize: 5-10 mg/kg/24 hr) given PO for 6 wk (hair) or 3 mo (nails). Ultramicrosize is better absorbed. Culture before instituting griseofulvin therapy. Griseofulvin should be supplemented by twice weekly shampooing with selenium sulfide suspension.
3. Kerion. Requires prednisone 1-2 mg/kg/24 hr for 1 mo

Diaper dermatitis and candidiasis

Diaper dermatitis is a result of prolonged contact with urine or feces, leading to chemical irritation and associated dampness and maceration. Candidiasis secondary to *Candida albicans* is usually associated with prolonged dermatitis in the diaper region.

DIAGNOSTIC FINDINGS

Diaper dermatitis has a clinical presentation of diffuse erythema with vesiculation and isolated erosions in the diaper area. Satellite papules on an erythematous base caused by *C. albicans* usually develop when the dermatitis has been present for over 3 days (also called *Monilia*). This may be associated with white plaques on an erythematous base on the buccal mucosa, which is known as **thrush.**

DIFFERENTIAL DIAGNOSIS

Other entities that must be distinguished include contact dermatitis (p. 435), atopic dermatitis (p. 431), and bullous impetigo (p. 439).

MANAGEMENT

1. Remove the irritant.
   a. Change diapers frequently.
   b. Leave the baby without a diaper as much as possible. Naps are a particularly good time. Overnight, use triple diapers and rubber pad.
   c. Fasten diapers loosely.
      (1) If cloth diapers are used, double rinse them. Alkalinity may be reduced in dilute vinegar (1 cup in ½ washer tub of water or 1 oz in 1 gallon). Do not use plastic pants.
      (2) If disposable diapers are used, punch a few holes in the plastic liner.
   d. Keep the skin clean, washing gently with warm water. Superfatted or nonirritating soaps (Neutrogena, Basis, Lowila) may be used sparingly. Cetaphil lotion cleanser may also be used.
2. If there is any evidence of satellite lesions associated with candidiasis, initiate application of nystatin cream to the involved area during diaper changes. Continue for 2-3 days after resolution of the diaper dermatitis.
   a. With marked erythema mix hydrocortisone cream (1%) with the nystatin and apply to the diaper area until the erythema has decreased. Other alternatives to nystatin include miconazole and clotrimazole. Do not use fluorinated steroid preparations.
   b. Treat oral white plaques (thrush) with nystatin oral suspension: 1 ml in each side of the mouth 4 times/day for 2-3 days after clearing.

Complication

A complication is secondary bacterial infection.

DISPOSITION

Patients may be sent home.

Parental education

1. Initiate more frequent diaper changes and avoid skin-sensitizing agents.
2. Expose the diaper area to air when possible and avoid airtight occlusion caused by such things as rubber pants.
3. Do not use cornstarch or ointments in the diaper area.
4. Call physician if
   a. Satellite lesions develop in the diaper area
   b. White plaques develop in the mouth
   c. There is evidence of bacterial infection, including crusting, pustules, or large blisters
   d. There is no resolution in 1 wk

Erythema multiforme

Erythema multiforme is a self-limited, hypersensitivity reaction with a broad spectrum of presentations, including toxic epidermal necrolysis and Stevens-Johnson syndrome.

ETIOLOGY: PRECIPITANTS

1. Infections
   a. Viral: herpes simplex, EB virus—infectious mononucleosis, enterovirus
   b. Other: group A streptococci, *mycoplasma pneumoniae*
2. Intoxications: sulfonamides, penicillin, barbiturates, phenytoin

DIAGNOSTIC FINDINGS

Classically, erythema multiforme is a monomorphous eruption.
1. Initially it presents as symmetric, concentric, and erythematous lesions, primarily on the dorsal surfaces of the hand and extensor surfaces of the extremities. The palms and soles are often involved while the trunk is spared. The lesions become papular with an intense erythematous periphery and cyanotic center appearing as target or iris lesions. They may become bullous.
2. There may be a prodrome of fever, headache, sore throat, cough, rhinorrhea, and lymphadenopathy.
3. The skin lesions evolve over 3-5 days with resolution over 2-4 wk. They may recur.

Toxic epidermal necrolysis (Lyell's disease)

1. Drug induced, it represents a severe form of erythema multiforme with cleavage of the skin below the epidermis and dermal layer, resulting in full thickness necrosis of the epidermis.
2. Rarely, the lesions progress to produce severe confluent erythema and bullae with subsequent shedding of the epidermis, predominantly over the extremities, face, and neck.
3. Patients have a positive Nikolsky's sign at the site of the lesions, whereby minor rubbing results in desquamation of underlying skin.
4. Extensive loss of superficial epidermis may occur, with subsequent fluid losses and complications paralleling those of a second-degree burn.
5. Patients are usually toxic, with high fever, malaise, and anorexia.

Stevens-Johnson syndrome

1. A variant of erythema multiforme, the cutaneous lesions extensively involve the mucosal membranes and affect at least two sites (conjunctivae or mucosa of mouth, genitalia, or nose).
2. Blisters form and subsequently unroof with formation of extensive hemorrhagic crusts on the mucosal surface.
3. Patients are usually toxic and have difficulty with fluid intake.
4. A prodrome 1-14 days before the onset of mucocutaneous lesions is noted, including malaise, nausea, vomiting, sore throat, cough, myalgia, and arthralgia.

Complications

1. Dehydration from surface losses or poor fluid intake
2. Secondary bacterial infections

Ancillary data

1. Throat culture to rule out Group A streptococci
2. Data related to fluid status if dehydration is present (Chapter 7)
3. Other tests related to defining precipitants

DIFFERENTIAL DIAGNOSIS

1. Toxic epidermal necrosis: staphylococcal scalded-skin syndrome or Ritter's syndrome in newborn (pp. 443 and 540). Patients are sick with fever.
2. Differential considerations of Stevens-Johnson syndrome: Kawasaki disease (mucocutaneous lymph node syndrome) (p. 538)

MANAGEMENT

1. Supportive care is essential: fluid management, antipruritics, and analgesics.
2. For toxic epidermal necrolysis, see Chapter 46 on burns for discussion of management of fluids, etc. (steroids have no value in therapy).
3. For Stevens-Johnson syndrome careful attention to fluid management, oral hygiene, and eye care are important.
   a. If fluid intake is a problem, discomfort may be decreased by having patient gargle with a solution containing equal parts of Kaopectate, diphenhydramine (Benadryl), and 2% viscous lidocaine (Xylocaine). The dose of the 2% viscous lidocaine (Xylocaine) should not exceed 15 ml q 3 hr or 120 ml in 24 hr in the adult (proportionately less in child). The patient should not eat or drink for 1 hr after application because of the danger of aspiration. Antacids such as Maalox or Mylanta are equally effective.
   b. Mouth washes with half-strength peroxide, if tolerated, are useful.
   c. If there is extensive involvement of the eye, an ophthalmologist should be consulted.

If possible the precipitant should be identified.

DISPOSITION

Patients with uncomplicated illness may be followed as outpatients, with instructions to watch for more extensive involvement.

Patients with toxic epidermal necrolysis should be hospitalized for fluid and skin management unless there is very minimal involvement and follow-up is excellent. Dermatologic consultation should be obtained.

The ability to maintain hydration and the extent of involvement dictate the disposition of patients with Stevens-Johnson syndrome.

Impetigo

ETIOLOGY: INFECTION

Impetigo is a bacterial infection caused by group A streptococci or *S. aureus* (bullous impetigo).

DIAGNOSTIC FINDINGS

An erythematous area evolves into numerous thin-walled vesicles, often overlying areas of abrasion or trauma. The vesicles are quickly unroofed, leaving a superficial ulcer that becomes covered with a thick, honey-colored crust. These spread centrifugally and may coalesce into larger lesions.

Less commonly, the vesicles become bullae that coalesce. When ruptured, they leave a discrete round lesion. This is **bullous impetigo**, usually caused by *S. aureus*.

Lesions most commonly occur on the face and extremities or in areas of trauma.

Complications

1. Acute glomerulonephritis secondary to nephrogenic strains of streptococci
2. Ecthyma: streptococcal infection with extension through all layers of the epidermis resulting in a firm, dark crust with surrounding erythema and edema

Ancillary data

Very rarely, a culture of the lesion is indicated if there is doubt about the diagnosis.

MANAGEMENT

Local skin care may be helpful. Soaking with water combined with some abrasion is useful in removing the crusts.

Antibiotics are indicated for all patients.

1. For lesions that consist primarily of erythema and crusts (the most likely causative organism is group A streptococci):
   a. Penicillin V 25,000-50,000 units/kg/24 hr q 6 hr PO for 10 days **or**
   b. Benzathine penicillin G (Bicillin C-R), usually given 900:300, IM as a single injection according to the schedule listed at the bottom of the page:
2. For bullous impetigo (resulting from *S. aureus* infection): dicloxacillin 50 mg/kg/24 hr q 6 hr PO for 10 days
3. Alternative antibiotics include:
   a. Erythromycin 30-50 mg/kg/24 hr q 6 hr PO for 10 days **or**
   b. Cephalexin (Keflex) or cephradine (Velosef) 25-50 mg/kg/24 hr q 6 hr PO for 10 days

DISPOSITION

All patients may be sent home.

Parental education

1. Have child take all medication.
2. Remove the crust with soaking and minimal abrasion.
3. Minimize sharing of towels, sheets, etc.
4. Bring any other children with similar lesions in for treatment.

Patients are not infectious 24 hr after initiating treatment.

Lice (pediculosis)

Lice or crabs primarily affect the head or pubic areas and are transmitted by person-to-person spread. They cannot live beyond 3 days without human contact.

DIAGNOSTIC FINDINGS

Excoriated papules or pustules are noted in the scalp or perineum. The louse is frequently seen in the hair or on hats or underwear. Gelatinous nits are often noted as tightly adherent white specks on the shaft of the hair.

Intense nocturnal pruritus may be present.

Complications

Complications consist of secondary bacterial infection such as impetigo (p. 439).

MANAGEMENT

Two pediculicides are commonly available:
1. Lindane (Kwell): Apply about 1 oz (adult) of

Weight (lb)	Benzathine penicillin G	Bicillin C-R (900,000 benzathine:300,000 procaine)
<30	300,000	300,000:100,000
31-60	600,000	600,000:200,000
61-90	900,000	900,000:300,000
>90	1,200,000	NA

Kwell shampoo to either the scalp or pubic region and work into a lather, frequently adding small amounts of water. Scrub the hair well for 4 min and rinse thoroughly. Removal must be thorough because of the potential for contact dermatitis or CNS toxicity. One treatment is usually adequate but some prefer to retreat in 10 days. For an adult, 1-2 oz is enough; prescribe smaller amounts for children. Do not give extra medication or use in pregnant women.

2. RID (purified pyrethrins): Apply about 1 oz undiluted to infested area until entirely wet and allow to remain for 10 min. Wash thoroughly. A second treatment is usually needed in 7-10 days.

If the nits are present in the eyelashes or eyebrows, apply petrolatum (Vaseline) carefully to the area overnight once. Do not have the parents mechanically remove them because this tends to produce eye trauma.

Although the nits are dead in the hair, they may stay tightly adherent. Remove by washing the hair with warm vinegar for about 30 min to loosen the nits and then mechanically remove them with a fine-toothed comb.

Treat symptomatic contacts, for example, all nonpregnant sexual contacts.

All the child's bed linens and clothes that have been recently worn should be machine washed. Hats and other headgear that are difficult to wash should be put away for 4 days. Children may return to school after one treatment.

Antihistamines may be necessary for pruritus: diphenhydramine (Benadryl) 5 mg/kg/24 hr q 6 hr PO **or** hydroxyzine (Atarax, Vistaril) 2 mg/kg/24 hr q 6 hr PO.

Pinworms

Enterobius vermicularis are ½-inch, white, threadlike worms that infect the perianal region.

DIAGNOSTIC FINDINGS

1. Children complain of perianal itching. Rarely, with persistent irritation, an associated vulvovaginitis may be present.
2. Worms may be seen by parents.

Ancillary data

A piece of transparent adhesive tape or special kit is gently touched to the perianal region. The sticky side is applied to a glass slide for examination for ova by light microscopy. The highest yield is at night.

DIFFERENTIAL DIAGNOSIS

Pinworms should be distinguished from irritation, fissures, or contact dermatitis in the perianal region.

MANAGEMENT

1. One of two drugs should be used:
   a. Mebendazole (Vermox) for children over 2 yr: 100 mg chewable tablet PO once (repeat in 1 wk) **or**
   b. Pyrantel (Antiminth) 11 mg (~0.2 ml)/kg/dose (maximum: 1 g) PO once (repeat in 1 wk)
2. Family members or contacts with perianal irritation or itching should be similarly examined and treated. Asymptomatic contact need not be treated.

Parental education

Children are usually infected by other children, many of whom carry pinworms but are asymptomatic. Good personal hygiene, with particular attention to hand washing, may reduce the chance of infection.

Pityriasis rosea

Pityriasis rosea affects children and adolescents and is of unknown etiology.

DIAGNOSTIC FINDINGS

1. Initially, a round, scaly, erythematous patch (2-4 cm) with central clearing develops, usually on the trunk. This herald patch precedes the generalized eruption by an average of 10 days and may be confused with tinea corporis.
2. Multiple erythematous macules develop and progress to small, rose-colored papules, primarily over the trunk. The individual lesions are oval shaped, 1-2 cm in size, and follow the wrinkle or cleavage lines of the skin. This creates a "Christmas tree" distribution on the back.
3. In black children, the distribution varies, being primarily on the proximal extremities, inguinal and axillary areas, and the neck.
4. Patients may initially have pruritus but later become asymptomatic.
5. The rash may last for several months, marked by resolution and recurrences.

MANAGEMENT

1. Reassurance is of primary importance. Contact irritants should be avoided.
2. Antihistamines may be useful if itching is severe:
   a. Diphenhydramine (Benadryl) 5 mg/kg/24 hr q 6 hr PO **or**
   b. Hydroxyzine (Atarax, Vistaril) 2 mg/kg/24 hr q 6 hr PO
3. Ultraviolet light (either natural or sunlamp) may hasten the resolution.

Scabies

Scabies is caused by the mite *Sarcoptes scabiei* and requires close person-to-person contact for transmission. The female mite cannot live beyond 2-3 days without human contact.

DIAGNOSTIC FINDINGS

1. The lesions appear as erythematous papules associated with S-shaped linear burrows.
   a. They are primarily located on the dorsum of the hand, interdigital web spaces, elbows (extensor surface), wrists, anterior axillary fold, abdomen, and genitalia. The head and neck are rarely involved.
   b. There is intense nocturnal pruritus, which may continue for up to 1 wk after successful treatment.
2. Infants often have an associated acute dermatitis with excoriations and crusting. In addition to the normal distribution, they also have involvement of the head, neck, palms, and soles.

Complications

Impetigo (p. 439) is a secondary bacterial infection.

Ancillary data

Microscopic examination for mites, eggs, or feces may be done by placing a drop of mineral oil at the advancing end of a burrow and unroofing the burrow with a scalpel. The specimen is then placed on a microscope slide, a coverglass applied, and the material examined by light microscopy.

MANAGEMENT

Two scabicides are primarily used although Lindane is preferred.
1. Lindane (Kwell lotion) is applied to dry skin in a thin layer from the neck down. The lotion is left on for 8 hr and the patient is then bathed thoroughly to remove residual lotion. Removal must be complete because of the potential of contact dermatitis and CNS toxicity. It should not be used in pregnant women or children under 1 yr old. One treatment is usually adequate, although a retreatment is sometimes necessary 1 wk later, particularly in infants and children with many lesions. In adults, 1-2 oz is usually adequate with proportionately smaller volumes in children.
2. Crotamiton 10% (Eurax cream) is applied

from the neck down, with particular attention to folds and creases, and repeated in 24 hr. After 48 hr, the child should be thoroughly bathed.

All members of the household and sexual contacts should be treated (Lindane should not be used in pregnant women). All the child's bed linens and clothes that have recently been worn should be machine washed. Blankets and other items that are difficult to clean should be put away for 4 days. After one treatment, children can return to school.

Antihistamines may be necessary for pruritus: diphenhydramine (Benadryl) 5 mg/kg/24 hr q 6 hr PO **or** hydroxyzine (Atarax, Vistaril) 2 mg/kg/24 hr q 6 hr PO. Itching may continue for 1 wk after treatment.

Seborrheic dermatitis

Seborrheic dermatitis is caused by the overproduction of sebum in areas rich with sebaceous glands, including the scalp, face, midchest, and perineum. It is commonly seen during the first few months of life and in adolescents at puberty.

DIAGNOSTIC FINDINGS

1. The involved areas are minimally erythematous, dry, and scaly with a greasy sensation. Lesions have more intense color and periphery, with clearing at center. Edges are sharply demarcated. Weeping and edema are not present.
2. Newborns particularly have problems with the scalp and may develop "cradle cap."

MANAGEMENT

1. In infants the scalp may be treated by washing with minimal abrasion (washcloth or soft brush) in an effort to remove the scales. Do not use oils.
2. In children and adolescents, shampoos such as Sebulex or those containing selenium sulfide, combined with abrasion, may be helpful.
3. Hydrocortisone cream (1%) is used in markedly involved areas, except for the scalp.
4. Resolution usually occurs within 1 wk. Recurrences may be noted.

Staphylococcal scalded skin syndrome

ETIOLOGY: INFECTION

Staphylococcus aureus, phage group II, produces an exotoxin (exfoliatin) in the patient. The bacteria typically colonize the patient without overt infection.

DIAGNOSTIC FINDINGS

1. Staphylococcal scalded skin syndrome may be generalized in the newborn (Ritter's disease) and the child. Patients may be febrile and irritable.
2. An erythematous eruption develops primarily on the face (perioral and periorbital), the flexor area of the neck, and the axilla and groin, with accompanying tenderness of the skin, progressing to a tender scarlatiniform rash over 1-2 days.
   a. Edema of the face develops, with crusting around the eyes and mouth and sparing of mucous membranes.
   b. Patients have a positive Nikolsky's sign, whereby the epidermis separates with only minor trauma.
3. If the erythema does not progress but desquamates, the patient merely has a scarlatiniform rash.
4. Some patients develop only a localized involvement with the evolution of large bullae with clear or purulent fluid. This is bullous impetigo (p. 439).

Complications

1. Dehydration from fluid losses
2. Systemic infection with *S. aureus*

Ancillary data

Bacterial culture of involved areas may be done.

DIFFERENTIAL DIAGNOSIS

1. Erythema multiforme, toxic epidermal necrolysis (p. 438)
2. Group A streptococcal infection: impetigo or scarlatiniform rash (p. 439)

MANAGEMENT

1. Patients require support with fluids and analgesia.
2. Local treatment with warm compresses may be helpful. However, if the loss of epidermis is extensive, the protocol for management of burns should be implemented (Chapter 46).
3. Antibiotics should be initiated for all patients:
   a. Dicloxacillin 50 mg/kg/24 hr q 6 hr PO for 10 days
   b. Parenteral antibiotics (nafcillin or equivalent) for toxic patients

DISPOSITION

The majority of patients should be hospitalized for local skin care, monitoring of fluids, and antibiotics.

Sunburn

Sunburn results from overexposure to ultraviolet (UV) light. Phototoxic agents that sensitize skin to sun include sulfonamides, tetracycline, hydantoin, barbiturates, chlorpromazine, chlorothiazide, coal tar derivatives, perfumes, celery, and parsnips.

DIAGNOSTIC FINDINGS

1. The exposed skin is erythematous and tender in the first few hours. With significant burns, it will become erythematous and edematous over the next 6-12 hr and ultimately blister by 24 hr.

2. Patients may have concomitant chills, headache, and malaise (Chapter 50).
3. Photosensitizing agents should be considered, including sulfonamides, diphenhydramine, phenothiazines, and tetracyclines.

MANAGEMENT

1. Cool baths or wet compresses are helpful in relieving the pain and burning.
2. Aspirin or indomethacin (1-3 mg/kg/24 hr q 6-8 hr PO in children over 14 yr) is useful in the management of severe sunburn if begun within 12 hr.
3. Steroids have no proven role.

DISPOSITION

Patients may be sent home.

Parental education

1. Avoid overexposures in the future, particularly if your child is taking a photosensitizing agent.
2. Use sunscreens with a skin-protective factor (SPF) of 15 before exposure in the future.
3. Push fluids to maintain hydration.

Urticaria

ETIOLOGY

1. Allergy
   a. Drugs: penicillin, salicylates, narcotics
   b. Foods: nuts, shellfish, eggs
   c. Inhalants
   d. Insect bites (p. 232)
2. Infections
   a. Viral: hepatitis, EB virus (infectious mononucleosis)
   b. Parasites
3. Trauma: mechanical, thermal (cold and heat), sun or solar
4. Autoimmune: systemic lupus erythematosus, inflammatory bowel disease
5. Neoplasms

DIAGNOSTIC FINDINGS

1. Eruption is a rapidly evolving, erythematous, raised wheal with marked edema. The edema is well circumscribed and tense. The lesions are markedly pruritic.
2. Subcutaneous extension of the edema, known as angioedema, occurs in as many as 50% of children with acute urticaria.
3. If associated with anaphylaxis, there may be respiratory or circulatory compromise.

Ancillary data

No tests are indicated initially except to define the etiology.

MANAGEMENT

1. Avoiding etiologic conditions
2. Ensuring that there is no associated respiratory compromise. If present, begin therapy immediately as outlined in Chapter 12.
3. Antihistamines and epinephrine are the hallmarks of therapy:
   a. Diphenhydramine (Benadryl) 5 mg/kg/24 hr q 6 hr PO, IM or IV **or**
   b. Hydroxyzine (Atarax, Vistaril) 2 mg/kg/24 hr q 6 hr PO (causes less associated fatigue)
   c. With poor response, addition of pseudoephedrine (Sudafed) 4-5 mg/kg/24 hr q 6 hr PO
   d. Epinephrine (1:1,000) 0.01 ml/kg/dose (maximum: 0.35 ml/dose) SQ q 20 min prn up to three doses if rapid clearing of rash is desired
4. Referral for a more complete evaluation of patients with recurrent or persistent urticaria beyond 4-6 wk

Warts and molluscum contagiosum

Warts are viral-induced, intraepidermal tumors caused by human papovavirus. They are often asymptomatic, although those on pressure-

TABLE 72-4. Categories of warts and appropriate management

	Common	Filiform	Flat	Plantar	Venereal
DIAGNOSTIC FINDINGS	Solitary papule, irregular scaly surface; found anywhere	Projection from skin on narrow stalk; lip, nose, or eyelids	Flat-topped, skin-colored papule; face or extremity	Smooth papule level with skin surface on weight-bearing surfaces	Multiple confluent papules, irregular surface; genital mucosa or adjacent skin (condylomata acuminata)
MANAGEMENT	Cryotherapy, salicylic acid paint, (periungual: cantharidin, salicylic acid paint)	Surgery	Retinoic acid, salicylic acid paint	Salicylic acid plaster, salicylic acid paint	Podophyllin, cryotherapy

bearing surfaces may be painful. Spontaneous resolution occurs in 9-24 mo. Warts may be categorized by their appearance and location (Table 72-4).

MANAGEMENT TECHNIQUES (listed in Table 72-4)

1. Cryotherapy. Cotton swab is dipped in liquid nitrogen, applied to the center of the wart until it is white, and maintained for 20-30 sec.
2. Salicylic acid paint. Salicylic acid in concentration >10% is applied to wart twice a day for 2-4 wk. On thick surfaces salicylic acid 16.7% and lactic acid 16.7% in flexible collodion are used. Weaker concentration (10%) is used on flat warts.
3. Salicylic acid plaster. Cotton plaster with salicylic acid (40%) is cut to size of wart and taped to skin to remain for 3-5 days and replaced. Wart is treated for 2-3 wk.
4. Retinoic acid (0.1% cream) is applied once or twice a day with resolution in 2-4 wk.
5. Cantharidin is applied directly to periungual warts and covered with tape for 24 hr.
6. Podophyllin (25%) is applied to venereal warts and washed off thoroughly in 4 hr. May need to be repeated in 1 wk. Because it is neurotoxic, it must not be used on an extensive area or at home.

Molluscum contagiosum is a white or whitish-yellow papule with central umbilication caused by a poxvirus. Grouped genital lesions are common, often surrounded by an area of dermatitis. Wright's stain of the contents of the papule will reveal epidermal cytoplasmic viral inclusions.

Sharp dermal curettage is the treatment of choice if removal is desired. This may leave a small scar. Spontaneous resolution occurs in 2-3 yr.

REFERENCES

Rasmussen, J.E., editor: Pediatric dermatology, Pediatr. Clin. North Am. **30**:417, 1983.

Weston, W.L.: Practical pediatric dermatology, ed. 2, Boston, 1985, Little, Brown & Co.

73 Ear, nose, and throat disorders

Dentoalveolar infections

PAUL S. CASAMASSIMO
GARY K. BELANGER

Toothaches and associated dentoalveolar infections usually are caused by untreated dental caries, although they may be related to failing dental restorations.

DIAGNOSTIC FINDINGS

1. Patients usually complain of local or generalized dental or facial pain, often exacerbated by heat, cold, sweets, air, and chewing pressure.
2. Affected tooth usually has obvious defect such as dental caries or broken or lost restoration.
3. Facial swelling is commonly noted. Dentoalveolar swelling or fistula also may be present.

Complications

1. Facial cellulitis (p. 432)
2. Bacteremia
3. Loss of tooth

Ancillary data

Dental x-ray film, if available, is helpful.

DIFFERENTIAL DIAGNOSIS

1. Dentoalveolar or periodontal abscess
2. Newly erupting tooth
3. Traumatic dental injury
4. Broken dental restoration
5. Foreign object embedded in tissue
6. *Dental stains* may be mistaken for caries in a tooth. Normal teeth have some color vari-

ation. Stains also may be caused by external agents that can be removed with cleaning; such stains (green, orange or black in color) result from poor hygiene or from excessive use of certain foods, beverages, smoking, or liquid medications (iron). Intrinsic conditions that lead to dental staining include problems in the neonatal period (biliary atresia, hepatitis, erythroblastosis or maternal tetracycline ingestion), trauma, excessive flouride, or tetracycline ingestion between 3 mo and 8 yr of age.

MANAGEMENT
Toothache without infection

1. Evaluation of legitimate need for analgesics, which children rarely require
2. Dental referral within 24 hr

Toothache with localized infection

1. Initiation of antibiotics: penicillin 25,000-50,000 units (15-30 mg)/kg/24 hr q 6 hr PO for 7-10 days
2. Consideration of analgesics
3. Dental referral within 24 hr

Dental infection with cellulitis

1. Hospitalization
2. Initiation of antibiotics
   a. Nafcillin (or equivalent) 150 mg/kg/24 hr q 4 hr IV
   b. A switch to dicloxacillin (once parenteral therapy is no longer indicated): 50 mg/kg/24 hr q 6 hr PO for a total course of 10 days
3. Dental consultation to evaluate need for in-

cision and drainage, extraction of tooth, or open drainage. Dentist will attempt to relieve pain, treat infection, and provide appropriate follow-up as necessary for extraction or root canal treatment, restoration, or dental prosthesis.

REFERENCE

Josell, S.D., and Abrams, R.E.: Common oral and dental emergencies and problems, Pediatr. Clin. North Am. **29:**705, 1982.

Epistaxis (nosebleed)

Nasal bleeding normally originates in the anterior portion of the nasal septum (Kiesselbach's area), which accounts for 90% of cases.

ETIOLOGY

1. Trauma: nose picking, foreign body, repeated hard blowing with associated upper respiratory infection, nasal fracture
2. Allergic rhinitis or polyp
3. Bleeding dyscrasia, aspirin ingestion, anticoagulants, leukemia
4. Vascular: telangiectasia, hemangioma. Hypertension is an unusual association.

DIAGNOSTIC FINDINGS

There is active bleeding from one or both nostrils. Examination of the nose reveals an inflamed area at Kiesselbach's plexus. Predisposing causes should be defined.

Complication

Although epistaxis is usually self-limited, extensive bleeding may cause anemia or shock.

Ancillary data

Rarely are any laboratory data indicated unless there are suggestions of systemic disease. A bleeding screen (CBC, platelet count, PT, and PTT) for recurrent epistaxis is indicated if there is a history of significant bleeding with lacera-tions, circumcision, etc., spontaneous bleeding at other sites, or a positive family history (Chapter 29).

MANAGEMENT

1. Apply constant pressure over the anterior nares for a minimum of 10 min. Preceding this, the patient should blow the nose to remove clots. Optimally the patient should be kept sitting with head forward to avoid draining blood posteriorly into airway or esophagus.
2. If pressure is unsuccessful, place in the nose a piece of cotton soaked in 0.25% phenylephrine (Neo-Synephrine) or epinephrine (1:1000) and 1% cocaine, and then apply pressure for 10 min.
3. If anterior bleeding continues or the problem is recurrent, cauterize the bleeding site with application of silver nitrate stick for 3 sec. Do not cauterize children with bleeding problems.
4. Apply petrolatum (Vaseline) daily for 4-5 days to decrease friability of anterior nasal mucosa.

If posterior bleeding is present, a posterior pack may be inserted by an otolaryngologist.

DISPOSITION

Patients can usually be discharged. If posterior pack is inserted, patient must be admitted. Admission should be seriously considered if bilateral anterior packs are used. Appropriate allergy management, if indicated, should be instituted. Hematologic or otolaryngologic consultation is rarely indicated.

Parental education

1. Increase home humidity. Minimize nose trauma and picking.
2. Apply Vaseline daily to anterior nares for 4-5 days.
3. If bleeding recurs, apply pressure for a full 10 min, compressing the soft and bony parts of the nose, pressing downward toward the

cheeks with thumb and forefinger.
4. Call physician if there are unexplained bruises, if large amounts of blood are lost, or if bleeding cannot be controlled by pressure.

Foreign bodies in the nose and ear

Foreign bodies found in the nose or ear commonly include inanimate matter, vegetable materials, and insects.

DIAGNOSTIC FINDINGS

1. Patient with *nasal* foreign bodies have nasal obstruction or unilateral foul-smelling discharge. The object often may be visualized.
2. Patients with foreign bodies in the *ear* often have pain or discharge from the external ear canal. Frequently there is a history either of inserting an object into the ear or of a buzzing sound associated with an insect. The object may be visualized.

MANAGEMENT

Cooperation is essential through immobilization, sedation, or anesthesia. Good visualization, an excellent light source, and proper equipment are necessary.

Nasal foreign bodies

Have child blow nose vigorously, then try suction. If unsuccessful, proceed with other techniques.
1. Vasoconstriction. Use topical epinephrine (1%) applied with a cotton-tipped swab, sprayed phenylephrine (0.25%), or cocaine (1%) before instrumentation.
2. Use forceps if the object can be grasped. Suction and hook or loop may be useful for larger objects.

If these maneuvers are unsuccessful and there is room, a lubricated no. 8 Foley catheter may be passed beyond the object and inflated with 2-3 ml of water (with patient in reverse Trendelenburg's position). Then the Foley catheter is withdrawn.

Ear foreign bodies

Several techniques are useful in attempting to remove objects.
1. If insect, kill it before removal by inserting alcohol.
2. Irrigation. Direct the stream of water beyond the object to flush it out. Do not use with vegetable matter (the material may swell) or if tympanic membrane is perforated.
   NOTE: A useful irrigation technique is to cut off the needle of a large butterfly (18-gauge) catheter, leaving a pliable section of tubing. The ear is then easily irrigated with water and the fluid aspirated from the canal. A pulsating water device also may be used.
3. Mechanical removal: use forceps for small objects, hooks, or loops.

DISPOSITION

If the foreign body cannot be removed, patients should be referred to an otolaryngologist for ambulatory management.

REFERENCE

Stool, S.E., and McConnell, C.S.: Foreign bodies in pediatric otolaryngology: some diagnostic and therapeutic points, Clin. Pediatr. **12**:113, 1973.

Acute necrotizing gingivitis

This is an acute, contagious oral infection of adolescents and young adults involving the gingival tissues.

ETIOLOGY: INFECTION

It is caused by spirochete *Borrelia vincentii.*

DIAGNOSTIC FINDINGS

1. History of recent emotional or physical stress (rarely epidemic). Fatigue may be a factor.

2. Classic triad of intense, unremitting pain; punched-out interdental papillae covered with a white pseudomembrane; and foul odor from mouth
3. Rare associated regional lymphadenopathy, malaise, and fever

Complications

Without treatment there is bone loss and loosening of teeth.

DIFFERENTIAL DIAGNOSIS

1. Infection: acute viral and bacterial infections
2. Leukemic gingivitis

MANAGEMENT

1. Pencillin 25,000-50,000 units (15-30 mg)/kg/24 hr q 6 hr PO for 10 days
2. Dental referral and close follow-up for tissue debridement. Surgery may be necessary.

Cervical lymphadenopathy

The cervical lymph nodes course along the carotid sheath and drain the head and neck. The superior node group has afferents from the tongue, tonsils, nose, teeth, and the back of the head and neck. It becomes inflamed with potential suppuration from infections in these areas.

ETIOLOGY: INFECTION

1. Bacterial: group A streptococci, *S. aureus,* typical and atypical mycobacteria
2. Viral: infectious mononucleosis, enterovirus, rubella
3. Other: cat scratch fever, toxoplasmosis, mucocutaneous lymph node syndrome (Kawasaki disease)

DIAGNOSTIC FINDINGS

1. History should be obtained for rapidity of progression, recent travel, exposure to tuberculosis, contact with cats, and concurrent systemic signs and symptoms.
2. Pyogenic lesions have a unilateral, visible, firm, tender, discrete swelling early in the disease, which may progress to generalized swelling, erythema, and tenderness that becomes fluctuant. Patients usually are febrile and become increasingly toxic with extension of the process. There may be pain on neck movement.
3. Nonpyogenic organisms have a more insidious course.
4. Palpable head and neck nodes are detected in 45% of normal children. Younger children most commonly have nodes in the occipital and postauricular areas whereas older children have them predominantly in the cervical and submandibular regions.

Complications

Suppuration and spontaneous drainage of the lymph node occurs.
1. Exteriorly, this is a problem for cosmetic reasons.
2. Nodes caused by atypical mycobacteria may chronically drain.
3. Interior drainage may involve multiple neck structures, with significant morbidity.

Ancillary data

1. WBC with differential (shift to left)
2. Throat culture for group A streptococci
3. Monospot and Streptozyme
4. Intermediate-strength purified protein derivative (PPD) test (usually <10 mm with atypical disease but may be negative)
5. Aspiration of the node with an 18-gauge needle if there is no resolution of signs and symptoms in 48 hr
   a. Care should be exercised if atypical mycobacteria are considered because of the potential for chronic drainage.
   b. Culture for bacteria and mycobacteria should be done, as well as Gram's and acid-fast stains.

c. If incision and drainage (I and D) are performed, similar cultures should be obtained.

DIFFERENTIAL DIAGNOSIS

1. Infection: parotitis (most commonly mumps). Obliterates the angle of the jaw, is associated with parotid tenderness, and is often bilateral
2. Neoplasm: lymphoma, leukemia, metastatic carcinoma
3. Congenital: bronchial cleft or thyroglossal duct cyst
4. Hemangioma or cystic hygroma

MANAGEMENT

Management of cervical lymphadenopathy must proceed in an orderly fashion, and other etiologies should be considered if the patient's initial response is slow. Total resolution may occur over many weeks.

1. Antibiotics should be initiated after appropriate cultures are obtained.
   a. Penicillin 80,000 units (50 mg)/kg/24 hr q 6 hr PO is given for 48 hr if the node is not fluctuant initially. This is a relatively high dose.
   b. If clinical improvement is noted, the therapy is continued.
   c. If a therapeutic response has not occurred after 48 hr or the patient worsens:
      (1) The drug is changed to dicloxacillin 50 mg/kg/24 hr q 6 hr PO **or**
      (2) Cephalexin (Keflex) or cephradine (Velosef): 25-50 mg/kg/24 hr q 6 hr PO
      (3) Other antibiotics should be considered if the Gram's stain or culture of the node aspirate reveals less common organisms, such as *H. influenzae*.
2. I and D are indicated if fluctuance is present. Whether this can be done on an outpatient or inpatient basis depends on the child's toxicity, comfort, and cooperation as well as surgical experience. Most physicians prefer inpatient management with parenteral antibiotics (nafcillin or equivalent 150 mg/kg/24

hr q 4 hr IV) in the immediate postoperative period.

Treatment of atypical mycobacterial infections is controversial. Excision provides the best cure rate. Some clinicians treat with rifampin after surgery.

DISPOSITION

1. Patients may be followed at home unless there is significant toxicity or I and D are required. Close follow-up is essential.
2. Surgical consultation is necessary for patients with fluctuant nodes.

Parental education

Lymphadenopathy may require several *months* for complete resolution. For children followed at home, the parent should understand that

1. Treatment requires very high-dose antibiotics. The child should take all doses.
2. Call physician if
   a. Swelling increases or becomes more red, tender, or fluctuant
   b. Systemic toxicity develops

Acute mastoiditis

The middle ear communicates with the mastoid air cells, leading to concurrent infections if acute otitis media (AOM) is improperly treated.

ETIOLOGY

Acute mastoiditis is caused by bacterial infection, identical to those organisms causing AOM, most commonly *Streptococcus pneumoniae*, *Haemophilus influenzae*, and group A streptococci. *H. influenzae* is rare in children over 8 yr of age.

DIAGNOSTIC FINDINGS

AOM is followed by pain, edema, and tenderness over the mastoid area. Postauricular swelling resulting from a subperiosteal abscess may cause severe pain and displace the pinna forward, making the ear prominent.

Complications

1. Infection: meningitis and intracranial abscess
2. Paralysis of facial nerve
3. Sensorineural hearing loss

Ancillary data

1. Mastoid x-ray film show clouding of the septa of the mastoid bone. Bony destruction and resorption of air cells eventually occur.
2. Tympanocentesis, culture, and Gram's stain of aspirated material may be useful.

DIFFERENTIAL DIAGNOSIS

Acute mastoiditis should be differentiated from other infections. Postauricular lymphadenitis is difficult to differentiate.

1. Postauricular tenderness and erythema overlie a distinct node and do not diffusely involve the mastoid.
2. There is often an associated external otitis media.

MANAGEMENT

1. Antibiotics should be initiated pending culture and sensitivity results.
   a. For children 8 yr and younger.
      (1) Ampicillin 100-200 mg/kg/24 hr q 4 hr IV **and** chloramphenicol 100 mg/kg/24 hr q 6 hr IV; **or**
      (2) Cefotaxime 50-150 mg/kg/24 hr q 6 hr IV; **or** cefuroxime 100 mg/kg/24 hr q 6-8 hr IV; **or** ceftriaxone 50-75 mg/kg/ 24 q 12 hr IV
   b. For children over 8 yr: ampicillin 100-200 mg/kg/24 hr q 4 hr IV
      NOTE: Once the illness begins to resolve, oral antibiotics may be continued for a total course of 4 wk of treatment.
2. Analgesia may be given, including codeine 0.5 mg/kg/dose q 4-6 hr PO **or** meperidine (Demerol) 1 mg/kg/dose q 3-4 hr IM as indicated.

3. If the patient's condition worsens or a subperiosteal abscess develops, a postauricular I and D with a mastoidectomy should be performed by an otolaryngologist.

DISPOSITION

Hospitalization and consultation with an otolaryngologist usually are required.

REFERENCE

Hawkins, D.B., Dru, D., House, J.W., et al.: Acute mastoiditis in children: a review of 54 cases, Laryngoscope **93**:568, 1983.

Acute otitis media

ALERT: **Extreme irritability or lethargy may imply concurrent meningitis or other systemic infection.**

Acute otitis media is a suppurative effusion of the middle ear accounting for one third of office visits of children who are ill.

ETIOLOGY: INFECTION

Infection often follows evidence of eustachian tube dysfunction caused by either obstruction or abnormal patency. Pathogens include:

1. Bacteria (Table 73-1). No bacteria are isolated in 30% of patients studied, whereas *Streptococcus pneumoniae* (25%-30%) and *Haemophilus influenzae* (20%) are the most common pathogens identified.
2. Viral: parainfluenza, respiratory syncytial virus, influenza, adenovirus, and enterovirus
3. *Mycoplasma pneumoniae*: associated with bullous myringitis, as are other pathogens
4. Other: tuberculosis

Predisposing factors include associated upper respiratory infection, nasotracheal intubation, and Down's syndrome. American Indians, Eskimos, and infants with straight eustachian tubes also are at higher risk.

TABLE 73-1. Acute otitis media: common pathogens and treatment

Age-group/condition	Common pathogens	Antibiotics*	Dosage† (mg/kg/24 hr)	Frequency/route	Minimum duration	Comments
<2 mo	S. pneumoniae, H. influenzae, group A streptococci, S. aureus, gram-negative enteric	Ampicillin **and**	100-200	q 4 hr IV	3-7 days, then appropriate PO	Appropriate if signs of systemic illness; tympanocentesis indicated; hospitalize; if no signs or symptoms, use 2 mo-8 yr regimen
		gentamicin	5.0-7.5	q 8 hr IV		
2 mo-8 yr	S. pneumoniae, H. influenzae, group A streptococci	Amoxicillin; **or**	30-50	q 8 hr PO	10-14 days	
		erythromycin *and*	30-50	q 6 hr PO	10-14 days	
		sulfisoxazole‡; **or**	100-150	q 6 hr PO	10-14 days	
		erythromycin *and*	30-50	q 6 hr PO	10-14 days	
		trimethoprim-sulfamethoxazole; **or**	8.0/40	q 12 hr PO	10-14 days	
		Augmentin; **or**	20-40 (Amox)	q 8 hr PO	10-14 days	
		cefaclor	20-40	q 8 hr PO	10-14 days	
9 yr and older	S. pneumoniae, group A streptococci§	Penicillin V; **or**	25,000-50,000 units/kg/24 hr	q 6 hr PO	10-14 days	
		erythromycin	30-50	q 6 hr PO	10-14 days	
Persistent		Sulfisoxazole; **or**	100-150	q 6 hr PO	14 days	Use after initial course of amoxicillin; if no resolution consider tympanocentesis
		trimethoprim-sulfamethoxazole; **or**	8.0/40	q 12 hr PO	14 days	
		Amoxicillin	20	q 8 hr PO	14 days	
Recurrent		Sulfisoxazole; **or**	50-75	q 12 hr PO	2-mo	Should be done in conjunction with otolaryngologist
		trimethoprim-sulfamethoxazole	8.0/40	q 24 hr PO	2-4 mo	
			4.0/20			

*Additional acceptable antibiotics are available but are either broader in spectrum or more costly.
†See Formulary (p. 660) for adult (maximum) doses.
‡Available as a single combination (Pediazole).
§There is increasing evidence that *H. influenzae* is an important pathogen in this age-group; therefore amoxicillin is also an appropriate therapy.

DIAGNOSTIC FINDINGS

1. Lethargy, irritability and other behavioral changes, ear pain, fever, and accompanying respiratory symptoms. Drainage may be present if the tympanic membrane has ruptured. In the older child, hearing loss may occur.
2. Tympanic membrane (TM)
   a. Full visualization is essential, often necessitating the removal of cerumen and debris, using irrigation (provided no perforation is present) or a cerumen spoon. The presence of cerumen does not preclude the diagnosis of AOM.

      A useful irrigation technique is to cut the needle off a large butterfly catheter (18 gauge), leaving only the pliable tubing. The ear then can be easily irrigated with subsequent aspiration of the fluid from the canal. A pulsating water device also may be useful.
   b. TM has increased vascularity and erythema with obscured landmarks.
   c. Pneumatic otoscopy is the only reliable means of determinig if an effusion is present. Decreased mobility accompanies AOM, often with bulging or retraction unless the TM is perforated.
   d. The optimal position of the child for the examination varies with the examiner and the child. Many prefer to have the child supine on the examining table, restrained by an adult or by specific pediatric restraints. In the partially cooperative child, the child may be seated in the parent's lap, face-to-face, and hugged tightly; the child's legs are wrapped around the parent's waist. One of the parent's arms embraces the child while the other holds the child's head.

Complications

1. Persistent AOM after an initial course of antibiotics occurs in 25% of patients. A second course of antibiotics is appropriate. If AOM persists after completion of a second course (or third course), referral to an otolaryngologist and tympanocentesis usually are indicated for diagnostic and therapeutic purposes. Based on culture results, an additional course of antibiotics is initiated and follow-up is arranged.
2. Recurrent AOM occurs when a child has had three episodes of AOM in 6 mo or 4 in 12 mo.
   a. It is particularly common in children who had their first episode of AOM before 1 yr of age. In children who have six or more episodes of AOM before 6 yr of age, 49% had their initial episode during the first year of life.
   b. Prophylactic antibiotics or pressure-equalizing tubes are indicated.
3. Perforations occur when sufficient pressure in the middle ear develops, which may produce external otitis media (p. 456) or a transient conductive hearing loss. Local and systemic therapy is indicated.
4. Serous otitis media (SOM) occurs in 42% of children following an episode of AOM and usually resolves without intervention. Temporary hearing losses may occur, and such children should be referred for audiologic evaluation if the loss persists beyond 2 mo.
5. Conductive hearing loss may be present with AOM and SOM. If persistent, intervention with pressure-equalizing tubes may be appropriate.
6. Mastoiditis, common before the antibiotic era, now is rare (p. 451).
7. Cholesteatoma, a sac-like structure lined by keratinized, stratified, squamous epithelium with accumulation of desquamating epithelium or keratin in the middle ear, may be caused by recurrent AOM. It may result in erosion of the bone and progressive enlargement of the otic antrum.

Ancillary data

1. Tympanocentesis is indicated in symptomatic

patients under 8 wk of age, in immunocompromised children, and in those with persistent AOM beyond two to three treatment courses. It is useful in defining pathogens, and the material should be Gram's stained and cultured. Rarely, tympanocentesis may be used to relieve severe pain. Puncture of the bullae associated with tense bullous myringitis results in immediate relief. Tympanocentesis often is done by an otolaryngologist.

2. Tympanometry with an electrical acoustic impedance bridge measures compliance of the tympanic membrane and middle ear. It is useful in confirming findings on examination of children over 7 mo.

3. Nasopharyngeal and throat cultures are not helpful.

DIFFERENTIAL DIAGNOSIS

AOM should be differentiated from ear pain caused by:
1. Infection
   a. External otitis media (p. 456)
   b. Mastoiditis (p. 451)
   c. Dental abscess (p. 447)
   d. Peritonsillar abscess
   e. Sinusitis
   f. Lymphadenitis
   g. Parotitis
2. Trauma: foreign body perforating the tympanic membrane or, if still present, external otitis media; barotrauma; instrumentation
3. Serous otitis media or eustachian tube dysfunction
4. Impacted third molar
5. Temporomandibular joint dysfunction

MANAGEMENT

The patient must be evaluated to be certain that a more significant infection such as meningitis is not present.
1. Antibiotics are indicated for all children with AOM. The choice of antibiotics varies with the child's age, allergies, the seriousness of the infection, compliance, and etiologic agents (Table 73-1).
   a. Children under 2 mo require broad-spectrum coverage, usually administered parenterally as an inpatient.
   b. Children under 9 yr of age need coverage for *H. influenzae* as well as *S. pneumoniae* and group A streptococci. There is increasing evidence that *H. influenzae* is an important pathogen in children over 9 yr and therefore broader coverage may be indicated (e.g., amoxicillin).
   c. Children with bullous myringitis, which is frequently associated with *Mycoplasma pneumoniae*, also require treatment for other organisms considered to be pathogens in the age-group. If pain is severe, myringotomy may be indicated.
   d. 60%-90% of patients improve within 72 hr of initiating therapy.
   e. Although there is some controversy regarding the ideal nature and length of treatment for AOM, until definitive data are available, standard practice as outlined previously should be followed.
2. Decongestants, given either systemically (antihistamines or vasoconstrictors) or nasally, are not effective in altering the course.
3. Eardrops may be useful in the treatment of external otitis media resulting from perforation (polymyxin B [Lidosporin] or cortisporin suspension) or to relieve pain (glycerin [Auralgan] or mineral oil).
4. Antipyretics and analgesics such as acetaminophen or aspirin should be initiated.
5. Recurrent AOM is initially treated with prophylactic antibiotics, including amoxicillin 20 mg/kg/24 hr q 12-24 hr PO **or** sulfisoxazole 50-75 mg/kg/24 hr q 12 hr PO **or** trimethoprim-sulfamethoxazole 4-20 mg/kg/24 hr q 24 hr PO.

DISPOSITION

1. Children may be followed at home if no other serious systemic infection is present, with a

follow-up appointment in 2-3 wk.

2. Children under 2 mo of age and those with significant toxicity or immunodeficiencies should be hospitalized.

3. Patients with persistent (after two courses) or recurrent AOM should be followed by an otolaryngologist.

Parental education

1. The entire course of antibiotics should be taken even if your child is better.

2. Antipyretics (acetaminophen or aspirin) may make your child feel better.

3. A return appointment in 2-3 wk should be made to evaluate the response.

4. Call physician if
   a. There is no improvement in 36 hr or if the fever continues beyond 72 hr. If the signs and symptoms continue, the antibiotic may have to be altered to ensure treatment of resistant *H. influenzae* (change to sulfisoxazole or trimethoprim with sulfamethoxazole).
   b. Your child becomes increasingly irritable or lethargic
   c. Your child develops vomiting or diarrhea

REFERENCES

Cantekin, E.I., Mandel, E.M., Bluestone, C.D., et al.: Lack of efficacy of a decongestant-antihistamine combination for otitis media with effusion in children, N. Engl. J. Med. **308**:297, 1983.

Kramer, I.I., and Kramer, A.M.: The phantom earache: temporomandibular joint dysfunction in children, Am. J. Dis. Child. **139**:943, 1985.

Neu, H.C.: Contemporary antibiotic therapy in otolaryngology, Otolaryngol. Clin. North Am. **17**:745, 1984.

Paradise, J.L.: Otitis media in infants and children, Pediatrics **65**:917, 1980.

Perrin, J.M., Charney, E., MacWhinney, J.B., et al.: Sulfisoxazole as chemoprophylaxis for recurrent otitis media, N. Engl. J. Med. **291**:664, 1974.

Roberts, D.B.: The etiology of bullous myringitis and the role of mycoplasma in ear disease: a review, Pediatrics **65**:761, 1980.

vanBuchem, F.L., Dunk, J.H.M., and van't Hof, M.A.: Therapy of acute otitis media: myringotomy, antibiotics or neither, Lancet **2**:883, 1981.

Schwartz, R.H., and Rodriquez, W.J.: Acute otitis media in children eight years old and older: a reappraisal of the role of *Haemophilus influenzae*, Am. J. Otolaryngol. **2**:19, 1981.

External otitis media

External otitis media is an inflammatory reaction of the external ear canal.

ETIOLOGY

1. Infection
   a. Perforated tympanic membrane with drainage of pus
   b. Impetigo
   c. Herpes simplex
   d. Furunculosis associated with *S. aureus*
2. Dermatitis referred to as "swimmer's ear," causing irritation and damage
3. Foreign body

DIAGNOSTIC FINDINGS

1. Severe pain (particularly on movement of the tragus) and drainage are common.
2. Systemic signs are uncommon.
3. The external ear canal is swollen with drainage, erythema, and edema. The tympanic membrane is intact and mobile with normal color (unless caused by perforation).

Complications

Malignant external otitis media (caused by *Pseudomonas* organisms) is uncommon.

Ancillary data

Culture of the discharge is not helpful since it often grows *Pseudomonas* or *S. aureus* organisms, not necessarily reflecting true pathogens.

DIFFERENTIAL DIAGNOSIS

Ear pain from external otitis media should be differentiated from pain caused by infections such as:

1. AOM (p. 452)
2. Dental infection (p. 447)
3. Mastoiditis (p. 451)
4. Posterior auricular lymphadenopathy

MANAGEMENT

1. If no perforation is present, the ear may be irrigated with saline.
2. Eardrops (suspension if perforated) such as polymyxin B (Lidosporin or Cortisporin) should be initiated: 2-3 drops 4-6 times/day inserted into the ear. If significant swelling is present, a cotton wick should be inserted after soaking in an otic-drop suspension until direct application is possible. Many ear solutions and suspensions contain neomycin, which may cause contact dermatitis in 1 out of every 1,000 patients.
3. Systemic antibiotics are not indicated unless the underlying condition requires such treatment.
4. Foreign bodies, if present, should be removed.

DISPOSITION

Children may be followed at home and re-evaluated if there is no resolution in 4-5 days.

Acute parotitis

ETIOLOGY: INFECTION

1. Viral (nonsuppurative)
   a. **Mumps** (the most common etiologic agent)
   b. Other: coxsackievirus and parainfluenza virus
2. Bacterial (suppurative)
   a. *S. aureus* and *S. pneumoniae*
   b. Obstruction from stricture, calculi, or foreign material (food) often present
3. Fungi: *Candida* organisms

DIAGNOSTIC FINDINGS

1. Nonsuppurative parotitis (e.g., mumps) is an insidious disease with slow onset of fever and earache accompanied by tenderness and enlargement of the parotid.
   a. The ear lobe is pushed upward and outward, and the angle of the mandible is obscured.
   b. The orifice of Stensen's duct is edematous and erythematous and exudes a clear fluid.
2. Suppurative parotitis is caused by an anatomic stricture.
   a. Systemic toxicity is present.
   b. The area of the parotid is painful and tender with overlying erythema.
   c. A purulent discharge is noted at Stensen's duct.

Complications

1. Mumps may have an associated encephalitis or orchitis.
2. Suppurative parotitis may occur following an episode of nonsuppurative infection.

Ancillary data

1. Serum amylase is elevated in acute infectious parotitis and normal in recurrent parotitis.
2. Culture of the drainage from Stensen's duct may be helpful if the suppurative parotitis is unresponsive to antibiotics.
3. Sialogram is rarely helpful.

DIFFERENTIAL DIAGNOSIS

1. Infection: cervical lymphadenopathy (p. 450)
2. Recurrent parotitis. Usually unilateral and may occur as many as 10 times before spontaneous resolution
3. Neoplasm
4. Hemangioma

MANAGEMENT

1. Nonsuppurative parotitis, most commonly mumps, resolves without therapy. Discom-

fort may be reduced by avoiding citrus fruits such as oranges and lemons.
2. Suppurative parotitis requires antibiotic therapy:
   a. For nontoxic children: dicloxacillin 50 mg/kg/24 hr q 6 hr PO
   b. For systemically ill children: nafcillin (or equivalent) 100 mg/kg/24 hr q 4 hr IV
3. If suppurative parotitis is present, surgical consultation should be sought early, since early I and D is desirable to avoid damage to the facial nerve.

DISPOSITION

All patients may be followed at home unless they are toxic or have fluctuant parotitis requiring parenteral therapy.

Parental education

Mumps is contagious until the swelling has disappeared, usually 6 days into the illness.
1. Avoid citrus fruits.
2. Call physician if
   a. The swelling has not resolved in 7 days
   b. Erythema, increasing tenderness, or pain develops over the parotid gland

Peritonsillar abscess

Tonsillar infections occasionally suppurate beyond the tonsillar capsule into surrounding tissues.

ETIOLOGY

Bacterial infection is caused:
1. Most commonly by group A streptococci
2. Uncommonly by *H. influenzae*, *S. pneumoniae*, *S. aureus*
3. By normal mouth flora, including anaerobes (occasionally implicated)

DIAGNOSTIC FINDINGS

These infections have a rapid onset.
1. Toxicity accompanied by fever, severe sore throat, progressive trismus, drooling, alteration in speech ("hot potato voice"), and dysphagia are common.
2. Tonsil is unilaterally displaced medially with erythema and edema of the soft palate. Uvula deviates to the opposite side. The abscess may be fluctuant.

Complications

1. Extension beyond the tonsillar regions into the retropharyngeal or mediastinal spaces
2. Upper respiratory obstruction as a result of edema and swelling
3. Aspiration pneumonia secondary to spontaneous rupture.

Ancillary data

1. Aspirate cultures and Gram's stain
2. WBC. Usually elevated with a shift to the left

DIFFERENTIAL DIAGNOSIS

Peritonsillar abscess should be differentiated from infection caused by:
1. Severe pharyngotonsillitis from group A streptococci or infectious mononucleosis
2. Parapharyngeal abscess with erythema and swelling of the lateral pharyngeal wall and brawny induration of the neck. Neck spasms and torticollis occur in children usually under 5 yr.
3. Peritonsillar cellulitis without definite abscess or displacement of the uvula. This can usually be treated with high doses of penicillin and close follow-up.
4. Tetanus
5. Dental infection

MANAGEMENT

If there is any compromise of the airway, intervention should be an immediate priority.
1. Antibiotics should be initiated early in treatment: ampicillin 100-200 mg/kg/24 hr q 4 hr IV.
   a. If resolution is slow: nafcillin (or equivalent) 100-150 mg/kg/24 hr q 4 hr IV should be started
   b. Antibiotics may be altered when results

of culture and sensitivity are available.

2. Analgesia may be given: meperidine (Demerol) 1-2 mg/kg/dose q 4-6 hr IM.

3. I and D are required if abscess is fluctuant or if there is no resolution after 48 hr of therapy.
   a. Needle aspiration may initially be both diagnostic and therapeutic.
   b. Definitive I and D should be carried out in the operating room.

4. Tonsillectomy is indicated on an elective basis 3-4 wk after resolution of the inflammation unless improvement is slow, in which case it may be done on an emergent basis.

DISPOSITION

Patients should be admitted to the hospital for antibiotics and drainage. An otolaryngologist should be involved in the management.

REFERENCE

Schuit, K.E., and Johnson, J.T.: Infection of the head and neck, Pediatr. Clin. North Am. **28**:965, 1981.

Pharyngotonsillitis (sore throat)

Acute pharyngitis is commonly associated with tonsillitis resulting from inflammation of the throat, with associated soreness, fever, and minimal nasal involvement.

ETIOLOGY: INFECTION

1. Bacterial
   a. Group A streptococci
   b. Less common pathogens, including *Neisseria gonorrhoeae*, *Haemophilus influenzae*, *Neisseria meningitidis*, other streptococci, and *Corynebacterium diphtheriae*

2. Viral
   a. Adenovirus: patient may have accompanying conjunctivitis
   b. Enterovirus: *herpangina* with associated fever, sore throat, dysphagia, vomiting, and small vesicles on soft palate, tonsil, or pharynx
   c. Influenza, parainfluenza, EB virus (infectious mononucleosis), and herpes simplex (less frequent)

3. *M. pneumoniae:* common in schoolage children

DIAGNOSTIC FINDINGS (Table 73-2)

Clinically, patients have a range of symptoms, which make it difficult to differentiate group A streptococci from viral infections.

1. Infants with streptococcal infections commonly have excoriated nares and are listless.

2. Streptococcal infections in schoolage children produce complaints of sore throat accompanied by headache, vomiting, and abdominal pain.

3. Adults with streptococcal infections have tonsillar findings similar to the schoolage group but rarely have abdominal pain or a history of contact.

4. A scarlatiniform rash is diagnostic of streptococcal infection (infants rarely have this eruption).

5. Viral pharyngotonsillitis usually has associated conjunctivitis, cough, congestion, and hoarseness. Less toxicity is present.

6. Exudative pharyngitis accompanies group A streptococci, EB virus (infectious mononucleosis, p. 542), *Corynebacterium diphtheriae*, and adenovirus infections; soft-palate petechiae are found with group A streptococcal and EB virus infections; vesicles or ulcers on the posterior tonsillar pillars with enterovirus infection; and ulcers anterior with adenopathy in herpes infections.

Complications

1. Group A streptococci: acute rheumatic fever (p. 426) and acute glomerulonephritis (p. 607)
2. Otitis media (p. 452)
3. Cervical lymphadenopathy (p. 450)
4. Recurrent pharyngitis (histories rarely reliable). Culture documentation is important.

TABLE 73-2. Pharyngotonsillitis: diagnostic signs and symptoms

	Group A streptococci			Viral
	Infant	**Schoolage**	**Adult**	**Viral**
ONSET	Gradual	Sudden	Sudden	Gradual
CHIEF COMPLAINT	Anorexia, rhinitis, listlessness	Sore throat	Sore throat	Sore throat, cough, rhinitis, conjunctivitis
DIAGNOSTIC FINDINGS				
Sore throat	+	+ + +	+ + +	+ + +
Tonsillar erythema	+	+ + +	+ + +	+ +
Tonsillar exudate	+	+ +	+ + +	+
Palatal petechiae	+	+ + +	+ + +	+
Adenitis	+ +	+ + +	+ + +	+ +
Excoriated nares	+ + +	+	+	+
Conjunctivitis	+	+	+	+ + +
Cough	+	+	+	+ + +
Congestion	+	+	+	+ + +
Hoarseness	+	+	+	+ + +
Fever	Minimal	High	High	Minimal
Abdominal pain	+	+ +	+	+
Headache	+	+ +	+ +	+
Vomiting	+	+ +	+ +	+
Scarlatiniform rash	+	+ + +	+ + +	+
Streptococcal contact	+ + +	+ + +	+ + +	+
ANCILLARY DATA				
Positive streptococcal culture	+ + +	+ +	+ + +	+
Elevated WBC	+ +	+ +	+ + +	+

Ancillary data

Throat cultures are indicated for patients with sore throat with or without fever.

1. Cultures should normally be evaluated only for group A streptococci.
2. Infants should have their noses rather than their throats cultured.
3. Positive cultures with low colony counts may be indicative of the carrier states. To investigate this possibility, a Streptozyme must be ordered. Low titers are consistent with the chronic carrier state.
4. Symptomatic family members should have cultures.
5. If suggestive, culture for *C. diphtheriae*.
6. Rapid simple diagnostic tools to identify group A streptoccocci make immediate diagnosis possible, simplifying management. Some of the available tests include Culturette, Patho-Dx, Q-Test Stat, and Directigen.

MANAGEMENT

Symptomatic relief may be obtained by gargling with warm water, sucking hard candy, and initiating aspirin or acetaminophen (40-50 mg/kg/24 hr q 6 hr PO).

If the infection is streptococcal, antibiotic therapy should be administered for a total of 10 days of therapy (unless given IM):

1. Penicillin 25-50 (40,000-80,000 units) mg/kg/24 hr q 6 hr PO **or**
2. Benzathine penicillin G administered IM once (usually given as 900:300 Bicillin C-R—which is 75% benzathine—because it hurts less). Dosing should be calculated by the amount of benzathine required (see material at the bottom of the page).
3. An alternative antibiotic: erythromycin 30-50 mg/kg/24 hr q 8 hr PO. It has the additional benefit of treating other potential pharyngeal pathogens such as *Chlamydia* organisms.

Symptomatic improvement is noted following early therapy with antibiotics. Treatment also allows children to return to school or daycare sooner, thereby decreasing the associated family disruption. Patients may return to school (work or day-care) 24 hr after beginning medication. The risk of developing acute rheumatic fever and acute glomerulonephritis is not increased if antibiotics are started within 7 days of the onset of symptoms.

Indications for tonsillectomy for recurrent sore throats are controversial, and the procedure should be considered only in selected cases.

Evidence would suggest that the child with *problematic* group A streptococcal carriage may be treated with benzathine penicillin G as outlined above and rifampin 10 mg/kg/dose q 12 hr for 8 doses PO.

DISPOSITION

Patients may be followed at home.

Parental education

1. Medication should be taken for the full 10 days (unless given IM).
2. Symptomatic treatment may be helpful.
   a. Gargle with warm salt water (1 tsp. in 8 oz glass).
   b. Suck hard candy.
   c. Take aspirin or acetaminophen (10-15 mg/kg/dose q 6 hr prn PO).
3. Family members who are symptomatic with fever, sore throat, anorexia, or headache should have cultures.
4. Children may return to school in 24 hr.
5. Call physician if
   a. Your child develops severe pain, drooling, difficulty swallowing or breathing, or big, swollen lymph nodes
   b. There is evidence of infection elsewhere
   c. Fever lasts over 48 hr

REFERENCES

Berkowitz, C.D., Anthony, B.F., Kaplan, E.L., et al.: Cooperative study of latex agglutination to identify group A streptococcal antigen on throat swabs in patients with acute pharyngitis, J. Pediatr. **107**:89, 1985.

Breese, B.R.: A simple scorecard for the tentative diagnosis of streptococcal pharyngitis, Am. J. Dis. Child. **131**:514, 1977.

Krober, M.S., Bass, J.W., and Michels, G.N.: Streptococcal pharyngitis: placebo controlled double blind evaluation of clinical response to penicillin therapy, JAMA **253**:1271, 1985.

Nelson, J.D.: The effect of penicillin therapy on the symptoms and signs of streptococcal pharyngitis, Pediatr. Inf. Dis. **3**:10, 1984.

Weight (lb)	Benzathine pencillin G	Bicillin C-R (900,000 benzathine:300,000 procaine)
<30	300,000	300,000:100,000
31-60	600,000	600,000:200,000
61-90	900,000	900,000:300,000
>90	1,200,000	NA

Paradise, J.L., Bluestone, C.D., and Bachman, R.Z.: History of recurrent sore throat as an indication for tonsillectomy, N. Engl. J. Med. **298**:409, 1978.

Paradise, J.L., Bluestone, C.D., and Bachman, R.A.: Efficacy of tonsillectomy for recurrent throat infection in severely affected children: results of parallel randomized and nonrandomized clinical trials, N. Engl. J. Med. **310**:674, 1984.

Randolph, M.F., Gerber, M.A., DeMeo, K.K., and Wright, L.: Effect of antibiotic therapy on the clinical course of streptococcal pharyngitis, J. Pediatr. **106**:870, 1985.

Tanz, R.R., Shulman, S.T., Berthel, M.J., et al.: Penicillin plus rifampin eradicates pharyngeal carriage of group A streptococci, J. Pediatr. **106**:876, 1985.

Wannamaker, L.W.: Perplexity and precision in the diagnosis of streptococcal pharyngitis, Am. J. Dis. Child. **124**:352, 1972.

Retropharyngeal abscess

ALERT: Retropharyngeal abscess requires immediate intervention to prevent respiratory obstruction.

Otitis media and nasopharyngeal infections may lead to suppurative adenitis of the small lymph nodes between the buccopharyngeal and prevertebral fascia. If untreated, this can lead to abscess formation, particularly in children under 5 yr of age.

ETIOLOGY

Retropharyngeal abscess results from bacterial infection commonly caused by group A streptococci or *S. aureus*. It occurs by direct spread from nasopharyngitis, otitis media, or vertebral osteomyelitis or from wound infection following a penetrating injury of the posterior pharynx or palate.

DIAGNOSTIC FINDINGS

1. Nasopharyngitis or otitis media usually precedes the development of fever, difficulty swallowing, drooling, and severe throat pain. Meningismus may result from irritation of the paravertebral ligaments. Some complain of pain in the back of the neck or shoulder, precipitated or aggravated by swallowing.
2. Labored respirations with gurgling and hyperextension of the head are evidence of potential respiratory obstruction.
3. A definite unilateral posterior pharyngeal wall mass is present, often becoming fluctuant.

Complications

1. Obstruction of the trachea, esophagus, or nasal passages
2. Aspiration pneumonia if abscess ruptures. Possible dissection of purulent material into mediastinum
3. Sudden death if abscess erodes into major blood vessel

Ancillary data

1. Lateral neck x-ray film. Demonstrates increased soft tissue mass between the anterior wall of the cervical spine and the pharyngeal wall. In a child the retropharyngeal soft tissue should not be >5 mm at the level of C3 or 40% of the AP diameter of the body of C4 at that level.
2. WBC. Increased with shift to left
3. Cultures and Gram's stain of purulent material. Obtained from I and D

DIFFERENTIAL DIAGNOSIS

1. Infection: croup or epiglottitis
2. Trauma: foreign body

MANAGEMENT

1. Stabilization of the airway, if necessary
2. Antibiotics initiated immediately: nafcillin (or equivalent) 100-150 mg/kg/24 hr q 4 hr IV
3. Analgesia: meperidine (Demerol) 1-2 mg/kg/dose q 4-6 hr IM
4. I and D. Indicated immediately if obstruction is present or becomes fluctuant
   a. It is normally done in the operating room
   b. The head is positioned down and hyperextended to minimize aspiration.

DISPOSITION

All patients require hospitalization, antibiotics, and immediate otolaryngologic consultation.

REFERENCE

McCook, T.A., and Felman, A.H.: Retropharyngeal masses in infants and young children, Am. J. Dis. Child. 133:41, 1979.

Rhinitis (common cold)

Nasopharyngitis or rhinitis is common among children and represents what is usually a self-limited process.

ETIOLOGY: INFECTION

1. Viral: rhinovirus, respiratory syncytial virus (RSV), adenovirus, influenza, and parainfluenza
2. Bacterial: *C. diphtheriae, H. influenzae, S. pneumoniae, N. meningitidis*

DIAGNOSTIC FINDINGS

Patients have nasal congestion, sneezing, and, commonly, a clear watery discharge. Throat irritation and pharyngitis may be associated. There are minimal constitutional symptoms.

Associated clinical findings may include lymphadenopathy, otitis media, sinusitis, pneumonia, croup, and bronchiolitis. Allergic rhinitis is usually accompanied by pale, swollen, and boggy nasal mucosa.

Ancillary data

Nasal cultures should not be done since there is no way to interpret them unless nares are excoriated (group A streptococci).

MANAGEMENT

Symptomatic therapy is indicated by removing the discharge and attempting to decrease congestion.

1. In younger children, bulb syringe. May also use Neo-Synephrine nosedrops (⅛%) q 4 hr
2. In older children, bulb syringe or prescribe blowing and decongestants. Oxymetazoline (Afrin) nosedrops (0.025%-0.05%) q 8-12 hr may be useful. Routine antibiotic treatment of purulent nasopharyngitis is not useful.

Parental education

1. Place 2-3 drops of water or fresh salt water (½ tsp of salt in a cup of water) in each nostril with the child lying on the back.
   a. If old enough, have the child blow the nose.
   b. With a baby, use a rubber bulb syringe to remove the mucus.
2. Use a vaporizer in your child's room during napping and sleeping
3. For children over 18 mo of age, use decongestants such as pseudoephedrine and chlorpheniramine (can be obtained over the counter without prescription).
4. Call physician if
   a. Your child develops a fever and is under 3 mo of age
   b. The fever lasts over 24-48 hr
   c. Child develops difficulty breathing, is wheezing, or has croup or any other evidence of infection such as red eye or ear pain
   d. The skin under the nose becomes crusty

REFERENCES

Karlin, J.M.: The use of antihistamines in allergic disease, Pediatr. Clin. North Am. **22**:157, 1975.

Todd, J.K., Todd, N., Damato, J., Todd, W.A.: Bacteriology and treatment of purulent nasopharyngitis: a double blind, placebo controlled evaluation, Pediatr. Inf. Dis. 3:226, 1984.

Acute sinusitis

ALERT: Sinusitis may be associated with intracranial and extracranial infections.

Swelling of the nasal mucosa and obstruction of the meatus result in an acute inflammatory reaction within the sinuses.

ETIOLOGY

1. Infections
   a. Common bacterial. *H. influenzae* accounts for 19-32% of positive aerobic cultures; *S. pneumoniae* 9%-28%; group A streptococci 17%-27%; and *S. aureus* 6%-21%.
   b. Fungal infections in diabetics and immunocompromised patients
      NOTE: Cultures are nondiagnostic in as many as a third of patients.
2. Impairment of normal nasal physiology with poor ventilation and increased secretions secondary to adenoidal hypertrophy, polyps, cleft palate, or allergies
3. Trauma
4. Dental infections with contiguous spread

DIAGNOSTIC FINDINGS

1. Rhinorrhea is present in 78% of patients, 64% having a purulent discharge. Cough, often worse at night (50%), sinus pain or headache (12%), and temperatures over 38.5° C (101° F) (19%) are reported. Concurrent upper respiratory tract infections are common. Malodorous breath (fetor oris) may be noted.
2. Only 8% of patients have tenderness overlying the frontal, ethmoid, or maxillary sinuses, whereas 76% have unequal or poor transillumination. Transillumination is of limited value in children because of the variable development of sinuses before age 8-10 yr. Sphenoid sinusitis is associated with occipital pain and is rare in children. Swelling may be present over involved sinus.

Complications

These occur in 4.5% of patients:
1. Periorbital infections, particularly ethmoid (p. 432)
2. Osteomyelitis of the sinus wall, most commonly the frontal (this appears as Pott's puffy tumor, a midfrontal swelling)
3. Brain, subdural, or epidural abscesses
4. Meningitis

Ancillary data

1. Radiologic examination has variable reliability in young children. Normal sinus films are helpful. Abnormal sinus films are difficult to interpret, although after 6 yr of age the interpretation can be more definitive. Sinusitis appears as clouding, mucosal thickening, or air fluid levels within the sinuses, the latter being most helpful in defining an acute infection. Tomograms and, rarely, CT scan may be required in difficult cases.

   Radiographs are indicated if the child is seriously ill, had had recurrent episodes, or has chronic disease or suspected suppurative complications.
2. Antral puncture by an otolaryngologist is indicated if there is severe pain unresponsive to medical management, sinusitis in a seriously ill, toxic child, an unsatisfactory response, suppurative complications or if the patient is an immunocompromised host. A Gram's stain and an aerobic and anaerobic culture should be done on the aspirated material.

DIFFERENTIAL DIAGNOSIS

1. Allergy
2. Foreign body in nose (p. 449)
3. Neoplasm or polyp
4. Functional organic causes of headache (Chapter 36)

MANAGEMENT

The symptoms in bacterial sinusitis usually resolve in 48-72 hr. Up to 20% of patients have a persistent nasal discharge after a 2 wk course of antibiotics:
1. Antibiotics treatment for 2-3 wk total course
   a. Amoxicillin 50 mg/kg/24 hr q 8 hr PO; **or**
   b. Augmentin (amoxicillin with clavulanic acid) 20-40 mg/kg/24 hr q 8 hr PO; **or**
   c. Erythromycin 30-50 mg/kg/24 hr q 6 hr PO **and** sulfisoxazole (Gantrisin) 150 mg/kg/24 hr q 6 hr PO (available as a combination drug: Pediazole); **or**
   d. Erythromycin, (as in *c*) and trimethoprim/

sulfamethoxazole (8 mg/40 mg)/kg/24 hr
q 12 hr PO
NOTE: Failure to respond justifies the addition of dicloxacillin 50 mg/kg/24 hr q 6 hr PO.
2. Decongestants and antihistamines are of controversial value.
3. Desensitization rarely may be helpful if allergies are a contributory factor.
4. Sphenoid sinusitis requires aggressive antibiotic therapy (often parenteral), sometimes in conjunction with surgical drainage.

DISPOSITION

1. Patients usually may be discharged and instructed to take oral antibiotics at home for 2-3 wk. If symptoms do not resolve, patients should be referred to an otolaryngologist for assessment and possible irrigation of the antrum.
2. Patients with sphenoid sinusitis usually are hospitalized for parenteral therapy.

Parental education

The parent should call physician if
1. Symptoms worsen or patient develops a fever or toxicity
2. Symptoms have not improved markedly in 1 wk and disappeared in 2-3 wk

REFERENCES

Bluestone, C.D.: Medical and surgical therapy of sinusitis, Pediatr. Inf. Dis. **3**:513, 1984.
Kogutt, M.S., and Swischuck, L.E.: Diagnosis of sinusitis in infants and children, Pediatrics **52**:121, 1973.
Kovatch, A.L., Wald, E.R., Ledesma-Medina, J., et al.: Maxillary sinus radiographs in children with nonrespiratory complaints, Pediatrics **73**:306, 1984.
Lew, D., Southwick, F.S., Montgomery, W.W., et al.: Sphenoid sinusitis: a review of 30 cases, N. Engl. J. Med. **309**:1149, 1983.

Acute stomatitis

Acute stomatitis is generalized inflammation of the oral mucosa.

ETIOLOGY AND DIAGNOSTIC FINDINGS
Infection

1. Herpes simplex causes distinct multiple small ulcers of the oral mucosa and generalized inflammation. Rarely, other viruses (coxsackievirus) may cause diffuse ulceration, primarily on the palate, that lasts 7-10 days.
2. Thrush is caused by *Candida albicans*. The white plaques are predominantly on the buccal mucosa and tongue with generalized erythema.

Aphthous stomatitis or "canker sores"

These are erythematous, indurated papules that quickly erode to become painful circumscribed necrotic lesions of the mucosa that do not involve the lips. Their onset is often related to physical or emotional stress, and they resolve spontaneously in 1-2 wk.

Complication

Dehydration may result if oral intake is impaired by painful ulcers.

DIFFERENTIAL DIAGNOSIS

1. Infection: necrotizing ulcerative gingivitis (Vincent's angina) (p. 449)
2. Trauma
   a. Acid, alkali, or other caustic agents (p. 282)
   b. Mechanical or thermal injuries

MANAGEMENT

1. These entities are self-limited but occasionally cause discomfort and interfere with intake so that some intervention is appropriate. Approaches to local analgesia include:
   a. Antacid (Maalox or Mylanta) gargles or swallowed to coat the mucosa; **or**
   b. 1%-2% viscous lidocaine (Xylocaine) gargled or applied directly prn; **or**
   c. Mixture (1 part each) of lidocaine (2% viscous Xylocaine), diphenhydramine (Benadryl), and kaolin-pectin (Kaopectate), gargled prn
   NOTE: The dose of the 2% viscous lido-

caine (Xylocaine) should not exceed 15 ml q 3 hr or 120 ml in 24 hr in the adult (proportionately less in children). The patient should not eat or drink for 1 hr after application because of the danger of aspiration.

2. Frequent mouthwashes and alteration of diet to bland foods may help.

3. Thrush may be treated with nystatin (100,000 units/ml), using 1 ml (½ dropper) in each side of mouth 4 times/day, and continued 3-4 days after resolution.

DISPOSITION

Patients should be followed at home unless the hydration status requires inpatient therapy.

74 Endocrine disorders

Adrenal insufficiency

ETIOLOGY

1. Congenital: enzymatic defects, hemorrhage (birth injury), and hypoplasia
2. Infection
   a. Waterhouse-Friderichsen syndrome (adrenal hemorrhage), *Neisseria meningitidis, Streptococcus pneumoniae*
   b. Tuberculosis, histoplasmosis
3. Autoimmune disease
4. Withdrawal of steroid therapy or unusual stress in patient taking pharmacologic dosage of glucocorticosteroids (surgery, infection, etc.)

DIAGNOSTIC FINDINGS

See Table 74-1.

DIFFERENTIAL DIAGNOSIS

1. Acute insufficiency: infection, poisoning, diabetic ketoacidosis, hemorrhage
2. Addison's disease: CNS disease such as tumor or anorexia nervosa

MANAGEMENT

1. Initial management: restoration of intravascular volume with normal saline (0.9%NS), initially 20 ml/kg and then at a rate reflecting vital signs. Correction, when appropriate, of electrolytes, glucose, and acid-base status should be achieved. Hypotension may require pressor agents.
2. Adrenal corticosteroid replacement therapy (Table 74-2)

   a. Acute crisis:
      (1) Hydrocortisone (Solu-Cortef) 2 mg/kg/dose q 4-6 hr IV **and**
      (2) Cortisone 1-5 mg/kg/24 hr q 12-24 hr PO to allow tapering of intravenous medications. Intramuscular cortisone therapy often is recommended initially to facilitate the transition to oral therapy once stabilization has occurred.
   b. Addison's disease
      (1) Glucocorticoid
         (a) Hydrocortisone 0.5 mg/kg/24 hr (15-20 mg/m²/24 hr) q 6-8 hr PO **or**
         (b) Cortisone 0.5-0.75 mg/kg/24 hr (20 mg/m²/24 hr) q 6-8 hr PO **or**
         (c) Prednisone 0.1-0.15 mg/kg/24 hr (4-5 mg/m²/24 hr) PO

TABLE 74-1. Adrenal insufficiency

Clinical manifestation	Acute	Chronic (Addison's disease)
Nausea/vomiting	+ + +	+ + +
Abdominal pain	+ +	+ +
Hypothermia	+	±
Hypotension	+ + +	+ + +
Dehydration	+ +	±
Failure to thrive	−	+
Fatigue/weakness	+ + +	+ + +
Confusion, coma	+	−
Hyperpigmentation	−	+ +
Hypoglycemia	+ +	+ +
↓ Na⁺/↑ K⁺	+ + +	+ + +

TABLE 74-2. Adrenal corticosteroids

Drug	Availability	Dose*	Frequency (hr)	Glucocorticoid effect†	Mineralocorticoid effect††
GLUCOCORTICOIDS					
Cortisone	IM: 25,50 mg/ml PO: 5,25 mg	0.25 mg/kg/24 hr 0.5-0.75 mg/kg/24 hr	q 12-24 q 6-8	100 mg	100 mg
Hydrocortisone (Solu-Cortef)	PO: 5,10,20 mg IV/IM: 100,250,500 mg	0.5 mg/kg/24 hr Shock‡: 50 mg/kg/dose (maximum: 500 mg) Asthma§: 4-5 mg/kg/dose	q 8	80 mg	80 mg
Prednisone	PO: 1,5,10,20 mg, 5 mg/5 ml	0.1-0.15 mg/kg/24 hr Asthma: 1-2 mg/kg/24 hr	q 6 q 12 q 6	20 mg	Little effect
Methylprednisolone (Solu-Medrol)	IV: 40,125,500,1,000 mg	Shock: 30-50 mg/kg/dose Asthma: 1-2 mg/kg/dose	q 6	16 mg	No effect
Dexamethasone (Decadron)	IV/IM: 4,24 mg/ml	Shock: 3 mg/kg/dose Cerebral edema: 0.25-0.5/kg/dose Croup: 0.25 mg/kg/dose	q 6 q 6	2 mg	No effect
MINERALOCORTICOIDS					
Fludrocortisone (Florinef)	PO: 0.1 mg	0.05-0.1 mg/24 hr	q 24	5 mg	0.2 mg
Desoxycorticosterone (DOCA)	IM: 5 mg/ml (in oil)	1-5 mg/24-48 hr	q 24-48	No effect	2 mg

With long-term therapy, dose requires adjustment. Attempt q.o.d. dosing when employing pharmacologic doses. Long-acting preparations for physiologic replacement are available with monthly (or longer) activity.
*Physiologic replacement unless otherwise indicated.
†Equivalent doses required for same clinical effect.
‡Use of steroids controversial for shock and septic shock.
§Asthma, Status asthmaticus.

(2) Mineralocorticoids
    (a) Fludrocortisone (Florinef) 0.05-0.1 mg/24 hr PO **or**
    (b) Desoxycorticosterone 1-5 mg/24-48 hr IM
3. Antibiotics when indicated
4. Corticosteroids to patients with adrenal insufficiency who are undergoing surgery
    a. Administer hydrocortisone (Solu-Cortef) 1-2 mg/kg IV (or equivalent) before surgery. In emergency, administer as preanesthetic drug. If elective, administer in 4 doses over 48 hr.
    b. During anesthesia, administer hydrocortisone 25-100 mg IV.
    c. Following surgery, give hydrocortisone 0.5-1.0 mg/kg/dose q 6 hr IV for 3 days and then taper to presurgical levels (if any).

DISPOSITION

Patients with acute adrenal crisis should be admitted to an ICU. In cases of chronic illness, disposition must be determined by clinical status and ease of follow-up, which is essential.

Diabetic ketoacidosis

ALERT: Start treatment early with hydration. Insulin may be given once a glucose determination has been made. Always look for a precipitating cause.

Diabetes mellitus has certain unique features in the pediatric age-group. Children are more subject to infection, emotional and environmental stresses, increased caloric requirements, and extremes of activity and dietary patterns. These place the child with diabetes at risk of developing ketoacidosis.

Diabetic ketoacidosis (DKA) requires attention when a patient is hyperglycemic (>300 mg/dl), ketonemic (serum ketones large at $>1:2$ dilution), or acidotic (pH <7.1 or HCO_3 <12 mEq/L) and is experiencing glycosuria and ketonuria.

ETIOLOGY: PRECIPITATING FACTORS

1. Infection: virus, bacteria (group A streptococci or abscess is common)
2. Intrapsychic: emotional or environmental stresses at home or school. Adolescents often manipulate their surroundings by becoming ill.
3. Drugs and diet: alteration of normal insulin dosage (poor compliance), steroids, birth control pills. Major change in diet
4. Trauma: major trauma or surgery
5. Endocrine: pregnancy, Cushing's syndrome, hyperthyroidism

DIAGNOSTIC FINDINGS

DKA is marked by tachypnea with Kussmaul's respiration (deep, rapid pattern), tachycardia, orthostatic blood pressure changes, acetone on the breath, vomiting, dehydration, and mental status changes, which may lead to obtundation and coma. Abdominal pain is a common finding, often mimicking an acute surgical condition, which resolves with treatment of the acidosis.

It is imperative to document the history of diabetes mellitus, standard insulin regimen, past management, duration of symptoms, estimated weight loss, and presence of precipitating factors.

Patients not previously diagnosed may give a history of excessive or poor food intake, weight loss, or dehydration in the face of large urinary output. A dehydrated child with a normal or large urine flow must be considered diabetic until proved otherwise.

Those whose diabetes is in poor control have polyuria, polydipsia, polyphagia, and weight loss. Recurrent episodes of DKA often are associated with psychosocial dysfunction.

Complications

1. Dehydration with metabolic acidosis (differential of metabolic acidosis: p. 277)
2. Coma and seizures, possibly caused by cerebral edema. Many patients have subclinical brain swelling from cerebral vasodilation or cerebral edema, often noted following volume expansion.

3. Death from CNS or metabolic complications
   Hyperosmolar nonketotic coma with glucose between 800-1,200 mg/dl rarely occurs in children; it occurs more frequently in adults. Patients may not be acidotic, but they do have hyperglycemia, hyperosmolality, and dehydration. They also may be comatose, presumably because of a relative water deficiency. This has been reported in children under 2 yr and in children with preexisting neurologic damage.

Ancillary data

1. Electrolytes may be abnormal with an anion gap (p. 53) and must be monitored q 2-4 hr during stabilization.
   a. Hyponatremia resulting from urinary losses. Sodium may be artificially depressed by hyperglycemia and hyperlipidemia. An estimate of the true serum sodium may be derived as follows:

Corrected serum Na$^+$ (mEq/L) = Measured serum Na$^+$
   (mEq/L) + (Plasma glucose [mg/dl] − 100 × 0.016)

   b. A total body potassium deficit (the serum level may be normal). Serum potassium increases 0.5 mEq/L for each 0.1 decrease in pH.
   c. Acidosis with a low bicarbonate and pH, the degree of decrease reflecting the severity of disease
   d. BUN is usually elevated
2. Glucose is elevated above 300 mg/dl with glucosuria and must be monitored q 1-2 hr until stable. Screening by Dextrostix or Chemstrip may provide a bedside estimate. Serum osmolarity should be determined if the glucose is >1,000 mg/dl.
3. Serum ketones are large at a dilution of ≥1:2 with ketonuria. Ketone measurements

reflect acetoacetate but not beta-hydroxybutyrate. Since the latter dissociates to acetoacetate with clinical improvement, ketonemia may persist despite clinical resolution and should be checked q 2-4 hr until clear.
4. Urinalysis will reveal glucosuria and ketonuria. The normal renal glucose threshold is about 180 mg/dl.
5. Arterial blood gas demonstrates a respiratory alkalosis superimposed on a metabolic acidosis.
6. Amylase may be elevated; WBC is variable.
7. ECG may be used to rapidly assess serum potassium levels (p. 37).
8. Cultures of throat, blood, urine, and cervix are done as indicated.
9. Glycosylated hemoglobin gives an excellent measure of the degree of long-term control.

MANAGEMENT
Initial management

Initial stabilization must include intravenous fluids, cardiac monitoring, and determination of serum electrolytes, glucose, acetone, BUN, and venous (or arterial) pH. A bedside Dextrostix or Chemstrip test may facilitate management. Laboratory data should be repeated every 1-2 hr during the initial treatment periods. Vital signs, fluids, insulin, and urinary output must be monitored and followed on a flow sheet.

Initial therapy should begin with aggressive hydration, infusing 0.9%NS at a rate of 20 ml/kg over 30 min, with partial reconstitution of vascular space and expected improvement in blood pressure, pulse, and respiration. If there is no response, this is repeated.

Following the initial bolus, fluid and electrolyte therapy must reflect maintenance and deficit requirements. Patients typically have an isotonic 10% dehydration (Chapter 7):

1. Summary of fluid requirements*

	H_2O (ml)	Na (mEq)	K (mEq)
Maintenance	1,500 (50-100 ml/kg)	60 (3 mEq/kg)	40 (2 mEq/kg)
Deficit			
(100 ml/kg)			
ECF (60%)	1,200	168 (140 mEq $\times$ 1.2)	
ICF (40%)	800		60 (150 mEq $\times$ 0.8 $\times$ 50% correction)
TOTAL	2,000	168	60

2. Fluid schedule

		Fluids	
Time	**Calculation**		**Administered**
0-1 hr	20 ml/kg		400 ml 0.9%NS over 45 min
1-9 hr	½ deficit: 1,000 ml with 84 mEq NaCl and 30 ml KCl		1,500 ml (~200 ml/hr) of 0.45%NS with 30 mEq KCl/L
	⅓ maintenance: 500 ml with 20 mEq NaCl and 13 mEq KCl		
	Total: 1,500 ml with 104 mEq NaCl and 43 mEq KCl		
9-25 hr	½ deficit		2,000 ml (~125 ml/hr) of 0.45%NS with 30 mEq KCl/L
	⅔ maintenance		

These calculations facilitate care, and the rates often need to be increased because of the obligate excessive urinary losses. If the patient is significantly acidotic with pH <7.0 or HCO_3 <10 mEq/L, sodium bicarbonate can be given in conjunction with normal (0.9%NS) or half-normal (0.45%) saline. The bicarbonate deficit should be only partially corrected. In patients requiring sodium bicarbonate therapy, administer 1-2 mEq/kg over 30 min while monitoring the response. Normally, the pH does not need to be actively corrected above 7.1-7.15, since correction of intravascular volume will facilitate the return to normal values and excessive administration of sodium bicarbonate may lead to alkalosis.

Potassium must be added to the infusion early (after initial flush) because of the total body deficit. Potassium acetate may be substituted for

potassium chloride if the patient is highly acidotic. Some clinicians prefer KPO_4 because of a relatively common phosphorus depletion, but there is no evidence that this is beneficial.

Glucose should be added to the IV fluid infusion when the glucose is <250 mg/dl (without stopping the infusion of insulin). One unit of insulin will cause intracellular movement of 2-4 g of glucose.

Those with mild to moderate disease who respond rapidly to the initial fluid management can be given oral hydration if vomiting has ceased and vital signs are stable with normovolemia.

Patients with only mild diabetes and without significant acidosis may be managed by oral hydration if vomiting is not a problem. Patients with nonketotic hyperosmolar diabetic coma respond to hydration, replacement of electrolyte deficits, and reduction of serum glucose and hyperosmolarity. Fluid therapy is primary.

---

*For a 20 kg (pre-illness weight) patient with a 10% (100 ml H_2O/kg) isotonic dehydration.

Insulin

Insulin is the second major component of therapy. Infusion must be related to the state of hydration, fluid management, and laboratory data. Several routes of administration are available. U100 preparations are commonly used.

1. Continuous regular insulin IV infusion causes a smooth fall in glucose, with lower incidence of hypoglycemia and hypokalemia and better ongoing control of therapy. Optimally, glucose falls 50-100 mg/dl/hr.
   - Method: 50 units of regular insulin are mixed in 250 ml of 0.9%NS (0.2 units/ml) and infused at a rate of 0.1-0.2 units/kg/hr. Run insulin solution through IV tubing before initiating therapy.
2. Intramuscular injection of regular insulin is an acceptable alternative, 0.1-0.2 units/kg/hr injected intramuscularly.

Insulin administration should not be stopped when the glucose is <250 mg/dl. The hourly insulin dose is lowered and glucose is added to the fluid to maintain a serum glucose around 200-250 mg/dl. Insulin infusion or IM injections should be stopped and SQ insulin begun when the patient has negative serum acetone at a dilution of 1:2.

SQ insulin is initiated at the rate of 0.25-0.5 units/kg q 6 hr. It is sometimes useful to establish a sliding scale based on the glucose and acetone in the urine (Table 74-3). The scale must be individualized.

Long-acting insulin should be initiated as soon as possible. This therapy should be coordinated with the primary care provider. Typically, patients require 0.5-1.0 unit/kg/day divided so that ⅔ dose is administered in the morning and ⅓ in the evening. A common insulin mixture is ⅔ NPH insulin and ⅓ regular insulin to provide a smooth pattern (Table 74-4).

NOTE: Patients with newly diagnosed diabetes have a low initial insulin requirement. At time of initial diagnosis, insulin requirement is high (≤1 unit/kg/24 hr). This requirement falls rapidly ("honeymoon period") to as little as 0.1-0.3 units/kg/24 hr for the next few weeks to months.

Recently, insulin pumps have been introduced with the potential for markedly improved control.

DISPOSITION

Patients with significant DKA require hospitalization unless prolonged observation with monitoring equipment, personnel, and expertise is available in the ambulatory setting. Patients with pH <7.0, and HCO_3^- <10 mEq/L, or altered mental status should be hospitalized early in treatment. In addition, those with intercurrent infections often require admission. Those with their first episode usually should be hospitalized for control and education.

Insulin therapy on discharge should be coordinated with the primary care provider. All diabetic patients require close follow-up. This must be ensured before discharge.

REFERENCES

Chase, H.P.: Office management of diabetes mellitus in children, Postgrad. Med. 59:243, 1976.

Fisher, J.N., Shahshahani, M.N., and Kitabchi, A.E.: Diabetic ketoacidosis: low-dose insulin therapy by various routes, N. Engl. J. Med. 297:238, 1977.

Krane, E.J., Rockoff, M.A., Wallman, J.V., and Wolfsdorf, J.I.: Subclinical brain swelling in children during treatment of diabetic ketoacidosis, N. Engl. J. Med. 312:1147, 1983.

Owens, D.R., Hayes, T.M., Alberti, K.G., et al.: Comparative study of subcutaneous, intramuscular and intravenous administration of human insulin, Lancet 118:121, 1981.

Sperling, M.A.: Diabetic ketoacidosis, Pediatr. Clin. North Am. 31:591, 1984.

White, K., Kolman, M.L., Wexler, O., et al.: Unstable diabetes and unstable families: a psychosocial evaluation of diabetic children with recurrent ketoacidosis, Pediatrics 73:749, 1984.

Thyroid disease

THYROIDITIS

Chronic lymphocytic thyroiditis (Hashimoto's disease) is an autoimmune disease. It accounts

TABLE 74-3. Sliding scale for 4 hr insulin

Urine sugar* (g/dl)	Insulin (units) required by body weight†			
	10 kg	15-30 kg	30-45 kg	>45 kg
5%†	3-5	8-12	15-20	20-25
4%	2-3	5-8	10-15	15-20
3%	1-2	2-5	5-10	10-15
2%	1	2	5	5-10

*2-drop Clinitest method on double-voided urine.
†Maximum dose: 0.5 units/kg.

TABLE 74-4. Insulin preparations

Insulin product by rapidity of onset of action	Hypoglycemic effect (hr)			Compatible with regular insulin
	Onset	Peak	Duration	
RAPID				
Regular crystalline	$\frac{1}{2}$	2-4	6-8	Yes
Semilente	$\frac{1}{2}$	2-4	10-12	Yes
INTERMEDIATE				
NPH	2	8-10	16-20	Yes
Lente	2	8-10	20-26	Yes
DELAYED				
Ultralente	4-8	14-24	≥36	No

for the majority of nontoxic goiters, with a peak incidence between 8-15 yr and a female predominance of 4:1.

Diagnostic findings

Thyroid enlargement is noted in over 85% of patients—the thyroid usually being firm and nontender and having a cobblestone sensation. Patients rarely are symptomatic.

Ancillary data (Table 74-5)

Thyroglobin and microsomal antibodies may be elevated. Function studies are usually normal.

Differential diagnosis

1. Simple colloid goiter
2. Infection. Suppurative thyroiditis has an acute onset of fever, dysphagia, sore throat, and painful, tender swelling in the area of the thyroid. Commonly it results from mixed aerobic and anaerobic organisms, with *Staphylococcus aureus* rarely being cultured. Antibiotics (penicillin or dicloxacillin) or surgical drainage is required.

Management

Patients with documented hypothyroidism should be treated with replacement doses of sodium L-thyroxine (100 μg/m²/24 hr). Patients with euthyroidism are usually treated, because some patients develop hypothyroidism. Such treatment ordinarily reduces the goiter size.

Disposition

All patients should be followed at home for at least 6 mo. If treatment was not initiated, they

TABLE 74-5. Thyroid function tests: common disorders of thyroid function

Disorder	Serum thyroxine (T₄)	Triiodothyronine resin uptake	Serum thyrotropin	Comments
Chronic lymphocytic thyroiditis				
Euthyroid	WNL	WNL to ↑	WNL to ↑	Thyroglobin/micromal antibody increased
Hypothyroid	↓	WNL to ↓	↑	
Hyperthyroid	↑	↑	↓	
Hyperthyroid	↑ *	↑	↓	
Hypothyroid				
Primary	↓	↓	↑	
Secondary	↓	↓	↓	Decreased response TRH
TBG				
↓ TBG	↓	↑	WNL	Free thyroxin index normal
↑ TBG (pregnancy, birth control pills)	↑	↓	WNL	Free thyroxin index normal

Modified from Fisher, D.A.: Advances in the laboratory diagnosis of thyroid disease, J. Pediatr. **82**:187, 1973.
TRH, Thyroid-releasing hormone. TBG, Thyroid-binding globulin.
*May be normal or low in triiodothyronine toxicosis.

should be reevaluated at 6 mo intervals to assess thyroid function.

HYPERTHYROIDISM
Etiology

1. Autoimmune (Graves' disease). Often associated with other autoimmune diseases. About 10% of patients with chronic lymphocytic thyroiditis develop hyperthyroidism.
2. Hypothalamic or pituitary dysfunction. Rare
3. Congenital. Present in children of mothers who have or have had Graves' disease. May persist to 6-12 mo and may have postneonatal onset.

Diagnostic findings

Patients usually have a gradual onset of symptoms, with an enlarged thyroid gland and associated decreasing school performance, weight loss, tachycardia, eye prominence and exophthalmos, motor hyperactivity with tremor, and increased sweating. Atrial fibrillation can be present.

Thyroid storm is very rare in children. It is manifested by acute onset of hyperthermia, tachycardia, sweating, and nervousness. It occurs almost exclusively in patients with preexisting hyperthyroidism, secondary to a diffuse toxic goiter (Graves' disease).

Complications

Hyperthyroidism can cause an elevated metabolic rate, with delirium, coma, and, potentially, death.

Ancillary data
See Table 74-5.

Differential diagnosis

Hyperthyroidism should be differentiated from a neoplasm such as pheochromocytoma.

Management

Several management options exist.

1. Most clinicians inhibit synthesis of thyroid hormone and initiate oral antithyroid medication (propylthiouracil 5 mg/kg/24 hr up to 300 mg/24 hr) for 3-4 yr unless remission occurs earlier.
2. Surgery is indicated for patients whose com-

pliance is poor, for those whose glands are 3-4 times their normal size, and for those with adenomas or carcinomas. Patients must be euthyroid before surgery. The use of radioactive iodides in children is controversial.

3. Propranolol 10-20 mg/dose q 6-8 hr PO is useful initially for patients in a hypermetabolic state. In patients with thyroid storm, immediate therapy with propranolol 1-2 mg/dose IV initially, followed by oral therapy, is indicated. Propranolol is contraindicated in patients with congestive heart failure. Fluid deficits, hyponatremia, and hyperthermia should be corrected.

Disposition

Patients generally can be followed clinically and chemically at home, with frequent visits for at least 3-4 yr. Patients with thyroid storm require hospitalization.

HYPOTHYROIDISM

1. Congenital: aplasia, hypoplasia, errors of metabolism, autoimmune disease, maternal ingestion of drugs or goitrogens during pregnancy
2. Autoimmune: chronic lymphocytic thyroiditis (Hashimoto's thyroiditis)
3. Intoxication: iodides, radiation
4. Hypothalamic or pituitary dysfunction
5. Trauma: neck injury or surgery
6. Infection: viral (rarely aerobic or anaerobic bacteria)
7. Neoplasm: primary (carcinoma) or secondary infiltration

Diagnostic findings

Clinical presentation is variable, depending on the patient's age and duration of illness. Although a large majority of patients with congenital hypothyroidism are asymptomatic, they may be lethargic and eat poorly. Less commonly, hypotonia, prolonged jaundice, umbilical hernia, wide fontanel, or delayed growth is noted. Most states require neonatal screening, and the diagnosis should be made early.

In later childhood, patients exhibit growth retardation, delays in dentition, edema, poor performance (school and play), hoarseness, delayed tendon reflexes with flabby muscles, and a dull, placid expression.

Complications

Myxedema coma (usually caused by autoimmune [Hashimoto's] thyroiditis, ^{131}I therapy, or surgery) is extremely rare but may accompany coma, hypothermia, hypoglycemia, and respiratory failure. Therapy is initiated parenterally.

Ancillary data
See Table 74-5.

MANAGEMENT

Hormone replacement is initiated after obtaining laboratory specimens to evaluate function. Levothyroxine (Synthroid) is a stable, synthetic hormone that can be given once a day. Dosage should be adjusted to maintain the serum thyroxine (T_4) between 10-12 µg/dl.

Age	Dosage (µg/kg/24 hr)	Average levothyroxine/24 hr
<6 mo	8-10	25-50 µg
6-12 mo	6-8	50-75 µg
1-5 yr	5-6	75-100 µg
6-12 yr	4-5	100-150 µg
>12 yr	2-3	100-200 µg

In older children, there is usually less urgency, and the child should be started on a low dose (25 µg/24 hr) and increased every 2-4 wk until full replacement is achieved. Patients should be monitored closely.

Therapy for myxedema coma should be initiated parenterally. The adult dose is 200-500 µg levothyroxine IV, followed by 50 µg/24 hr IV.

Disposition

Patients without complications should have therapy initiated and be followed as outpatients with laboratory tests repeated in 2 wk. Serum thyroxine and serum thyrotropin are the tests of choice. Because excessive therapy in the infant may cause cranial synostosis and brain dysfunction, infants should be monitored at 3 mo intervals in the first year of life.

75 Eye disorders

James Sprague

Chalazion and hordeolum

A *chalazion* is an inflammatory granulomatous nodule of the meibomian gland on an otherwise normal eyelid. It results from retained secretions of a gland. There may be physical discomfort as well as some disfigurement, from the mass effect of the nodule.

Hot compresses are used initially to encourage drainage. The chalazion may be incised and curetted by an ophthalmologist. It also may respond to steroid injection.

A *hordeolum (stye)* is a painful, tender, erythematous infection of the hair follicle of the eyelashes, usually resulting from *Staphylococcus aureus*. A hordeolum usually points and drains and may occur in multiple sites. Very rarely is it complicated by periorbital cellulitis (p. 432).

Hot compresses are useful; if a stye does not drain spontaneously, incision and drainage may be done. Topical medications probably are not helpful, and recurrent multiple lesions may respond to systemic antistaphylococcal agents.

Conjunctivitis

Conjunctivitis is by far the most common cause of red eyes in children. The etiology and management vary with the age of the child.

ETIOLOGY AND DIAGNOSTIC FINDINGS

1. Infection
   a. Bacterial
      (1) *Haemophilus influenzae*. Bilateral and purulent
      (2) *Streptococcus pneumoniae*. Purulent
      (3) *Neisseria gonorrhoeae*. Occurs in the first few weeks of life; large amount of hyperacute mucopurulent discharge; also occurs in sexually active individuals
      (4) *S. aureus*. Rare
      (5) *Pseudomonas* organisms secondary to contact lens
   b. Viral
      (1) Adenovirus. Serous discharge with associated pharyngitis
      (2) Herpes simplex. Possible dendritic spreading, with corneal ulcer and keratitis; unilateral; vesicle on eyelid may be present
      (3) Varicella. Vesicle on lid; conjunctivitis
   c. *Chlamydia trachomatis*. Purulent discharge beginning at 5-15 days of life; possible associated pneumonia; primary infectious cause in infants
2. Allergy
   a. Watery discharge with chemosis and edema of the conjunctiva
   b. Bulbar conjunctivitis
   c. Rhinorrhea

d. Seasonal allergy
3. Foreign body, irritative or chemical (Chapter 59)
   a. Unilateral with acute onset and variable history of exposure
   b. Fluorescein staining positive with foreign body or marked irritation
   c. Chemical conjunctivitis. May occur bilaterally in newborns after delivery if silver nitrate drops are not well irrigated; in older children it is secondary to cosmetics, drugs, eyedrops, or air pollution.

DIFFERENTIAL DIAGNOSIS (Tables 75-1 and 75-2)

In addition to various distinguishing etiologic agents that cause infectious conjunctivitis, a number of other entities must be considered:
1. Foreign body: usually associated with pain, photophobia with normal visual acuity; fluorescein positive (p. 334)
2. Acute glaucoma: vision impaired with minimal conjunctival injection; photophobia; small or midsize fixed pupil; rare
3. Acute uveitis: impaired vision; photophobia; small, irregular pupil; rare, often secondary to trauma, herpes, or conjunctivitis
4. Iritis: blurred vision with severe acute unilateral pain; photophobia; flush around limbus
5. Allergic conjunctivitis: vision normal, watery discharge, seasonal

MANAGEMENT

1. Foreign body, if present, should be removed (p. 334).
2. Allergic conjunctivitis may be treated, if significantly symptomatic, with antihistamines: diphenhydramine (Benadryl) 5 mg/kg/24 hr q 6 hr PO for 3-5 days **or** hydroxyzine (Vistaril, Atarax) 2 mg/kg/24 hr q 6 hr PO
3. Infectious conjunctivitis
   a. *Chlamydia* organisms may be treated with oral erythromycin (30-50 mg/kg/24 hr q 6-8 hr PO) **or** sulfisoxazole (Gantrisin) (150

mg/kg/24 hr q 6 hr PO)
   b. Herpes conjunctivitis should be referred to an ophthalmologist. Treatment is controversial and constantly evolving.
   c. Bacterial and viral conjunctivitis should in general be treated with sulfacetamide or sulfisoxazole ophthalmic ointment or solution for 2 days beyond clearing.
      (1) Sulfacetamide (10%-15%) or sulfisoxazole (4%) solution (drops) q 2-4 hr in eye; **or**
      (2) Sulfacetamide (10%) or sulfisoxazole (4%) ointment q 4-6 hr in eye
   d. Gonococcal ophthalmia requires systemic antibiotics. Full-term infants may be treated with aqueous penicillin G 50,000 units/kg/24 hr q 8 hr IV for 7 days.

DISPOSITION
Parental education

1. Before using topical medication, remove the yellow discharge and dried matter from the eye with a wet cotton ball and warm water.
2. Place 2 drops of sulfacetamide drops in each eye every 2-4 hr (or as often as possible) while your child is awake until the eye is improving, when you can decrease the frequency.
   a. For younger children, you will receive an ointment only, which may be used 4 times/day but which blurs vision. It also may be used for bad infections at bedtime in conjunction with the drops.
   b. Continue the medication until your child has awakened for 2 mornings without discharge.
3. Your child may infect other people. The use of separate towels and washcloths, as well as careful handwashing, are helpful.
4. Call physician if
   a. Infection has not responded in 72 hr
   b. Eyelids become red or swollen
   c. Eyeball becomes cloudy or sores develop on it
   d. Vision becomes blurred
   e. Eye becomes painful or develops photophobia

TABLE 75-1. Infective conjunctivitis: diagnostic findings and management

Etiology	Epidemiology	Diagnostic findings						Management*
		Vision	Pain	Photophobia	Discharge	Cornea	Conjunctiva	
BACTERIA (a,d)								
S. pneumoniae H. influenzae	Bilateral, history of exposure	WNL	None	None	Purulent; PMN on smear	WNL	Injected papillary	Topical antibiotics
VIRAL (d)								
Adenovirus (b) types 8, 19, 3, and 7	Incubation: 5-14 days; history of exposure; systemic symptoms; preauricular node	Often decreased	FBS	±	Mucoid; mononuclear on smear	Punctate keratopathy	Injected follicles	Topical antibiotics
Herpes (c)	Unilateral; often secondary	±	FBS	+	Mucoid; mononuclear on smear	Dendrite	Injected follicles	Refer to ophthalmologist
Varicella (chickenpox)	"Pox" may involve lid, rarely cornea	WNL	±	±	Mucoid; mononuclear on smear	±	Injected follicles	Follow
CHLAMYDIA	May be recurrent if inadequately treated	WNL	±	None	Inclusion bodies on Giemsa	WNL	Injected follicles	Erythromycin for 2-3 wk

FBS, Foreign body sensation.

*Do not prescribe topical analgesics for *prn* use.

a. "Bacterial" conjunctivitis unresponsive to topical antibiotics more often results from viral agents or from insensitivity to antibiotics.

b. Adenoviral conjunctivitis also is known as epidemic keratoconjunctivitis. Children should be kept out of school until resolution.

c. Herpes simplex can be difficult to diagnose. Since steroids dramatically worsen herpes keratitis, they should *not* be prescribed without clear indications.

d. Prolonged treatment with neomycin-containing antibiotics can cause local sensitivity.

TABLE 75-2. Neonatal ophthalmia: diagnostic findings

Etiology	Incubation period	Diagnostic findings	Management
CHEMICAL Silver nitrate	24 hr	Diffuse injection; culture: negative	Wait and watch
GONOCOCCAL *Neisseria gonorrhoeae*	24-72 hr	Hyperpurulent; history of infected birth canal or infected contact; smear: typical gonococcus	Systemic and topical antibiotics
CHLAMYDIA (inclusion conjunctivitis) *Chlamydia trachomatis*	7-10 days	Indolent, although often purulent; history of infected birth canal; may have had partial response to topical antibiotics; no follicles in infant; smear: cytoplasmic inclusion; culture: negative	Systemic erythromycin or sulfonamides; exclude systemic disease
OTHER BACTERIA	2-5 days	Purulent or hyperpurulent	Topical antibiotics

REFERENCES

Gigliotti, F., Williams, W.T., Hayden, F.G., et al.: Etiology of acute conjunctivitis in children, Pediatrics **98**:531, 1981.

Heggie, A.D., Jaffe, A.C., Stuart, L.A., et al.: Topical sulfacetamide vs oral erythromycin for neonatal chlamydial conjunctivitis, Am. J. Dis. Child. **139**:564, 1985.

76 Gastrointestinal disorders

Acute infectious diarrhea

ALERT: Rapid assessment of the patient's state of hydration, complications, and likely etiologic agents is imperative.

Acute infectious diarrhea is accompanied by an increase in stool number or water content. Commonly, a host of viral and bacterial agents and parasites is associated with unique epidemiologic and clinical characteristics (Chapter 32).

ETIOLOGY AND DIAGNOSTIC FINDINGS
(Table 76-1)
Rotavirus (or *Reovirus* organisms)

This accounts for 39% of patients requiring hospitalization for diarrheal disease. It occurs commonly in the cooler months, usually affecting children 6-18 mo of age. Vomiting is a prominent early symptom, often preceding the onset of diarrhea, which is loose, relatively frequent (>5 stools/day), and rarely associated with mucus or blood. Respiratory symptoms may accompany the GI symptoms that last for 2-3 days.

Norwalk agent

This is a viral agent associated with epidemic disease. Symptomatically, patients have nausea, vomiting, abdominal cramps, lethargy, and fever associated with diarrhea.

Salmonella organisms

Multiple animal reservoirs (cattle, poultry, shellfish, rodents, and turtles) facilitate trans-mission. This is more common in warm months.

1. Gastroenteritis is the most common clinical presentation.
   a. It primarily affects children under 5 yr of age.
   b. Symptoms of fever, vomiting, and diarrhea begin 24-48 hr after exposure, diminishing over 3-5 days. Older children may have abdominal pain, often confused with an acute appendicitis.
2. Septicemia may occur because of the potential of penetrating the lamina propria. Meningitis, osteomyelitis, septic arthritis, endocarditis, pneumonia, and urinary tract infections (UTI) have been reported. Children under 1 yr of age and those who have sickle cell disease or other hemoglobinopathies or who are immunocompromised are at increased risk.
3. *Salmonella typhi* causes severe, prolonged disease with gastroenteritis associated with fever, malaise, headache, and myalgias. Hepatosplenomegaly and rose spots (2 mm maculopapular lesions) may appear.

   Prolonged shedding of *Salmonella* organisms in the stool is a common finding, stools being positive for several months.

Shigella organisms

1. These are commonly spread by person-to-person transmission, occurring most frequently in children under 5 yr of age.
2. Patients have rapid onset of fever, crampy abdominal pain, and diarrhea. Stools are wa-

TABLE 76-1. Clinical features of acute diarrheal disease

	Viral	Salmonella organisms	Shigella organisms
Age	Any age	Any age	6 mo-5 yr
Onset	Abrupt	Variable	Abrupt
Incubation	Variable	12-36 hr	24-72 hr
Signs and symptoms			
Vomiting	Common	Common	Uncommon
Fever (>102° F)	Uncommon	Variable	Common
Respiratory	Common (URI)	Uncommon	Common
Convulsion	Rare	Rare	Common
Stools			
Consistency	Loose	Loose, slimy	Watery
Odor	Unpleasant	Foul	Odorless
Blood	Rare	Rare	Common
Color	Variable	Green	Yellow-green
Mucus	Absent	Variable	Present
Polymorphonuclear leukocytes	Rare	Common	Common
Laboratory			
High WBC	Rare	Common	Variable
Left shift	Rare	Variable	Common
Pos blood culture	Absent	Variable (<1 yr)	Rare
Diarrhea in household	Variable	Variable	Common (>50%)
Carrier	?	Common	Rare

Modified from Nelson, J.D., and Haltalin, K.C.: J. Pediatr. **78**:519, 1971.

tery and usually contain mucus and blood.
3. Febrile convulsions are common, with a peak between 6 mo-4 yr, particularly in children with a family history of seizures or a high peak temperature (p. 564). Meningismus and respiratory symptoms may be present.
4. WBC usually is <10,000/mm³ with a marked shift to the left.

Campylobacter organisms

1. These are transmitted by contaminated food and person-to-person contact. Incubation period is 2-7 days, with a peak in children under 6 yr during warm months.
2. Although the patient may be asymptomatic, the onset of illness can be marked by high fever, myalgia, headache, abdominal cramps, and vomiting. Diarrhea is profuse, watery, mucousy, and bloody. Leukocytes are common. Resolution occurs in 2-5 days.

Yersinia enterocolitica

1. It occurs in sporadic cases in toddlers and teenagers during the cooler months following exposure to contaminated food or water or by person-to-person transmission. Incubation is 3-4 days.
2. In younger children, acute diarrhea, with fever and abdominal pain, is common. Stools contain rare leukocytes and blood. Older children with mesenteric adenitis have fever and right lower quadrant (RLQ) pain.

Enterotoxigenic or invasive Escherichia coli

1. It may cause disease by production of an enterotoxin or by tissue invasion. Classification of the mechanism by serogroup of the organism is unreliable.
2. Diarrhea is particularly severe in infants and young children. It may produce symptoms similar to those caused by cholera (profuse,

watery diarrhea) or *Shigella* organisms (fever and systemic symptoms). Mucus, blood, and polymorphonuclear (PMN) leukocytes are found in the stool.

Food poisoning

1. Staphylococcal food poisoning results from a common-source food that is usually poorly refrigerated. Vomiting, marked prostration, and diarrhea occur within 12-16 hr of ingestion.
2. *Clostridium perfringens* may produce abdominal pain and diarrhea within 12-24 hr of ingestion of contaminated food. Fever, nausea, and vomiting are rare. Resolution occurs in 24-48 hr.
3. *Clostridium botulinum*, although it does not cause diarrhea, may produce clinical symptoms within 12-36 hr of ingestion of foods—usually home-preserved vegetables, fruit, or fish. Honey may cause infantile botulism. Patients develop nausea, vomiting, diplopia, dysphagia, dysarthria, and dry mouth. Ptosis, miosis, nystagmus, and paresis of extraocular muscles may be noted. (p. 537).

Parasites

1. *Giardia lamblia* is the most commonly identified intestinal parasite. It is usually asymptomatic but may cause nausea, flatulence, bloating, epigastric pain or cramps, and watery diarrhea. The patient rarely has right upper quadrant (RUQ) pain and tenderness.
2. Other diarrheal diseases associated with parasites are usually chronic in nature and are associated with multisystem disease and weight loss.

Clostridium difficile

This is associated with pseudomembranous colitis and with many cases of antibiotic-related diarrhea in adults and children. Children may be asymptomatic or have chronic diarrhea. Stools are bloody with very rare leukocytes.

Traveler's diarrhea

This is a nonspecific term used to define diarrhea that often occurs during travel in foreign countries and that is not associated with a known pathogen. *E. coli* that produces a heat-labile enterotoxin is probably causative. Symptomatically, patients have abdominal cramps, tenesmus, vomiting, nausea, chills, anorexia, and watery diarrhea.

Complications

1. Dehydration (Chapter 7)
2. Postinfectious malabsorption
   NOTE: Children often experience a temporary lactose intolerance and develop watery diarrhea when challenged with lactose (dairy) products. Lactose-free soy formulas should be used for 2-4 wk
3. Hemolytic uremic syndrome (p. 608)
4. Acute tubular necrosis (p. 376)
5. Systemic extension of infection (meningitis, septic arthritis, etc.)

Ancillary data

Cultures of the stool

Cultures are useful in determining the bacterial etiology of the acute diarrhea but should be reserved for those patients in whom the results will have a therapeutic or epidemiologic impact. Rectal swabs handled expeditiously provide a good culture source if stool is unavailable. Cultures should be routinely done in children under 1 yr of age who are febrile or toxic on arrival with diarrhea and who have PMN leukocytes in their stool. Cultures are also important if multiple members of the same family are ill, if any member of the family is a food handler, or if symptomatic children are immunosuppressed or have hemoglobinopathy.

Fecal leukocytes (methylene blue smear of stool)

This is a reliable test to determine the etiologic agent, since >90% of diarrhea resulting from *Salmonella* or *Shigella* organisms have

PMN leukocytes in the stool. Fecal leukocytes also are found in patients with *Campylobacter* organisms, *Y. enterocolitica*, invasive *E. coli*, and *Vibrio parahaemolyticus*.

A small amount of mucus is placed on a clear glass slide and mixed with 2 drops of methylene blue. A coverglass is placed on the slide and nuclear staining occurs over 2 min. Microscopic examination for PMN leukocytes is performed.*

Rotavirus test

This may be identified by electron microscopy, radioimmunoassay, or the easier enzyme-linked immunosorbent assay (ELISA) test, which is commercially available.

Blood tests

These are important if there is a significant abnormality of intake or output and should include electrolytes, BUN, and a CBC with differential. All patients with any degree of dehydration or a prolonged course should have these studies performed. When the ratio of band forms over total neutrophils (segmented plus bands) is >0.10, *Shigella*, *Salmonella*, or *Campylobacter* organisms should be suspected. The WBC is usually under 10,000/mm^3, with a marked shift to the left in patients with *Shigella* infection. In *Salmonella* infection, WBC is increased, with a mild shift to the left. A high WBC count is also found in patients with *Campylobacter* and *Yersinia* infections.

Ova and parasites

Cultures are important if *Giardia* or other parasites are suspected. With *Giardia* organisms, cysts are present in formed stools and trophozoites in watery stool or duodenal aspirates.

Blood cultures

These are indicated for infants and young children with high fever and significant toxicity.

DIFFERENTIAL DIAGNOSIS

See Chapter 32.

---

*Harris, J.C., Dupont, H.L., and Hornick, R.B.: Fecal leukocytes in diarrheal illness, Ann. Intern. Med. **76**:699, 1972.

MANAGEMENT

The initial assessment of the patient must focus on the magnitude and type of dehydration. Rapid correction of deficits as outlined in Chapter 7 is imperative.

Antibiotics (Table 76-2)

Antibiotics must be restricted to specific etiologic agents, especially *Shigella* infection. In general they are not useful in the majority of diarrheal illnesses. The ultimate choice should reflect culture and sensitivity results, the patients' clinical status, and epidemiologic considerations.

Antibiotic therapy in patients with proved or suspected *Salmonella* infection is controversial because it prolongs the carrier state; however, it should be initiated in toxic patients under 6 mo, in those with suspected bactermia, and in children who are immunosuppressed or have a hemoglobinopathy.

C. difficile pseudomembranous colitis rarely requires antibiotic therapy but, on the contrary, cessation of previous antibiotics. If indicated, vancomycin 10-40 mg/kg/24 hr q 6 hr IV **or** metronidazole 15-40 mg/kg/24 hr q 8 hr PO may be useful.

Antidiarrheal agents

Agents like kaolin and pectin suspensions have no defined value. Diphenoxylate (Lomotil) will relieve abdominal cramping but should not be used for children. It may have a detrimental effect on recovery from *Shigella* organisms. Although these agents may reduce output, they merely increase third spacing of fluid.

Antispasmodics

Their role is controversial, and they are rarely indicated.

Bile acids

In children with prolonged diarrhea, primarily of a secretory nature that does not respond

TABLE 76-2. Antibiotic indications in infectious diarrhea

Etiologic agent	Drug of choice	Dose mg/kg/24 hr (adult: g/dose)	Route/ frequency	Comments
Salmonella	Ampicillin **and** chloramphenicol*	200-400 (1 g) 75-100 (1 g)	IV q 4-6 hr IV q 6 hr	Only in toxic patient where bacteremia is a concern; prolongs carrier status
Shigella	Trimethoprim-sulfamethoxazole **or**	8-10/ 40-50 (double strength)	PO q 12 hr	Preferred, depending on sensitivity; treat 5 days
	Ampicillin	50-100 (0.5 g)	PO q 6-8 hr	Do not use amoxicillin; may give parenterally for very toxic patients
Campylobacter	Erythromycin	30-50 (0.5 g)	PO q 6-8 hr	Effectiveness unproved; reduces length of excretion
Yersinia enterocolitica	Trimethoprim-sulfamethoxazole	8-10/ 40-50	PO q 12 hr	With severe toxicity, may use tetracycline and aminoglycoside
Giardia	Furazolidone **or**	6-8 (0.1 g)	PO q 6 hr	7-10 days; suspension available
	Quinacrine **or**	6 (0.1 g)	PO q 8 hr	5-10 days; poorly tolerated under 5 yr
	Metronidazole	15 (0.25 g)	PO q 8 hr	5-10 days

*Controversial. Other approaches include ampicillin and gentamicin; trimethoprim-sulfamethoxazole (IV). Drug must reflect local sensitivity patterns and treatment approaches.

to a clear liquid or NPO regimen, bile acids may contribute to GI irritation. A short course of aluminum hydroxide (Amphojel) 2.5-5.0 ml (½-1 tsp) q 6 hr or with meals PO for 2-4 days may be useful in recalcitrant diarrhea. Cholestyramine (Questran), available in 4 g packages, also absorbs and combines with bile acids when 1 g/24 hr is administered to infants under 1 yr (up to 4 g/24 hr in older children). Both also bind bacterial enterotoxins and fatty acids.

Prostaglandin inhibitors

Hormonally or prostaglandin-mediated secretory diarrhea may be treated pharmacologically if traditional dietary manipulations are ineffective. Aspirin, indomethacin, and nonsteroidal antiinflammatory agents may be indicated empirically.

Traveler's diarrhea prophylaxis

Treatment should focus primarily on support, including fluid management and restricted diet. Recent guidelines recommend against routine prophylaxis, because adverse reactions occur in 2%-5% of patients. The decision to employ prophylaxis must be individualized, reflecting the underlying health of the patient and the circumstances of the prospective travel. For mild diarrhea in adolescents and adults, antimotility agents such as diphenoxylate with atropine (Lomotil) may have a very limited role, supplementing fluid therapy. More severe diarrhea (>3 stools in 8 hr with nausea, vomiting, or fever) is treated with doxycycline (children over 8 yr) or trimethoprim-sulfamethoxazole. Drugs normally are prescribed for the patient, who carries them along in the event of illness. They are not given prophylactically. Oral hydration must be simultaneously instituted.

DISPOSITION

All patients with serious toxicity, dehydration, abnormal electrolytes, or a history of significant noncompliance should be hospitalized for IV therapy. In addition, admission should be sought for patients with sickle cell disease, hemoglobinopathies, or compromised immune systems. Oral rehydration may be attempted in nontoxic children under close observation.

Once the deficit has been restored and abnormal losses reduced, clear liquids (Pedialyte or Lytren) should be initiated slowly. If an adequate response is noted, a soy formula can be tried with slow progression.

Patients with minimal or no dehydration may be followed at home with careful fluid management and close follow-up.

Parental education

1. Give only clear liquids; give as much as your child wants. The following may be used during the first 24 hr:
   a. Pedialyte RS, Lytren, or Infalyte (requires mixing)
   b. Jell-O water: one package strawberry/quart water (twice as much as usual)
   c. Gatorade
   d. Defizzed, room-temperature soda for older children (over 2 yr) if diarrhea is only mild
2. If child is vomiting, give clear liquids *slowly*. In younger children, start with a teaspoonful and slowly increase the amount. If vomiting occurs, let your child rest for awhile and then try again. About 8 hr after vomiting has stopped, child can gradually return to a normal diet.
3. After 24 hr, your child's diet may be advanced if the diarrhea has improved. If child is taking only formula, mix the formula with twice as much water to make up half-strength formula, which should be given over the next 24 hr. Applesauce, bananas, and strained carrots may be given if child is eating solids. If this is tolerated, the child may be advanced to a regular diet over the next 2-3 days.
4. If child has had a prolonged course of diarrhea, it is helpful in the younger child to advance from clear liquids to a soy formula (Isomil, ProSobee, or Soyalac) for 1-2 wk. Children over 1 yr should not receive cow's

milk products (milk, cheese, ice cream, or butter) for several days.
5. Do not use boiled milk. Kool-Aid and soda are not ideal liquids, particularly for younger infants, because they contain few electrolytes.
6. Call physician if
   a. The diarrhea or vomiting is increasing in frequency or amount
   b. The diarrhea does not improve after 24 hr of clear liquids or resolve entirely after 3-4 days
   c. Vomiting continues for more than 24 hr
   d. The stool has blood or the vomited material contains blood or turns green
   e. Signs of dehydration develop, including decreased urination, less moisture in diapers, dry mouth, no tears, weight loss, lethargy, or irritability

REFERENCES

Barkin, R.M.: Acute infectious diarrheal disease in children, J. Emerg. Med. **3**:1-9, 1985.

Drachman, R.H.: Acute infectious gastroenteritis, Pediatr. Clin. North Am. **24**:711, 1974.

Kapikian, A.Z., Whakin, H., Whatt, R.G., et al.: Human Reovirus-like agent as the major pathogen associated with "winter" gastroenteritis in hospitalized infants and young children, N. Engl. J. Med. **294**:965, 1976.

Listernick, R., Zieseri, E., and Davis, A.T.: Outpatient oral rehydration in the United States, Am. J. Dis. Child. **140**:211, 1986.

Santosham, M., Daum, R.S., Dillman, L., et al.: Oral rehydration therapy of infantile diarrhea, N. Engl. J. Med. **306**:1070, 1982.

Gastrointestinal foreign bodies

Although most foreign bodies inadvertently swallowed by the inquisitive child pass without incident, they may lodge at points of physiologic narrowing, including the cricopharyngeal muscle, the carina or aortic arch, Schatzki's ring, or the cardioesophageal junction. They also may get stuck at the ligament of Treitz. Children rarely insert foreign bodies into the rectum.

DIAGNOSTIC FINDINGS

Most patients are asymptomatic and the foreign body passes without difficulty. When the foreign body does lodge in the esophagus, the patient may be anxious and have difficulty in swallowing.

Physical examination usually is unremarkable. It is important to be certain that there is no evidence of any airway foreign body.

X-ray films are indicated if there is any question of an airway foreign body or if the patient is symptomatic.

1. Coins that are in the esophagus lie in the fontal plane (full circle can be seen) while those in the trachea lie sagitally and appear end-on in a PA chest film.
2. A lateral chest view may be helpful if there is any question of localization.
3. If the foreign body is not found on the chest films, an abdominal film should be obtained. If it still cannot be located, a contrast study may be indicated.
4. For reference, a dime is 17 mm, a penny is 18 mm, a nickel is 20 mm, and a quarter is 23 mm in diameter.

DIFFERENTIAL DIAGNOSIS

Foreign bodies in the trachea are differentiated by history, physical examination, and x-ray film (p. 600).

MANAGEMENT

Historically, asymptomatic patients have been managed without intervention or diagnostic studies and with reassurance. Most foreign bodies, whether round, irregular, or sharp (such as pins) will pass without difficulty. Recent evidence, however, has suggested that 17% of patients with coin ingestions were without symptoms. Therefore it is appropriate to consider chest radiographs, including the cervical esophagus, in patients ingesting coins if there is any question of symptoms, poor compliance, or if follow-up will be difficult.

All patients should be instructed to watch for fecal passage of the object and report any symptoms including pain, tenderness, obstruction, or signs of perforation immediately to permit further diagnostic and therapeutic steps.

1. Esophageal foreign bodies
   a. If the object is sharp or has sharp projections and it is lodged, it should be removed by endoscopy. Endoscopy also may be used for other types of objects.
   b. Other foreign bodies that become lodged in the esophagus in the asymptomatic patient for <24 hr may be removed by passing a Foley catheter beyond the foreign body, blowing up the balloon with a radiopaque substance, and gently pulling out the material.
   The procedure should be done under fluoroscopic control, with an NG tube having been passed initially to empty the stomach. Preparations should be made in the event that the patient aspirates the foreign body, a risk that is minimized by placing the patient in Trendelenburg's position.
2. Foreign bodies lodged in the stomach (usually distal antrum) usually can be watched for 2-3 wk unless they have corrosive potential such as button batteries.
3. Foreign bodies lodged at the ligament of Treitz
   a. Round objects may be watched for up to 1 wk, awaiting passage, unless the patient has evidence of obstruction or perforation.
   b. Elongated objects such as pencils should be observed for 6-8 hr and, if no movement is noted, removed either by endoscopy or surgery.
4. Rectal foreign bodies
   a. If large, they usually require general anesthesia to facilitate removal.
   b. Small objects can be removed through an anoscope. Preparation of the patient with PO or PR mineral oil may be useful.
5. Although without proved efficacy, some clinicians continue to believe that glucagon (0.03-0.1 mg/kg/dose IV; adult: 1 mg/dose)

may have some value in the management of esophageal foreign bodies.

DISPOSITION

Asymptomatic patients may be discharged with close follow-up if the foreign body is lodged in an anatomic site not requiring urgent removal. Symptomatic patients and those requiring removal should be hospitalized.

REFERENCES

Hodge, D., Tecklenburg, F., and Fleisher, G.: Coin ingestion: does every child need a radiograph? Ann. Emerg. Med. **14**:443, 1985.

Nixon, G.W.: Foley catheter method of esophageal foreign body removal: extension of application, Am. J. Radiol. **132**:441, 1979.

O'Neill, J.A., Holcomb, G.W., and Neblet, W.W.: Management of tracheobronchial and esophageal foreign bodies in childhood, J. Pediatr. Surg. **18**:475, 1983.

Viral hepatitis

Acute viral hepatitis commonly is classifed as hepatitis A (predominantly fecal-oral transmission), hepatitis B (largely parenteral), and non-A/non-B (transfusion related) on the basis of serologic and clinical data.

DIAGNOSTIC FINDINGS (Table 76-3)

Epidemiologic and diagnostic findings are variable.

TABLE 76-3. Acute viral hepatitis

	Hepatitis A	Hepatitis B	Hepatitis non-A/non-B
EPIDEMIOLOGIC FEATURES			
Incubation (weeks)	2-7	6-27	2-22
Onset	Acute	Insidious	Insidious with relapses
Cluster	Epidemic	Sporadic	Sporadic
Transmission	Fecal-oral, common source; rarely parenteral	Parenteral; rarely nonparenteral	Transfusions, very rarely nonparenteral
Age distribution	Children	Adolescents, adults	Adolescents, adults
Duration	Weeks	Weeks to months	
DIAGNOSTIC FINDINGS			
Fever	High	Moderate	Minimal
Nausea, vomiting	Common	Rare	Rare
Serum sickness (arthralgia, rash)	Rare	Common	Variable
Severity	Mild	Severe	Moderate
Carrier state	No	Yes	Yes
ANCILLARY DATA			
Transaminase elevation	1-3 wk	Months	
Bilirubin elevation	Weeks	Months	
PROPHYLAXIS	IG	HBIG	IG

IG, Immune serum globulin; HBIG, hepatitis B immunoglobulin.

1. Patients generally have a prodromal, preicteric phase with malaise and anorexia.
2. Jaundice develops, accompanied by scleral icterus (bilirubin >2.5 mg/dl) and pruritus.
3. The abdomen may be distended. Palpation of the right upper quadrant over the liver demonstrates the greatest tenderness. Splenomegaly is variably present.
4. Evidence of serum sickness is present with hepatitis B. Arthralgia, myalgia, erythematous or maculopapular rash, and fever are noted. Patients may develop myocarditis or pericarditis, with symptoms of pleuritic chest pain and friction rubs.

Complications

1. Fulminant hepatitis. A poor prognosis is seen with hepatitis B when associated with a prolonged PT (>4 over control) unresponsive to large doses of vitamin K, elevated bilirubin$_3$ (>20 mg/dl), leukocytosis (>12,500 WBC/mm^3), and hypoglycemia.
2. Chronic active hepatitis
3. Hepatorenal syndrome with edema and ascites
4. Hepatic encephalopathy marked by altered mental status, seizures, and coma. Tremor, asterixis, and hyperreflexia may be present.
5. Bleeding diathesis

Ancillary data

1. WBC usually is normal.
2. Prothrombin time is prolonged. Other bleeding studies are normal.
3. Liver functions are elevated. Transaminases and bilirubin are elevated for weeks in hepatitis A and months in hepatitis B. Bilirubin >20 mg/dl is consistent with severe disease. Glutamyl transferase level >300 units/L is consistent with biliary atresia or alpha$_1$ antitrypsin deficiency.
4. Urine is dark with urobilinogen and bilirubin.
5. Serologic studies are important in differentiating the type of hepatitis.
   a. Hepatitis A antibody (IgM) is diagnostic of an acute infection, whereas hepatitis A[n] antibody (IgG) is evidence of previous infection.
   b. Serologic tests for hepatitis B are listed at the bottom of the page.
6. If indicated, other studies should be done to exclude other causes of hepatitis.

DIFFERENTIAL DIAGNOSIS

1. Infection/inflammation
   a. Viral: infectious mononucleosis (EB virus), cytomegalovirus, herpes simplex
   b. Toxoplasmosis
   c. Cholangitis
2. Metabolic disorders
   a. Cholelithiasis
   b. Wilson's disease
   c. Gilbert's disease and Dubin-Johnson syndrome
3. Drugs
   a. Alcohol
   b. Analgesic: aspirin, acetaminophen
   c. Anesthetic: halothane
   d. Antibiotic: erythromycin estolate, sulfonamides, tetracycline, rifampin, carbenicillin

Test	Description	Interpretation
HbsAg	Hepatitis B surface antigen	Active infection, carrier state, or chronic active hepatitis
Anti-HBs	Antibody to hepatitis B surface antigen	Convalescence, persistent infection, or past infection
Anti-HBc	Antibody to hepatitis B core antigen	Active infection or past infection
HBeAg	Hepatitis B "e" antigen	Highly infectious patient with increased risk of chronic active hepatitis; fetus or newborn at risk
Anti-HBe	Antibody to hepatitis B "e" antigen	Noninfectious; fetus and newborn not at risk

e. Antituberculosis: isoniazid, rifampin

f. Others: phenytoin, phenothiazine, morphine

4. Congenital disorder: biliary atresia (infants)

MANAGEMENT

The majority of patients need careful follow-up and monitoring to ensure that their liver functions are normalizing and that hydration is maintained.

Patients with impending liver failure require a host of supportive measures:

1. Respiratory and cardiovascular support
   a. Oxygen and active airway management if necessary
   b. Maintenance of intravascular volume
2. CNS support, if encephalopathy is present
   a. Decrease of protein intake
   b. NG tube with administration of neomycin 50-100 mg/kg/24 hr q 6 hr via tube
   c. Treatment of cerebral edema
      (1) Fluid restriction: 75% of maintenance
      (2) Steroids: dexamethasone 0.25 mg/kg/dose q 6 hr IV. Controversial
      (3) Mannitol: 0.25-1.0 g/kg/dose q 6 hr IV
      (4) Hyperventilation (if ventilatory support is necessary)
3. Other
   a. Give diuretics for fluid overload.
      (1) Furosemide (Lasix) 1-2 mg/kg/dose q 2-6 hr IV or PO
      (2) Spironolactone (Aldactone) 1-3 mg/kg/24 hr q 6-8 hr PO
   b. Maintain glucose at 100-150 mg/dl.
   c. Support nutrition.
   d. For bleeding, administer fresh frozen plasma (10 ml/kg/dose q 12-24 hr IV) and vitamin K (infants: 1-2 mg/dose IV slowly; children and adults: 5-10 mg/dose IV).
   e. Treat infections and GI bleeding appropriately.
   f. Isolate patient.
      NOTE: Other modalities that have been attempted without proved benefit include exchange transfusions and dialysis.

Preventive measures

Hepatitis A

Those with *household contacts* should receive 0.02 ml/kg IM of immune serum globulin (IG) as soon after exposure as possible. IG is not indicated beyond 2 wk after exposure. Administration of IG also should be considered in the following circumstances:

1. Children and staff of day-care centers where there are children in diapers and in which there have been cases in parents or other household contacts of children in day-care, especially those under 3 yr.

   If the outbreak is well developed by the time intervention is begun (three families with cases or two cases if both in diapered children), then IG should be administered to household contacts of children 3 yr or under. If hepatitis A occurs in a center without diapered children, IG should be given only to age-group contacts at the center and household contacts.

2. Those who have personal contact with individuals with hepatitis in an institutional setting

3. Exposure in classrooms or other places in schools has not generally posed a significant risk of infection. Hospital personnel caring for patients with hepatitis A are not routinely treated. Emphasis should be on good hand-washing technique.

Hepatitis B

Preexposure prophylaxis is available from a vaccine prepared from inactivated virus obtained from the serum of patients with hepatitis B virus. A three-dose series is recommended, administering the vaccine at days 1, 30, and 180 to high-risk individuals. Children in this group include those from families with hepatitis B virus infection or chronic carriers, those in institutions for the mentally retarded, and those receiving large amounts of blood and blood products.

Postexposure prophylaxis must reflect the type of exposure (blood or percutaneous needle stick or mucousal membrane) and HBsAg of the donor.

1. For those with exposure to blood known to be HBsAg positive: Exposure may be percutaneous, ocular or through mucosal membrane. A single dose of hepatitis B immunoglobulin (HBIG) (0.06 ml/kg or 5.0 ml for adult) should be given as soon as possible after exposure and within 24 hr if possible. Hepatitis B vaccine 1 ml (20 μg) (children under 10 yr: 0.5 ml) should be given as an IM injection at a separate site as soon as possible but within 7 days of exposure, with second and third doses given at 1 mo and 6 mo after the first dose. If HBIG is unavailable, IG may be given at an equivalent dose (0.06 ml/kg or 5.0 ml for adult). For those choosing not to receive hepatitis B vaccine, give HBIG at time of exposure and 1 mo later.

2. For those with exposure to blood of unknown HBsAg status:
   a. High-risk patients (e.g., those with Down's syndrome who are institutionalized, dialysis patients, drug abusers)
      (1) If the results of HBsAg will be available within 7 *days:* IG 0.06 ml/kg IM immediately. If the test is positive, give HBIG 0.06 ml/kg (adult: 5.0 ml) IM immediately and 1 mo later. Also initiate hepatitis B vaccine three-dose regimen. If HBsAg is negative, no further treatment is necessary.
      (2) If the results will not be available within 7 days, the decision as to whether to give IG or HBIG and hepatitis B vaccine must be based on clinical and epidemiologic information.
   b. Low-risk patients (or if the source is unknown): either IG 0.06 ml/kg IM or nothing

Sexual contacts of persons with acute hepatitis B infections are at increased risk of acquiring the disease. A single dose of HBIG (0.06 ml/kg or 5.0 ml in adult) should be given to susceptible individuals who have had sexual contact with an HBsAg positive person if it can be given within 14 days of the last sexual contact. A second HBIG dose should be given in cases of heterosexual exposures if the index patient remains HBsAg positive 3 mo after detection. Hepatitis B vaccine should be considered for homosexual men and for those with ongoing contact to carriers.

Newborns of mothers who are HBsAg positive are at risk of hepatitis B virus transmission. HBIG (0.5 ml) IM should be administered within 12 hr of birth. Additionally, hepatitis B vaccine IM in a dose of 0.5 ml should be administered within 7 days of birth and again at 1 mo and 6 mo of age. HBsAg testing should be done at 6 mo in consultation with appropriate experts.

Hepatitis non-A/non-B

Management is the same as for hepatitis A.

REFERENCES

Centers for Disease Control: Postexposure prophylaxis of hepatitis B. Morb. Mort. Week. Rep. **33**:285, 1984.

Centers for Disease Control: Recommendations for protection against viral hepatitis, Morb. Mort. Week. Rep. **34**:314, 1985.

Hadler, S.C., Erbon, J.J., Matthews, D., et al.: Effect of immunoglobulin on hepatitis A in day-care centers. JAMA **249**:48, 1983.

Lemon, S.M.: Type A viral hepatitis: new developments in an old disease, N. Engl. J. Med **313**:1059, 1985.

Pancreatitis

ETIOLOGY

1. Infection
   a. Viral: mumps, hepatitis, coxsackie virus
   b. *Mycoplasma pneumoniae*
2. Trauma: blunt, penetrating, or surgical
3. Intoxication
   a. Diuretics: thiazides, furosemide
   b. Prednisone, oral contraceptive agents
   c. Antibiotics: rifampin, tetracycline, isoniazid
4. Congenital: biliary tract anomalies

DIAGNOSTIC FINDINGS

1. Abdominal pain is the primary complaint, either of insidious or sudden onset. Upper quadrant or epigastric constant or intermittent pain is reported. It may radiate to the back or neck. Relief is obtained in the knee-chest position.
2. Abdominal tenderness and distension are noted, with decreased bowel sounds and ascites. Cullens' (bluish periumbilical discoloration) and Grey Turner's (discoloration of the flank) signs are indicative of pancreatic necrosis and only occur late.
3. Low-grade fever, nausea, vomiting, and lethargy may be present.

Complications

1. Hypotension and shock secondary to third-space losses and intravascular volume depletion
2. Acute respiratory distress syndrome with left-sided pleural effusions and pneumonitis
3. Pancreatic pseudocyst or abscess, usually with delayed onset
4. Disseminated intravascular coagulation

Ancillary data

1. Electrolytes are normal. Glucose may be increased.
2. Hypocalcemia is a bad prognostic sign.
3. Elevation of amylase peaks at 12-24 hr, which may return to normal in 48-72 hr. Lipase rises early and normalizes less rapidly. A determination that is useful for patients whose serum amylase is not diagnostic is clearance values calculated from spot urine and serum vales:

$$\frac{C_{amylase}}{C_{creatine}} = \frac{Amylase\ (serum)}{Amylase\ (urine)} \times \frac{Creatinine\ (serum)}{Creatinine\ (urine)} \times 100$$

This ratio is normally equal to 1%-4%. A larger value is indicative of pancreatitis.
NOTE: Amylase may be elevated in abdominal trauma and infection, not specifically causing pancreatitis.

4. Liver functions are elevated, particularly bilirubin.
5. X-ray films may demonstrate pleural effusions, atelectasis, pneumonitis, and an intestinal ileus or sentinel loop.

DIFFERENTIAL DIAGNOSIS

1. Infection
   a. Peritonitis and other causes of surgical abdomen
   b. Pneumonia
2. Trauma. It is essential to differentiate pancreatitis from other abdominal organic involvement. Peritoneal lavage may be necessary. Consider child abuse.

MANAGEMENT

1. Stabilization is of primary importance, with initial attention to fluid therapy, usually requiring IV replacement of deficits (Chapter 7). In cases of trauma, it is imperative to be certain that other organs are not involved. Glucose and calcium abnormalities may require intervention.
2. An NG tube attached to suction should be begun and the patient made NPO until pain has subsided for several days.
3. Analgesia may be used. Meperidine (Demerol) 1 mg/kg/dose q 4-6 hr IM or IV is the drug of choice.
4. When the patient can tolerate food, a bland, low-fat diet should be used, often requiring pancreatic enzyme supplements. Until that time, IV alimentation is appropriate.
5. Once the patient is stabilized, antacids or cimetidine may be useful.

DISPOSITION

1. Patients require hospitalization for IV fluids, gastric suction, and monitoring.
2. Long-term follow-up is essential because of the delayed onset of pancreatic pseudocyst and abscess.

REFERENCES

Jordan, S.C., and Ament, M.E.: Pancreatitis in childhood and adolescents, J. Pediatr. **91**:211, 1977.

Moossa, A.R.: Current concepts: diagnostic tests and procedures in acute pancreatitis, N. Engl. J. Med. **311**:639, 1984.

Reye's syndrome

ALERT: Vomiting and behavior changes following an acute illness require rapid evaluation and intervention.

Reye's syndrome is an acute, noninflammatory encephalopathy with altered level of consciousness, cerebral edema without perivascular or meningeal inflammation, and fatty metamorphosis of the liver, probably secondary to mitochondrial dysfunction. It is a multisystem disease with a biphasic history marked by an infectious phase followed by an encephalopathic stage. There have been reports of the syndrome in children between 4 mo and 14 yr, with an average age of 7 yr and a peak occurrence at 4 and 11 yr. It often follows a viral infection: influenza B and chickenpox are particularly implicated. Salicylate ingestion may be a predisposing factor.

DIAGNOSTIC FINDINGS

1. A prodrome of respiratory or GI symptoms is consistently present for 2-3 days.
2. Vomiting develops and is followed in 24-48 hr by an encephalopathic phase with marked behavioral changes, including delirium and combativeness, disorientation and hallucination. The deteriorating level of consciousness reflects increasing intracranial pressure. Obtundation and coma may follow, associated with seizures, hyperventilation, and hypothermia. Five stages have been outlined, based on progression of findings in cephalocaudal progression of brainstem dysfunction (Table 76-4).
3. Hepatomegaly and pancreatitis may be present.
4. In children under 1 yr of age, vomiting is mild and the predominant findings are apnea, hyperventilation, seizures, hepatomegaly, and hypoglycemia.

Complications

Children in stages IV or V and those progressing rapidly from stage I to III have a poor prognosis.
1. Acute respiratory failure
2. Cerebral edema with herniation, reflecting progression of increased ICP (10%)

TABLE 76-4. Staging of Reye's syndrome

	I	II	III	IV	V
Level of consciousness	Lethargy; follows verbal commands	Combative/stupor; verbalizes inappropriately	Coma	Coma	Coma
Posture	Normal	Normal	Decorticate	Decerebrate	Flaccid
Response to pain	Purposeful	Purposeful/nonpurposeful	Decorticate	Decerebrate	None
Pupillary reaction	Brisk	Sluggish	Sluggish	Sluggish	None
Oculocephalic reflex (doll's eyes)	Normal	Conjugate deviation	Conjugate deviation	Inconsistent or absent	None

3. Cardiac dysrhythmias
4. Death (10%)

Ancillary data

1. Plasma ammonia levels are usually $\geq 1\frac{1}{2}$ times normal values (normal: 40-80 μg/dl). Transiently present for 24-48 hr after the onset of mental status changes. A level >300 μg/dl is associated with a poor prognosis.
2. Elevated serum transaminases (usually 3 times normal) and other liver function tests, osmolality, and amylase. Normal or slightly elevated bilirubin. Variable BUN and electrolytes. Decreased glucose, particularly in children under 4 yr.
3. Decreased liver-dependent clotting factors (II, VII, IX, and X), with prolonged prothrombin time and partial thyromboplastin time. Fibrinogen may be decreased. Normal platelets.
4. ABG, lumbar puncture (assuming no evidence of increased ICP), blood cultures, and toxicology screen to exclude other potential etiologies and to monitor the patient.
5. CT scan to exclude intracranial lesions (e.g., abscess) if diagnosis is uncertain. Scan will demonstrate cerebral edema.
6. Percutaneous liver biopsy may be useful in patients with an atypical presentation, including infants under 1 yr, in recurrent episodes and familial cases, and in nonepidemic cases without an antecedent infection or vomiting.

DIFFERENTIAL DIAGNOSIS (Chapter 15)

1. Infection
   a. Meningitis/encephalitis (p. 549)
   b. Sepsis
   c. Viral: chickenpox or hepatitis
2. Endocrine/metabolic disorders
   a. Hypoglycemia (Chapter 38)
   b. Hypoxia
   c. Amino/organic-acid inborn errors of metabolism

3. Intoxication: salicylates, acetaminophen, ethanol, lead camphor (Table 54-3)
4. Trauma: head
5. Vascular: intracranial hemorrhage

MANAGEMENT (Table 76-4)

1. General supportive care is crucial in determining the ultimate outcome. Dehydration may be present but should not be fully corrected because of the concurrent cerebral edema. Serum glucose should be kept between 125-175 mg/dl, with a serum osmolality <310 mOsm/kg water.
2. Stages I and II require frequent monitoring of vital and neurologic signs, IV infusion of D10W-D20W, and correction of fluid and electrolyte abnormalities.
3. Stages III-V require aggressive support and intervention:
   a. Supportive measures
      (1) Monitoring of venous and arterial pressures; NG tube; and urinary catheter for intake and output measurement
      (2) Respiratory support including intubation, mechanical ventilation, and hyperventilation, if indicated
      (3) IV infusion of D15W at two-thirds maintenance after cardiovascular stabilization to maintain urine output at 1 ml/kg/hr
      (4) Seizure control: phenytoin (Dilantin) loading with 15-20 mg/kg/dose, with maintenance at 5 mg/kg/24 hr q 6 hr IV; does not cause sedation; monitor level
      (5) Control of temperature
   b. Metabolic abnormalities. Maintenance of glucose between 125-175 mg/dl, using glucose and insulin (1 unit/5 g of glucose given) infusion
   c. For coagulation abnormalities:
      (1) Fresh frozen plasma 10 ml/kg/dose q 12-24 hr IV or prn

(2) Vitamin K 1-10 mg/dose IV slowly

(3) Exchange transfusion rarely indicated

d. Intracranial monitoring to measure efficacy of a number of therapeutic modalities. Maintain ICP ≤15-18 mm Hg and the CPP >50 mm hg. Measures may be tried individually or concurrently, depending on patient response.

(1) Mannitol 0.25-0.5 g/kg/dose IV infusion over 20 min. May repeat q 2 hr as needed. Monitor osmolality of serum, keeping <210 mOsm/kg water.

(2) Hyperventilation to maintain $PaCO_2$ at 20-25 mm Hg

(3) Furosemide (Lasix) 1-2 mg/kg/dose q 4-6 hr IV

(4) Head elevation

(5) Muscular paralysis: pancuronium (Pavulon) 0.05-0.1 mg/kg/dose q 1-2 hr prn IV. Patient must be intubated with respiratory support.

(6) Pentobarbital (Nembutal) 3-20 mg/kg by IV slowly while monitoring blood pressure. Maintain level at 25-40 µg/dl by maintenance infusion of 1-2 mg/kg/hr. Barbiturate coma is maintained for 2-3 days while monitoring other parameters if alternative approaches have not been successful (Chapter 57).

4. Treatment of complications

DISPOSITION

All patients require admission to an ICU capable of intracranial monitoring. Appropriate consultation should be sought.

REFERENCES

Committee on Infectious Diseases (AAP): Aspirin and Reye's syndrome, Pediatrics **69**:810, 1982.

Hurwitz, E.S., Barrett, M.J., Bregman, D., et al.: Public health service study on Reye's syndrome and medications, N. Engl. J. Med. **313**:849, 1985.

Rogers, M.F., Schonberger, L.B., Hurwitz, E.S., et al.: National Reye's syndrome surveillance, Pediatrics **75**:260, 1985.

Conditions requiring surgery

Ronald D. Lindzon

James C. Mitchiner

APPENDICITIS

ALERT: Severe right lower quadrant (RLQ) pain requires urgent surgical consultation.

Inflammation of the appendix usually results from obstruction of the lumen. It is the most common cause of an acute surgical abdominal condition in older children.

Diagnostic findings

Classically, patients have a low-grade fever and loss of appetite. Symptoms quickly progress to include pain, vomiting, and changes in bowel habits. Clinical signs and symptoms vary, depending on the degree of inflammation and whether perforation has occurred. The hydration status of the patient also may affect the clinical presentation, most patients being 5%-10% dehydrated.

1. The cramping abdominal pain initially is in the area of the umbilicus but gradually, over the ensuing 4-12 hr, shifts to the RLQ. The maximum intensity is over McBurney's point, located 1½-2 inches from the iliac crest, along the line drawn between the iliac crest and the umbilicus.

a. With rupture of the appendix, there is initial relief but subsequent progression to peritonitis.

b. The patient is most comfortable lying down with the legs flexed.

2. The abdomen has diminished bowel sounds and associated tenderness, rebound, and guarding the RLQ. With perforation there is less localization, and more generalized peritoneal signs are present.

a. Rectal examination demonstrates tenderness, greatest on the right.

b. Psoas sign: pain is produced with the right thigh extended and the patient lying on the left side, indicative of peritoneal or pelvic inflammation.

   c. Obturator sign: pain is produced when the right thigh is flexed and internally rotated, with the patient in the supine position—consistent with pelvic inflammation.

3. In children under 2 yr of age, the diagnosis is particularly difficult because of the non-specific nature of the clinical picture, and 94% of such patients are not diagnosed until perforation has occurred.

   a. Vomiting, diffuse pain, lethargy or irritability, nausea, and feeding problems are noted.

   b. The abdomen is tender, with absent bowel sounds, guarding and a positive rectal examination. Patients are febrile, and urinary retention may occur.

Complications

1. Peritonitis. Perforation is associated with delay in treatment and with younger children
2. Intrabdominal or pelvic abscess
3. Ileus or obstruction
4. Pyelophlebitis
5. Sepsis and shock

Ancillary data

1. WBC. Elevated >15,000 in about 40% of patients, with 93% having a shift to the left (percentage of neutrophils: >50% for 1 to 5-year-olds, >65% for 5 to 10-yr-olds, and >75% for 10 to 15-year-olds)
2. Urinalysis. May demonstrate minimal pyuria secondary to ureteral irritation (must exclude UTI). It also will assist in assessment of hydration.
3. Chest x-ray film to exclude pneumonia
4. Abdominal x-ray film (three-way view includes supine and upright abdomen and AP chest)

   a. Abnormal gas pattern with decreased gas, air-fluid levels, or diffuse small-bowel dilation

   b. Free peritoneal air

   c. Thickening of abdominal wall

   d. Fecalith

   e. Abscess in RLQ

5. Barium enema. Rarely done at present but an appendix that fills is good evidence against appendicitis
6. Laparoscopy. Indicated for patients with relative contraindications to surgery and an equivocal examination

Differential diagnosis (Table 76-5)

Management

1. Focus initial management on stabilization of the patient.

   a. IV hydration, initially with 20 ml/kg of D5W.9%NS or D5WLR over 1 hr if any deficit exists (Chapter 7)

   b. NG tube

   c. Oxygen if patient is in marked distress

   d. Lowering of temperature by cooling blanket or antipyretics

2. Involve surgical consultant early.
3. If there is any evidence of peritonitis or perforation, begin antibiotics:

   a. Ampicillin 100-200 mg/kg/24 hr q 4 hr IV **and**

   b. Clindamycin 30-40 mg/kg/24 hr q 6 hr IV **and**

   c. Gentamicin 5.0-7.5 mg/kg/24 hr q 8 hr IV or IM

4. Give analgesia, if necessary, but only after diagnosis is certain and decision to operate has been made: meperidine (Demerol) 1-2 mg/kg/dose IM (maximum: 50-100 mg/dose)
5. Perform surgery.

Disposition

All patients require admission for surgical management.

Patients for whom the diagnosis is uncertain may often benefit from 12-24 hr of observation to allow the disease to progress and define itself.

REFERENCES

Blair, G.L., and Gaisford, W.D.: Acute appendicitis in children under six years, J. Pediatr. Surg. 4:445, 1969.

TABLE 76-5. Right lower quadrant pain: diagnostic considerations

	Infection/inflammatory	Neoplasm	Congenital
Systemic	Influenza		
Skin	Herpes zoster Cellulitis		
Abdominal wall			Inguinal hernia
Pulmonary	Pneumonia		
Gastrointestinal tract	**Mesenteric adenitis** **Gastroenteritis** (Sal- monella, Shigella, Yersinia, typhoid) **Appendicitis** Diverticulitis Peritonitis Meckel's syndrome Cholecystitis Duodenal ulcer Hepatitis	Hodgkin's disease Carcinoma	Intussusception Obstruction Meckel's diverticulum
Kidney/ulcer	**Pyelonephritis** **Cystitis** Perinephric abscess	Wilms' tumor	Hydronephrosis
Ovary/tubes/pelvis	**Pelvic inflammatory disease** **Salpingitis** Tubal-ovarian abscess Pelvic abscess	Endometriosis	Testicular torsion
Spine	Osteomyelitis		

Brender, J.D., Marcuse, E.K., Koepsell, T.D., et al.: Child-
hood appendicitis: factors associated with perforation. Pe-
diatrics **76**:301, 1985.
Grosfeld, J.L., Weinberger, M., and Clatworthy, H.W.:
Acute appendicitis in the first two years of life, J. Pediatr.
Surg. **8**:285, 1973.

HIRSCHSPRUNG'S DISEASE

JAMES C. MITCHINER

**ALERT: Intestinal obstruction in the newborn or in-
fant requires a careful and expeditious evaluation.**

Hirschsprung's disease or congenital megacolon results from congenital aganglionosis of the
distal colon and rectum, leading to failure of
effective peristalsis through the aganglionic segment. It is a cause of partial intestinal obstruction in early infancy and occasionally in childhood.

Diagnostic findings

Infants may fail to pass meconium in the first
24 hr of life. They also may be constipated, often
not until 2-3 wk of age. Paradoxically, diarrhea
caused by mucosal ulcerations in the proximal
dilated segment may develop. Vomiting may
occur.

Bowel obstruction usually is present, with a
distended, tympanitic abdomen, hyperactive or
high-pitched bowel sounds, and a history of
vomiting. Rectal examination reveals an absence
of stool in the ampulla, often followed by evacuation of gas and liquid stool after the examiner's
finger is withdrawn.

Autoimmune	Trauma	Intrapsychic	Vascular	Endocrine/metabolic
	Black widow spider bite	Functional		Diabetic ketoacidosis Acute porphyria
	Contusion Muscle rupture			
Regional enteritis	**Impacted feces**		Mesenteric infarct	
Ulcerative colitis				
				Renal calculi
				Mittelschmerz **Dysmenorrhea** Ovarian cyst Threatened abortion Ectopic pregnancy

Complications

1. Acute necrotizing enterocolitis with cecal perforation, pneumoperitoneum, and pericolic abscess
2. Acute appendicitis
3. Malnutrition
4. Reversible urinary tract obstruction (hydronephrosis, hydroureter, and recurrent urinary tract infections)
5. Septicemia, particularly in newborns

Ancillary data

1. CBC and electrolytes as indicated by clinical condition
2. Abdominal x-ray film. Demonstrates distended, gas-filled proximal segment, associated with small lucent rectum. May be normal
3. Barium enema. Shows a normal diameter in the aganglionic segment associated with a dilated proximal segment tapering at the rectosigmoid. Once the dilated segment is defined, it is not necessary to complete the study and, in fact, it may be dangerous. A postevacuation film taken 12-48 hr later shows residual barium.
4. Rectal biopsy. Ideally performed in the stable patient whose diagnosis is uncertain; often follows an equivocal barium enema and is performed proximal to the anorectal junction, 2-3 cm above the rectal columns. Specimen must be of sufficient depth to include both the mucosal and muscular layers for proper diagnosis. General anesthesia is usually necessary. Acetylcholinesterase activity,

which is high in Hirschsprung's disease, should be obtained from the biopsy material.

5. Manometry

Differential diagnosis

1. Congenital disorders
   a. Colonic or ileal atresia
   b. Hypoplastic left colon syndrome
2. Infection/inflammation: neonatal sepsis, megacolon, ulcerative colitis
3. Endocrine disorders: hypothyroidism and adrenal insufficiency
4. Trauma: anal fissure
5. Intoxication: drug-induced hypomotility (anticholinergics, narcotics)
6. *Acquired constipation* usually occurs after 2 yr of age, with associated incontinence, abdominal pain, and obstruction. Stools usually are large in caliber, with increased stool in the ampulla. Barium enema shows a diffuse megacolon.

   In contrast, Hirschsprung's disease may occur in the newborn period with symptoms of failure to thrive but only rarely with associated incontinence or abdominal pain. The stool is thin and ribbonlike, with decreased frequency and little stool in the ampulla. Barium enema demonstrates a localized constriction with proximal dilation.

Management

1. Initial hydration and gastric decompression with an NG tube to suction are essential in the management of acute obstruction.
   a. Fluids: D5W.9%NS at 20 ml/kg over the first hour, then deficit and maintenance replacement
   b. With evidence of obstruction: institution of NG decompression
   c. Surgical consultation
2. After stabilization, a barium enema is indicated if enterocolitis and perforation are not present and, if suggestive, a rectal biopsy performed by a pediatric surgeon or gastroenterologist.

3. In general, surgery is the definite treatment if the biopsy shows no ganglion cells and high acetylcholinesterase (ACE) activity.
   a. The goal is to place normal ganglion-containing bowel within 1 cm of the anal opening.
   b. Acute surgical therapy decompresses the bowel obstruction by a loop colostomy. The stoma must contain normal bowel.
   c. Following the colostomy, the bowel can be adequately cleansed and definitive procedure done electively at a later date.
   d. Staging is not necessary in a relatively well child.

REFERENCES

Kleinhaus. S.: Hirschsprung's disease: a survey of the members of the surgical section of the American Academy of Pediatrics. J. Pediatr. Surg. 14:588, 1979.

Swenson, O., Sherman, J.O., and Fisher, J.H.: Diagnosis of congenital megacolon: analysis of 501 cases, J. Pediatr. Surg. 8:587, 1973.

INTUSSUSCEPTION

ALERT: Classic signs of abdominal pain, vomiting, and bloody stool with mucus are not always present.

Intussusception occurs when the proximal bowel invaginates into the distal bowel, resulting in infarction and gangrene of the inner bowel. It commonly occurs in children under 1 yr of age and is usually of the ileocolic type.

A leading point is more commonly found in older children with conditions such as Meckel's diverticulum, polyp, duplication, lymphoma, and Henoch-Schönlein purpura or following surgery.

Diagnostic findings

1. Typically, patients have an acute onset of intermittent fits of sudden intense pain with screaming and flexion of the legs. The episodes occur in 5-20 min intervals. Vomiting, often bilious, commonly occurs, accompanied by passage of blood and mucus ("currant jelly stool") via the rectum. This classic triad

is present in less than half of patients.

2. The abdomen is often distended and swollen, with a palpable mass and absent cecum in the right iliac fossa. Peristaltic waves may be present. The rectal and bimanual examinations may reveal bloody stool and a palpable mass.

3. Altered mental status may occur, marked by lethargy, behavioral changes, irritability, somnolence, and listlessness. These changes may precede abdominal findings.

Complications

1. Perforation of bowel with peritonitis
2. Shock and sepsis
3. Reintussusception

Ancillary data

1. Abdominal x-ray film are positive in 35%-40% of patients.
   a. Decreased bowel gas and fecal material in the right colon
   b. An abdominal mass
   c. The apex of the intussusception outlined by gas
   d. Small-bowel distension and air-fluid levels secondary to mechanical obstruction
2. Barium enema is both diagnostic and therapeutic and is up to 75% successful at achieving reduction.
   a. A nonlubricated catheter is inserted into the rectum. Under fluoroscopic observation the barium solution flows, filling by means of gravity. The intussusception is identified and reduction is manifest by free filling of the small intestine past the point of obstruction. The procedure should be performed only by an experienced radiologist after surgical consultation.
   b. Up to three attempts of 3 min each may be tried. Sedation of the patient may be helpful in successfully performing the procedure. The abdomen should not be palpated or compressed during the study.
   c. Underlying lesions should be sought, particularly in children over 1 yr of age,

where a lead point may be detected.
   d. Contraindications to performing a barium enema include necrotic, gangrenous bowel or an unstable patient with shock, anemia, or acidosis.
3. Sonography may be useful as a noninvasive screening technique in the stable patient with an uncertain diagnosis.

Differential diagnosis (Chapters 24 and 35)

1. Infection
   a. Acute gastroenteritis
   b. Appendicitis
2. Infantile colic
3. Intestinal obstruction or peritonitis (e.g., volvulus, postoperative complication, tumor)
4. Incarcerated hernia
5. Testicular torsion

Management

1. Once intussusception is suspected, patients should have an IV line established and rehydration initiated. A bolus of D5W.9%NS 20 ml/kg over 45-60 min should be given if there is any evidence of a deficit.
2. Surgical consultation should be obtained.
3. An abdominal x-ray film should be taken and, if indicated, a barium enema.
4. If the barium enema is successful at reducing the intussusception, the patient should be hospitalized for observation because of the risk of recurrence and for continuous IV therapy. Since there is also a small risk of reducing the necrotic bowel, the child should be observed by serial physical examinations and monitoring of vital signs and WBC.
5. Surgery is indicated immediately if the barium enema is unsuccessful or contraindicated. If there is evidence of peritonitis or perforation, initiate antibiotics, including ampicillin 100-200 mg/kg/24 hr q 4 hr IV **and** clindamycin 30-40 mg//kg/24 hr q 6 hr IV **and** gentamicin 5.0-7.5 mg/kg/24 hr q 8 hr IV before surgery. Adults and children over 4 yr of age commonly need surgery because

of the high incidence of pathologic lead points.

REFERENCES

Hutchison, I.F.: Intussusception in infancy and childhood, Br. J. Surg. **67**:209, 1980.

Liu, K.W., MacCarthy, J., Guiney, E.J., and Fitzgerald, R.J.: Intussusception: current trends in management, Arch. Dis. Child. **61**:75, 1986.

Rachmel, A., Rosenbach, Y., Amir, J., et al.: Apathy as an early manifestation of intussusception, Am. J. Dis. Child. **137**:701, 1983.

MECKEL'S DIVERTICULUM

JAMES C. MITCHINER

ALERT: Meckel's diverticulum must be considered in patients with rectal bleeding or RLQ pain.

Meckel's diverticulum is the most common congenital malformation of the GI tract, resulting from the persistence of the vitelline duct remnant. Symptomatic diverticula usually contain gastric mucosa and are proximal to the ileocecal valve. The majority of cases occur by 2 yr of age, a third of which are symptomatic during infancy.

Diagnostic findings

1. Although many patients remain asymptomatic with a diverticulum, patients with diverticulitis have crampy, RLQ abdominal pain associated with nausea, vomiting, and anorexia. Symptoms are caused by narrowing of the diverticular mouth as a result of peptic strictures, fecal material, granulomas, foreign bodies, tumors, etc.
2. Perforation or obstruction may be present, the former associated with abdominal guarding, decreased bowel sounds, and fever. Obstruction produces distension with abdominal pain.
3. Lower GI hemorrhage may be present in 40% of patients with Meckel's diverticulum. Children have painless rectal bleeding, which may be episodic. The stool blood is usually bright red or dark but rarely tarry.

Complications
1. Perforation of the diverticulum with peritonitis
2. Massive GI bleeding
3. Small bowel obstruction, often from obstruction of the ileum

Ancillary data
1. WBC is often elevated and the Hct decreased if significant bleeding has occurred.
2. Stool has bright-red or dark-red blood without PMN leukocytes.
3. X-ray films
   a. Abdominal flat plate is not diagnostic but may demonstrate free air if perforation has occurred or distension and air fluid levels if obstruction is present.
   b. Technetium sodium pertechnetate study (done before barium enemas) is diagnostic. False positive x-ray findings are rare, whereas false negative x-ray findings may occur in as many as 30% of cases.

Differential diagnosis

1. Rectal bleeding, most commonly resulting from intestinal polyps, intussusception, volvulus, and anal fissures (Chapter 35)
2. RLQ pain: appendicitis (p. 494)
3. Small bowel obstruction caused by intussusception or volvulus
4. Other causes of peritonitis

Management

1. Depending on the degree of rectal bleeding and obstruction, patients may require resuscitation and blood products. An NG tube should be inserted for gastric decompression.
2. A rapid evaluation of the patient, including a surgical consultation, is usually required.
   a. Laboratory studies (CBC, electrolytes, type and crossmatch, and urinalysis) should be rapidly obtained.
   b. If the etiology of the bleeding is uncertain, a rapid radiologic evaluation of the patient should be completed, including abdomi-

nal flat plate, sigmoidoscopy, technetium scan, and barium enema, depending on likely causes and the patient's clinical status.

3. If there is evidence of peritonitis or perforation, antibiotics should be initiated:
   a. Ampicillin 100-200 mg/kg/24 hr q 4 hr IV **and**
   b. Clindamycin 30-40 mg/kg/24 q 6 hr IV **and**
   c. Gentamicin 5.0-7.5 mg/kg/24 hr q 8 hr IV
4. Surgical laparotomy is the definitive diagnostic and therapeutic procedure. A wedge diverticulectomy, which includes excision of the diverticulum and a wedge of ileum, should be performed in the majority of symptomatic cases.

Disposition

1. All patients should be admitted for evaluation and treatment.
2. A surgical consultation is required.

REFERENCES

Kilpatrick, Z.M., and Aseron, C.A.: Isotope detection of Meckel's diverticulum causing acute rectal hemorrhage, N. Engl. J. Med. **287:**653, 1972.

Rutherford, R.B., and Akers, D.R.: Meckel's diverticulum: a review of 148 pediatric patients, with special reference to the pattern of bleeding and to mesodiverticular vascular bands, Surgery **59:**618, 1966.

PYLORIC STENOSIS

RONALD D. LINDZON

ALERT: Pyloric stenosis should be suspected in neonates 3 to 6 wk old with postprandial, nonbilious vomiting. Projectile vomiting is not always present.

Hypertrophic pyloric stenosis results from hypertrophy and hyperplasia of the circular antral and pyloric musculature, resulting in gastric outlet obstruction. Although it has been reported in infants from birth to 5 mo, it most commonly occurs at 3-4 wk of life. White males are more frequently affected, and there is a familial incidence.

Diagnostic findings

1. Gradual onset of vomiting between 3-4 wk is common. This progresses to forceful or projectile, nonbilious emesis. An associated esophagogastritis is present in 20% of children, producing blood-tinged vomitus. The child is hungry and easily refed. Constipation is common.
2. Visible peristaltic waves may be observed traveling from the left upper to the right upper quadrant. These are best visualized postprandially and before emesis.
3. A palpable pyloric "olive" or tumor is present below the liver edge and just lateral to the right rectus abdominis muscle. It is best felt after emesis or when an NG tube has been placed on low intermittent suction.
4. Dehydration with varying degrees of lethargy may be present. This is often a hypochloremic alkalosis.
5. Jaundice may be present (8%) secondary to glucuronyl transferase deficiency. It clears after surgery.

Complications

1. Dehydration with metabolic alkalosis and, rarely, shock
2. Esophagitis, gastritis, or gastric ulceration, with upper GI hemorrhage or perforation
3. Failure to thrive and secondary neurologic sequelae

Ancillary data

1. Electrolytes, BUN, and glucose to evaluate hydration and nutrition. Bilirubin if patient has jaundice. CBC to exclude infection
2. X-ray film
   a. Abdominal plain film will demonstrate gastric dilation.
   b. Barium swallow is indicated if suspected diagnosis is unconfirmed by physical examination. It reveals "string" or "beak" sign (fine elongated pyloric canal) and delayed gastric emptying. Rarely is there complete pyloric obstruction.
   c. Abdominal ultrasound

Differential diagnosis (Chapter 44)

1. Infection/inflammation
   a. Gastroenteritis or sepsis
   b. Esophagitis or gastritis
2. Endocrine disorders: adrenal insufficiency (adrenal-genital syndrome)
3. Congenital disorders: hiatal hernia, intestinal obstruction, atresia, malrotation
4. Chalasia or poor feeding technique

Management

1. Once the diagnosis is considered, patients should have an IV line inserted and fluid deficits corrected. Initially give D5W.9%NS at 20 ml/kg IV over 30-60 min, and then compute deficit and maintenance replacements. Aggressive management of the inevitable hypokalemia is essential in correcting the electrolyte imbalance and alkalosis.
2. An NG tube should be inserted and placed on intermittent low suction.
3. Surgical consultation should be obtained early in the work-up.
4. Surgery is indicated once the fluid and electrolyte status is stable.
   a. Rarely, conservative medical management has been attempted, but it results in prolonged hospitalization and significant morbidity.
   b. Pyloromyotomy is performed and is associated with low morbidity and mortality.

Disposition

All patients require hospitalization and surgery.

VOLVULUS

ALERT: Acute onset of abdominal pain and obstruction in the child over 1 yr of age requires evaluation for volvulus.

Volvulus is a closed-loop obstruction with massive distension resulting from the twisting of a section of intestine on its own axis. Although uncommon in children, the rare cases that are reported occur in the first few days of life and between 2 and 14 yr of age.

The condition may result from congenital malrotation, the presence of a long and freely mobile mesentery, Meckel's diverticulum, or surgical adhesions. Chronic constipation is a predisposing factor. Sigmoid volvulus is most frequently seen, although gastric (along axis joining lesser and greater curvatures), midgut, and transverse colon volvulus have been reported.

Diagnostic findings

1. Sudden onset of crampy abdominal pain, often greater in the lower quadrants, is common. Rarely, patients have progressive or intermittent pain over several days or weeks, associated with sporadic twisting. Pain increases with worsening distension.
2. Marked intestinal obstruction is present with sigmoid volvulus, the degree reflecting the competency of the ileocecal valve. Tenderness is present, but guarding and peritoneal signs appear only if complications of peritonitis develop.
3. The rectum is empty of stool. Bloody stool is uncommon.
4. Anorexia and vomiting occur frequently.
   Complications
1. Perforation with peritonitis
2. Dehydration
   Ancillary data
1. CBC and electrolytes
2. X-ray films
   a. Abdominal films show dilated, gas-filled loops with colonic distension. No gas is present in the rectum.
   b. Barium enema (very carefully performed) demonstrates in sigmoid volvulus that the sigmoid colon has a circular pattern and that barium stops at the junction of the sigmoid and left colon.

Differential diagnosis

1. Congenital disorders
   a. Intussusception (usually occurs in children under 1 yr of age)

b. Hirschsprung's disease
2. Inflammatory disorders
   a. Colitis with megacolon
   b. Peritonitis
3. Uremia

Management

1. Initial stabilization should provide for oxygen, replacement of fluid deficits, and surgical consultation.
2. Hydrostatic reduction of the volvulus during the performance of the barium enema is often successful in children. This must be done carefully after surgical consultation.

3. If peritonitis is present, if it develops, or if reduction is not achieved, immediate surgical repair is necessary.
4. The necessity for surgical repair on a semi-elective basis of a sigmoid volvulus in a child whose volvulus has been hydrostatically reduced is controversial. Children, in contrast to adults, have a decreased risk of recurrence.

REFERENCE

Nadala, L.A., and Ramirez, H.: The successful hydrostatic reduction of sigmoid volvulus in an infant: case report and literature review, Milit. Med. **145:**132, 1980.

77 Genitourinary diseases

Epididymitis

ALERT: Testicular torsion must be excluded in patients with testicular pain.

ETIOLOGY: INFECTION

1. Common organisms
   a. *Neisseria gonorrhoeae*
   b. *Chlamydia trachomatis*
2. Uncommon organisms (in younger age-group): coliforms and *Pseudomonas* bacteria

DIAGNOSTIC FINDINGS

1. Usually, there is a gradual onset of scrotal and groin pain with edema.
2. Initially, the epididymis is tender and swollen, with a soft, normal testicle. This evolves to diffuse tenderness and edema of the epididymis and testicle, often involving the scrotal wall as well.
3. The patient may have a history of trauma, lifting, or heavy exercise.
4. Dysuria, frequency of urination, and urethral discharge may be present.

Ancillary data

1. WBC (may be elevated)
2. Urinalysis and urine culture
3. Gram's stain and culture of urethral discharge

DIFFERENTIAL DIAGNOSIS

See p. 507.

MANAGEMENT

The most important part of the management is to be certain of the diagnosis. If there is any question that a testicular torsion exists, immediate urologic consultation should be obtained.

1. For epididymitis, institute scrotal support, bed rest, and analgesia.
2. Start antibiotics (dose for boys >45 kg or 100 lb)
   a. Amoxicillin 3 g PO once *and* probenecid 1 g PO once; **or** ceftriaxone 250 mg once
   b. Follow (for boys over 8 yr of age) with tetracycline 500 mg q 6 hr PO **or** doxycycline 100 mg q 12 hr PO for 10 days
   c. If a specific organism is identified, alter antibiotics.

DISPOSITION

Patients may be sent home with supportive care and antibiotics.

Hernias and hydroceles

HERNIAS

Hernias result from persistence of the processus vaginalis.

Diagnostic findings

Patients usually have intermittent, localized swelling in the groin or labia, sometimes accompanied by irritability, pain, abdominal tenderness, or limp.

1. Incarcerated hernias occur when the intestine becomes trapped in the sac, usually before 3 yr of age.

2. Strangulated bowel has a compromised blood supply, leading to necrosis. It is tender and swollen, and the overlying skin is usually edematous with a red or violaceous color. It is very rare in pediatric patients for the hernia to strangulate. However, in female patients the ovary or uterus may incarcerate, preventing easy reduction.
3. Intestinal obstruction may occur.

Management

1. Uncomplicated hernias may be repaired electively.
2. Incarcerated hernias can usually be reduced manually, after sedation, with gentle, prolonged pressure and elevation of the foot of the bed. Such patients should be hospitalized for observation and then urgent repair 12-24 hr after edema has resolved.
3. Strangulated hernias require immediate surgical intervention.

HYDROCELES

Hydroceles occur with closure of the processus vaginalis at the abdominal end and fluid accumulation in the sac.

Diagnostic findings

1. The testicle appears large, surrounded by fluid-filled sac. This usually resolves by 6 mo of age. The sac is transilluminated.
2. If the size of the sac (or amount of fluid) changes from day to day, it is considered to communicate and is associated with a hernia.

Management

1. Noncommunicating hydroceles resolve by 6 mo of age.
2. Communicating hydroceles or those that are still present at 12 mo of age require surgical intervention for repair of the associated hernia.
3. Hydroceles of adolescents should be explored because of the potential for underlying neoplasm.

Penile disorders

See also Chapter 64.

PHIMOSIS

Phimosis is a narrowing of the foreskin with an inability to retract the prepuce over the glans because of poor hygiene or chronic infection. Normally, retraction is possible by 4 yr of age. If obstruction to urinary flow occurs, early circumcision (or dorsal slit) may be necessary.

PARAPHIMOSIS

Paraphimosis occurs when the foreskin retracts and is caught proximal to the coronal sulcus with subsequent swelling and venous congestion, with potential compromise of the vascular supply to the glans. It usually occurs with manipulation, masturbation, intercourse, or irritation.

After sedation, an ice and water mixture (usually in a rubber glove) is place over the foreskin and glans for 3-4 min. With gentle, continuous, circumferential pressure on the glans for 5 min, the foreskin usually slips over. If the foreskin does not slip easily, hold the shaft of the penis between the thumb and fingers of one hand (after 5-10 min of squeezing to reduce swelling) and push the glans down into the prepuce with a slow, steady pressure with the free thumb. Alternatively, the shaft may be held in both hands with the thumb on the glans and the foreskin pulled forward over the glans in a slow, steady motion. A dorsal slit with later circumcision rarely is indicated.

In newborns with a plastibell circumcision, the ring may slip behind the glans onto the shaft of the penis and cannot be slipped forward. In such event an attempt should be made to reduce the swelling with cold compresses and steady continuous circumferential pressure. The ring also can be cut off.

BALANITIS

Balanitis is a chronic irritation and inflammation of the foreskin and glans, usually secondary to poor hygiene. The foreskin is red and swollen with a collection of smegma. There is often a concurrent diaper dermatitis.

Hot baths and local care are usually sufficient for treatment.

Testicular torsion

ALERT: Acute onset of testicular pain and tenderness requires immediate urologic consultation.

ETIOLOGY

1. Congenital. A freely mobile testis suspended on a long mesorchium ("bell clapper") is usually present bilaterally.
2. Trauma. Scrotal trauma or exercise may precede the torsion, but torsion can occur at rest or may awaken the patient from sleep.

DIAGNOSTIC FINDINGS

Intermittent or constant testicular pain, which is sudden and intense in onset, occurs. Rarely, it may be gradual in onset with progression of severity. The testicle is tender, high riding, and often horizontal. Scrotal edema is present. Nausea may accompany the testicular pain.

Complications

Testicular necrosis will occur withing 6-8 hr of torsion.

Ancillary data

1. Doppler examination of the testicle demonstrates decreased pulsatile flow in the affected testicle. Normally, flow is equal in both testicles.
2. Technetium nuclear scan has decreased perfusion and is 90% sensitive and specific for testicular torsion but should not delay surgery inordinately.

DIFFERENTIAL DIAGNOSIS

Diagnostic considerations must be rapidly excluded in evaluating the patient with testicular pain. Table 77-1 summarizes significant findings.

For *acute scrotal swelling* a broader list of entities should be considered. *Painful* swelling with a tender testicle may be caused by testicular torsion, trauma with a hematocele, and epididymitis or orchitis. A nontender testicle and painful swelling may be secondary to an incarcerated hernia or torsion of the appendix testicle. In cases of *painless* swelling with an enlarged testicle a testicular tumor or antenatal testicular torsion must be considered. If the testis is normal, underlying pathology may include a hydrocele, an incarcerated hernia, Henoch-Schönlein purpura, or generalized edema or the swelling may be idiopathic.

MANAGEMENT

1. Testicular torsion is a urologic emergency. If there is any question regarding the diagnosis, immediate consultation is required. Doppler and nuclear scans should be performed.
2. Surgical detorsion is indicated immediately. If this is unavailable, local detorsion by outward twisting (toward the outer thigh) may be cautiously attempted. Edema usually precludes local detorsion from being successful. This procedure may be monitored by Doppler examination, verifying return of blood flow.
3. Analgesia is useful after the diagnosis is certain and the decision made to operate.

DISPOSITION

All patients require immediate hospitalization for surgical detorsion and bilateral fixation. Necrosis usually results if torsion has existed for several hours when the cord is twisted three to four complete turns. Various degrees of atrophy have been reported following detorsion.

TABLE 77-1. Testicular pain: diagnostic considerations

Condition	Diagnostic findings	Ancillary data
TESTICULAR TORSION	Sudden onset; may follow trauma or occur during sleep or vehicle ride Physical examination: tender testicle with horizontal lie; abdominal or flank pain	Urine: normal Technetium scan: decreased activity Doppler examination: decreased flow
TRAUMA	Sudden onset with history of trauma Physical examination: pain and swelling of testicle; hematoma may be present; findings reflect injury	Urine: normal Technetium scan: variable Doppler examination: variable
EPIDIDYMITIS	Usually gradual onset; uncommon in boys before puberty; groin pain; may be associated with trauma, lifting, exercise Physical examination: tender epididymis present early with a soft normal testicle whereas later, diffuse tenderness of epididymis and testicle is noted; febrile; prostatic tenderness	Urine: pyuria, bacteriuria Technetium scan: increased activity Doppler examination: normal or increased flow
TUMOR	Gradual onset unless hemorrhage Physical examination: hard, irregular, and usually painless testicle	Urine: normal Technetium scan: normal Doppler examination: normal

REFERENCES

Haynes, B.E., and Bessen, H.A.: Diagnosis of testicular torsion, JAMA **249**:2522, 1983.

Herzog, L.W., and Alvarez, S.R.: The frequency of foreskin problems in uncircumcised children, Am. J. Dis. Child. **140**:254, 1986.

May, D.C., Lesh, P., Lewis, S., et al.: Evaluation of acute scrotum pain with testicular scanning, Ann. Emerg. Med. **14**:696, 1985.

78 Gynecologic disorders

Gynecologic examination

The gynecologic examination of the prepubescent patient requires patience, sensitivity, and a modified approach to the examination. It is crucial to provide a careful explanation and to move slowly while constantly reassuring the patient and parents. This usually will avoid the necessity for an examination under anesthesia. The most shy children are often those in the 11- to 13-yr age-group who are just experiencing puberty.

Younger children are best examined in the presence of their mothers. Examination of the external genitalia by inspection and palpation can usually be accomplished while the child is on the mother's lap. If appropriate, having the child assist the examiner by separating the labia may be reassuring to the child. The examiner should simultaneously depress the perineum. Particular attention should be focused on observation for trauma, foreign bodies, lacerations, discharges, vesicles, ulcers, and adenopathy. *Labial adhesions* are common in young children, usually secondary to irritation or inflammation. They may spontaneously separate by 12 mo, but this process may be facilitated by topical application of Premarin cream nightly for 2 wk.

Next, the child should be placed in the knee-chest position with her buttocks held up in the air and apart by an assistant. The girl is asked to lie on her abdomen with bottom up and to let her stomach and back sag. Instrumentation is rarely necessary, the short vagina of the prepubertal girl allowing enough visualization to rule out foreign bodies and other lesions. Samples of secretions, discharges, and seminal fluid for culture, cell cytology, or forensic examination may be obtained by using a moistened Q-tip or an eye dropper. A small vaginoscope or small nasal speculum should be used if direct visualization is necessary.

All discharges should be evaluated both for *Candida (Monilia)* and *Trichomonas* organisms, using a wet saline and KOH preparation. Gram's stain and culture of all discharges on a minimum of Thayer-Martin or Transgrow medium also should be done.

Palpation may be required to establish abdominal tenderness and the position of the cervix and to exclude foreign bodies or other masses. A bimanual rectoabdominal or one-finger vaginal examination may be performed with the child on her back.

In the pubescent female a careful examination should be done with detailed explanations to maximize cooperation. The procedures should parallel those for the older female. A straightforward, noncondescending approach to the patient is crucial.

Menstrual problems

DYSMENORRHEA

Dysmenorrhea commonly has pain associated with menstruation, which is functional in over 95% of patients. It may result from an increased secretion of prostaglandins causing contractility of the myometrium during a period of falling progesterone levels. Emotional problems or sexual maladjustment may rarely be contributory. Infrequently, endometriosis (rare in children), chronic pelvic inflammatory disease (PID), or anomalies of the müllerian ducts or genitourinary tract may be present as a cause of dysmenorrhea. There is a high correlation with dysmenorrhea in the mother. As many as 29% of girls 12-17 yr have pain severe enough to interfere with normal activity; 14% of girls miss an average of 12-15 days of school per year because of cramps.

Diagnostic findings

Crampy abdominal pain in the lower to middle abdomen with radiation to the back and thighs commonly are associated with the menses, often beginning 6-18 mo after menarche. The discomfort normally commences within 1-4 hr of the menstruation, continues for up to 24 hr, and may vary in severity from month to month. Rarely, the pain begins before bleeding and continues for several days. Nausea, vomiting, and diarrhea may be noted. Emotional problems should be suspected if the pain occurs at menarche and begins with anticipation of menses. Patients may be anxious and irritable with edema and weight gain or a sense of bloating. Patients also may be fatigued and depressed.

Premenstrual syndrome (PMS), a distinct luteal-phase disorder, starts 7-10 days before menses and includes symptoms of weight gain, fatigue, headache, pelvic pain, and emotional lability. It is uncommon in adolescents, usually occurring in the late twenties and thirties.

With functional dysmenorrhea physical examination is usually normal. A pelvic examination is indicated to exclude organic etiologies.

Management

1. Organic etiologies should be appropriately treated.
2. If functional, reassurance is of primary importance. Hot baths, heating pads, and relaxation may be used. Mild analgesics may be helpful. Aspirin is particularly useful since it is also a prostaglandin inhibitor and should be tried first, but it may produce increased bleeding.
3. If further intervention is appropriate, a prostaglandin inhibitor should be initiated on the first day of menses and taken for 2-3 days as necessary for pain control. It may be more effective for some patients to begin medication a day before onset of menstruation. Several options exist:
   a. Naproxen (Naprosyn): 500 mg initially, followed by 250 mg q 6-8 hr PO (maximum: 1,250 mg/24 hr)
   b. Ibuprofen (Motrin): 400 mg q 6 hr PO. Available as over-the-countrer medication (Nuprin or Advil 200 mg). Give 200-400 mg q 4-6 hr PO (maximum: 1200 mg/24 hr). Many find an initial dose of 800 mg to be useful.
4. If discomfort continues to be significant, oral contraceptives may be initiated for 3-6 mo. If the patient is sexually active, oral contraceptives (if there are no contraindications) are particularly useful.
5. Follow-up every 2-3 mo should be arranged to provide reassurance and monitor the clinical response.

PREMENSTRUAL EDEMA

Edema, bloating, and irritability may precede the onset of menstruation. Management includes mild salt restriction, and if the condition is severe, some clinicians suggest initiating diuretic therapy 3-4 days before the onset of menses and continuing for a total of 5-7 days. Hydrochlorothiazide (HydroDiuril) 25 mg/24 hr PO is appropriate.

MITTELSCHMERZ

Mittelschmerz is thought to be caused by ovulatory bleeding into the peritoneal cavity. It is typically dull and aching, occurring midcycle and predominantly in one lower quadrant. It sometimes lasts 6-8 hr but may be severe and cramping, lasting for several days. Distinguishing it from pain caused by appendicitis, torsion or rupture of an ovarian cyst, ectopic pregnancy, etc., may be difficult.

1. Physical examination usually will be normal.
2. Therapy includes reassurance, mild analgesia, and local application of heat.

DYSFUNCTIONAL UTERINE BLEEDING (HYPERMENORRHEA OR MENORRHAGIA)

Dysfunctional uterine bleeding is related to anovulatory cycles resulting in hyperplasia of the endometrium from continuous estrogenic stimulation. It often is associated with irregular menses and results when flow is frequent, heavy, and prolonged. It usually is painless. It may result from dietary changes, stress, diabetes mellitus, as well as from a number of endocrine conditions (hypothyroidism or hyperthyroidism, ovarian tumor, or adrenal insufficiency). Other etiologies of vaginal bleeding (Chapter 43) must be excluded before treatment. Patients should have a hematocrit to assess the severity of bleeding, as well as routine and orthostatic vital signs.

Management

Management depends on the significance of the bleeding.

1. **Minimal bleeding** with little discomfort may be treated with reassurance.
2. **Moderate bleeding** often requires pharmacologic intervention:
   a. Medroxyprogesterone (Provera) 10 mg/24 hr PO for 5 days
      (1) This is the most common approach, and usually bleeding stops in 3-5 days.
      (2) If bleeding persists with subsequent menses, the patient takes 10 mg/24 hr for 5 days at the beginning of expected menstruation for 3 cycles, at which time normal cycles should resume.
   b. A high estrogenic cyclic hormone may al-
   ternatively be used—mestranol and norethindrone (Ortho-Novum 2 mg) **or** mestranol and norethynodrel (Enovid-E 2.5 mg) for 2 mo
3. **Severe bleeding** requires hospitalization, treatment of anemia, and high-dose conjugated estrogens such as premarin 40 mg/dose q 4 hr IV for up to 24 hr (maximum: 6 doses) until bleeding stops.
   a. Once bleeding has stopped, a high estrogen-progestin oral preparation is begun: Ortho-Novum 5 mg; 2 tablets are given initially, followed by 1 tablet 4 times/day and gradually tapered over 1 mo. The patient is placed on a cycle of Ortho-Novum 2 mg or Enovid-E 2.5 mg for 2-3 mo.
   b. Gynecologic consultation is required.

Iron deficiency anemia in menstruating adolescents often can be prevented by treating with supplemental iron and vitamin C (enhances oral iron absorption) and by monitoring response.

Pelvic inflammatory disease
(vulvovaginitis and vaginal discharge-p. 514)

Pelvic inflammatory disease (PID) encompasses a spectrum of illnesses that are seen with increasing frequency in adolescents. Asymptomatic or uncomplicated genital infections may involve only the urethra, vagina, or cervix, but they may become disseminated, resulting in generalized PID.

Although PID is normally considered a sexually transmitted disease and pelvic disease occurs almost exclusively in sexually active women, nonsexual transmission is possible, particularly in children. Factors contributing to sensitivity include foreign bodies such as an intrauterine device (IUD), instrumentation and other trauma, pregnancy, and menstruation.

The majority of cases of gonococcal disease occur within 7 days of the onset of menses.

ETIOLOGY: INFECTION

1. *Neisseria gonorrhoeae*
2. Nongonococcal (often mixed) infection
   a. *Chlamydia trachomatis* (probably most common of nongonococcal etiologies)
   b. Anaerobes: *Bacteroides, Peptostreptococcus,* and *Peptococcus* organisms
   c. Aerobes: *Escherichia coli, Proteus* organisms, *Gardnerella vaginalis (Haemophilus vaginalis)*
   d. *Mycoplasma hominis* or *Ureaplasma urealyticum*

DIAGNOSTIC FINDINGS

Uncomplicated PID: cervicitis or urethritis

1. Gonococcal organisms
   a. Cervicitis in postpubertal females is marked by purulent discharge, dysuria, and dyspareunia. The cervix is hyperemic and tender on touch but not on movement.
   b. Urethritis occurs in boys and, rarely, girls and is associated with a purulent discharge and dysuria.
   c. Vaginitis in prepubertal females is associated with dysuria and purulent discharge. The vulva is erythematous, edematous, and excoriated (p. 514).
   d. Potential child abuse should be considered in the evaluation of gonococcal disease in prepubertal children.
2. Nongonococcal organisms
   a. Cervicitis with mucopurulent discharge is often caused by *Chlamydia* organisms.
   b. Urethritis in men and, rarely, women, with associated dysuria, frequency, and pyuria, is usually caused by *Chlamydia* organisms.
   c. Women may develop a vaginitis with associated nonirritating, odorous, thin, grayish-white discharge. Small refractile coccobacillus *(G. vaginalis)* may be seen near epithelial cells ("clue cells").

Complicated PID: endometritis, salpingitis, parametritis, or peritonitis

Complicated PID may be divided into acute, subacute, and chronic categories on the basis of the onset of symptoms, severity of findings, and number of previous episodes. In general, *N. gonorrhoeae* produces more severe symptoms and a more acute onset, and it usually is associated with the menstrual cycle, whereas *Chlamydia* infection is more commonly associated with an insidious course of pelvic pain. However, the differentiation from nongonococcal disease is not reliable for the individual patient.

Acute PID
1. Patients usually have high fever. Vital signs reflect the severity of abdominal inflammation, including endometritis, salpingitis, parametritis, or peritonitis.
2. Abdominal pain is continuous, usually bilateral, and most severe in the lower quadrants. Peritonitis with rebound, guarding, and decreased bowel sounds may be present. Liver tenderness may result from perihepatitis (Fitz-Hugh–Curtis syndrome).
3. Cervical and adnexal tenderness is present and increases with movement. Uterine bleeding and vaginal discharge may be noted.

Subacute PID
1. Patients often have low-grade fever and few systemic signs.
2. Moderate abdominal, cervical, and adnexal tenderness are present.

Chronic PID
Patients have recurrent episodes of abdominal pain, backaches, vaginal discharge, dysmenorrhea, and menorrhagia.

Complications

1. Infection/inflammation
   a. Peritonitis

b. Tubo-ovarian abscess
c. Endometriosis
d. Salpingitis
2. Endocrine disorders
  a. Infertility
  b. Ectopic pregnancy (risk increased in sub-sequent pregnancies)

Ancillary data

1. WBC and ESR are elevated. Hematocrit may be decreased with extensive bleeding. A normal ESR makes PID unlikely.
2. Culdocentesis or laparoscopy for patients with acute abdomens and potential pelvic pathology is the procedure of choice. It permits rapid assessment for blood and provides culture material.
3. Cultures of cervix or discharge
  a. Gram's stain in females is unreliable unless there are ≥3 WBC with intra-cellular gram-negative diplococci, which increases the chance of recovery of gonococci. Gram's stain of urethral discharge is reliable in males.
  b. Thayer-Martin (or Transgrow) culture and, if complicated, anaerobic cultures
4. Ultrasound to define masses, exclude ectopic pregnancy, or localize IUD if indicated
5. Pregnancy test, if indicated
6. Direct immunofluorescence staining of *Chlamydia* organisms using fluorescein-labeled monoclonal antibody
7. Serologic test for syphilis

DIFFERENTIAL DIAGNOSIS

1. Infection/inflammation
  a. Urethritis
  b. Urinary tract infection (p. 620)
  c. Appendicitis, diverticulosis (p. 494)
  d. Peritonitis
  e. Gastroenteritis
  f. Mesenteric lymphadenitis
  g. Pancreatitis
  h. Inflammatory bowel disease
  i. Endometriosis

2. Endocrine disorders
  a. Ovarian cyst, torsion, tumor
  b. Ectopic pregnancy (p. 519)
  c. Spontaneous abortion
  d. Diabetic ketoacidosis

MANAGEMENT

Prescribed doses in the following sections are for *adolescents (>45 kg or 100 lb) and adults*.

Uncomplicated PID: cervicitis or urethritis
Gonococcal disease

1. Ampicillin (3.5 g) PO; *or* amoxicillin (3 g) PO; *or* aqueous procaine penicillin G 4.8 million units IM (one half given at each of two separate sites); *or* ceftriaxone 250 mg IM. An alternative is cefoxitin 2 g IM.
   • Ampicillin, amoxicillin, penicillin, cefoxitin (but not ceftriaxone) are accompanied by probenecid 1 g PO. Patient should be observed for 30 min after administration.
2. Tetracycline 500 mg q 6 hr PO for 7 days; *or* doxycycline 100 mg q 12 or PO for 7 days; do not use for children under 9 yr of age or pregnant women.
3. To cover all potential pathogens and because of the prevalence of *C. trachomatis*, com-*bined* therapy is usually recommended. The single dose regimen for gonorrhea is appropriate if there is no coinfection with *C. trachomatis*. However, since this often is difficult to determine, gonorrhea treatment usually is followed by the tetracycline or doxycycline course in those over 8 yr who are not pregnant.
4. Homosexual males with rectal gonococcal infection should be treated with ceftriaxone 250 mg IM; *or* aqueous procaine penicillin G 4.8 million units IM *and* probenecid 1 g PO. With allergy to penicillin, use spectinomycin 2 g IM. Anal gonorrhea in females is treated with combined therapy. Pharyngeal gonorrhea should be treated with ceftriaxone, aqueous procaine penicillin G, or tetracycline, as in *1* and *2*.

5. Treatment of gonococcal infections in pregnancy requires modification of the regimen. Ampicillin 3.5 g PO; *or* amoxicillin 3 g PO; *or* aqueous procaine penicillin G 4.8 million units IM; *or* ceftriaxone 250 mg IM; **and** erythromycin 500 mg q 6 hr PO for 7 days.

Nongonococcal disease

C. trachomatis commonly causes urethritis or cervicitis.

1. Tetracycline 500 mg q 6 hr PO for 7 days; *or* doxycycline 100 mg q 12 hr PO; do not use for children under 9 yr of age
2. Alternative is erythromycin 500 mg q 6 hr PO for 7 days

NOTE: One of these regimens should be combined with adequate treatment for gonococcal disease.

Disposition

Follow-up cultures from the infected sites should be obtained 4-7 days after treatment. Positive cultures often are caused by new exposures. If gonorrhea persists, administer *one* IM injection of spectinomycin 2 g *or* ceftriaxone 250 mg.

Complicated PID: endometritis, salpingitis, parametritis, or peritonitis

Support includes parenteral fluids, analgesics, NG tube (if ileus is present), and bed rest, as indicated. The following combination regimens of antibiotics are for *inpatient* adolescents (>45 kg or 100 lb) and adults who are not pregnant:

1. Doxycycline 100 mg q 12 hr IV slowly **and** cefoxitin 2 g q 6 hr IV; continue drugs IV for at least 4 days and at least 48 hr after improvement, then continue doxycycline 100 mg q 12 hr PO to complete a 10-14 day total course; **or**
2. Gentamicin 2 mg/kg followed by 1.5 mg/kg q 8 hr IV in patients with normal renal function; **and** clindamycin 600 mg q 6 hr IV; continue drugs IV for at least 4 days and at least 48 hr after improvement, then continue clindamycin 450 mg q 6 hr PO to complete a 10-14 day total course

When a patient does not require hospitalization and may be treated as an *outpatient*, the following regimens my be considered for adolescents (>45 kg or 100 lb) and adults:

1. Ampicillin 3.5 g PO; *or* amoxicillin 3 g PO; *or* aqueous procaine penicillin G 4.8 million units IM (administered in two separate sites); or cefoxitin 2 g IM; *or* ceftriaxone 250 mg IM; **and**
2. Doxycycline 100 mg q 12 hr PO for 10-14 days (tetracycline 50 mg q 6 hr PO may be substituted but is less active against certain anaerobes). Do not use in children under 9 yr of age or pregnant women.)

Ampicillin, amoxicillin, penicillin, and cefoxitin also must be accompanied by probenecid 1 g PO. Patients should be observed for 30 min after administration.

Prepubertal children should be treated as follows:

1. Cefuroxime 150 mg/kg/24 hr q 24 hr IV; **or** ceftriaxone 100 mg/kg/24 hr q 24 hr IV for at least 4 days or 2 days after improvement; **and**
2. Erythromycin 40 mg/kg/24 hr q 6 hr IV; **or** sulfisoxazole 100 mg/kg/24 hr q 6 hr IV; **or** (in children over 8 yr) tetracycline 30 mg/kg/24 hr q 8 hr IV: continue oral therapy for at least 14 days

Disposition

Hospitalization is indicated under the following circumstances:

1. Uncertain diagnosis, requiring further evaluation
2. Possibility of surgical emergencies such as appendicitis, ectopic pregnancy, or peritonitis
3. Moderate to severe disease with fever, nausea, vomiting, peritonitis, and leukocytosis
4. Suspicion of a pelvic mass or abscess
5. Pregnancy
6. Poor compliance
7. Failure to respond to outpatient therapy
8. Recurrent episodes consistent with chronic PID

Many clinicians recommend that all patients with PID, particularly younger women, should be hospitalized to reduce complications and maximize long-term fertility. Indwelling IUDs commonly are removed. A single episode of tubal infection results in tubal closure in 14% of women, and the rate of ectopic pregnancies is five times greater than in women without a pelvic infection.

Vulvovaginitis and vaginal discharge (pelvic inflammatory disease—p. 510)

Vulvovaginitis and vaginal discharges are common problems of the prepubertal and pubescent females, although the common etiologies vary with age.

A careful history should focus on the presence of accompanying pruritus and odor, and it should define the quality, duration, and volume of the discharge. Other illnesses (diabetes, infections) should be excluded, medications defined (i.e., contraceptives, deodorant sprays, douches, antibiotics), and menstrual history, sexual activity, previous infections, and symptoms in sexual partners clarified. Vaginal discharge associated with cervical motion or adnexal tenderness usually is associated with PID (p. 510).

PREPUBESCENT FEMALE
Nonspecific etiologies

Poor hygiene or an allergic reaction usually are causative. Cultures show a variety of organisms, most of which are normal flora. Substances responsible for allergic responses in younger children include bubble bath and, in adolescents and adults, sanitary napkins, chemical douches, and deodorant and contraceptive sprays.

Diagnostic findings

The discharge is thin and mucoid, and the introitus is painful, erythematous, and swollen. Patients may have a positive history of contact with an irritant.

Management

1. Improved perineal hygiene with particular attention to ensure that child wipes from front to back after bowel movements
2. Frequent changes of white cotton underpants
3. Avoidance of bubble baths and other irritating substances
4. Sitz baths. May be useful 2-4 times/day, washing the area with a very mild soap and allowing to air dry
5. For severe cases: 1% hydrocortisone cream for 2-3 days
6. If there is no resolution in 2-3 wk: systemic ampicillin 250-500 mg q 6 hr PO for 10 days

Foreign body

Articles commonly found in the vagina include paper products, vegetable matter and, in older patients, forgotten tampons. The discharge is blood tinged and foul smelling. Physical examination should reveal the foreign body. It often can be palpated on rectal examination.

Pinworms (p. 441)

Vulvovaginitis is secondary to irritation and itching of the perineum.

Physiologic leukorrhea

A clear, sticky, nonirritating discharge may develop at the onset of puberty secondary to estrogen stimulation and irritation; it ceases once menarche occurs.

It is common for children in the first few days of life to have a thin vaginal discharge. This discharge may become bloody at 5-10 days because of withdrawal of maternal estrogens.

Infection

The infectious etiologies specified for the pubescent female may cause vulvovaginitis in the younger child and should be diagnosed and treated with weight-specific doses of drugs as outlined in the discussion of the postpubescent female.

Nonsexual transmission of sexually transmitted disease is uncommon in prepubescent females beyond the neonatal period. In general, sexual abuse should be considered, particularly in the presence of gonorrhea, *Chlamydia trachomatis, Trichomonas vaginalis*, and condyloma accuminatum.

Although uncommon, *Shigella* organisms can cause a chronic, purulent, blood-tinged discharge that is foul smelling. There may be no associated diarrhea. *E. coli* and group A *streptococci* also have been associated with vulvovaginitis.

POSTPUBESCENT FEMALES

Etiologies specified for the prepubescent female also occur after puberty, although the infectious agents discussed here are more common.

Gonorrhea

Although *N. gonorrhoeae* may cause vaginitis in prepubescent girls, it is more often associated with cervicitis and salpingitis in the pubescent female (p. 511).

Diagnostic findings

1. Patients have a vaginal (urethral in males) discharge that is yellow-green and purulent or mucopurulent. However, 60%-80% of females (and 10% of males) are asymptomatic. Infection is most likely to occur in proximity to menses. Symptomatic patients have discharge, dysuria, frequency, variable cervical tenderness, and proctitis.
2. Complications
   a. PID (p. 510)
   b. Disseminated gonorrhea, often associated with polyarthritis or polytenosynovitis. Endocarditis and meningitis are rare.
   c. Polyarthritis, most frequently the wrist, ankle, or knee (Chapter 27)

d. Monoarticular arthritis
3. **Ancillary data**
   a. Swab or aspirate of discharge (and also of rectum and pharynx, when appropriate) is cultured on Thayer-Martin, Transgrow, or similar medium. Urethral or cervical discharge may reveal intracellular gram-negative diplococci on Gram's stain. Rectal cultures should be done in females (and males if appropriate), since rectal culture is positive in 5% of cases with negative cervical cultures.
   b. Syphilis serologic tests should be obtained (VDRL or equivalent).

Management

Antibiotics therapy should be initiated and may include any of the following (doses are for adolescents >45 kg or 100 lb and for adults):
1. Ampicillin 3.5 g PO; *or* amoxicillin 3 g PO; *or* aqueous procaine penicillin G, 4.8 million units IM (one half in each of two separate sites and observe patient for 30 min after administration); or ceftriaxone 250 mg IM; **and**
2. Tetracycline 500 mg q 6 hr PO for 7 days; *or* doxycycline 100 mg q 2 hr PO for 7 days; do not use for children under 9 yr; for patients in whom tetracycline is contraindicated or not tolerated: erythromycin 500 mg q 6 hr PO for 7 days
   NOTE: Ampicillin, amoxicillin, and penicillin are accompanied by probenecid 1 g PO
3. Anal gonorrhea in females is treated with combined therapy. Pharyngeal gonorrhea should be treated with ceftriaxone, aqueous procaine penicillin G (and probenecid), or tetracycline.
4. Spectinomycin 2 g IM may be used in patients failing to respond to appropriate therapy, for those with infections of penicillinase-producing *N. gonorrhoeae*, or for those allergic to pencillin for whom tetracycline is not desired.
5. Disseminated gonorrhea requires high dose

penicillin: 150,000 units/kg/24 hr (adults: 10 million units/24 hr) q 4 hr IV. These patients obviously must be hospitalized.

6. After 1 wk of treatment, patients should have another culture to ensure a satisfactory response.

Disposition

Patients who have evidence of peritoneal signs or sepsis (e.g., arthritis, liver tenderness) should be hospitalized. Others may be followed at home.

Candida albicans (Monilia)

This is an oval-budding fungus. Patients predisposed to this infection include diabetic individuals, those with recent antibiotic or oral contraceptive use, and those who are pregnant or use nylon undergarments.

Diagnostic findings

1. The discharge is thick and white and resembles cottage cheese, often occurring 1 wk before menses. There often is associated dysuria, intense pruritis, and dyspareunia. The vulva is red and edematous, with excoriations secondary to the intense itching.
2. A slide prepared by placing 1 drop of KOH (10%) on a small amount of discharge and covering with a cover glass will reveal branching filaments, yeast like budding hyphae, or both.

Management

1. Sitz baths may provide symptomatic relief.
2. Topical treatment may include any of the following:
   a. Miconazole (Monistat): 1 applicator full before bed for 7-14 days. Also available as miconazole 200 mg suppository (Monistat 3) that requires only 3 days of therapy.
   b. Clotrimazole (Gyne-Lotrimin) 100 mg vaginal tablet before bed for 7 days
   c. Nystatin cream or suppository (Mycostatin or Nilstat): 2 applications/day until symptoms are relieved; then before bed for a total of 10 days

   d. Ketoconazole (Nizoral) 200 mg q 12 hr PO for 5 days
3. Discontinue oral antibiotics or contraceptives, if possible.

Trichomonas vaginalis

Diagnostic findings

1. Discharge is thin, frothy, malodorous, and yellow-green. Commonly, patients have itching, erythema, pain, and burning of the vulvovaginal area, with cystitis or urethritis. The cervix typically has red, punctate hemorrhages. Rarely (10%), patients have abdominal pain.
2. A wet mount, with saline, of the cervical discharge will reveal motile, flagellated organisms, slightly larger than a leukocyte.

Management

1. Sitz bath or wet compresses for symptomatic relief
2. Metronidazole (Flagyl): 250 mg 3 times per day PO for 7 days *or* 2 g as single dose PO. The sexual partner should be treated with metronidazole, 2 g PO as a single dose.
   a. Younger children may receive 15 mg/kg/24 hr, divided into 3 doses for 10 days.
   b. Patients must not drink alcohol during the course of therapy. Do not give during pregnancy. Use clotrimazole 2-100 mg vaginal tablet before bed for 7 days.

Haemophilus vaginalis (gram-negative pleomophic coccobacilli) *(Gardnerella vaginalis)*

Diagnostic findings

1. Discharge is gray or clear, with a fishy smell. Gram's stain shows multiple organisms and PMN leukocytes. Pruritus and burning may be present.
2. Microscopic examination will reveal epithelial cells coated with small refractile bacteria ("clue cells"). PMN leukocytes are frequent. Mixing the discharge with 10% KOH liberates a fishy, aminelike odor.

Management

Systemic treatment is most effective. Topical treatment can be used for symptomatic relief only.

1. Systemic
   a. Metronidazole (Flagyl) 500 mg given 2 times/day for 7-10 days **or**
   b. Ampicillin 500 mg, 4 times/day for 7-10 days
2. Topical
   a. Sultrin (triple sulfa): 1 applicator full (or tablet), 2 times/day for 4-6 days **or**
   b. AVC cream: 1 applicator full, 2 times/day for 4-6 days
3. The sexual partner should be treated concurrently.

Herpes simplex, type 2

Although both types 1 and 2 can cause infections of the vagina, vulva, and cervix, type 2 is the more common.

Diagnostic findings

1. Grouped vesicles progress to ulcers in the perineal area, associated with bilateral tender inguinal nodes, pain, burning, and itching. Systemic illness may be present. Each episode of infection is usually self-limited but may last for a prolonged period with recurrence. It is particularly important to determine if the patient is pregnant because of the fetal risk.
2. Wright's stain of a vesicle has giant multinucleated cells and inclusion bodies.

Management

1. Sitz baths or wet compresses
2. Analgesics, if necessary
3. Acyclovir (Zovirax)
   a. *Oral* therapy shortens the symptomatic period by reducing the number of new lesions and duration of pain, dysuria, and constitutional symptoms while shortening the shedding of virus. This efficacy

has been documented in primary herpes when treatment is initiated early in the first episode.

- Dose: 200 mg q 4 hr while patient is awake (5 doses per day) PO for 10 days.

Treatment of the initial infection does not prevent recurrences.

Treatment of recurrent episodes may shorten the healing time.

- Dose: 200 mg 5 times per day for 5 days initiated within 2 days of onset

Suppression of recurrences with long-term therapy has been useful in severe disease. The frequency of episodes decreases, but once the drug is discontinued, the frequency returns to the pretreatment level, with a first episode after medication that is often severe. Dose: 200 mg q 8 hr PO for up to 6 mo.

   b. *Topical* (5% ointment) is less effective in decreasing symptoms.

REFERENCES

Abramowicz, M.: Treatment of sexually transmitted diseases, Med. Lett. Drugs Ther. **26**:5, 1984.

Abramowicz, M.: Oral acyclovir for genital herpes simplex infection, Med. Lett. Drugs Ther. **27**:41, 1985.

Centers for Disease Control: 1985 STD treatment guidelines, Morb. Mort. Week. Rep. **34**:755, 1985.

Corey, L., and Spear, P.G.: Infections with herpes simplex viruses, N. Engl. J. Med. **314**:686, 1986.

Cowell, C.A., editor: Pediatric and adolescent gynecology, Pediatr. Clin. North Am. **28**:245, 1981.

Emans, S.J., and Goldstein, D.P.: Pediatric and adolescent gynecology, ed. 2. Boston, 1982. Little, Brown & Co.

Guinan, M.E.: Oral acyclovir for treatment and suppression of genital herpes simplex virus infection, JAMA **255**:1747, 1986.

Rice, R.J., and Thompson, S.E.: Treatment of uncomplicated infections due to *Neisseria gonorrhoeae*, JAMA **255**:1739, 1986.

Sanders, L.L., Harrison, H.R., and Washington, A.E.: Treatment of sexually transmitted chlamydial infections, JAMA **255**:1750, 1986.

Shafer, M.B., Irwin, C.E., and Sweet, R.L.: Acute salpingitis in the adolescent female, J. Pediatr. **100**:339, 1982.

Complications of pregnancy

BENJAMIN HONIGMAN

The diagnosis of pregnancy is based on clinical presentation and a host of urine or serum pregnancy tests. Pregnancy causes secondary amenorrhea. Women also have breast fullness and tenderness, darkening of the areola, enlargement of the nipples, and protrusion of Montgomery's glands. Fatigue, lassitude, nausea, and vomiting are commonly present early in pregnancy. Urinary frequency may be reported. Approximately 6 wk after the last menses, early changes of softening of the uterine isthmus and violaceous coloration of the vulva, vagina, and cervix become evident. At about 8 wk the uterus is enlarged with early changes of softening of the cervix (Hegar's sign), and a bluish hue of the mucosa of the cervix and vagina (Chadwick's sign) is present.

A number of pregnancy tests are available to the clinician.

1. Latex agglutination-inhibition (LAI) test for human chorionic gonadotropin in urine is a 2½ min test that is 90% accurate at 45 days after the last menstrual period. Errors occur from not using first morning urine (concentrated urine), from excessive liquid intake, from proteinuria or hematuria, from intake of psychotropic drugs, and from technical problems. This test should not be relied on early in pregnancy if a complication is suspected. It is useful in the diagnosis of a routine pregnancy.
2. Radioimmunoassay (RIA), which uses antisera against the beta-subunit of human chorionic gonadotropin or the chemically modified beta-subunit, can detect pregnancy 8-13 days after conception (shortly before missed period) with 99% specificity. This is presently the "gold standard."
3. Monoclonal antibody agglutination test to the beta-subunit of HCG in urine or serum is an easy test to perform and correlates well with the RIA. Cheaper and easier to do, it

is becoming the preferred test. In addition, it can detect levels of HCG as low as 5-40 mIU/ml.

The emergency physician most commonly is faced with one of a number of complications of pregnancy that must be considered in the differential diagnosis of a host of presenting complaints.

All of these patients require monitoring of vital signs with orthostatic blood pressure readings and a hematocrit.

ABORTION
Threatened abortion
Diagnostic findings
1. Painless vaginal bleeding during the first trimester of pregnancy
2. Enlarged and nontender uterus, appropriate for dates. The cervix is closed.
3. **Inevitable abortion:** the os is open without tissue

Management
1. Reassurance. 75% of these patients will carry pregnancy to term.
2. Bed rest with bathroom privileges at home. Any blood pooled in the vagina during rest will become apparent when the patient stands, giving the impression of profuse bleeding.

NOTE: Patients with an open os will abort eventually and should be under continuing observation. An outpatient dilation and curettage (D & C) may be indicated in patients in whom the os is open (inevitable abortion).

Incomplete abortion

ALERT: If pain is constant and lateralizes, consider ectopic pregnancy.

Diagnostic findings
1. First trimester bleeding accompanied by cramps and cervical dilation
2. Enlarged, mildly tender uterus. The cervix admits a ring forceps beyond the internal os

without resistance. Products of conception may be visible in the os. Bleeding may be profuse.

Management

1. Remove any material from the cervical os. This should reduce bleeding.
2. Place oxytocin (Pitocin) 20 units in 1,000 ml of D5W, and infuse over 1-2 hr.
3. Consult a gynecologist for an outpatient D & C.
4. With Rh incompatibility administer Rh_0 (D antigen) immune globulin (RhoGAM). Normally, an Hct and blood type determination should be obtained.

Complete abortion

Diagnostic findings

1. Complete expulsion of products of conception during the first trimester
2. Small, firm, and nontender uterus. The cervix admits a ring forceps beyond the internal os. Products of conception are in the vagina or previously have been expelled.
3. Hct with CBC and type and hold. Rh determination must be done.

Management

1. Gynecologic consulation for D & C. (Some clinicians are now deferring this procedure.)
2. RhoGAM for Rh incompatibility.

Missed abortion

Diagnostic findings

1. Threatened or incomplete abortion followed by decrease in bleeding to a brownish discharge. Symptoms of pregnancy decrease.
2. Small uterus for gestational date and variably will admit ring forceps
3. Hematocrit with CBC and type and hold. Rh determination

Management

1. If ≤12 wk: D & C
2. If > 12 wk: oxytocin drip (see above) and hematologic monitoring for hypofibrinogenemia and DIC.
3. With Rh incompatibility, administration of RhoGAM

ECTOPIC PREGNANCY

ALERT: Amenorrhea, abdominal pain, and vaginal bleeding accompanying symptoms of pregnancy must be rapidly investigated. The triad of abdominal pain, abnormal vaginal bleeding, and mass is present in only 45% of patients.

Ectopic pregnancies are normally tubal. Less than 3% are cornual, ovarian, or abdominal. Predisposing factors include PID, previous tubal surgery or ectopic pregnancy, an IUD, or endometriosis.

Diagnostic findings

Ruptured ectopic pregnancy

Abdominal pain is invariably present. Sudden onset of pain associated with vaginal spotting in a pregnant female is very suggestive of a ruptured ectopic pregnancy. The pain may be described as sharp, dull, or aching, and it may be continuous or intermittent, reflecting episodes of intraperitoneal bleeding. Shoulder and back-pain suggests peritonitis.

1. Rebound tenderness is present and, rarely, a bluish ecchymotic area round the umbilicus (Cullen's sign) may develop if there has been a rupture.
2. The cervix is usually tender and the cul-de-sac full. Adnexal tenderness is present and, variably, a mass. The uterus is smaller than expected for gestational age.
3. Vaginal bleeding can range from spotting to heavy flow.
4. Patients often experience vomiting and nausea (morning sickness), amenorrhea, and, rarely, breast engorgement and other suggestions of pregnancy.
5. Patients often demonstrate hypotension, tachycardia, and dyspnea.

Unruptured ectopic pregnancy

Unruptured ectopic pregnancies are difficult to diagnose since abdominal pain may be the only symptom. A pelvic mass is present in one half of patients. Thus women of child bearing age with abdominal pain should have a pregnancy test.

Complications
1. Disseminated intravascular coagulation (p. 522)
2. Fertility problems and recurrent ectopic pregnancies
3. Death secondary to hemorrhagic shock

Ancillary data
1. Hematocrit with CBC and type and cross-match
2. Pregnancy test. The test used should reflect the days since the last menses. RIA and monoclonal antibody to beta-subunit of HCG in urine or serum are sensitive early in the pregnancy. Although ectopic pregnancy usually has a range of HCG of 150-800 mIU/ml, it may be as low as 10 mIU/ml. In selected cases, serial determinations may be useful.
3. Ultrasonography. A valuable diagnostic aid, it is particularly useful in identifying an intrauterine gestation. An adnexal mass may sometimes be visualized.
4. Culdocentesis. A useful diagnostic test that is indicated if there is a question of ectopic pregnancy or infection or to differentiate abdominal from pelvic pathology before surgery for an acute abdomen. The aspirate results are categorized as follows:
   a. Normal tap: straw-colored fluid
   b. Dry tap: nondiagnostic, requiring a repeat tap or other diagnostic procedure (may occur with ectopic pregnancy before rupture)
   c. Positive diagnostic tap: bloody (nonclotting) aspirate with an Hct > 15%
5. Laparoscopy. Useful, particularly if available on an emergent basis

Differential diagnosis
1. Infection: PID, appendicitis, etc.
2. Neoplasm
3. Endocrine disorders: ovarian cyst, follicular or twisted; threatened or incomplete abortion

Management
1. For the unstable patient, IV fluids (crystalloid and blood), MAST suit, NG tube, and urinary catheterization for treatment and monitoring should be initiated.
2. Diagnostic evaluation should include ultrasonography, culdocentesis, or laparoscopy.
3. If diagnosis is confirmed, surgery is indicated to remove ectopic pregnancy and to ligate tube. Rarely, a tuboplasty is indicated for a single remaining tube in a nulliparous female.
4. For the stable patient with unconfirmed but suspected ectopic pregnancy, hospitalization usually is indicated for further diagnostic evaluation.

ABRUPTIO PLACENTAE AND PLACENTA PREVIA

ALERT: Third trimester vaginal bleeding requires urgent evaluation.

Abruptio placentae is the premature separation of a normally implanted placenta, with peak incidence between 20-29 wk and again at 38 wk.

Placenta previa occurs when the attachment of a placenta is located over or near the internal os. Its classification as total or partial is dynamic because of the changing location of the placenta with the progression of pregnancy.

Predisposing factors include abdominal trauma (abruptio placentae), hypertension, high parity, maternal age over 35 yr, and smoking.

Diagnostic findings
Abruptio placentae

Patients classically have vaginal bleeding and abdominal pain. The extent of pain reflects the degree of disruption of the myometrial fibers and intravasation of blood at the site of bleeding. Vaginal bleeding is variable and may be concealed. The uterus is uniformly tender but should be examined only when preparations have been made to perform a cesarean section using a double setup.

Hypotension is usually present. The decrease in blood pressure is often disproportionate to the amount of hemorrhage because of the concealed nature of the blood loss.

Placenta previa

Vaginal bleeding is the prominent sign, varying from repeated episodes to profuse bleeding. The initial bleeding episode is classically minimal; the second episode may have profuse bleeding. The bleeding is painless. The cervix is boggy and easily admits a finger, but examination should be done only when preparations have been made to perform a cesarean section.

Hypotension is present, reflecting the amount of blood loss.

Complications

1. Disseminated intravascular coagulation (p. 522)
2. Acute tubular necrosis (p. 376)
3. Fetal death

Ancillary data

1. Hematocrit is decreased. Type and cross-match should be sent to the laboratory.
2. Fibrinogen is decreased along with thrombocytopenia and coagulation abnormalities.
3. Ultrasonography will localize the placenta and is appropriate for the stable patient.

Differential diagnosis

1. Trauma: laceration or other perineal injury
2. Endocrine disorders: complications of pregnancy including uterine rupture or marginal sinus bleeding, premature labor, or abortion

Management

1. Stabilization should include IV fluids and blood, MAST suit, NG tube, and urinary catheterization. DIC should be treated, if present.
2. With a diagnosis of placenta previa, an attempt to stop labor should be made with a beta-adrenergic agent such as terbutaline (0.25 mg).
3. Fetal heart tones and status should be monitored continuously.

The examination of the patient should be done only in the obstetric or operating suite where double setup precautions are available and an immediate cesarean section can be performed. If the mother and fetus are stable, an ultrasound image may be useful in the initial assessment. The decision regarding vaginal delivery of the fetus is best done by the obstetric and pediatric consultants involved in the examination. Cesarean section usually is indicated if there is any evidence of fetal distress. Support personnel must be available to assist in the management of the unstable or potentially unstable patient.

79 Hematologic disorders

Disseminated intravascular coagulation

Disseminated intravascular coagulation (DIC) is an acquired coagulopathy that may occur in a variety of clinical settings in which the clotting mechanism is triggered. This results in the deposition of thrombi within the microcirculation, consumption of coagulation factors (I, II, V, VIII) and platelets, and, ultimately, bleeding. The severity and clinical significance of DIC varies grately between patients.

ETIOLOGY

The following are common triggers of DIC:
1. Infection
   a. Bacterial
      (1) Gram-negative sepsis
      (2) Meningococcemia (p. 541)
      (3) Gram-positive sepsis: *Streptococcus pneumoniae* and *Staphylococcus aureus*
   b. Viral
      (1) Herpes simplex
      (2) Measles
      (3) Chickenpox
      (4) Cytomegalovirus
      (5) Influenza
   c. Rocky Mountain spotted fever
2. Shock (Chapter 5)
3. Respiratory distress syndrome and asphyxia
4. Trauma
   a. Burns (Chapter 46)
   b. Multiple trauma (Chapter 56)
   c. Snake bites (p. 235)

d. Heat stroke (Chapter 50)
   e. Head injury
5. Complications of pregnancy (p. 518)
6. Neoplasms
7. Necrotizing enterocolitis
8. Hemangioma
9. Intravascular hemolysis
   a. Incompatible blood transfusion
   b. Autoimmune hemolytic anemia

DIAGNOSTIC FINDINGS

The primary determinant of the clinical presentation is the triggering condition. In addition to the signs and symptoms related to that disease, a number of specific findings may be present with DIC.
1. Simultaneous evidence of diffuse bleeding and thrombosis, including petechiae, purpura, peripheral cyanosis, ischemic necrosis of the skin and subcutaneous tissues, hematuria, and melena.
2. Prolonged bleeding from venipuncture and other sites of injury

Complications

1. Organ damage as a result of bleeding and infarction. May include GI hemorrhage, hematuria, CNS bleeding first appearing as mental status changes, apnea, seizures, and coma
2. Purpura fulminans. Occurs as patchy hemorrhagic infarction of the skin and subcutaneous tissue

3. Complications of the precipitating event
4. Death from hemorrhage

Ancillary data (Table 29-2)

1. CBC and peripheral blood smear
    a. Evidence of hemolysis with fragmented red cells resulting from microangiopathy
    b. Anemia may occur as a result of bleeding or hemolysis
    c. Thrombocytopenia is usually present
2. Coagulation studies. Typical findings include the following:
    a. Prolonged PTT as a result of decreased consumable clotting factors (fibrinogen, II, V, VIII)
    b. Increased fibrin split (degradation) products
    c. Increased fibrin monomer
    d. Once the consumption of coagulation factors has ceased, values will normalize (fibrinogen and factor VIII in 24-48 hr; platelet count in 7-14 days)

DIFFERENTIAL DIAGNOSIS

1. Bleeding (Chapter 29)
2. Precipitating conditions

MANAGEMENT

   Initial attention must be toward stabilizing the patient and treating the underlying condition triggering DIC. If this precipitating event can be quickly relieved (e.g., shock, hypoxia, endotoxin release), further therapy is often unnecessary.

1. Administration of fresh whole blood or packed red cells if there is significant hemorrhage
2. Replacement of depleted coagulation factors is usually necessary with active or impending bleeding (Table 79-1 and Fig. 79-1 for management of bacterial septicemia)
    a. Fresh frozen plasma (FFP): fibrinogen (I) and other clotting factors (II, V, and VIII)
       (1) Usually deficient if hypoxia or acidosis is present
       (2) Administration of 10-15 ml/kg/dose IV repeated as indicated by follow-up coagulation studies
    b. Cryoprecipitate: fibrinogen (1) and factor VIII. Indicated only with no response to FFP. Does not correct deficiencies of other coagulation factors.
       (1) For infants: 1 bag cryoprecipitate/3 kg. For older children: 1 bag cryoprecipitate/5 kg
       (2) Will usually raise fibrinogen to greater than 100 mg/100 ml, a level sufficient to promote hemostasis
    c. Platelet concentrate: platelets plus aged plasma
       (1) Usually deficient if triggered by infection

TABLE 79-1. Recommendations for hematologic treatment

Bacterial septicemia	Platelets (1 pack/ 5 kg)	Vitamin K (1-10 mg IV)	Fresh frozen plasma (10-15 ml/kg)	Cryoprecipitate (1 bag/3-5 kg)	Heparin (10-15 units/kg/ hr IV)
Normotensive	±	±	±	0	0
Hypotensive					
Blood pressure restorable	±	±	±	±	0
Blood pressure not restorable					
Bleeding	+	±	+	+	+
Not bleeding	0	±	0	0	±

Modified from Corrigan, J.J.: J. Pediatr. **91:**695, 1977.
+, Recommended; 0, not recommended; ±, may be necessary in certain circumstances.

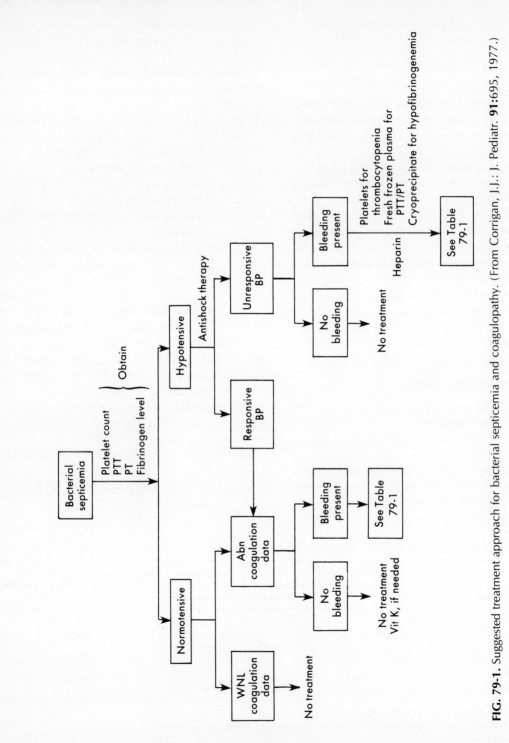

FIG. 79-1. Suggested treatment approach for bacterial septicemia and coagulopathy. (From Corrigan, J.J.: J. Pediatr. **91**:695, 1977.)

(2) Administration of 1 platelet pack/5-6 kg or, for infants, 10 ml/kg should increase platelet count by 50,000 - 100,000/mm³

d. Vitamin K (infants: 1-2 mg/dose IV slowly; children and adults: 5-10 mg/dose IV)

3. Heparin. Indicated in the presence of widespread thrombosis or active bleeding that cannot be controlled by replacement of clotting factors and platelets coupled with aggressive treatment of the triggering disorder. In this setting, the intent of heparin therapy is to block further consumption of clotting factors. It is not recommended until other therapies have failed. Heparin should be used early in the course of DIC associated with meningococcemia because of the frequent occurrence of fulminant thrombosis and tissue necrosis.

• Heparin is administered preferentially by continuous IV infusion.

a. Load with 50 units/kg IV.

b. Give continuous drip of 10-15 units/kg/hr IV.

c. With purpura fulminans, give higher dose if necessary: 20-25 units/kg/hr IV.

d. If bolus infusion is used, give 4 times the hourly dose q 4 hr IV.

  • Replacement therapy with FFP and platelet concentrate should be continued following the initiation of heparin therapy in order to minimize bleeding risk.

  • The efficacy of heparin therapy is monitored, measuring fibrinogen level and, later, platelets and watching for increase and return to normal.

e. Unresponsive neonates. Exchange transfusion may occasionally be indicated for those who do not respond to normal medical management.

DISPOSITION

1. Most patients require admission to an ICU for treatment of the underlying disease as well as the DIC.

2. Emergency care is required with involvement of a hematologist and those with expertise in the management of the underlying pathology.

REFERENCES

Corrigan, J.J., Jr.: Disseminated intravascular coagulation, Pediatrics **64**:37, 1979.

Feinstein, D.I.: Diagnosis and management of disseminated intravascular coagulation: the role of heparin therapy, Blood **60**:284, 1982.

Hemophilia

ROCHELLE A. YANOFSKY

ALERT: Minor pain often signifies deep muscle or joint bleeding requiring factor replacement. Any head trauma requires urgent intervention.

Hemophilia, an X-linked recessive condition, most commonly results from factor VIII (classical) or factor IX (Christmas) deficiency. Patients are classified as mild (5%-25%), moderate (2%-5%), or severe (0%-2%) on the basis of the percentage of coagulation factor, which is determined by assay.

DIAGNOSTIC FINDINGS

Bleeding commonly occurs in deep muscles or joints, either spontaneously or as result of minor trauma. Pain is often the first sign of bleeding. Sites typically involved include:

1. Musculoskeletal

   a. Joints most commonly involved are the elbow, knee, and ankle. Joint tenderness, swelling, and limitation of range of motion are present in the involved joint. Septic arthritis may occur.

   b. Muscle bleeding is common. This is particularly significant in the forearm flexor group and the gastrocnemius and may cause a compartment syndrome. Bleeding in the iliopsoas muscle results in local tenderness accompanied by hip or back pain, limp, and weakness.

2. Subcutaneous. May present with hematomas and ecchymoses
3. Intracranial. Bleeding may be subdural, subarachnoid, intraventricular, cerebellar, or cerebral in location. Without provocation, or following seemingly minor head trauma, patients may experience headache, vomiting, altered mental status, or seizures. With severe bleeding, signs of increased intracranial bleeding may develop (Chapter 57).
4. Spinal cord hematomas. May cause paralysis, weakness, back pain, and asymmetric neurologic findings
5. Upper or lower GI bleeding. May be associated with hematemesis, melena, abdominal tenderness and distension, and shock. Intussusception is rare. Intraperitoneal or retroperitoneal hemorrhage may be present.
6. Retropharyngeal hematomas. May produce dyspnea, dysphagia, and potential GI or respiratory obstruction
7. Mild hematuria is a common finding.

Complications

1. Hepatitis secondary to repeated factor replacement, usually non-A and non-B is common. Cryoprecipitate has reduced this complication if only rare transfusions are needed. However, the risk after multiple transfusions is similar to that of concentrates.
2. A factor VIII (A) or factor IX (B) IgG inhibitor may develop, making management exceedingly difficult.
3. Death is usually secondary to intracranial bleeding, underlining the necessity of rapid intervention in patients with head trauma (even minimal).
4. Acquired immune deficiency syndrome (AIDS) has been described in a small percentage of hemophiliacs; it results from HTLV-III presumably acquired by transfusion of blood products. Evidence of immune dysfunction (AIDS-related complex or ARC) is seen more commonly than full-blown AIDS in transfused hemophiliacs. Hepatosplenomegaly, lymphadenopathy, lymphopenia,

high levels of IgG, thrombocytopenia, and Coombs' positivity may be seen as part of the ARC.

Treatment with cryoprecipitate instead of commercial concentrates in patients with mild factor VIII deficiency appears to decrease the risk of infection with the AIDS agent. Ideally, improved screening of plasma donors and the recent availability of heat-treated factor VIII concentrates will decrease the incidence of AIDS in hemophiliacs.

Ancillary data

1. CBC with Hct, if significant bleeding has occurred
2. Blood coagulation studies including partial thromboplastin time (PTT), prothrombin time (PT), thrombin time (TT), and bleeding time (BT). A platelet count is helpful. Assays for factors VIII and XI will define the deficiency. These are useful in the initial evaluation (Table 29-2).
   a. PTT is prolonged. Specific factor level will be abnormally low.
   b. Treatment of major bleeding or bleeding during surgical procedures is guided by factor levels (Table 79-2).
3. Urinalysis. Mild hematuria is common. Moderate or severe hematuria requires factor replacement therapy.
4. X-ray studies are indicated for specific signs and symptoms. Skeletal films are useful for specific complaints but are not used to assess acute hemarthroses. They are helpful to look for degenerative joint changes or fractures. If symptoms of retropharyngeal hematomas develop, a soft-tissue lateral neck view will define the degree of swelling.
5. CT scan is indicated for anyone with head trauma and any neurologic symptoms, even if minimal. Evolving neurologic deficits require immediate intervention.
6. Contrast studies of the GU and GI tracts are indicated for evaluation of serious bleeding.
7. Ultrasound is useful in defining the extent of

a hematoma and differentiating it from other mass lesions. It is particularly helpful for retroperitoneal bleeding.

8. Aspiration of involved joints is indicated only if the etiology is uncertain and infection suspected. Hematologic consultation should be obtained before the procedure.

DIFFERENTIAL DIAGNOSIS

See Chapter 29.

MANAGEMENT

1. Stabilization of the patient requires IV fluids or blood for major hemorrhages. Airway management, if obstruction is present, must receive first priority.
2. Factor replacement should be initiated immediately as outlined in Tables 79-2 and 79-3.
   a. One unit of factor VIII or IX equals the activity of factor contained in 1 ml of plasma.
   b. The number of units of factor VIII required = $0.5 \times$ weight (kg) $\times$ desired increment (%) of factor VIII level. The half-life is 12 hr.
   c. The number of units of factor IX required = $1.0 \times$ weight (kg) $\times$ desired increment (%) in factor IX level. The half-life is 24 hr.
   d. Cryoprecipitate should be used in the treatment of mild hemophilia A and in children with hemophilia A who are under 5 yr of age.

TABLE 79-2. Factor levels for bleeding episodes in patients with hemophilia

Site of bleeding	Factor level (%) desired	Comments
Common joint	20-40	Phone follow-up at 24 and 48 hr
Joint (hip or groin)	40	Repeat transfusion in 24-48 hr
Soft tissue or muscle	20-40	No therapy if small and not enlarging; transfuse if enlarging
Muscle (calf or forearm)	30-40	Admit if impending or actual anterior compartment syndrome; surgical consultation
Muscle: deep (thigh, hip, or iliopsoas)	40-60	May require admission; transfusion, then another at 24 hr, then prn
Neck or throat	50-80	Admit; consider airway management
Mouth, lip, tongue, or dental work	40	Aminocaproic acid (Amicar)
Laceration	40	Transfuse until wound is healed; if sutured, continue transfusions until 24 hr after suture removal
Hematuria		Mild: prednisone (controversial), rest, hydration
	40	Moderate to severe: transfuse to 40% plus prednisone (controversial), rest, hydration
Gastrointestinal	60-80	Admit
Head trauma (no evidence of CNS bleeding)	50	Very close follow-up
Head trauma (probable or definite CNS bleeding—headache, vomiting, neurologic signs)	100	Admit: transfuse and then investigate (CT scan, etc.); maintain peak and trough factor levels at 100% and 50%, respectively, for 14 days if documented CNS bleeding
Surgery	80-100	At time of surgery; maintain peak and trough factor levels at 60% and 30%, respectively, for 1 wk postoperatively; add aminocaproic acid for mouth surgery.

The minimum hemostatic level for factors VIII and IX is 10%-20%.

TABLE 79-3. Therapeutic concentrates used for factor replacement

Product	Available forms	Coagulation factors	Average units/ bag or unit	Half-life (hr)	Comments
Cryoprecipitate		III Fibrinogen	60-125 (average: 100)	12	Use for mild hemophilia and those <5 yr; less hepatitis risk; inconvenient
Factor VIII	Hemofil Humafac Koate Profilate	VIII	280-300	12	Convenient; hepatitis risk; expensive
Factor IX	Konȳne Proplex	IX II, VII, X	400-600	24	Convenient; hepatitis risk; useful for factor VIII inhibitor

3. Aminocaproic acid (Amicar) is given in conjunction with factor replacement for oral (mouth, lip, and tongue) bleeding. It is given in an initial dose of 200 mg/kg (maximum: 6 g) PO and then 100 mg/kg/dose (maximum: 6 g/dose) q 6 hr PO for 2-5 days or until healing occurs.

4. Prednisone 1-2 mg/kg/24 hr q 6 hr PO may be indicated for hematuria, although this is controversial.

5. Patients who have a poor response to factor replacement may have an inhibitor. The inhibitor level to factor VIII is measured by the Bethesda Unit Titer. To determine the appropriate therapy for patients with inhibitors, one must know the severity of the bleed, the actual inhibitor level, and the inhibitor response to transfused factor VIII (that is, a high responder has a marked rise in his inhibitor level about 5 days after the factor VIII is given). Factor VIII concentrate may be used in the treatment of minor bleeding episodes if the patient has a low titer inhibitor (less than 2 on the Bethesda Unit Titer) and is a low responder. Factor IX concentrate at a dose of 50-100 units/kg should be used for treatment of minor bleeding episodes in all other patients. Splinting the affected limb and analgesia are useful adjuncts.
   a. If a life-threatening hemorrhage and a low titer of inhibitor (less than 10 on the Be-
   thesda Unit Titer and especially less than 5 on the Bethesda Unit Titer) are present, massive doses of factor VIII may be helpful.
   b. If a life-threatening hemorrhage and a high titer of inhibitor (greater than 10 on the Bethesda Unit Titer) are present, activated factor IX concentrates such as Feiba or Autoplex products are unsuccessful, plasmapheresis plus factor replacement may be necessary.
   c. A hematologist usually should be consulted.

6. In some patients with mild classic hemophilia, vasopressin (desmopressin [DDAVP]) has been shown to increase factor VIII to hemostatic levels and alleviate the need for further replacement. In patients with levels of factor VIII >5%, desmopressin may be mixed with saline and infused slowly over 30 min in a dose of 0.3 μg/kg q 48 hr (adult: 20-25 μg/dose) in consultation with a hematologist.

7. Other considerations include the following:
   a. Hematology consultation
   b. Immobilization and rest for 12-24 hr for acute muscle and joint bleeding. Analgesia is often required.
   c. Immediate surgical consultation for anterior compartment syndrome or any evidence of intracranial bleeding

DISPOSITION

1. The majority of patients may be treated and discharged. Those who require admission have:
   a. Head trauma, acute onset of headache, or spinal cord hematoma
   b. Retropharyngeal hematoma
   c. Muscle bleeding with impending or actual compartment syndrome
   d. GI bleeding
   e. Retroperitoneal or severe iliopsoas bleeding
   f. Poor patient compliance
2. Immediate consultation with a hematologist should be obtained under the following circumstances:
   a. Before any surgical or invasive procedure
   b. Intracranial, retropharyngeal, or GI bleeding
   c. Bleeding in patients with inhibitors
3. Other consultants should be involved for specific indications.
4. All patients should be followed in a comprehensive hemophilia clinic.
5. Early treatment of joint and muscle bleeding, coupled with an aggressive physical therapy program, helps to prevent prolonged disability. Home transfusion programs can expedite early intervention.

REFERENCES

Buchanan, G.R.: Hemophilia, Pediatr. Clin. North Am. **27**:309, 1980.

Eyster, M.E., Gill, F.M., Blatt, P.M., et al. (hemophilia study group): Central nervous system bleeding in hemophiliacs, Blood **51**:1179, 1978.

Gill, F.H.: Congenital bleeding disorders: hemophiliac and Von Willebrand's disease, Med. Clin. North Am. **68**:601, 1984.

Idiopathic thrombocytopenic purpura

Idiopathic thrombocytopenic purpura (ITP) results from increased destruction of platelets on an autoimmune basis. It is associated with a spectrum of viral illnesses including measles, rubella, mumps, chickenpox, infectious mononucleosis, and the common cold. Most cases of childhood ITP are self-limited, between 70% and 90% resolving within 6 mo.

DIAGNOSTIC FINDINGS

1. An antecedent viral illness is reported in 50% of cases.
2. Symptomatic thrombocytopenia with abrupt onset of petechiae, purpura, and spontaneous bleeding of the skin and mucous membranes; epistaxis and hemorrhage of the buccal mucosa are common; bleeding usually responds to pressure.

Complications

1. Intracranial hemorrhage. Occurs in approximately 1% of patients, usually within the first 2-4 wk. May be life threatening. Patients with headache or altered level of consciousness require emergent care.
2. GI bleeding
3. Massive hematuria
4. Chronic ITP. Thrombocytopenia >6-mo duration. Most common in female children over 10 yr of age. Patients have a greater likelihood of associated autoimmune, collagen, vascular, or malignant disease.

Ancillary data

1. CBC, blood smear, and platelet count. Normal platelet count is 150,000-400,000 platelets/mm^3. In ITP patients, the platelet count is usually <100,000 platelets/mm^3 at the time of presentation. If the count falls below 20,000 platelets/mm^3, the patient is at risk of major hemorrhage.
2. Bone marrow puncture and analysis should be done early in the evaluation to confirm the diagnosis in patients with <50,000/mm^3 or when bone marrow disease is suspected. Normal or increased number of megakaryocytes are present in otherwise normal aspirate or biopsy.

DIFFERENTIAL DIAGNOSIS (partial)
Thrombocytopenia

1. Increased destruction of platelets
   a. Consumption
      (1) Microangiopathic state: hemolytic uremic syndrome (HUS), DIC, local ischemic disease (necrotizing enterocolitis [NEC])
      (2) Prosthetic heart valves
      (3) Hyaline membrane disease (HMD)
   b. Autoimmune: SLE, Evans' syndrome
2. Sequestration/maldistribution: splenomegaly or hypothermia
3. Decreased production of platelets
   a. Marrow infiltration: leukemia, lymphoma, storage disease, or solid tumor
   b. Marrow dysfunction
      (1) Congenital: Wiskott-Aldrich syndrome, etc.
      (2) Infection: viral
      (3) Drugs
         (a) Cytotoxic drugs
         (b) Anticonvulsants: phenytoin, carbamazepine, valproate
         (c) Antibiotics: sulfonamides, chloramphenicol, rifampin, trimethoprim with sulfamethoxazole

Platelet dysfunction (normal count)

1. Congenital: Von Willebrand's syndrome
2. Drugs: aspirin, antihistamines, antibiotics (carbenicillin), nonsteroidal antiinflammatory agents
3. Uremia

Purpura and petechiae without thrombocytopenia or platelet dysfunction

These conditions include vasculitides such as Henoch-Schönlein purpura (HSP) and systemic lupus erythematosus and connective tissue disorders such as Ehlers-Danlos syndrome.

MANAGEMENT

Once the diagnosis is comfirmed by bone marrow testing, expectant observation is indicated for several days with close monitoring for developing CNS signs and symptoms. Since the antibodies responsible for ITP react with both patient and donor platelets, platelet transfusions are generally of little help in managing these patients. ITP is usually self-limited, 80% recovering spontaneously within 6 mo.

Steroid therapy

If the platelet count is $<10,000\text{-}20,000/mm^3$ or if there are extensive bleeding manifestations, most authorities recommend starting steroid therapy:

- Prednisone 2 mg/kg/24 hr (maximum: 60 mg/24 hr) q 8 hr PO for 2-3 weeks; then taper at 5-7 day intervals.

Steroids lead to an increase in the platelet count by blocking reticuloendothelial consumption of antibody-coated platelets. They may also lessen the fragility of capillary membranes, causing a further decrease in bleeding.

The effects of steroid therapy are usually apparent by 48-72 hr, and over 50% of children with ITP respond to steroids. However, the effect is transient and may only last as long as therapy is continued. If there is no initial response to steroids or if the platelet count falls when they are discontinued, some suggest repeating a 4 wk course after steroids have been discontinued for a month and the patient has been watched during that period. This should be done after consultation.

Emergent intervention

If there is severe GI bleeding, epistaxis, hematuria, headache, or intracranial hemorrhage, emergent intervention is essential.

1. RBC transfusion for hypotension and anemia should be initiated.
2. Steroids are administered: hydrocortisone (Solu-Cortef) 4-5 mg/kg/dose q 6 hr IV.
3. Hematuria may respond to pushing fluids.
4. Emergency splenectomy is usually necessary. There is an increased risk of infection following surgery.

5. Intravenous infusions of gamma globulin (1 g/kg/dose IV over 4-8 hr up to 3 doses) may be indicated in patients requiring a rapid rise in platelet count (surgery, trauma, or life-threatening mucosal or internal hemorrhages).
6. Platelet transfusions may be used with massive bleeding unresponsive to pressure. Adolescents and adults require 5-10 units depending on size, age of platelet packs, and response. The half-life of transfused platelets is very short and usually fails to provide prolonged hemostasis.

Chronic ITP

This requires a sequential therapeutic plan:
1. Steroids: prednisone, as above
2. If no improvement: splenectomy. The patient whose count does not improve with splenectomy should be evaluated for an accessory spleen, by checking the blood smear for Howell-Jolly bodies and performing spleen scan.
3. Immunosuppressive drugs such as vincristine and cyclophosphamide and intravenous immunoglobulins have been tried with some success
4. Danazol may have a role in long-term management of chronic ITP, but its use requires further study.

DISPOSITION

1. Patients with platelet counts <50,000/mm^3 should be admitted for initial evaluation, monitoring, education, treatment. A hematologist should be involved to perform a bone marrow and assist in management.
2. If no complications develop, the patient may be discharged after 3 days with close follow-up to ensure that there is resolution of the thrombocytopenia and that there are no complications. Activity should be restricted and close follow-up assured.

Parental education

1. Watch for bleeding or any evidence of CNS abnormality.
2. Contact sports as well as high-risk endeavors (skiing, diving, etc.) should be avoided.
3. Seat belts should be worn when the child travels in a car.
4. Young children (under 4 yr) can be fitted with padded helmets to decrease risk of head trauma.
5. Aspirin and other drugs that inhibit platelet function should be avoided. Use soft toothbrush, stool softener, and limit activity.

REFERENCES

Ahn, Y.S., Harrington, W.J., Simon, S.R., et al.: Danazol for the treatment of idiopathic thrombocytopenic purpura, N. Engl. J. Med. **308**:1396, 1983.

Bussel, J.B., Goldman, A., Imbach, P., et al.: Treatment of acute idiopathic thrombocytopenia of childhood with intravenous infusions of gammaglobulin, Pediatrics **106**:886, 1985.

Crain, A.M., and Choudhury, A.M.: Thrombotic thrombocytopenic purpura: a reappraisal, JAMA **246**:1243, 1981.

Humbert, J.R., Sills, R., editors: Controversies in treatment of idiopathic thrombocytopenic purpura in children, Am. J. Pediatr. Hematol./Onc. **6**:147, 1984.

Lightsey, A.L.: Thrombocytopenia in children, Pediatr. Clin. North Am. **27**:293, 1980.

Stuart, M.J., and McKenna, R.: Diseases of coagulation: the platelet and vasculature. In Nathan, D.G., and Oski, F.A., editors: Hematology of infancy and childhood, Philadelphia, 1981, W.B. Saunders Co.

Sickle cell disease

ROGER H. GILLER

Sickle cell anemia (SS disease) is an inherited disorder of hemoglobin synthesis, resulting from a single amino acid substitution (valine for glutamate) in the beta-subunit of the hemoglobin chain. Homozygotes for the sickle gene produce a predominance of sickle hemoglobin and develop symptomatic SS anemia, which occurs in approximately 1 in 500 American blacks and occasionally may be seen in other racial groups from the Mediterranean region, the Middle East, and India. Sickle cell–hemoglobin C (SC) disease and sickle cell-thalassemia are less common variants with similar but less severe clinical manifestations. Heterozygotes (AS) for the sickle gene produce both sickle (S) and normal adult (A) hemoglobin and remain asymptomatic carriers of the sickle trait except under conditions of severe hypoxia.

DIAGNOSTIC FINDINGS (Table 79-4)

The clinical course is one of chronic illness punctuated by acute episodes ("crises") that threaten the life or comfort of the patient.

Anemia crises

Sickling of erythrocytes results in chronic hemolytic anemia. Any process that further decreases the circulating red cell mass may produce a profound degree of anemia.

Splenic sequestration crisis

Young children with SS disease may suddenly pool a large portion of their peripheral blood volume in the spleen. This results in massive splenomegaly, severe anemia, and hypovolemic shock evolving over a period of hours to days. It occurs most commonly between 6 mo and 6 yr of age, before autoinfarction of the spleen. It may be precipitated by infection.

Aplastic crisis

Impaired red cell production in the bone marrow causes exacerbation of the chronic hemolytic anemia. Profound anemia may lead to high-output congestive heart failure. Hematocrit and reticulocyte counts are decreased relative to baseline values. Impaired erythropoiesis can be related to infection or folic acid deficiency. Recent evidence suggests that human Parvovirus infection is the predominate cause of aplastic crises in SS disease.

Hyperhemolytic crisis

Acceleration of the rapid rate of red cell destruction may be related to concurrent G6PD deficiency, hereditary spherocytosis or mycoplasmal infection.

Vasoocclusive crises

Gelation of the abnormal hemoglobin within erythrocytes causes them to sickle, making them less deformable and leading to recurrent thromboses of the microvasculature. Local ischemia and tissue infarction result. Sickling is enhanced by dehydration, hypoxemia, acidosis, and hypertonicity. Bones, pulmonary parenchyma, abdominal viscera, and the CNS are the sites most often affected by the vasoocclusive process.

Musculoskeletal system

1. Bone pain, particularly of the extremities
2. Dactylitis (hand-and-foot syndrome): symmetric, nonpitting edema of the hands and feet, accompanied by warmth and tenderness. Most common in children under 4 yr of age. Frequently the first manifestation of SS disease and should alert the clinician to evaluate the patient for this underlying disorder.
3. Aseptic necrosis of bone, particularly of the femoral or humeral head
4. Leg ulcers

Gastrointestinal tract

1. Abdominal pain that is caused by a crisis is usually without peritoneal signs or decreased bowel sounds. In addition, the patient usually has experienced this pain previously and there is no significant fever nor increase in WBC or band count.
2. Autosplenectomy by 5 yr of age

Central nervous system

These crises consist of cerebral vascular accidents with an incidence of about 8%. Patients develop severe headache, nuchal rigidity, focal neurologic findings, coma, and xanthochromic spinal fluid.

Pulmonary infarction (acute pulmonary syndrome)

Patients initially appear with chest pain, infiltrate, fever, leukocytosis, and rub or effusion. Pulmonary infarction must be differentiated

TABLE 79-4. Sickle cell disease: clinical manifestations

Category	Infant (5 mo-5 yr)	Child (5-12 yr)	Adolescent (13-18 yr)	Management
VASOOCCLUSIVE	Dactylitis	Painful crisis →		Pain control, hydrate
		Stroke →		Pain control, hydrate
				Hospitalize, hydrate, and replace sickled cells with normal RBC
		Hematuria →		Observe
		Hyposthenuria →		Observe
		Autosplenectomy		Observe for infection
			Aseptic necrosis of bone	Conservative treatment; arthroplasty
			Acute pulmonary syndrome	Hospitalize, hydrate, O_2; possibly replace sickled cells with normal RBC
INCREASED RED CELL DESTRUCTION	Aplastic crisis →			Hospitalize, transfuse to restore RBC mass
		Impaired growth →	Delayed puberty	Observe
			Psychosocial problems	Observe
				Counseling
SEQUESTRATION AND STASIS	Splenomegaly			Observe
	Splenic sequestration crisis			Hospitalize, hydrate, support intravascular volume, transfuse to replace sequestered RBC
		Hepatomegaly →		Observe
		Priapism →		If severe, hospitalize; hydrate; possibly replace sickled cells with normal RBC; pain control
FUNCTIONAL ASPLENIA	Sepsis			Hospitalize
	Pneumonia →			Give antibiotics
	Meningitis			
	Osteomyelitis			

from pneumonia. Infarction usually occurs in children over 5 years and is associated with a painful crisis. The chest x-ray film is initially clear with a positive V/Q scan and lower lobe disease involvement.

Other diagnostic findings

Infection
1. Functional asplenia leads to increased risk of serious bacterial infection. Sepsis, meningitis, pneumonia, and osteomyelitis occur with increased frequency and severity. Common causative organisms are listed in Table 79-5.
2. The likelihood of bacterial infection is increased with over 1,000/mm^3 nonsegmented neutrophils (bands) in the CBC.

Gastrointestinal tract
1. Cholelithiasis caused by chronic hemolysis is increasingly prevalent after 10 years of age. Cholelithiasis may cause acute or insidious right upper quadrant pain and jaundice.
2. Hepatomegaly. A mild degree of enlargement is usually present, but it may progress because of one of the following:

a. Acute hepatic sludging/right upper quadrant syndrome. Sickling may obstruct blood flow within the liver, leading to noncolicky right upper quadrant pain, progressive hepatomegaly, malaise, and jaundice.
b. Viral hepatitis
c. Hepatic sequestration, following infarction of the spleen
d. Congestive heart failure

Genitourinary tract
1. Irreversible renal hyposthenuria is present in all patients by 5 years of age.
2. Hematuria may occur in both SS disease and sickle trait. There is an increased risk of urinary tract infections.
3. Priapism is caused by obstruction of the venous drainage of the corpus cavernosum.

Other
1. Impaired growth and delayed puberty are common
2. Congestive heart failure (Chapter 16)
3. Psychosocial problems
4. Retinopathy secondary to sequestration of

TABLE 79-5. Sickle cell disease: infections

Infection	Common organisms	Initial antibiotic therapy
Sepsis (no focus)	S. pneumoniae H. influenzae	Ampicillin 300 mg/kg/24 hr q 4 hr IV
Meningitis	S. pneumoniae H. influenzae	Ampicillin as above **and** chloramphenicol 100 mg/kg/24 hr q 6 hr IV (10 days); **or** cefotaxime 150 mg/kg/24 hr (adult: 4-12 g/24 hr) q 6 hr IV; **or** ceftriaxone 100 mg/kg/24 hr (adult 4 g/24 hr) q 12 hr IV; **or** cefuroxime 200 mg/kg/24 hr (adult: 9 g/24 hr) q 6-8 hr IV
Pneumonia	S. pneumoniae H. influenzae M. pneumoniae	Ampicillin 200 mg/kg/24 hr q 4 hr IV (10 days) If Mycoplasma—**add** erythromycin 30-50 mg/kg/24 hr q 6 hr PO (10 days)
Osteomyelitis	Salmonella S. aureus S. pneumoniae	Ampicillin (IV) as above **and** nafcillin 100 mg/kg/24 hr q 4 hr IV **and** gentamicin 5.0-7.5 mg/kg/24 hr q 8 hr IV

In critically ill children, more broad-spectrum antibiotics may be initiated. Therapy should be altered when culture and sensitivity data are available.

blood in the conjunctival vessels. Marked by dilated and tortuous retinal vessels, microaneurysms, and retinal hemorrhage.

5. Premature births and spontaneous abortions are common during pregnancy.

Ancillary data

1. CBC and reticulocyte count: abnormal. Baseline values for an individual patient are particularly important in the evaluation of acute problems (Table 79-6).
2. Hemoglobin electrophoresis. Confirms diagnosis. Solubility tests (e.g., Sickledex) will not distinguish between disease and trait. Available as newborn screen.
3. Unconjugated bilirubin is elevated (range: 1.5-4.0 mg/dl) because of chronic hemolysis. Other LFTs are normal unless there is supervening hepatobiliary disease (hepatitis, cholelithiasis, hepatic sludging, etc.)
4. ABG. Helpful in the evaluation of pneumonia, pulmonary infarction, acute pulmonary syndrome, CHF, and metabolic acidosis
5. Cultures: blood, urine, bone, CSF as indicated
6. X-ray studies
   a. Chest x-ray study: acute pulmonary syndrome, infarction, infection, CHF
   b. Abdominal x-ray study: cholelithiasis
   c. Bone x-ray study: infarction, infection, aseptic necrosis
   d. CT scan: stroke
7. Abdominal ultrasound: cholelithiasis

8. ECG: biventricular hypertrophy is common. Cor pulmonale may result from recurrent pulmonary infarcts.

MANAGEMENT
Fluids

1. Administer 1½-2 times maintenance fluids IV or PO during vasoocclusive crisis.
2. Monitor patient for dehydration, fluid overload, and high output CHF.

Adequate fluids must be given to counterbalance the renal hyposthenuria. In splenic sequestration crisis, emergent fluid resuscitation with isotonic crystalloid, colloid, or whole blood is necessary to treat potential vascular collapse.

Blood products

• Restore circulating RBC during aplastic or hyperhemolytic crises by administering packed RBC, 5-10 ml/kg over 3-4 hr.

If more rapid replacement of sickle erythrocytes is required (e.g., stroke, acute pulmonary syndrome, priapism), if CHF is present, or if there is concern about augmenting sickling because of increased blood viscosity following transfusion, partial exchange transfusion can be used.

• Reduction of cells containing sickle hemoglobin to ≤40% of the total circulating red cells will effectively prevent further sickling. Adequacy of transfusion therapy can be assessed using the sodium metabisulfite sickling test.

TABLE 79-6. Hematologic values in sickle cell anemia

	Normal values	Sickle cell disease	
		Average	Range
Hemoglobin (g/dl)	12	7.5	5.5-9.5
Hematocrit (%)	36	22	17-29
Reticulocytes (%)	1.5	12	5-30
WBC count (/mm³)	7,500	20,000	12,000-35,000

From Pearson, H.A., and Diamond, L.K.: In Smith, C.A., editor: The critically ill child, Philadelphia, 1977, W.B. Saunders Co., p. 320.

Sodium bicarbonate

Acidosis precipitates sickling. If present it should be corrected with sodium bicarbonate 1-3 mEq/kg/dose IV initially and repeated as required by acid-base status.

Oxygen

Hypoxia precipitates sickling and should be corrected when present, particularly in pulmonary disease, stroke, severe anemia, and CHF. Oxygen is not required for treatment of all vasoocclusive crises.

Analgesia

1. Codeine 3 mg/kg/24 hr q 4-6 hr PO
2. Hydromorphone (Dilaudid) 1-4 mg/dose q 4-6 hr PO (or IM). Not recommended for children under 10 yr of age.
3. Morphine 0.1-0.2 mg/kg/dose q 1-4 hr IV or IM. Maximum dose: 10 mg/dose
   NOTE: Prolonged use of meperidine (Demerol) should be avoided because of risk of seizures.

A useful analgesic routine for inpatient management of severe pain may include:
1. First 24 hr: Morphine sulfate 0.15 mg/kg/dose (maximum: 10 mg/dose) q 2½ hr IM. May supplement with aspirin q 4 hr PO
2. After 24-48 hr or when acute pain has diminished: taper parenteral dose by 20% daily but do not change interval. When one half of the starting parenteral dose is achieved, switch to oral analgesics q 4 hr and then slowly decrease interval to a prn basis.

Antibiotics

Antibiotics (Table 79-5) should be given if there is any evidence of bacterial infection.
1. Cultures should be obtained before initiating treatment and should determine the ultimate choice of antibiotics.
2. A bacterial infection is more likely if there are >1,000 bands/mm^3.
3. The route of administration of antibiotics and the necessity of hospitalizing the patient are

determined by the degree of toxicity and nature of systemic involvement.

Surgery

1. Cholecystectomy: symptomatic cholelithiasis
2. Splenectomy: recurrent splenic sequestration crises
3. Arthroplasty: aseptic necrosis of femoral or humeral head

DISPOSITION

1. Hospitalization is indicated for patients with splenic sequestration crisis, aplastic crisis with severe anemia, stroke, pulmonary infarction, suspected bacterial infection, severe or prolonged priapism, and severe vasoocclusive pain crisis in which parenteral analgesia or IV hydration is required. It is important not to prolong ambulatory management of such patients in the ED. Patients not responding in the first 2 hr with appropriate pain medication and hydration should usually be admitted.
2. Long-term follow-up is essential. Health maintenance considerations should include:
   a. Prophylactic antibiotics
   b. Pneumococcal and *H. influenzae* vaccine
   c. Folic acid therapy (1 mg/day PO)
   d. Chronic transfusion therapy
   e. Genetic counseling
   f. Ophthalmologic examination for sickle retinopathy
   g. Psychosocial counseling

REFERENCES

Alavi, J.B.: Sickle cell anemia: pathophysiology and treatment, Med. Clin. North Am. **68**:545, 1984.

Buchanan, G.R., and Glader, B.E.: Leukocyte counts in children with sickle cell disease, Am. J. Dis. Child. **132**:398, 1978.

Davis, J.R., Vichinsky, E.P., Lubin, B.H.: Current treatment of sickle cell disease, Curr. Probl. Pediatr. **10**:1, 1980.

Mills, M.L.: Life-threatening complications of sickle cell disease in children, JAMA **254**:1487, 1985.

Powars, D.R.: Natural history of sickle cell disease: the first ten years, Semin. Hematol. **12**:267, 1975.

Scott, R.B.: Advances in the treatment of sickle cell disease in children, Am. J. Dis. Child. **139**:1219, 1985.

80 Infectious disorders

Botulism

Botulism results from the ingestion of pre-formed toxins (canned vegetables, etc.), ingestion of spores in infant botulism (honey), or spore contamination of open wounds. *Clostridium botulinum* produces a neurotoxin that blocks the presynaptic release of acetylcholine. The incubation period is 12-48 hr.

DIAGNOSTIC FINDINGS

1. A symmetric descending paralysis is noted, with weakness and equal deep tendon reflexes (DTR).
   a. Pupils are fixed and dilated with oculomotor paralysis, blurred vision, diplopia, ptosis, and photophobia.
   b. Slurred speech, dysphagia, and sore throat are reported.
   c. Nausea, vomiting, vertigo, dry mouth, constipation, and urinary retention occur.
   d. Dyspnea and rales are commonly noted. Rarely, secondary bacterial infection and total respiratory failure occur as a result of paralysis.
2. The sensorium and sensory examinations are normal.
3. If a wound is present, it may suppurate with gas formation.

Ancillary data

1. *C. botulinum* toxin assay, if available
2. Lumbar puncture (LP) (may have increased protein)
3. Chest x-ray film and ABG as indicated

DIFFERENTIAL DIAGNOSIS

Botulism should be distinguished from intoxication (Chapter 54) caused by heavy metals or organophosphates (p. 297).

MANAGEMENT

1. Initially, attention must focus on airway management as well as other aspects of cholinergic blockage. An NG tube and urinary catheter should be placed. All patients require intensive monitoring.
2. Any wound should be irrigated and debrided.
3. Trivalent ABE antitoxin should be administered. Available from the Centers for Disease Control (days: [404]329-3111; nights: [404] 329-2888) or a state health department
4. Individuals exposed to the source by ingestion should receive antitoxin.
5. Botulism may be prevented by boiling all foods adequately (over 10 min). Children under 1 yr of age should not eat honey.

Diphtheria

Corynebacterium diphtheriae, a club-shaped, gram-positive, pleomorphic bacillus, produces an exotoxin that accounts for much of the systemic disease and its complications. The incubation period is 2-5 days.

DIAGNOSTIC FINDINGS

Four distinct clinical presentations have been described:

1. Pharyngeal-tonsillar: sore throat, fever, vomiting, difficulty swallowing, and malaise associated with a gray, closely adherent pseudomembrane. It may progress to respiratory obstruction.
2. Laryngeal: less common. Initially occurs with hoarseness, loss of voice, and may extend into the pharynx
3. Nasal: serosanguineous nasal discharge that may persist for weeks
4. Cutaneous: sharply demarcated ulcer with membranous base. Common in the tropics

Complications

These are primarily the result of effects of exotoxin on organs beyond the respiratory tract.
1. Cardiac: myocarditis, endocarditis (p. 423). dysrhythmias (AV block, left bundle branch block) (Chapter 6)
2. Respiratory obstruction and failure
3. Palatal and oculomotor palsy and peripheral polyneuritis (Chapter 41)
4. Death, usually secondary to respiratory or cardiac complications

Ancillary data

1. Cultures (Loeffler medium and tellurite agar) and Gram's stain
2. CBC (variable, platelets decreased)
3. Cardiac enzymes, ECG, and ABG as needed

DIFFERENTIAL DIAGNOSIS

See p. 459.

MANAGEMENT

1. Initially, management should focus on stabilization of the airway and treatment of cardiac dysfunction.
2. Exposed, immunized, asymptomatic contacts should receive a Td booster. Asymptomatic, unimmunized individuals should receive erythromycin (as below) for 7 days and begin immunization schedule.
3. Corticosteroids have no proven beneficial role in preventing ECG changes or neuritis.

Antitoxin

1. Intradermal and conjunctival tests for horse-serum sensitivity should be done, using 0.1 ml of 1:1,000 dilution. Desensitization may be required.
2. If the membrane has not extended beyond the tonsils and with only mild disease, administer 20,000 units IM or IV.
3. With extensive disease, administer 80,000-100,000 units IV.

Antibiotics

• Penicillin G 100,000 units/kg/24 hr q 4 hr IV for 7-10 days
  Once parenteral therapy is no longer required, a 10-day course of oral penicillin (or, with allergic patient, erythromycin) is begun:
1. Penicillin V 25,000-50,000 units (15-30 mg)/kg/24 hr q 6 hr PO **or**
2. Erythromycin 30-50 mg/kg/24 hr q 6 hr PO

DISPOSITION

Patients should be hospitalized for close observation and respiratory isolation.

Parental education

Active immunization should be encouraged.

REFERENCE

Thisyakorn, U.S.A., Wongvarich, J., and Kumpeng, V.: Failure of corticosteroid therapy to prevent diphtheritic myocarditis or neuritis, Pediatr. Inf. Dis. 3:126, 1984.

Kawasaki's syndrome

Kawasaki's syndrome is a multisystem disease affecting young children often under 5 yr and primarily in the late winter and early spring. It is also known as *mucocutaneous lymph node syndrome* (MCLS). Although it is self-limited, the major involvement of the coronary arteries results in significant morbidity. The etiology is unknown but may be related to some infectious agents. There has been a reported association with house dust, mites, and rug shampoo.

DIAGNOSTIC FINDINGS

The syndrome is triphasic in clinical presentation. An *acute* febrile episode lasts for 7-10 days with the appearance of the six major diagnostic criteria. The *subacute* stage lasts 10-14 days up to 25 days from the onset with associated anorexia, desquamation, and cardiovascular complications and the highest risk of death. *Convalescence* lasts 6-8 wk, and may be a continuing period of high risk of death.

Six major criteria have been established in diagnosing the syndrome, at least five of which are required for confirmation of the diagnosis.
1. Fever > 38.5° C (usually 38.5°-40° C) for at least 5 days. The fever begins abruptly and may last as long as 23 days (average: 11 days).
2. Discrete bilateral, nonexudative conjunctival injection, usually within 2 days of the onset of fever and sometimes lasting 1-2 wk.
3. Mouth changes appear 1-3 days after onset and may last 1-2 wk.
   a. Erythema, fissuring, and crusting of the lips
   b. Diffuse, oropharyngeal erythema
   c. Strawberry tongue
4. Peripheral changes beginning after 3-5 days and lasting 1-2 wk
   a. Induration of the hands and feet. May be edematous
   b. Erythema of the palms and soles
   c. Desquamation of the tips of fingers and toes 2-3 wk after onset of illness
   d. Transverse nail grooves are common during convalescence
5. Erythematous, polymorphous rash concurrent with the fever and spreading from the extremities to the trunk. May be pruritic. Rash usually disappears in less than 1 wk but during the second wk of illness may get desquamation at the junction of the nails and the tips of fingers and toes
6. Enlarged lymph nodes, usually cervical and over 1.5 cm.

Other findings may include urethritis, arthritis, irritability, meningismus, diarrhea, pneumonia, photophobia, aseptic meningitis, obstructive jaundice, gall bladder hydrops, pericardial effusion, uveitis, and iritis.

Complications

Coronary artery disease caused by arteritis, aneurysm, or thrombosis occurs in as many as 20% of patients with onset as long as 45 days after the first fever. It may be asymptomatic but accounts for the mortality of 1%-2%. The risk is greatest during the subacute and convalescent periods, 70% of all deaths occuring 15-45 days after the onset of fever.

Congestive heart failure is frequently observed, accompanied by carditis with complications such as dysrhythmias, pericarditis, mitral insufficiency, myocardial ischemia, or myocardial infarction.

Ancillary data

1. CBC is usually elevated >20,000/mm^3 with a predominance of neutrophils. Hct may be reduced.
2. Platelets are significantly increased, often as high as million/mm^3.
3. ESR is elevated with a mean of 55 mm/hr. Serial monitoring may be useful.
4. Sterile pyuria and proteinuria may be present.
5. ECG is not diagnostic. Echocardiography and arteriography are often needed to define the extent of coronary artery disease and should routinely be dose initially and at 7-12 days into the illness.
6. Gallium citrate Ga^{67} scanning may be useful in demonstrating myocardial inflammation.
7. LP is indicated if meningismus is present.

DIFFERENTIAL DIAGNOSIS

Differentiating Kawasaki's (Table 80-1) syndrome from other entities is particularly important for both acute care and the determination of the need for close, long-term follow-up.
1. Infection (Table 80-1)
   a. Scarlatiniform rash: group A streptococci and *Staphylococcus aureus*
   b. Measles

TABLE 80-1. Kawasaki's syndrome: diagnostic considerations

Condition	Etiology	Diagnostic findings
Scarlatiniform rash (p. 219)	Group A streptococcus S. aureus	Diffuse erythroderma, prominent flexion creases; fingertip desquamation; pharyngitis; strawberry tongue
Scalded skin syndrome (Ritter's syndrome in newborn) (p. 443)	S. aureus	Painful erythroderma with bullae and positive Nikolsky's sign; toxic; may have fluid loss
Toxic epidermal necrolysis (Erythema multiforme) (Lyell's syndrome) (p. 438)	Drug reaction	Confluent erythema with bullae desquamation prominent over extremities, face, and neck; positive Nikolsky's sign; usually toxic with fever
Kawasaki's disease Mucocutaneous lymph node syndrome (MCLS) (p. 538)	Unknown	Polymorphous erythroderma; desquamation of tips of fingers and toes; fever; conjunctival injection; red fissured lips; lymphadenopathy
Toxic shock syndrome (p. 547)	S. aureus	Diffuse erythroderma; desquamation, especially of palms and soles; fever; shock; multisystem involvement
Leptospirosis	Leptospira	Erythematous, macular, papular petechial or purpuric rash; fever, conjunctivitis, pharyngitis, lymphadenopathy multisystem (renal, liver, CNS) involvement

   c. Leptospirosis and rickettsial disease
   d. Staphylococcal scalded skin syndrome (p. 443) and toxic shock syndrome (p. 547)
2. Autoimmune: juvenile rheumatoid arthritis (JRA) and SLE
3. Intoxication: acryodynia (mercury)
4. Erythema multiforme and Stevens-Johnson syndrome (p. 438)

MANAGEMENT

1. Supportive care is essential, focusing on fluids, antipyretics and treatment of CHF, if present (Chapter 16).
2. Aspirin therapy is antiinflammatory, inhibits platelet function and may reduce the tendency toward thrombosis. Initiate 100 mg/kg/24 hr q 4-6 hr PO until fever subsides and then maintain on at least 5-10 mg/kg/24 hr q 12-24 hr PO for 2-3 mo when the platelet count and ESR should return to normal. Because of the impaired aspirin absorption, higher doses may be required and it is imperative to monitor serum level and maintain it at 20-25 mg/dl initially.
3. Steroids and antibiotics are not indicated. Steroids may actually increase the incidence of aneurysms.
4. High-dose intravenous gamma globulin for 5 days combined with aspirin may decrease the frequency of coronary artery disease. It has been shown to do so in preliminary studies.
5. A cardiologist should be involved in the management to ensure immediate assessment and long-term follow-up.

DISPOSITION

1. All patients should be hospitalized early in their course for initial stabilization, in addition to ensuring an adequate and rapid assessment to exclude other diagnostic possibilities.
2. Patients require follow-up for several years after the illness, with particular attention to coronary artery disease; 50% of aneurysms

occur within 1-2 yr. Many recommend delayed catheterization.

REFERENCES

Bell, D.M., Morens, D.M., Holman, R.C., et al.: Kawasaki syndrome in the United States, Am, J. Dis. Child **137**:211, 1983.

Crowley, D.C.: Cardiovascular complications of mucocutaneous lymph node syndrome, Pediatr. Clin. North Am. **31**:1321, 1984.

Koren, G., Rose, V., Lavi, S., et al.: Probable efficacy of high-dose salicylates in reducing coronary involvement in Kawasaki disease, JAMA **254**:767, 1985.

Melish, M.E., Hicks, R.V., and Reddy, V.: Kawasaki syndrome: an update, Hosp. Pract. **17**:99, March 1982.

Rogers, M.F., Kochel, R.L., Hurwitz, E.S., et al.: Kawasaki syndrome: is exposure to rug shampoo important? Am. J. Dis. Child. **139**:777, 1985.

Meningococcemia

Neisseria meningitidis is a gram-negative diplococcus responsible for a spectrum of clinical infections. Meningococcemia is life threatening and presents a diagnostic dilemma. Rarely, *H. influenzae* can produce a comparable clinical picture.

DIAGNOSTIC FINDINGS

1. The onset is variable, ranging from insidious to fulminant.
2. Patients have fever, malaise, headache, weakness, lethargy, vomiting, and arthralgia, as well as signs and symptoms of complicating conditions.
3. Two patterns of skin eruptions are noted:
   a. Pink maculopapular and generalized petechial rash including palms and soles
   b. Purpuric and ecchymotic (often in a centrifugal distribution) associated with a very high mortality
4. Prognostically, unfavorable factors include:
   a. Presence of petechiae for <12 hr before hospitalization
   b. Shock
   c. Absence of meningitis (<20 WBC/mm^3 CSF)
   d. WBC normal or low (<10,000/mm^3)
   e. ESR normal or low (<10 mm/hr)
5. Survival is usually determined in the first 12 hr after treatment has begun.

Complications

1. Meningitis or meningoencephalitis (Chapter 81)
2. Pericarditis (p. 425)
3. Cervicitis
4. DIC (p. 522)
5. Hypotension (Chapter 5), cardiac collapse, and death

Ancillary data

1. WBC, platelet count, and bleeding screens
2. Cultures of blood, spinal fluid, nasopharynx, and other involved organs
3. Skin scraping of the purpuric lesion may have positive culture.

DIFFERENTIAL DIAGNOSIS
(See Table 42-1.)

One study of children with fever and petechiae demonstrated that 20% had bacterial infections. Of these, 50% were caused by *N. meningitidis*, 30% by *H. influenzae* and the remainder by a variety of agents.

MANAGEMENT

Patients require immediate resuscitation (fluids, ventilation and airway support, and pressor agents, if necessary), supportive care, and treatment of complications.

Antibiotics

• Penicillin 20,000 units/kg/24 hr q 4 hr IV (maximum: 20 million units/24 hr) for 10 days. Chloramphenicol for allergic patients

Treatment of contacts

Contacts are those who have slept or eaten in the same household as the index case or hospital personnel with intimate respiratory contact such as would occur with mouth-to-mouth resuscitation.

Contacts should be clinically monitored.
Rifampin
1. Children: 10 mg/kg q 2 hr PO for 2 days
   • To administer to children, open capsule and mix contents with known volume of applesauce, custard, etc. Make fresh mixture with each dose.
2. Adult: 600 mg q 12 hr PO for 2 days

DISPOSITION

1. All patients with systemic disease require admission to an ICU with provision for respiratory isolation.
2. Contacts require treatment and should notify primary physician if fever, headache, stiff neck, or malaise develops.

REFERENCES

Leibel, H.L., Fangman, J.J., and Ostrovsky, M.C.: Chronic meningococcemia in childhood: case report and review of the literature, Am. J. Dis. Child. **127**:94, 1974.
Toews, W.H., and Bass, J.W.: Skin manifestations of meningococcal infection: an immediate indicator of prognosis, Am. J. Dis. Child. **127**:173, 1974.

Infectious mononucleosis

An acute viral illness caused by EB virus, infectious mononucleosis most frequently occurs in adolescents and young adults.

DIAGNOSTIC FINDINGS

1. Although the severity varies, most patients have a prodrome of 3-5 days with malaise, anorexia, nausea, and vomiting.
2. Patients rapidly develop high fevers, pharyngitis, lymphadenopathy, particularly cervical, and splenomegaly. Lymph nodes are usually symmetrical, firm, discrete and mildly to moderately tender.
3. The symptoms may persist for weeks, particularly those associated with prodrome.
4. Young children may have fever, diarrhea, pharyngitis, otitis media, pneumonia, lymphadenopathy, hepatomegaly, and splenomegaly.

5. An erythematous, maculopapular rash may develop, commonly with the use of ampicillin. It is most prominent on the trunk and proximal extremities.

Complications

1. Upper airway obstruction from marked tonsillar hypertrophy
2. Splenic rupture, often preceded by abdominal pain secondary to splenomegaly. Risk is greatest between 14 and 28 days of illness.
3. Hepatitis (p. 487)
4. Autoimmune hemolytic anemia, leukopenia, and thrombocytopenia
5. Encephalitis or Landry-Guillain-Barré syndrome (Chapter 41). Oculomotor paralysis
6. Pericarditis (p. 425)

Ancillary data

1. WBC. Elevated, with a marked predominance of lymphocytes, 50%-90% of which will be atypical
2. Thrombocytopenia
3. Monospot test. Heterophil rarely indicated. Both usually negative in children under 5 yr (EB virus titer may be needed). In adolescents and adults, positive test is found during the second week of illness.
4. Throat culture for group A streptococci
5. Liver function tests with RUQ tenderness
6. ECG and ABG rarely indicated

DIFFERENTIAL DIAGNOSIS

1. Infection
   a. Pharyngitis: group A streptococci, diphtheria, or viral
   b. Toxoplasmosis
   c. Infectious hepatitis
   d. Meningoencephalitis, viral
2. Neoplasm: leukemia or lymphoma

MANAGEMENT

1. Support and symptomatic care are required.
   a. Establishment of an airway, if obstructed
   b. Bedrest, fluids, and antipyretics
2. Steroid may be indicated for patients

with complications of severe disease (severe hemolytic anemia, airway obstruction, secondary to tonsillar hypertrophy, thrombocytopenia, etc.): prednisone 1-2 mg/kg/24 hr q 6 hr PO for 7 days and then tapering over 2 wk

DISPOSITION

Patients with significant symptomatology and complications require hospitalization. Others may be sent home if hydration, observation, and support are adequate.

Pertussis (whooping cough)

Pertussis (whooping cough) is caused by *Bordetella pertussis* and occurs in all age-groups, although its greatest morbidity is in children under 1 yr of age. It peaks in late summer and early fall. Incubation period is 7-10 days.

DIAGNOSTIC FINDINGS

Three stages categorize the progression of pertussis in children.
1. Catarrhal: minor respiratory complaints of fever, rhinorrhea, and conjunctivitis lasting up to 2 wk
2. Paroxysmal: severe cough associated with hypoxia, unremitting paroxysms, and vomiting. As many as 40 episodes/day may occur and may go on for 2-4 wk. Rarely, it is associated with apnea.
3. Convalescent: residual cough
The infant often has only a paroxysmal cough and rhinorrhea. Stages are indistinct. Adults often only have rhinorrhea, sore throat, and persistent cough.

Partially immunized children will have less severe disease.

Complications

1. Pneumonia caused by secondary infection
2. Crepitus from subcutaneous or mediastinal emphysema

3. Pneumothorax
4. Seizures and encephalitis
5. Hypoxia
6. Apnea

Ancillary data

1. WBC. Markedly increased with a tremendous shift to the right (lymphocytosis)
2. Chest x-ray study. Peribronchial thickening, infiltrates, and "shaggy" heart border
3. Culture. Nasopharyngeal or cough plate on a Bordet-Gengou medium
4. Fluorescent antibody (FA) stain of nasopharyngeal swab (a rapid diagnostic technique)

DIFFERENTIAL DIAGNOSIS

Pertussis should be differentiated from other causes of pneumonia (p. 601).

MANAGEMENT

1. Of primary importance is pulmonary support, which may include oxygen, postural drainage, and, very rarely, intubation with sedation. Patients with severe paroxysms should be monitored to ensure that hypoxia and bradycardia are treated.
2. Antibiotics decrease the contagiousness of the patient: erythromycin 30-50 mg/kg/24 hr (adult: 250 mg/dose) q 6 hr PO (if possible) for 14 days. It may also decrease the symptomatic course if given early in the catarrhal phase. Additional antibiotics should be given if there is evidence of superinfection.
3. Patients should be isolated. Those exposed may be treated with erythromycin, as above, for 10 days.
4. Pertussis immune globulin is not effective.

DISPOSITION

1. Patients under 1 yr of age or those with any complication should be hospitalized for careful monitoring and pulmonary support.
2. Older children in the catarrhal phase or those experiencing only minor paroxysms may be discharged.

PARENTAL EDUCATION

1. Importance of active immunization in disease prevention.
2. Prophylaxis of household and other close contacts of pertussis cases should be considered.
   a. All household or other close contacts younger than 1 yr (regardless of DTP immunization status) should receive 14 days of oral erythromycin (40 mg/kg/24 hr q 6 hr PO)
   b. All household or other close contacts between 1 and 7 years of age who have had less than 4 DTP doses or whose last DTP was more than 3 years ago should receive 14 days of oral erythromycin, and many recommend a DTP immunization.
   c. Asymptomatic household or other close contacts need not be excluded from school if they are taking antibiotics or have up-to-date DTP immunization (4 DTPs, the last within 3 yr).
   d. Persons who have a positive laboratory test for pertussis should be excluded from school or work until they have taken antibiotics for 14 days.
   e. Adults and children with early symptoms who are household contacts should be excluded from school or work until they have completed 5 days of antibiotics.
   f. All household contacts aged 7 or older should receive antibiotics if the last DTP was 3 yrs or greater.
3. If patient has been discharged, the parent should call the physician immediately if
   a. Breathing difficulty recurs or worsens
   b. Color of lips or skin turns blue
   c. Restlessness or sleeplessness develops
   d. Fluid intake decreases
   e. Medicines are not tolerated

Rabies

Although very rare, rabies in humans is a fatal viral disease resulting from skin or mucous membrane contact with an infected animal. The incubation is 10 days to several months after the initial exposure, the length reflecting the site and severity of the wound. The primary goal must be prevention.

DIAGNOSTIC FINDINGS

Initially, hypoesthesia or paresthesia is noted at the site of injury. There is rapid progression of symptoms including hydrophobia, apprehension, and hyperexcitability associated with a clear sensorium. Seizures, delirium, and lethargy are noted in the period before death in 5-7 days. Cardiovascular, respiratory, and CNS instability may be noted in the interim.

Ancillary data

Rabies virus may be isolated from the saliva or brain of infected individuals. Examination of the biting animal's brain by fluorescent antibody or Negri body identification and confirmed by viral isolation provide additional confirmation.

MANAGEMENT

Although the mortality rate is extremely high, there have been several cases of survival with intense, supportive care.

Prevention of rabies
Risk factors
1. Bites and wounds inflicted by animals must be individually considered with regard to the risk of rabies. Skunks, foxes, coyotes, raccoons, wild dogs and cats, and bats are most commonly infected. Rodents (mice, rats, squirrels, chipmunks), rabbits, and hares are not normally considered to be risks.
2. Circumstances of the biting incident must be considered. Unprovoked attacks are more likely to indicate that the animal was rabid than are provoked attacks.
3. Type of exposure is a factor. Rabies is transmitted by the introduction of virus into open cuts or wounds in skin or via mucous membranes:
   a. Bite: any penetration of the skin by teeth

b. Nonbite: scratches, abrasions, open wounds, or mucous membrane contaminated with saliva
4. Epizootic conditions of rabies in the area should be considered.

Management of the biting animal
1. Healthy domestic dogs and cats should be confined and observed for 10 days. If any suggestive signs develop, the animal should be killed and the head removed and shipped under refrigeration to the designated health department, provided there is risk of rabies in that area. Stray and wild dogs and cats should be killed and examined.
2. Wild animals that bit or scratched a person should be killed and the brain examined.

Local treatment of wound
1. Immediate and thorough washing and debridement are appropriate.
2. Tetanus prophylaxis should be given, if indicated.

Immunization (Table 80-2)

Antirabies immunization after exposure should include both passively administered antibody *and* vaccine, unless the patient has been immunized before exposure.
1. Read instructions for administration carefully on inserts of products. If immune globulin or vaccine is unavailable, call the Centers for Disease Control ([404]329-3095 during working hours or [404]329-2888 on nights, weekends, and holidays).
2. Human rabies immune globulin (RIG) is supplied in 2 ml and 10 ml (150 IU/ml) vials. It should be administered at a dose of 20 IU/ kg. If anatomically feasible, approximately half the dose is used to infiltrate the wound and the remainder is given IM.
3. Human diploid cell rabies vaccine (HDCV) is administered IM in five 1 ml doses; the first dose is administered at the time of ex-

TABLE 80-2. Rabies postexposure prophylaxis guide

Species of animal	Condition of animal at time of attack	Treatment of exposed human*
DOMESTIC		
Dog and cat	Healthy or unknown	None: consult public health officer†
	Rabid or suspected rabid	RIG and HDCV
WILD		
Skunk, bat, fox, coyote, raccoon, bobcat, and other carnivores	Regard as rabid unless proved negative by laboratory test‡	RIG and HDCV
OTHER		
Livestock, rodents, rabbits, hares	Consider individually. Squirrels, hamsters, guinea pigs, gerbils, chipmunks, rats, mice, rabbits, and hares are not considered to be rabid.	

From Morb. Mort. Week. Rep. **33:**393, 1984. These recommendations are only a guide. They should be applied in conjunction with information about the animal species involved, the circumstances of the exposure, the vaccination status of the animal, and the presence of rabies in the region.
*All bites and wounds should immediately be thoroughly cleansed with soap and water. If antirabies treatment is indicated, both RIG and HDCV should be given as soon as possible, regardless of the interval from exposure.
†During the usual holding period of 10 days, begin treatment with RIG and HDCV at first sign of rabies in the animal. The symptomatic animal should be killed immediately and examined.
‡The animal should be killed and tested as soon as possible. Holding for observation is not recommended. Discontinue treatment if tests are negative.

posture, followed at 3, 7, 14, and 28 days by the remaining doses.

Tetanus

Tetanus results from puncture or other wounds with the introduction of *Clostridium tetani,* which produces a neurotoxin. Severe skeletal muscle hypertonicity occurs. The incubation period ranges from 3 days to 3 wk (average: 8 days). Generally, the shorter the incubation period, the more severe the clinical presentation.

DIAGNOSTIC FINDINGS

1. A wound is present in 80% of patients.
2. The onset of symptoms is marked by increased tone of the skeletal muscles initially involving the jaw and neck. This becomes generalized over the next 24-48 hr with spasms increasing in frequency and intensity.
   a. Trismus: inability to open the mouth secondary to spasms of the masseter muscles
   b. Peculiar, sustained facial distortion: risus sardonicus
   c. Opisthotonic posturing from spasms of neck and back
   d. Boardlike abdomen
   e. Stiff and extended extremities
3. A low-grade fever, headache, tachycardia, and anxiety are often present. The sensorium is totally normal.
4. Tetanus neonatorum occurs in the first 3-10 days of life, marked by muscle rigidity, particularly of the jaw and neck, difficulty swallowing, and irritability.

Complications

1. Respiratory: laryngospasm, pneumonia, pulmonary edema, and respiratory failure
2. Compression or subluxation injuries of the vertebrae

Ancillary data

1. WBC. Variably increased
2. LP. Normal

3. ABG. Indicated if there is respiratory compromise
4. Vertebral x-ray films. For patients with pain and severe opisthotonic posturing

DIFFERENTIAL DIAGNOSIS

1. Trauma: head and neck
2. Infection: dental abscess, peritonsillar abscess
3. Intoxication: phenothiazines, strychnine
4. Endocrine/metabolic: hypocalcemia (tetany)
5. Intrapsychic: hysteria, conversion reaction

MANAGEMENT
At time of exposure

1. Tetanus and diphtheria (Td) toxoid and tetanus immune globulin (TIG) are indicated (see schedule in Table 80-3 and Appendix C-7). DT (pediatric) may be used for children younger than 6 yr.
2. Wound cleansing and debridement must be done.

Treatment of acute disease

1. The patient must have immediate evaluation and support of the airway with oxygen and active intervention, when indicated.
2. Muscle spasms and associated pain must be controlled with:
   a. Diazepam (Valium) 0.1-0.3 mg/kg/dose q 4-8 hr IV or 0.1-0.8 mg/kg/24 q 6-8 hr PO **or**
   b. Phenobarbital 5 mg/kg/24 hr q 6-8 hr PO, IM, or IV (after loading)
   c. Minimizing external stimuli
3. Tetanus immune globulin antitoxin should be administered:
   a. 250-500 units IM
   b. 500 units IM for newborns
4. An antibiotic should be given: penicillin G 100,000 units/kg/24 hr q 4 hr IV for 10-14 days

Prevention

Active immunization (Appendix C-7) is recommended.

TABLE 80-3. Schedule for Td toxoid and TIG at time of exposure

History of tetanus immunizations (doses)	Clean, minor wounds		All other wounds	
	Td	TIG*	Td	TIG*
Uncertain	Yes	No	Yes	Yes
0-1	Yes	No	Yes	Yes
2	Yes	No	Yes	No†
3 or more	No‡	No	No§	No

Adapted from Report of the Committee on Infectious Diseases, American Academy of Pediatrics, 1982.
*250 units IM (under 5 yr) to 500 units IM in adults.
†Unless wound is > 24-hr-old.
‡Unless >10 yr have elapsed since the last dose.
§Unless >5 yr have elapsed since the last dose.

DISPOSITION

1. All patients with tetanus require admission to an ICU.
2. Those individuals with tetanus exposure may be discharged after appropriate immunologic therapy.

REFERENCE

Brand, D.A., Acampora, D., Gottlieb, L.D., et al.: Adequacy of antitetanus prophylaxis in six hospital emergency rooms, N. Engl. J. Med. **309**:636, 1983.

Toxic shock syndrome

Toxic shock syndrome (TSS) primarily affects menstruating young women; however, nonmenstruating females, men, and premenarcheal girls have also had the syndrome usually associated with a definable site of infection.

ETIOLOGY: INFECTION

1. Although the pathophysiology remains unclear, a toxin elaborated by coagulase-positive *S. aureus* (phage group I) is absorbed through the vaginal mucosa, causing systemic signs and symptoms.
2. There is a temporal relationship between tampon use, menstruation, and the onset of the syndrome.

DIAGNOSTIC FINDINGS

Clinically, TSS must include:
1. Fever (>39.9° C)
2. Rash (diffuse, blanching macular, erythematous, nonpruritic); erythroderma
3. Desquamation 1-2 wk after the onset of illness, particularly on the palms and soles
4. Hypotension (systolic BP <90 mm Hg for adults or <5% by age for children or orthostatic changes)
5. Involvement of three or more of the following organ systems:
   a. Gastrointestinal (vomiting or diarrhea usually at the onset of illness)
   b. Muscular (severe myalgia)
   c. Mucous membrane (vaginal, oropharyngeal, or conjunctival hyperemia)
   d. Renal (BUN or creatinine at least twice elevated or >5 WBC/HPF with no UTI)
   e. Hepatic (bilirubin, SGOT, or SGPT at least twice normal)
   f. Hematologic (platelets <100,000/mm³)
   g. Central nervous system (disorientation or alteration in consciousness without focal signs)
6. Negative results on the following tests, if obtained: serologic tests for Rocky Mountain spotted fever, leptospirosis, or measles
   NOTE: Blood culture may grow *S. aureus* (variable)

Patients often have a 2-day prodrome, comprised of fever, vomiting, diarrhea, and myalgia. Sore throat is a prominent complaint.

Complications

1. Cardiovascular collapse and shock with myocardial failure
2. Adult respiratory distress syndrome with pulmonary edema. More common in children younger than 10 yr.
3. Coagulopathy with DIC is usually mild
4. Recurrence

Ancillary data

1. Hematology. Increased WBC with shift to left, thrombocytopenia, and variable coagulation studies
2. Chemistry: electrolytes, BUN, creatinine, and calcium. May be abnormal. Liver function and bilirubin elevations are common.
3. Urinalysis. Proteinuria and pyuria
4. Cultures. Vaginal culture for *S. aureus*. Blood, throat, and CSF cultures are variable.
5. Chest x-ray study and ABG with any respiratory distress

MANAGEMENT

General supportive care is essential because of the multisystem involvement of the disease and the progressive nature of organ involvement.

1. Fluids for hypotension and abnormal loss from vomiting and diarrhea. Often very large volumes of fluids are required with 2-5 times normal maintenance fluids being necessary. Fluids should not be restricted or diuretics administered without being able to maintain an adequate filling pressure.
2. Pressor agents may be required for significant hypotension unresponsive to fluid therapy: dopamine, 5-15 µg/kg/min IV constant infusion, often in combination with other pressors after volume deficits have been replaced. Echocardiography and Swan-Ganz catheter monitoring are indicated if myocardial failure is noted.
3. Ventilatory support with PEEP, particularly

if adult resiratory distress syndrome (ARDS) with pulmonary edema is present.
4. If incriminated, removal of tampon and irrigation of vagina. Aggressive drainage of sites of staphylococcal infection must be achieved. Abscesses and empyemas always require surgical drainage.
5. Antibiotics should be initiated although their role is unclear. They decrease the incidence of recurrence but do not clearly alter the illness. The patient is given:
   a. Nafcillin 100-200 mg/kg/24 hr (adult: 1 g/dose) q 4 hr IV (or equivalent beta-lactamase–resistant penicillin) for at least 7 days **or**
   b. Cephalosporin: cephalothin (Keflin) 75-150 mg/kg/24 hr (adult: 1 g/dose) q 4 hr IV
6. Corticosteroids reduce the severity of illness and duration of fever if initiated within 2-3 days of illness: Methylprednisolone (Solu-Medrol) 30 mg/kg/dose q 6 hr IV
7. Calcium supplementation is usually required.
8. Renal dialysis may be required if renal failure develops.

DISPOSITION

Hospitalization is required of all patients with definite TSS because of the progression of findings. An ICU is usually indicated.

On discharge, long-term monitoring for renal and neuromuscular sequelae is essential.

REFERENCES

Centers for Disease Control: Toxic-shock syndrome, United States, 1970-1982, Morb. Mort. Week. Rep. **31:**210, 1982.
Chesney, P.J.: Toxic-shock syndrome: a commentary and review of the characteristics of *Staphylococcus aureus* strains, Infection **11:**181, 1983.
Garbe, P.L., Arko, R.J., Reingold, A.L., et al.: *Staphylococcus aureus* isolates from patients with nonmenstrual toxic shock syndrome: evidence for additional toxins, JAMA **253:**2538 1985.
Todd, J.K., Ressman, M., Caston, S.A., et al.: Corticosteroid therapy for patients with toxic-shock syndrome, JAMA **252:**3399, 1984.
Wiesenthal, A.M., and Todd, J.K.: Toxic-shock syndrome in children aged 10 years or less, Pediatrics **74:**112, 1984.

81 Neurologic disorders

Breath-holding spells

Breath-holding spells may result after prolonged crying, producing cyanosis and, ultimately, loss of consciousness. They most commonly begin after 6 mo of age and may continue until 4 yr.

DIAGNOSTIC FINDINGS

1. Vigorous crying is precipitated by a fall or injury or by anger. The child subsequently becomes cyanotic, unconscious, and limp. The episodes are self-limited, lasting <1 min.
2. Some evidence of disturbance at home or in the maternal-child interaction is usually evident. Youth of parents, maternal depression, or difficulty in setting limits can usually be detected.

Complications

Tonic-clonic seizures may be noted as a result of cerebral anoxia.

DIFFERENTIAL DIAGNOSIS

It is usually easy to differentiate breath-holding spells from a seizure. Patients with seizures lose consciousness and then become cyanotic; the reverse is true with breath-holding spells, which rarely occur at night. It is important to note that cerebral anoxia may cause brief seizures with breath-holding spells.

MANAGEMENT

1. Reassurance and calmness on the part of the parents must be emphasized. The episodes are self-limited. There must be neither support of the behavior patterns that initiate breath-holding spells nor secondary gain from that behavior.
2. Anticonvulsants are not indicated. The focus must be on behavior modification.

Parental education

1. Minimize the events or factors that trigger the spells.
2. Attempt to be firm and consistent in management of behavior problems.
3. Call if the nature, duration, or frequency of the breath-holding spells changes.

REFERENCE

Lombroso, C.T., and Lerman, P.: Breathholding spells: cyanotic and pallid infantile syncope, Pediatrics **39:**563, 1967.

Meningitis

ALERT: Infections elsewhere do not exclude the presence of meningitis. The younger the child, the less specific the presenting signs and symptoms.

ETIOLOGY: INFECTION

1. Bacterial
   a. The child's age is the predominant determinant of the common bacterial etiologies:

Age-group	Predominant organism
<2 mo	*Escherichia coli*, group B streptococci, *Listeria monocytogenes*, *Haemophilus influenzae*, *Neisseria meningitidis*, *Streptococcus pneumoniae*

2 mo-9 yr   *H. influenzae, N. meningitidis,*
             S. pneumoniae
>9 yr   *N. meningitidis, S. pneumoniae*

b. The relative importance of etiologic agents in children may be summarized as follows:

Etiologic agent	Cases	Mortality
H. influenzae	57%	5%
N. meningitidis	12%	7%
S. pneumoniae	8%	9%
Group A streptococci	7%	19%
Other	6%	

c. Ventriculoperitoneal (VP) shunt: 25% of patients with VP shunts have infections associated with alterations in the shunt, usually caused by *Staphylococcus epidermidis*.

2. Viral: most commonly enteroviral (Table 81-1)

3. Fungal and *Mycobacterium tuberculosis:* uncommon, but consider if endemic

DIAGNOSTIC FINDINGS: BACTERIAL MENINGITIS

1. In younger children the initial presentation is nonspecific, including fever, hypothermia, dehydration, bulging fontanel, lethargy, irritability, anorexia, vomiting, seizures, respiratory distress, or cyanosis (Table 81-2).
2. Older patients may have symptoms listed in *l*, as well as the more classic findings of nuchal rigidity, Kernig's sign (pain on extension of legs), Brudzinski's sign (flexion of the neck produces flexion at knees and hips), and headaches. Otitis media is often present.
3. Historically, the progression of illness, associated symptoms, exposures, and underlying health problems are important.

TABLE 81-1. Viral meningoencephalitis

Agent	Epidemiology	Clinical manifestations
Enterovirus	Epidemic, with summer and fall peak incidence; all ages affected, particularly <12 yr	Most common; usually mild; rash often present; rarely with focal findings or sequelae
Mumps	Epidemic, occurring year-round with increase in spring; all ages affected, particularly 2 to 14-yr-olds	Mild-to-moderate meningoencephalitis accompanied by parotitis (>50%); focal findings and sequelae rare
Herpes virus hominis	Year-round; most commonly affecting patients <1 yr and >15 yr	Severe and progressive encephalitis, 50%-75% having focal findings; severe motor and mental deficits occur in as many as 75% of survivors; high mortality rate
California	Occurs in rural areas with peak incidence in June-Oct; 5 to 9-yr-olds most commonly affected	Mild meningoencephalitis with accompanying seizures (50%) and focal findings (15%-40%); long-term behavioral problems (15%-20%)
St. Louis	Peaks in July-Oct; adults primarily involved	Commonly asymptomatic in children
Western equine	July-Oct peak incidence; primarily (20%-30%) affects infants	Sudden high fever with focal or generalized seizures, rare focal findings and coma; sequelae occur in >50% of children affected in first year of life

Modified from Menkes, J.H.: Hosp. Prac. **12**:101, 1977.

4. The distinction between a simple febrile seizure and a seizure-complicating meningitis is difficult to make in younger children and often requires a lumbar puncture (p. 564).

5. Patients with a ventriculoperitoneal or other shunt may have a somewhat different presentation, associated with a low-grade ventriculitis that includes headache, nausea, low-grade fever, and malaise.

The shunting device consists of three components. The ventricular catheter is passed into the anterior horns of the lateral ventricles through a right occipital or frontal burr hole. The catheter is attached subcutaneously to a reservoir that may be percutaneously tapped to obtain ventricular fluid. This reservoir is attached to a distal catheter containing a pump and one-way valve to regulate pressure and flow in the system. This distal catheter commonly passes into the peritoneum.

To assess shunt function, the reservoir is pumped and if it cannot be depressed there is a distal block, whereas if it pumps but does not refill, it is blocked proximally at the ventricular end. If it pumps poorly, there may be a relative dysfunction. Withdrawing fluid from the shunt for analysis or because of abnormal pumping requires consultation with a neurosurgeon.

NOTE: Aseptic (viral, fungal, mycobacterial) meningoencephalitis usually has a less toxic and acute clinical presentation. Encephalitis is often based on clinical evaluation.

Complications

1. Cerebral edema with potential for increased intracranial pressure and herniation
2. Septic shock and disseminated intravascular coagulation, particularly with *N. meningitidis*
3. Bacteremia with associated hematogenous involvement of joints (particularly the hip), pericardium, and myocardium
4. Inappropriate ADH with hyponatremia
5. Subdural effusions and empyema
6. Anemia, especially with *H. influenzae*
7. Of those patients with meningococcal or pneumococcal meningitis 90% are afebrile by the sixth day in contrast to only 72% of those with *H. influenzae* as the etiologic agent. Conditions associated with persistent fever include untreated disease, subdural effusion, nosocomial infection, phlebitis, and drug fever.
8. Neurologic findings, both transient and persistent, may include deficits in cranial nerves (particularly VI), hearing, vision, and retardation, as well as later behavioral problems.

TABLE 81-2. Bacterial meningitis: presentation by age

Diagnostic findings	Under 3 mo	3 mo-2 yr	Over 2 yr
Apnea/cyanosis	Common	Rare	Rare
Fever	Common	Common	Common
Hypothermia	Common	Rare	Rare
Altered mental status	Common	Common	Common
Headache	Rare	Rare	Common
Seizures	Early finding	Early finding	Late finding
Ataxia	Rare	Variable	Early finding
Jitteriness	Common	Common	Rare
Vomiting	Common	Common	Variable
Stiff neck	Rare	Late finding	Common
Bulging fontanel	Common	Common	Closed

Ancillary data

Lumbar puncture (Appendix A-4)

1. Cerebrospinal fluid (CSF) is the basis for evaluation of the patient with clinical signs of meningitis. Analysis of the fluid is essential (Table 81-3).
2. Partial treatment with antibiotics before lumbar puncture (LP) will rarely alter the CSF enough to interfere with an appropriate interpretation.
3. Although there is conflicting evidence regarding the potential risk of seeding the meninges with bacteria when performing an LP in the bacteremic patient, this consideration should *not* delay obtaining CSF in patients who are clinically at risk of having meningitis.
4. If it is difficult to distinguish bacterial from viral meningitis on the basis of the initial CSF, a repeat LP in 6-8 hr should demonstrate a marked decrease in the percentage of PMN leukocytes and an increase in lymphocytes in untreated patients with viral meningitis.
5. Repeat LP may be done at 36-48 hr and 10 days after initiating therapy if the clinical response has been slow or the therapy inadequate.
6. Bloody spinal taps create a diagnostic dilemma.

TABLE 81-3. Cerebrospinal fluid analysis

	Normal			Bacterial	Viral
	Preterm	Term	Over 6 months		
Cell count (WBC/mm³)*					
Mean	9	8	0	>500	<500
Range	0-25	0-22	0-4		
Predominant cell type	Lymph	Lymph	Lymph	80% PMN leukocyte	PMN leukocyte initially; lymphocyte later
Glucose (mg/dl)					
Mean	50	52	>40	<40	>40
Range	24-63	34-119			
Protein (mg/dl)					
Mean	115	90	<40	>100	<100
Range	65-150	20-170			
CSF/blood glucose (%)					
Mean	74	81	50	<40	>40
Range	55-150	44-248	40-60		
Gram's stain	Negative	Negative	Negative	Positive†	Negative
Bacterial culture	Negative	Negative	Negative	Positive‡	Negative

Modified from Sarff, L.D., Platt, L.H., and McCracken, G.H. Jr.: J. Pediatr. **88:**473, 1976; Portnoy, J.M. and Olson, L.C.: Pediatrics **75:**484, 1985.

*Total WBC/mm³ by age in the normal child can be further delineated as follows (mean ± 2 SD): <6 wk: 3.7 ± 6.8; 6 wk-3 mo: 2.9 ± 5.7; 3 mo-6 mo: 1.9 ± 4.0; 6-12 mo: 2.6 ± 4.9; >12 mo: 1.9 ± 5.4.

†If Gram's stain is negative, a methylene blue stain may distinguish intracellular bacteria from nuclear material.

‡85% of partially treated patients will have a positive Gram's stain and >95% have positive cultures. Counterimmunoelectrophoresis (CIE) may be helpful if the culture is negative.

   a. Hemorrhage into the subarachnoid space results in an equal number of RBC in the first and last samples of fluid. The fluid should be xanthochromic after centrifugation.

   b. Although the appraisal may be inexact and fraught with errors, the number of WBC in spinal fluid obtained after a traumatic tap may be estimated.

     (1) 1,000 RBC/mm^3 contribute 1-2 WBC/mm^3

     (2) Number of WBC introduced/mm^3 =
$$\frac{(\text{Peripheral WBC}) \times (\text{RBC in CSF})}{\text{Peripheral RBC count}}$$

     (3) The result is then compared with the actual number of WBC counted in the CSF.

     (4) 1,000 RBC/mm^3 in the CSF raises the protein about 1.5 mg/dl.

7. Cultures for tuberculosis or fungi may be done, if indicated.

8. Determinations of CSF lactic acid and LDH have not proved to be of value in the interpretation of the fluid.

9. Approximately 90% of children with ventriculoperitoneal shunts with CSF white count >100 cells/mm^3 will be infected. The CSF glucose is usually normal and the organisms are less pathogenic.

10. The infant's airway should never be compromised during an LP. This is particularly important in small infants who are held tightly, which could potentially cause suffocation or impaired central venous return.

11. LP should be performed only cautiously, if at all, in the patient with suspected papilledema or increased intracranial pressure or in patients who are uncooperative. Consultation usually is indicated.

Blood cultures

These may provide bacteriologic confirmation of the infecting organism and should always be obtained.

Cultures of infected sites

Aspirates of purpuric lesions, joints, and abscesses or middle ear infections should be obtained.

Counterimmunoelectrophoresis

Rapid bacteriologic diagnosis may be possible using antisera against capsular antigen to *H. influenzae*, type B; *S. pneumoniae;* and *N. meningitidis*.

Other blood studies

1. Blood glucose should be obtained before performing LP.
2. WBC and platelets
3. Electrolytes. Should be obtained every 1-2 days to monitor for inappropriate ADH

Chest x-ray film

A film should be taken if there are associated respiratory symptoms.

CT scan

A scan is indicated if there are focal neurologic signs or seizures or if there is clinical evidence of an intracranial mass effect.

Subdural taps

These should be done if there is evidence of increasing head circumference, expanding and bulging anterior fontanel, or continuing fever with poor clinical response (Appendix A-5).

DIFFERENTIAL DIAGNOSIS (Chapters 15, 34, and 39)

Differential considerations in the patient with a *stiff neck* include meningitis, adenitis, osteomyelitis, trauma with secondary fracture, hematoma or muscle injury, tumor, hysteria, torticollis, and oculogyric crisis from drugs such as phenothiazines (p. 299).

Infection

Because of the nonspecific signs and symptoms, particularly in younger children, it is often difficult, without an LP, to distinguish meningitis from a number of other infections, for instance:

1. Pneumonia
2. Acute gastroenteritis with dehydration, par-

ticularly if caused by *Shigella* organisms
3. Acute illness associated with a febrile seizure
4. Less commonly, brain abscess, subdural empyema, and acute obstruction of a VP shunt

Vascular disorder

Subarachnoid bleeding or a cerebrovascular accident may develop acutely and be associated with a systemic infection.

Intoxication

The stress of an acute infection may lead some individuals to overdoses, purposeful or accidental. Infection changes the kinetics of drugs like theophylline.

Trauma

Head trauma producing a subdural or epidural hematoma may be difficult to distinguish, sometimes necessitating a CT scan before the LP. Heatstroke may cause fever, dehydration, meningism, and marked changes in mentation.

MANAGEMENT

1. Initial management must focus on stabilizing the patient. Intravenous access should be ensured. Assessment of vital signs with concomitant evaluation for hypoxia, dehydration, increased intracranial pressure, acidosis, electrolyte abnormalities, and DIC, when appropriate, must be rapidly done.
2. An LP should be performed and rapidly analyzed.

Bacterial meningitis

This requires immediate intervention.
Antibiotics
Antibiotics should be initiated using the Gram's stain, patient's age, underlying disease, immunologic status of the patient, and allergy history as guides to selection. They should be altered once culture and sensitivity data are available. *H. influenzae* resistant to ampicillin, chloramphenicol, or both are important pathogens and require aggressive, broad initial coverage:

< 2 months

Unknown etiology	Ampicillin 100-200 mg/kg/24 hr q 4-6 hr IV *and* cefotaxime 100-150 mg/kg/24 hr q 8-12 hr IV (or ceftriaxone 50-100 mg/kg/24 hr q 12 hr IV)
E. coli	Chloramphenicol 50-100 mg/kg/24 hr q 6 hr IV; **or** cefotaxime *or* ceftriaxone, as above, *or* cefuroxime 150 mg/kg/24 hr q 8 hr IV
Group B streptococci	Penicillin G 150,000-250,000 units/kg/24 hr q 4-6 hr IV; *and* gentamicin 5.0-7.5 mg/kg/24 hr q 8-12 hr IV
L. monocytogenes	Ampicillin, as above

2 months-9 years

Unknown etiology	Ampicillin 200-400 mg/kg/24 hr q 4 hr IV *and* chloramphenicol 100 mg/kg/24 hr q 6 hr IV; **or** cefotaxime 200 mg/kg/24 hr q 6 hr IV (**or** ceftriaxone 100 mg/kg/24 hr q 12 hr IV **or** cefuroxime 200 mg/kg/24 hr q 6 hr IV)
H. influenzae	Ampicillin 200-400 mg/kg/24 hr q 4 hr IV *and* chloramphenicol, as above; **or** cefotaxime 200 mg/kg/24 hr q 6 hr IV (or ceftriaxone 100 mg/kg/24 hr q 12 hr IV or cefuroxime 200 mg/kg/24 hr q 6 hr IV)
S. pneumoniae	Penicillin G 250,000 units/kg/24 hr q 4 hr IV
N. meningitidis	Penicillin G 250,000 units/kg/24 hr q 4 hr IV

>9 years

Unknown etiology	Penicillin G 250,000 units/kg/24 hr q 4 hr IV*
S. pneumoniae	Penicillin G 250,000 units/kg/24 hr q 4 hr IV*
N. meningitidis	Penicillin G 250,000 units/kg/24 hr q 4 hr IV*

Serum concentration of chloramphenicol should be maintained at 10-25 μg/ml.
Duration of therapy in uncomplicated cases is 10-14 days except for children under 2 mo of age, who should be treated for 3 wk.
*Adult: 10-20 million units/24 hr q 4 hr IV.

Cerebral edema

An infrequent complication, it may develop with focal neurologic signs or evidence of herniation.

1. If patient is intubated, hyperventilate to maintain $PaCO_2$ at 20-25 mm Hg.
2. Give mannitol (20% solution) 0.5-1.0 g/kg/dose q 4-6 hr IV.
3. Give steroid: dexamethasone (Decadron) 0.25 mg/kg/dose q 4-6 hr IV. Controversial
4. Give diuretic: furosemide (Lasix) 1 mg/kg/dose q 4-6 hr IV.

NOTE: Most patients who have symptomatic increased intracranial pressure and who require aggressive treatment as above should have an intracranial monitor placed by a neurosurgeon. Prognosis is improved if the cerebral perfusion pressure (CPP = difference between ICP and BP) is >30 mm Hg.

Seizures

Seizures should be treated with diazepam (Valium) 0.2-0.3 mg/kg/dose q 5-10 min IV until seizures stop (maximum: 10 mg). Phenobarbital or phenytoin should be initiated for maintenance therapy (Chapter 21).

Physical examination

A complete examination, including head circumference, should be performed daily. Particular attention should be given to secondary complications such as septic arthritis or subdural effusion in performing daily examinations.

Fluid therapy

This should be conservative, reflecting hydration and vital signs. Following stabilization, fluids should be continued at 80%-100% of maintenance requirements. Serum sodium should be monitored and if decreased, spot urine and serum sodium, potassium, and osmolality should be measured. If hyponatremia secondary to inappropriate ADH secretion occurs, fluid should be further restricted.

Disposition

All patients require hospitalization. Those with high-risk features (under 1 yr of age or demonstrating shock, coma, seizures, petechiae for <12 hr, low CSF glucose, or very high CSF

protein) should be monitored very closely, often in an ICU.

If the patient is seen initially in a setting without facilities to perform an LP and has signs and symptoms highly suggestive of bacterial meningitis, blood cultures should be obtained and parenteral antibiotics (IV preferably) administered before transport.

Chemoprophylaxis is indicated in the following situations.

1. Individuals who have had intimate contact with a patient with meningitis caused by *N. meningitidis* should receive prophylaxis: rifampin 10 mg/kg/dose q 12 hr PO for 4 doses (adult: 600 mg/kg/dose q 12 hr PO for 4 doses; children under 1 mo, 5 mg/kg/dose q 12 hr PO for 4 doses).
2. Prophylaxis for exposure to systemic disease—especially meningitis caused by *H. influenzae*—is controversial but guidelines have been developed. Prophylaxis is recommended for all members of a household with children under 4 yr, who have systemic *H. influenzae* type B disease. The indications for prophylaxis in day-care settings include the following: (1) an index case that spent more than 4 hr in the center during the week before onset of disease, (2) 75% of the center's children are receiving prophylaxis, and (3) there is more than one case. Prophylaxis generally is not indicated if the exposure occurred over 7 days before the encounter. Dosage of rifampin is 20 mg/kg/dose (maximum: 600 mg/dose) q 24 hr PO for 4 doses (neonate: 10 mg/kg/dose q 24 hr PO). Efficacy is uncertain.

   Exposed children who develop a febrile illness should receive prompt medical evaluation and treatment should be initiated, if indicated.
3. Rifampin can be administered to children by opening the capsule and mixing contents with known volume of applesauce, custard, etc. Make fresh mixture with each dose. Do not give to patients with liver disease.
4. Parents should be warned of the increased

risk of children under 1 yr of age developing secondary cases of *H. influenzae* meningitis.

5. In epidemic *Neisseria* meningitis, immunization of potential contacts is indicated.

With good clinical response, patients may be discharged 24 hr after completion of antibiotic therapy. They should be followed closely, with particular attention to potential neurologic deficits and hearing loss. Immunization of children 24 mo or older with *H. influenzae* vaccine is indicated.

Viral meningitis or meningoencephalitis
(Table 81-1)

This requires supportive therapy.

1. If there is any concern regarding the reliability of the diagnosis, a repeat LP should demonstrate a marked decrease in the percentage of PMN leukocytes in 6-8 hr after the first study in untreated patients.
2. The majority of patients with viral meningitis should be hospitalized initially to ensure adequate fluid intake and pain management and to monitor patients for deterioration. Complications require aggressive management. Following an initial assessment and stabilization period, patients may be discharged with close follow-up.
3. Although a definite treatment is unavailable, patients should be monitored closely because of associated neurologic and learning deficits that may develop in subsequent months.

REFERENCES

Band, J.D., Fraser, D.W., Ajello, G., et al.: Prevention of Haemophilus influenzae type B disease, JAMA **251**:2381, 1984.

David, S.D., Hill, S.R., Feigl, P., et al.: Partial antibiotic therapy in *Haemophilus influenzae* meningitis: its effects on cerebrospinal fluid abnormalities, Am. J., Dis. Child. **129**:802, 1975.

Eichenwald, H.F.: Antimicrobial therapy in infants and children: update 1976-1985, J. Pediatr. **107**:161, 337, 1985.

Goitein, K.J., and Tanui, I.: Cerebral perfusion pressure in central nervous system infection in infants and children, J. Pediatr. **103**:40, 1983.

Jacobs, R.F., Wells, T.G., Steele, R.W., et al.: A prospective randomized comparison of cefotaxime vs ampicillin and chloramphenicol for bacterial meningitis in children, J. Pediatr. **107**:129, 1985.

Kaplan, S.L., Mason, E.O., Mason, S.K.: Prospective comparative trial of moxalactam versus ampicillin or chloramphenicol for treatment of *Haemophilus influenzae* type B meningitis in children, J. Pediatr. **104**:447, 1984.

Lin, T.Y., Chrane, D.F., Nelson, J.D., et al.: Seven days of ceftriaxone therapy is as effective as ten days' treatment for bacterial meningitis, JAMA **253**:3559, 1985.

Odio, C., McCracken, G.H., and Nelson, J.D.: CSF shunt infection in pediatrics, Am. J. Dis. Child. **138**:1103, 1984.

Rubenstein, J.S., and Yogev, R.: What represents pleocytosis in blood-contaminated ("traumatic tap") cerebrospinal fluid in children? J. Pediatr. **107**:249, 1985.

Taylor, H.G., Michaels, R.H., Maxur, P.M., et al.: Intellectual, neuropsychological and achievement outcomes in children six to eight years after recovery from *Haemophilus influenzae* meningitis, Pediatrics **74**:198, 1984.

Migraines

Migraines are recurrent headaches with initial intracranial vasoconstriction followed by extracranial vasodilation, producing a throbbing pain that may occur in any age-group. A positive family history commonly is present. The headache often is precipitated by stress and may first develop during puberty.

DIAGNOSTIC FINDINGS

1. The headaches are classically unilateral, but may be bilateral with a throbbing or pulsatile quality.
   a. They commonly are preceded by an aura, which may be visual (stars, spots, or circles), sensory (hyperesthesia), or motor (weakness), and they are accompanied by abdominal pain, nausea, vomiting, anorexia, vertigo, ataxia, and syncope.
   b. Headaches subsequently become recurrent.
2. Migraines may be hemicranial or generalized, without an aura—more common in younger children.

- Generalized malaise, dizziness, nausea, and vomiting are prominent.
3. Less commonly, specific migraine complexes may be present.
   a. Ophthalmoplegic migraines cause unilateral eye pain with limitation of extraocular movement involving cranial nerves III, IV, and VI.
   b. Basilar migraines involve the basilar artery, producing headaches, vertigo, ataxia, cranial nerve palsy, blindness, syncope, acute confusion without neurologic findings, cyclic vomiting, recurrent abdominal pain, and paroxysmal disequilibrium. Progressive mental status deterioration may be noted.
   c. Hemiplegic migraines primarily cause motor deficits.
4. Migraines are often relieved by rest.

Ancillary data

1. EEG (may show slowing but is not diagnostically or therapeutically useful)
2. Tests to exclude other causes of headaches.

DIFFERENTIAL DIAGNOSIS

See Chapter 36.

MANAGEMENT

1. Initial management must attempt to relieve pain. Many patients respond to mild analgesia such as acetaminophen or acetaminophen with codeine. Relief usually is achieved with sleep.
2. Once the diagnosis is established, treatment of the acute episode is best achieved when medication is initiated early in the course.
   a. If mild analgesics provide inadequate relief, aspirin, phenacetin, and caffeine combinations (Fiorinal or Fenbutal) should be initiated.
      - In the 5- to 12-year-old, 1 tablet is given and repeated 1 hr later if no relief is obtained. This may be doubled in older children.
   b. In the postpubertal child, Midrin (isometheptene mucate 65 mg, dichloralphenazone 100 mg, and acetaminophen 325 mg) given at the onset of pain with an additional tablet 1 hr later may be useful.
      - If relief from a severe migraine is not achieved, ergotamine preparations may be used with subsequent episodes. Ergotamine (1 mg with 100 mg caffeine) tables should be used at the onset of pain and repeated every 30 min up to 3 doses per headache in children under 12 yr and no more than 6 doses per headache, regardless of age. Suppositories are available if the patient is vomiting (1 suppository per headache for children under 12 yr and no more than 2 suppositories per headache for older patients).
      NOTE: Caffeine potentiates the ergotamine by increasing absorption, but it may prevent sleep.
3. Long-term prophylactic management of disabling migraines in adolescents and adults may include one of the following:
   a. Propranolol 20-60 mg (<35 kg: 10-20 mg) q 8 hr PO. Usually effective in 70% of patients
   b. Phenytoin (Dilantin) 5-7 mg/kg/24 hr q 12-24 hr PO
   c. Amitriptyline (Elavil) 1-2 mg/kg (adult: 50-100 mg)/24 hr q 6-8 hr PO (maximum: 150 mg/24 hr)
   d. Cyproheptadine (Periactin) 0.2-0.4 mg/kg (adult: 4-16 mg)/24 hr q 6-8 hr PO (maximum: 32 mg/24 hr)
   NOTE: Different medications may have to be attempted.
4. Therapy to reduce stress, including counseling and biofeedback, may be useful in decreasing the frequency of episodes.

DISPOSITION

1. Most patients may be sent home with appro-

priate acute and chronic medications and close follow-up.
2. Hospitalization is indicated only for severe pain.

REFERENCES

Diamond, S., and Medina, J.L.: Double-blind study of propranolol for migraine prophylaxis, Headache **16**:24, 1976.
Prensky, A.L.: Migraine and migrainous variants in pediatric patients, Pediatr. Clin. North Am. **23**:461, 1976.

Pseudotumor cerebri

Benign intracranial hypertension or pseudotumor cerebri occurs when there is increased intracranial pressure in the absence of a local, space-occupying lesion or there is acute brain swelling accompanying an identifiable infectious or inflammatory process.

ETIOLOGY

Although the pathogenesis is unknown, pseudotumor cerebri is associated with a host of clinical entities:
1. Infection: upper respiratory tract (URI) infection, acute otitis media (AOM), roseola infantum, sinusitis
2. Allergy
3. Deficiency: anemia, including iron deficiency, leukemia, vitamin A deficiency, or overdose
4. Endocrine/metabolic disorders: steroid medication, oral contraceptive pills, uremia, hyperthyroidism, hypothyroidism, Addison's disease, or galactosemia
5. Trauma: minimal head trauma
6. Vascular disorder: congenital or acquired heart disease
7. Intoxication: tetracycline, steroids, oral contraceptives, vitamin A
8. Idiopathic disorder

DIAGNOSTIC FINDINGS

1. Younger children may have only a bulging fontanel with some irritability or listlessness.
2. Older children have headache, nausea, vomiting, and dizziness. Eye examination may reveal papilledema, sixth nerve palsy, diplopia, blurred vision, and enlarged blind spot.
3. The level of consciousness is relatively normal, given the signs of intracranial pressure.

Ancillary data

1. LP: normal with the exception of increased pressure
2. CT scan: may be indicated to exclude mass lesion

DIFFERENTIAL DIAGNOSIS

1. Infection
   a. Meningitis or encephalitis: LP for evaluation
   b. Brain abscess: CT scan and subsequent LP
   c. Optic neuritis: slitlamp examination
2. Trauma (subdural effusion or hemorrhage): subdural tap or CT scan
3. Neoplasm: CT scan (may be diagnostic)

MANAGEMENT

Although pseudotumor cerebri is a benign entity with an excellent prognosis, it is a diagnosis of exclusion, and other entities must be considered. Once the diagnosis is confirmed, treatment of the underlying disease is appropriate.

Adjunctive therapy, implemented in conjunction with a neurologist, may include:
1. Acetazolamide (Diamox) 5 mg/kg/dose (maximum: 250-375 mg/dose) q 24-48 hr PO **or**
2. Serial LP

Uncontrolled, increased intracranial pressure and papilledema may result in visual loss. The patient should therefore be followed by an ophthalmologist with testing of visual fields if possible.

REFERENCE

Hagberg, B., and Sillanpea, M.: Benign intracranial hypertension, ACTA Pediatr. Scan. **59**:328, 1970.

Seizures

ALERT: If ongoing seizures are occurring, refer to status epilepticus (Chapter 21).

A seizure or convulsion is a paroxysmal disturbance in nerve cells resulting in abnormalities in motor, sensory, autonomic, or psychic function. (See febrile seizures, p. 564)

ETIOLOGY (Table 81-4)

The most common causes of acute onset of seizures in children are infection, trauma, poor compliance, intoxications, and idiopathic disorders. Epilepsy accounts for most chronic seizure disorders.

DIAGNOSTIC FINDINGS

Patients usually have a history of seizures, but if ongoing seizures are present, evaluation and management as described in Chapter 21 should be implemented. Commonly encountered seizure types as well as therapeutic approaches are outlined in Table 81-5.

1. The initial assessment must determine the characteristics of the seizure, defining its focality or generalized nature, frequency, associated sensory and autonomic function, and behavioral changes. Predisposing factors such as fever, intoxications, perinatal asphyxia, trauma, and preexisting abnormalities in growth and development require definition.
2. A complete neurologic examination is essential, differentiating long-standing from acute changes. Evidence of asymmetry of findings, increased intracranial pressure, or infection must be carefully assessed.

Ancillary data

Evaluation must reflect the nature of the seizure and potential etiologies.

Chemistries

A glucose should be performed on all patients: initially, Dextrostix or Chemstrip screening; electrolytes, Ca^{++}, Mg^{++}, and $PO_4^=$ as indicated.

Hematology

For febrile patients, a CBC and urinalysis should be done.

Lumbar puncture

An LP should be performed in febrile patients, if indicated (p. 566). Evaluation of the fluid must include Gram's stain (and methylene blue stain), culture, cell count, glucose, and protein.

X-ray film

1. A CT scan has a very low yield in generalized seizures without focal findings in the pediatric age-group and is usually not required. It may be useful in cases with preceding head trauma.
2. A skull roentgenogram is indicated with evidence of trauma preceding the seizure and where a CT scan is not readily available.

Drug levels

1. Evaluation for possibility of ingestion (Chapter 54)
2. Anticonvulsant medication levels if the patient is receiving chronic therapy. Subtherapeutic levels are a very common cause of seizures.

Subdural tap (Appendix A-6)

This may be indicated in the young child who has associated trauma or infection, particularly if the fontanel is full and the child is deteriorating.

Electroencephalogram

An electroencephalogram (EEG) is indicated to assess electrical seizure activity. The greatest yield in finding epileptiform abnormalities as a seizure focus is immediately after the seizure and declines with time. Nonspecific background changes may persist for 1-6 wk (at the extremes) after any type of seizure, including febrile or hypoxic breath-holding.

DIFFERENTIAL DIAGNOSIS

See Table 81-4.

Text continued on p. 564.

TABLE 81-4. Seizures: diagnostic considerations

Condition	Diagnostic findings	Comments
EPILEPSY	Variable seizure types as described in Table 81-5	Multiple etiologies, including idiopathic
INFECTION		
Febrile (p. 564)	Fever; grand mal seizure; variable focal seizure; self-limited; peak: 5 mo–5 yr; high association with *Shigella*; LP normal	Must distinguish from meningitis
Meningitis (p. 549)	Fever, stiff neck, headache, Kernig's, Brudzinski's; in young child, dehydration, bulging fontanel, lethargy, irritability, vomiting, cyanosis; LP diagnostic	May be viral or bacterial
Encephalitis (p. 550)	Headache, fever, vomiting, irritability, listlessness, stupor, variable focal neurologic signs; LP may be diagnostic or equivocal	Epidemiology important; usually viral
Intracranial abscess	Insidious onset; fever; variable focal neurologic findings; CT scan diagnostic	
S/P DTP immunization	History of immunization, fever; seizure within 48 hr	
Misc: pertussis, rabies, tetanus, syphilis	Disease-specific signs and symptoms	May have permanent sequelae
Subacute bacterial endocarditis (p. 420)	Fever; usually insidious; focal neurologic findings; splenomegaly; embolic phenomenon; variable heart disease; positive blood cultures	
TRAUMA (Chapter 57)		
Concussion	History of trauma, variable abnormal neurologic exam; focal or grand mal seizure within 24 hr; CT scan variably WNL	May be recurrent; close neurologic monitoring; may not require anticonvulsants
Acute Subdural	Variable focal neurologic signs; change in mental status; progression with increased intracranial pressure; positive CT scan	Immediate neurosurgical intervention
Epidural	Lucid period following trauma; eventual lapse into coma with herniation	Immediate neurosurgical intervention

CONGENITAL (Chapters 10 and 11)		
Birth asphyxia	History of perinatal injury; neurologic abnormality; premature; low Apgar	Infection, placental insufficiency, difficult birth
Neurocutaneous syndrome	Pathognomonic skin findings; variably abnormal neurologic exam; family history; CT scan may be useful	
INTRAPSYCHIC		
Breath-holding (p. 549)	Precipitated by crying, anger, injury, cyanosis, followed by loss of consciousness, may be opisthotonic; seizures rare and self-limited	Peak: 6 mo-4 yr; cyanosis precedes loss of consciousness; in seizures consciousness is lost first; usually maternal-infant problems
Hyperventilation		
Hysteria		
ENDOCRINE/METABOLIC		
Hypoglycemia (Chapter 38)	Sweating, pallor, syncope, vasovagal reaction; newborn: irritability, apnea, cyanosis, listlessness, poor feeding	Definition varies with age; glucose: newborn <2500 g (<20 mg/dl), term newborn (<30 mg/dl), older infant and child (<40 mg/dl)
Hyponatremia (Chapter 8)	Listlessness, vriable stupor; associated condition (dehydration, head trauma, inappropriate ADH, Addison's, intoxication, etc.)	Rarely causes seizures unless rapid rehydration
Hypernatremia (Chapter 8)	Listlessness or irritability; associated condition (dehydration)	
Hypocalcemia	Muscle cramps, pain, Chvostek's, Trousseau's, variable increased intracranial pressure, headache	Common in premature, parathyroid deficiency
Hypomagnesemia	Tetany, tremor, irritability	Difficult to determine true body deficit
Kernicterus (Chapter 11)	Jaundice, developmental delay	Rare at present
Inborn errors Phenylketonuria (PKU) Amino and organic acidemias	Neurologically abnormal; developmental delay; variable acidosis; need urine and blood screen	
Uremia (p. 615)	Signs and symptoms of renal failure	

Continued.

TABLE 81-4. Seizures: diagnostic considerations—cont'd

Condition	Diagnostic findings	Comments
INTOXICATION (Chapter 54)		
Aspirin	Signs and symptoms of associated drug intoxication or withdrawal	See Section VIII for complete listing
Amphetamine		
Anticholinergics (tricyclics, phenothiazines, etc.)		
Theophylline		
Carbon monoxide		
PCP, cocaine		
Propoxyphene		
Lead		
Drug withdrawal (alcohol, anticonvulsants, etc.)		
DEGENERATIVE/DEFICIENCY		
Pyridoxine deficiency or dependence	Mentally retarded, anemia, diarrhea	Responds well to pyridoxine (5-10 mg IV/IM), then 0.3-0.5 mg/24 hr
Tay-Sachs disease	Blind, spasms, floppy, cherry-red spot	Eastern European background
Juvenile Huntington's chorea	Rigidity, dementia	
Metachromatic leukodystrophy	Incoordination, upper and lower neurologic signs	
Other CNS diseases	Variable	
NEOPLASM	Often focal neurologic findings	Glioma, most common; supratentorial lesions more likely to cause seizure
VASCULAR (Chapter 18)		
Intracranial hematoma	Acute onset headache, neurologic findings; variable increased intracranial pressure	Associated with AV malformation, bleeding disorder (hemophilia, etc.), heart disease, sickle cell, trauma
Cerebral		
Extradural		
Subarachnoid		
Hypertensive encephalopathy (Chapter 18)	High blood pressure; vomiting, hyperpyrexia, ataxia, coma; facial paralysis	May be secondary to stroke
Embolism	Focal neurologic findings	Predisposing factors: heart disease, peripheral embolism
Transient ischemic attack infarct	Variable neurologic finding, dependent on site; fever; broad deficits; altered sensation	Differentiate from Todd's paralysis

TABLE 81-5. Common seizure types

Type of seizure	Etiology	Diagnostic findings	Treatment/comments
Grand mal (tonic-clonic)	Idiopathic, genetic, trauma, infection, intoxication, endocrine/metabolic, degenerative, tumor	Aura (50%): motor, sensory (smell, taste), visceral (abdominal pain); crying; loss of consciousness; tonic (stiffening)-clonic (rhythmic jerking, twitching); involuntary urination and defecation; postictal; rare transient paresis (Todd's paralysis)	Treat with Phenobarbital Phenytoin Carbamazepine Valproic acid
Psychomotor (temporal lobe), complex partial	Idiopathic, hypoxia, birth trauma, infection (herpes), temporal lobe mass	Aura: fear, abdominal pain, smell; automatisms: rubbing, chewing, staring, salivation; seizure occurs singly (minutes); psychic (fear, anger, hallucination), sensory (numbness, tingling), motor (purposeless movement)	Distinguish from petit mal and behavior disorder; treat with Carbamazepine Phenytoin Primidone Valproic acid
Petit mal (absence)	Idiopathic, genetic	No aura; transient (5-20 sec) lapses of consciousness, appearing to be day-dreaming, disinterested, staring, immobile; rhythmic blinking movement; not postictal; EEG 3 sec wave and spike; evoked by hyperventilation	Common in 4 to 10-year-olds; treat with Ethosuximide Valproic acid Clonazepam
Myoclonic Petit mal variant Lennox-Gastaut	Degenerative CNS, infection, lead, subacute sclerosing panencephalitis, retarded children	Sudden spasmodic contraction of extremities (few sec): single or repetitive; may also have akinetic spells (drop fits) with sudden loss of muscle tone	Very rare, usually accompanied by grand mal; treat with Valproic acid Clonazepam Ethosuximide

MANAGEMENT

1. Initial treatment of the patient with ongoing seizure activity (Chapter 21) must include oxygen, dextrose, and anticonvulsants.
2. In the absence of active seizure activity, efforts should focus on rapidly determining possible etiologic conditions and instituting specific treatment.
   a. Metabolic derangements require specific therapy to correct the abnormality.
   b. Seizures following trauma require immediate neurosurgical consultation and CT scan if the patient remains neurologically impaired.
   c. Infectious etiologies require antibiotics and supportive care.
3. If no etiology is determined, anticonvulsants should be considered after consultation with a neurologist. At present there is some controversy regarding the advisability of treating the first tonic-clonic seizure; many clinicians prefer to wait pending subsequent seizures when a more definite diagnosis of epilepsy can be made. If medication is begun, loading is required (Table 81-6).
   a. If the patient is taking medication, anticonvulsant dosages, if subtherapeutic, should be increased.
   b. If poor compliance is the basis for the low levels, the patient should be reloaded (in full or part, depending on the level) and educated about the importance of taking medications. Close follow-up with monitoring the levels is necessary.
   c. Anticonvulsants usually are continued for at least 2 years after the last seizures. They may be stopped at that time provided the child has been doing well.
4. Newborns require slightly different management (Chapter 11).

DISPOSITION

1. Patients with first seizures of unknown etiology are often admitted to the hospital for evaluation and control, as well as a response to parental anxiety.
2. After a period of observation, patients with chronic seizure disorders who are taking subtherapeutic doses or who require alteration in the therapeutic regimen can be discharged once the drugs are changed and follow-up arranged.
3. Patients with febrile seizures do not require hospitalization if no underlying life-threatening infection is detected as outlined below.
4. All patients with seizure disorders require close follow-up of clinical status and therapeutic response. Assessment of anticonvulsant levels is periodically indicated. Patients with complex recurrent seizures should routinely be referred to a neurologist.

Parental education

1. Give all medications as prescribed.
2. If a seizure does occur, institute seizure precautions to prevent your child from self-injury. Maintain airway.
3. Close follow-up is very important. Please keep all appointments.
4. Call physician if
   a. There is any change in the pattern or frequency of seizure
   b. There are behavior changes or problems with medication

REFERENCE

Oppenheimer, E.Y., and Rosman, N.P.: Seizures in childhood: an approach to emergency management, Pediatr. Clin. North Am. **26**:837, 1979.

Febrile seizures

ALERT: Meningitis must be considered as a potential etiology in the febrile child who has seizures.

Febrile seizures are generalized seizures occuring in children with febrile illnesses that do not specifically involve the central nervous system. They occur in 2%-5% of children between 5 mo and 5 yr of age, with the peak incidence between 8 and 20 mo.

TABLE 81-6. Common anticonvulsants

Drug/availability	Primary indications	Maintenance dosage (mg/kg/day) (PO)	Loading dose (mg/kg)	Serum half-life (hr)	Serum therapeutic range (µg/ml)
Phenobarbital Elix: 20 mg/5 ml Tab: 15, 30, 60, 90, 100 mg Vial: 65, 130 mg/ml	Grand mal	3-5	10-15 IV or IM* (<25-50 mg/min)	48-72	10-25 (may be higher)
Phenytoin (Dilantin) Susp: 30, 125 mg/5 ml Tab (chew): 50 mg Cap: 30, 100 mg Amp: 50 mg/ml	Grand mal, psychomotor	5-10	10-20 IV* (<40 mg/min)	6-30	10-20
Diazepam (Valium) Vial: 5 mg/ml	Status epilepticus	NA	0.2-0.3 IV (<1 mg/min)		
Carbamazepine (Tegretol)† Tab: 100 (chew), 200 mg	Grand mal, psychomotor	15-30		12	4-12 (varies with lab)
Ethosuximide (Zarontin) Syr: 250 mg/5 ml Cap: 250 mg	Petit mal	20-30		30	40-100
Valproic acid (Depakene) Syr: 250 mg/5 ml Cap: 250 mg	Petit mal, other minor motor, grand mal	15-60		6-18	50-100
Primidone (Mysoline) Susp: 250 mg/5 ml Tab: 50, 250 mg	Myoclonic, psychomotor	10-25		12	7-15 (or phenobarbital level)
Clonazepam (Klonopin; previously Clonopin) Tab: 0.5, 1, 2 mg	Minor motor	0.01-0.2		18-50	0.013-0.072

*Adult dose: phenobarbital—100 mg/dose IV q 20 min prn × 3; phenytoin maximum total dose—1250 mg IV. Oral loading of phenobarbital or phenytoin may be considered if patient's condition warrants. IM absorption of phenobarbital may be erratic.

†Patients with atypical absence seizures as well as other types of seizures may be predisposed to exacerbation of seizures when carbamazepine (Tegretol) is used.

ETIOLOGY: INFECTION

1. Upper respiratory tract infections are commonly present, representing >70% of underlying infections. Pharyngitis, otitis media, and pneumonitis are most frequent.
2. Gastroenteritis, urinary tract infections, measles, and immunizations (DTP) are less common.
3. Roseola (exanthema subitum) is associated with a high fever, often complicated by a seizure before the onset of the rash.
4. *Shigella* organisms produce high fevers and a neurotoxin. Seizures are common.
5. Meningitis occurs in about 2% of children with fevers and seizures.

DIAGNOSTIC FINDINGS

1. Typically, there is a preceding infectious illness and high fever (usually >39° C). Patients have signs and symptoms of the underlying systemic infection. Of obvious importance is to exclude meningitis; such patients commonly have lethargy, fever, headache, vomiting, etc. (p. 549).
2. Seizures are generalized tonic-clonic episodes lasting <15 min. Complex seizures occur when the episode lasts >15 min or it is focal or is followed by transient or persistent neurologic abnormalities.
3. Behavior and state of alertness are altered.
   a. Children are postictal.
   b. The underlying illness produces irritability, lethargy, and other changes in mental status.
4. Aggressive antipyretic therapy early in the management facilitates evaluation.

Complications

These are usually self-limited, although they may be recurrent or complex, resulting in hypoxia and self-injury.

Ancillary data

Lumbar puncture

LP is an essential part of the evaluation of the patient, particularly for those with a first febrile seizure (Appendix A-3). It should be done in the following children:
1. Under 1 yr of age
2. Under 2 yr of age with temperatures of 41.1° C or above
3. Those who, after aggressive antipyretic therapy, remain irritable, lethargic, or demonstrate other abnormal behavior
4. Where there is any question of the reliability of the examination, the caretaker, or follow-up

Evaluation of fluid should include Gram's stain, culture, cell count, protein, and glucose.

Blood glucose

This should be done immediately, either by quantitative methods or Dextrostix/Chemstrip.

CBC with differential

This is usually unreliable because of the demargination resulting from catecholamine release.

Electrolytes and BUN

These are indicated if there is a preceding problem with intake or output. Ca^{++}, $PO_4^=$, and Mg^{++} determinations are not indicated in previously normal children.

Other studies

Skull roentgenograms are obtained only if there is associated trauma. An EEG usually is not obtained because it has little or no prognostic value, although transient abnormalities may be noted.

DIFFERENTIAL DIAGNOSIS (p. 559)

1. Infection
   a. CNS infection including those caused by bacterial, viral, fungal or mycobacterial agents. LP is required for differentiation.
   b. Postinfectious encephalitis
   c. Brain abscess with fever, seizures, and variable spinal fluid
   d. Immunization, particularly DPT
2. Intoxication
   a. Hydrocarbon ingestion with aspiration pneumonitis, fever, and seizures

b. Salicylate overdose

3. Intrapsychic problem. Breath-holding spells may occur during intercurrent febrile illness.

MANAGEMENT (Chapter 21)

1. Patients with acute seizures require intervention with oxygen, suction, and maneuvers to minimize self-injury. Rarely is active airway management required. Venous access should be established for drug administration. By the time patients arrive, they rarely are having seizures. If they are, dextrose 0.5-1.0 g/kg/dose (2-4 ml D25W/kg/dose) IV should be given.

2. Anticonvulsants (Table 81-6) should be administered:
   a. Diazepam (Valium) 0.2-0.3 mg/kg/dose IV given over 2-3 min at a rate not to exceed 1 mg/min. May repeat every 5-10 min if seizures continue (maximum total dose: 10 mg). Used to stop seizures
   b. Phenobarbital 10-15 mg/kg/dose IV (25-50 mg/min) or IM, given as a loading dose is an alternative to diazepam. May be used as maintenance drug, as well as in the management of the patient who is having an acute seizure

3. Patients who are not having active seizures require rapid evaluation and antipyretic therapy. Questioning must focus on potential infectious sources, past history of seizures, neurologic deficits, developmental problems, family history, medications, precipitating events, and preceding illness.
   • Antipyretic therapy should include acetaminophen 10-15 mg/kg/dose q 4-6 hr PO and tepid water sponging. Aspirin may be used additionally if neither chickenpox nor influenza-like illness is present.

4. Laboratory data should be obtained, including an LP as appropriate.

5. Underlying infections should be treated as appropriate.

6. Long-term anticonvulsants reduce, but do not eliminate, recurrent febrile seizures and phenobarbital (5 mg/kg/24 hr q 12-24 hr PO after a loading dose) should be considered for certain patients (Table 81-6):
   a. Those with two or more of the following risk factors:
      (1) Abnormal neurologic or developmental history before the seizures
      (2) Complex seizure: >15 min in length or one that is focal or followed by transient or persistent neurologic abnormalities
      (3) Positive family history for afebrile seizures
   b. Children under 12 mo of age at the time of their first seizure
      NOTE: Anticonvulsants are continued for 2 yr if the patient remains seizure free, although this must be individualized. Intermittent use is of no value.
   • Family anxiety and other social factors may modify the decision to initiate anticonvulsants.
   • Learning disorders and hyperactivity may be associated with phenobarbital use. Anticonvulsants should be initiated only for appropriate reasons. Most children do not require medications.

DISPOSITION

1. Patients with simple febrile seizures may be discharged after appropriate fever control has been achieved. Underlying infections require treatment.

2. Patients requiring phenobarbital therapy may similarly be discharged with close follow-up and neurologic consultation after a loading dose has been given and maintenance therapy has been initiated. It is given normally for 2 yr when deemed appropriate with dosage adjustment to accommodate growth. Intermittent phenobarbital is of no value.

3. Approximately 40% of children with a simple febrile seizure will have a recurrence, half of which will occur within 6 mo of the first episode.

Parental education

Parental counseling is essential to provide reassurance. It is essential to discuss a number of issues:

1. Benign nature of febrile seizures in healthy children. Reassuring points include the high incidence (2%-5%), the only slightly increased incidence of epilepsy in those defined as high risk, the low frequency of recurrences, and the rare incidence of death or sequelae.
2. Home treatment, which must include first aid to protect the airway and minimize self-injury. Fever control must be reviewed.
3. The risks and benefits of anticonvulsant therapy. It may reduce recurrences, but it has adverse effects.
4. The parent should call physician after the initial evaluation if
   a. Fever continues >36 hr; behavioral changes develop; severe vomiting, headache, nonblanching rash, or stiff neck develops; or another seizure occurs
   b. If the child is on medication and becomes lethargic, hyperactive, or irritable or develops a rash from phenobarbital. Sedation early in the course of treatment is common.

REFERENCES

Bettis, D.B., and Ater, S.B.: Febrile seizures: emergency department diagnosis and treatment, J. Emerg. Med. 2:341, 1985.

Camfield, C.S., Chaplin, S., Doyle, A.B., et al.: Side effects of phenobarbital in toddlers: behavioral and cognitive aspects. J. Pediatr. 95:361, 1979.

Fishman, M.A.: Febrile seizures: the treatment controversy, J. Pediatr. 94:177, 1979.

Nelson, K.B., and Ellenberg, J.H.: Prognosis in children with febrile seizures, Pediatrics 61:720, 1978.

Wolf, S.M., Carr, A., and Davis, D.C.: The value of phenobarbital in the child who has had a single febrile seizure: a controlled prospective study, Pediatrics 59:378, 1977.

82 Orthopedic disorders

Septic arthritis

ALERT: Immediate drainage and antibiotics are indicated if the joint is to be salvaged.

Septic arthritis is an infection of the synovial membrane and joint space, resulting from either hematogenous spread or direct inoculation.

Predisposing factors include systemic bacterial infections, gonorrhea, and impaired immunologic status.

ETIOLOGY: INFECTION

1. *Staphylococcus aureus:* represents 20%-30% of isolates
2. *Haemophilus influenzae*
   a. Most common in children under 2 yr but found in older children
   b. Often associated with infections elsewhere (meningitis)
3. Streptococci: group A, B, anaerobic, *Streptococcus viridans*
4. *Streptococcus pneumoniae*
5. *Neisseria gonorrhoeae:* primarily knee, wrist, and hand
6. Uncommon
   a. Gram-negative enteric: neonates and immunosuppressed
   b. *Pseudomonas* organisms: neonates, immunosuppressed; those with puncture wounds

DIAGNOSTIC FINDINGS

1. Patients inconsistently have systemic illness with fever, anorexia, and listlessness.

2. Local findings include pain and tenosynovitis, particularly with gonorrhea. The joints are tender, with warmth, swelling, tenderness, effusion, and limitation of movement (Chapter 40). It is primarily a monoarticular disease, involving the large, weight-bearing joints of the knee, hip, shoulder, wrist, and elbow. The patient may have concurrent osteomyelitis.
3. In one series of *H. influenzae* septic arthritis, 35% had associated otitis media and 30% had meningitis.

Complications

These involve damage to growth plate and joint cartilage, leading to poor growth and a stiff or destroyed joint.

Ancillary data

1. WBC: variable; erythrocyte sedimentation rate (ESR): usually elevated and normalizes with recovery
2. Blood cultures: positive in 50% of cases of nongonococcal disease and 20% of gonococcal infections
3. Cultures of the cervix, rectum, and pharynx if gonorrhea is suspected: positive in 80% of patients with gonococcal disease
4. Arthrocentesis and analysis of the synovial fluid including glucose, cell count and differential, Gram's stain, and culture (Table 82-1 and Appendix A-2). Negative cultures in gonococcal arthritis are not uncommon.
5. X-ray films: plain films of joint

TABLE 82-1. Common synovial fluid findings

Category	Etiology	Appearance	Leukocytes (cells/mm³)	Percentage of neutro-phils	Percentage of glucose $\left[\dfrac{\text{synovial}}{\text{blood}}\right]$	Mucin* clot
Normal		Clear	<100	25	>50	Good
Bacterial	Septic arthritis	Turbid, purulent	>50,000	>75	<50	Poor
Inflammatory	Juvenile rheumatoid arthritis Rheumatic fever Mycobacterial, viral, and fungal arthritis	Clear or turbid	500-75,000	50	>50	Poor
Traumatic		Clear or bloody	<5,000†	<50	>50	Good

*For mucin clot: add 4 ml of water to 1 ml of synovial fluid supernatant. Mix in 2 drops of 5% glacial acetic acid. If normal, a tight rope of mucin will form. If infection or inflammation, clot will flake and shred.
†May have red cells.

a. Early changes include joint fluid with capsular distension. If difficult to interpret, comparison views may be helpful.

b. Bony demineralization and subsequent cartilaginous and bony destruction may develop; however, radiographs may be normal and therefore are not adequately sensitive to be used as a screen.

6. Nuclear scan

a. Indicated when joint tap is contraindicated (overlying infection, small joints, axial skeleton involved)

b. Technetium scan (Tc 99m): positive within 24 hr of symptoms and may remain positive. Three-phase study may be helpful in differentiating from osteomyelitis.

c. Gallium scan (Ga 67): positive within 24-48 hr of symptoms but reverts to normal with adequate treatment

DIFFERENTIAL DIAGNOSIS

See Chapter 27.

MANAGEMENT

1. Initial management must exclude other conditions in the differential diagnosis. Delay in treatment of septic arthritis exposes the patient to permanent joint damage.

2. Once septic arthritis is considered, the joint should be aspirated and the fluid analyzed (Table 82-1)

3. The joint should be immobilized and physical therapy initiated once recovery is partially achieved.

Antibiotics

Initial antibiotics are based on the Gram's stain of the fluid obtained from the arthrocentesis and drug allergies. Once final cultures and sensitivity data are available, these may be altered.

For known organism

S. aureus   Nafcillin 100-200 mg/kg/24 hr q 4 hr IV **or** an equivalent semisynthetic penicillin

H. influenzae   Ampicillin 150-200 mg/kg/24 hr q 4 hr IV **and** chloramphenicol 100 mg/kg/24 hr q 6 hr IV; **or** cefotaxime 150 mg/kg/24 hr q 6 hr IV; **or** ceftriaxone 75 mg/kg/24 hr q 12 hr IV

S. pneumoniae   Penicillin G 100,000 U/kg/24 hr q 4 hr IV

N. gonorrhoeae   Penicillin G

For unknown organism

All patients	Nafcillin
Neonates	**Add** gentamicin 5.0-7.5 mg/kg/24 hr q 8-12 hr IV or IM
Infants (under 5 yr)	**Add** ampicillin and chloramphenicol; **or** cefotaxime, **or** ceftriaxone

1. Although clinical trials have substantiated the value of third-generation cephalosporins in the treatment of joint infections, experience with children still is limited.
2. Traditionally, parenteral antibiotics are continued for a minimum of 2 (gonococci, streptococci, and *Haemophilus* organisms) to 3 (staphylococci, gram-negative enterics, and *Pseudomonas* organisms) wk. More recently, some investigators have used oral medications after 1 wk of parenteral drugs while carefully monitoring serum levels, which must have a bactericidal level of at least 1:8.

Joint drainage

1. Needle aspiration of the joint is attempted initially to relieve pressure and decompress the joint, unless surgical drainage is more appropriate.
2. Surgical drainage is indicated if:
   a. Hip, elbow, ankle, or shoulder are involved
   b. Thick, purulent material is obtained
   c. Adhesions are present or inadequate decompression is achieved after 2-3 days of repeated needle aspiration
   d. Response to therapy is poor after 36-48 hr of antibiotics
   e. Long delay in the initiation of treatment has occurred

DISPOSITION

All patients require hospitalization. Immediate orthopedic consultation should be obtained. The outcome is better in patients who are hospitalized and treated within 5 days of onset of symptoms.

REFERENCES

Goldenberg, D.L., and Reed, J.J.: Bacterial arthritis, N. Engl. J. Med. **312**:764, 1985.

Nelson, J.D., Bucholz, R.W., Kusmiesz, H., et al.: Benefits and risks of sequential parenteral-oral cephalosporin therapy for suppurative bone and joint infections, J. Pediatr. Orthop. **2**:255, 1982.

Rothbart, H.A., and Glode, M.P.: *Haemophilus influenzae* type b septic arthritis in children: report of 23 cases, Pediatrics **75**:254, 1985.

Volberg, F.M., Sumner, T.E., Abramson, J.S., and Winchester, P.M.: Unreliability of radiographic diagnosis of septic hip in children, Pediatrics **73**:118, 1984.

Osteomyelitis

ALERT: Acute onset of limp or local tenderness, warmth, or erythema requires a careful evaluation. A prolonged course of antibiotics is indicated.

Acute osteomyelitis is an infection of bone, occurring most commonly by hematogenous spread but also associated with direct inoculation, which is secondary to open fractures, penetrating wounds, or surgical procedures. The metaphysis of the long bones, particularly the femur and tibia, is most commonly involved.

Factors predisposing an individual to osteomyelitis include trauma, systemic bacterial disease, drug abuse, sickle cell disease, and impaired immunologic status.

ETIOLOGY: INFECTION

1. *S. aureus:* Accounts for 60%-90% of isolates
2. Streptococcal species: group A and B (in neonates usually B)
3. *Staphylococcus epidermidis*
4. *H. influenzae:* most common in children under 2 yr
5. Uncommon
   a. *Pseudomonas* organisms: common in drug abusers and with osteomyelitis caused by penetrating injury of the foot, usually through a rubber-soled shoe

b. *Salmonella* organisms: usually in patients with sickle cell disease

c. Gram-negative enterics: usually in newborns

d. Mycobacteria

e. Fungal: usually in immunocompromised patients

DIAGNOSTIC FINDINGS

1. The clinical findings are extremely variable, and a high index of suspicion is required. The majority of patients have a fever and occasionally report a predisposing factor. Systemic disease may be present.

2. Patients may have a limp (Chapter 40) and limitation of movement or merely a history of favoring the extremity.

3. Locally, patients inconsistently have tenderness, warmth, erythema, and pain over the involved site.

4. Children under 1 yr of age have little systemic toxicity.

Complications

1. Septic arthritis (p. 569). More common in infants

2. Growth disturbance of the limb if there is disruption of the epiphyseal growth plate

3. Chronic osteomyelitis with persistent infection, often secondary to inadequate treatment

Ancillary data

1. WBC. Often elevated, although the majority of patients have counts between 5,000 and 15,000 cells/mm^3

2. ESR. Commonly elevated; provides a useful parameter to assess the adequacy of treatment as it normalizes with resolution of inflammation

3. Blood cultures. Positive in >50% of patients

4. X-ray film: plain film of extremity
   a. Soft tissue findings develop 3-4 days after the onset of symptoms:

(1) Swelling of deep soft tissues next to metaphysis with displacement of fat lines

(2) Obliteration of lucent planes between muscles

(3) Subcutaneous edema

   b. Bony changes are noted 7-10 days after symptomatic onset:
   (1) Periosteal elevation
   (2) Lytic lesions
   (3) Sclerosis with new bone formation

5. Nuclear bone scan: technetium Tc 99m
   a. Often becomes abnormal 1-2 days after onset of symptoms with increased uptake in area of inflammation
   b. May be falsely negative in up to 25% of cases, particularly in newborns and children under 1 yr
   c. Uptake locally increased in osteomyelitis, septic arthritis, cellulitis, trauma, and neoplastic disease

6. Aspiration of involved bone (usually done by orthopedist). Provides definitive identification and sensitivity of etiologic organism.
   • Gram's stain of aspirate may provide initial etiologic information

7. Serum bactericidal titers are imperative in monitoring therapeutic regimens.

DIFFERENTIAL DIAGNOSIS

1. Infection
   a. Septic arthritis (p. 569)
   b. Cellulitis (p. 432)

2. Trauma
   a. Local soft tissue injury
   b. Fracture

3. Neoplasm: Ewing's tumor

MANAGEMENT

1. The key to appropriate management is early identification of the patient with osteomyelitis.

2. Cultures should be obtained before initiating therapy.

3. Aspiration of the lesions by an orthopedist is indicated. If pus is obtained, many clinicians recommend drainage and curettage. Open drainage also is indicated if there is poor response in the first 36-48 hr following initiation of therapy.
4. Immobilization of the involved extremity may minimize pain in the initial treatment stages during the initial evaluation and stabilization.

Antibiotics

1. Nafcillin (or other semisynthetic penicillin: methicillin or oxacillin) 100-200 mg/kg/24 hr q 4 hr IV should be given (assuming no allergy). Alternative regimens include cefazolin or cephalothin 100 mg/kg/24 hr q 4-6 hr IV.
2. Additional antibiotics should be administered if an organism other than *S. aureus* is suspected.
   a. If the patient has sickle cell disease or is a neonate, a *Salmonella* organism or gram-negative enteric may be etiologic
      • Give ampicillin 200 mg/kg/24 hr q 4 hr IV **and** gentamicin 5.0-7.5 mg/kg/24 hr q 8-12 hr IV or IM. Prolonged therapy is indicated.
   b. With puncture wound of the foot through a rubber-soled shoe or if patient is a drug abuser and routine management is not adequate, a *Pseudomonas* organism should be considered and treated with the following:
      (1) Surgical drainage, as needed
      (2) Carbenicillin 400-600 mg/kg/24 hr q 4 hr IV **and** gentamicin, as above
3. In the routine care of osteomyelitis caused by *S. aureus*, patients are normally treated parenterally for 5-7 days, assuming decreased local inflammation and normalization of the ESR.
4. After the initial parenteral course and resolution of signs and symptoms, patients may be switched to oral therapy for 3-6 wk:
   a. Dicloxacillin 75-100 mg/kg/24 hr q 6 hr PO
   b. If patient is allergic to penicillin: cephalexin 50-100 mg/kg/24 hr q 6 hr PO **or** clindamycin 15-25 mg/kg/24 hr q 6 hr PO
5. Antibiotics may be modified by the results of Gram's stain, culture, and sensitivity data.
6. During the phase of oral therapy, patients are often hospitalized to ensure continuing compliance.
7. Throughout the treatment course, serum bactericidal levels or serum antibiotic levels are monitored to ensure that adequate antibiotics are being administered. A bactericidal titer of 1:8 or greater is acceptable.

DISPOSITION

1. All patients should be hospitalized for therapy.
2. An orthopedic consultation should be obtained. Infectious disease consultants also may be useful in the evaluation and long-term management of the patient, particularly if an unusual organism is suspected or identified.

REFERENCES

Dich, V.Q., Nelson, J.D., and Haltalin, K.C.: Osteomyelitis in infants and children, Am. J. Dis Child. **129**:1273, 1975.

Eichenwald, H.F.: Antimicrobial therapy in infants and children: update 1976-1985, J. Pediatr. **107**:161, 337, 1985.

Fisher, M.C., Goldsmith, J.F., and Gilligan, P.H.: Sneakers as a source of *Pseudomonas aeroginosa* in children with osteomyelitis following puncture wound, J. Pediatr. **106**:607, 1985.

Tetzlaff, T.R., McCracken, G.H., and Nelson, J.D.: Oral antibiotic therapy for skeletal infections of children: therapy of osteomyelitis and suppurative arthritis, J. Pediatr. **92**:485, 1978.

Waldvogel, F.A., and Vasey, J.: Osteomyelitis: the past decade, N. Engl. J. Med. **303**:360, 1980.

Wolfson, J.S., and Swartz, M.N.: Serum bactericidal activity as a monitor of antibiotic therapy, N. Engl. J. Med. **312**:969, 1985.

83 Psychiatric disorders

WILLIAM V. GOOD

Management principles

The psychiatric examination of children and their families requires, above all else, sensitivity and a belief in one's own intuition. Data in the psychiatric evaluation may be "hard"—e.g., an admission by the patient that he or she is suicidal or homicidal—but it may also be "soft." At times the only clue to an adolescent's violent inclination may be an uneasiness or anxiety on the part of the evaluator. Such feelings in the examiner, termed *countertransference,* can be used with great acumen to diagnose a variety of psychiatric ailments. If used appropriately, such data complement the more objective data obtained in a history.

The evaluator also must be willing to ask probing and difficult questions. Objectivity in the history taking will maximize the chances of the patient responding honestly and candidly. The examiner who is in a hurry or does not want to hear about certain aspects of the patient's behavior will subtly encourage patients not to discuss their depression, suicidal ideation, or sexual perversions, for example. The examiner who is calm and maintains an empathic stance with patients will be amazed at how many describe really pressing psychiatric problems. The humbling statistic that nearly 50% of all patients who commit suicide have seen a physician sometime in the previous months speaks to the patient's wish to talk about problems and to get help, and, sadly, to the physician's frequent lack of responsiveness.

The approach to the preadolescent patient is usually different from that toward the adolescent. Initially, it is often appropriate to see the child's parents first and to gather as much history from them as possible. Then the child can be seen, usually alone, unless he or she is too stressed at being separated from the parents. The evaluator should first ask about the child's understanding of the evaluation. Clarifying that no shots will be given and that confidentiality will be maintained (unless information about the child being in danger emerges) can help loosen up a child. Even a 3-year-old can communicate. Toys and drawings (which may reveal unconscious problems) should be saved for last. Particular attention should be paid to how the child relates to the examiner (oblivious? clinging?), to the youngster's activity level, and to how he or she relates to the parents. The question "How do you get along with friends?" posed to parents and child is the best single screening question for major psychopathology. If the child is isolated or has major interactive problems, significant psychopathology can be expected. If not, the child usually is in reasonable shape.

In contrast the adolescent should always be seen first and alone. The typical adolescent bristles at the idea that the evaluator is the parents' agent and thus must understand that the examiner is there to help him or her. This can be achieved through honesty and *objectivity* (regardless of personal morals and values). Teenagers can usually see through any falseness in the evaluator, who should try to leave his or her

574

own adolescence in the waiting room and avoid the use of adolescent language that is not natural and who should not encumber the patient with personal feelings about such issues as marijuana, sex, and high school. Particular attention should be paid to such concerns as emancipation from family,* peer pressure, and heterosexual and homosexual exposure. These are the issues that dominate adolescent development and that lie at the root of an adolescent's psychiatric problems.

Conversion reactions

Classic conversion reactions are rare these days, but conversion components of true physical illness may exist and conversion reactions may occur concomitantly with other serious psychopathology. The *initial* approach to a patient with a possible conversion disorder ought to be *both* medical and psychiatric. Conversion reaction is not a diagnosis of exclusion. Conversely, even when no physical cause is found to explain the loss of functioning, medical care should not be dropped since a large percentage of cases are subsequently found to have etiologic organic pathology.

DIAGNOSTIC FINDINGS

1. Loss of physical functioning, suggesting a physical disorder
2. Psychologic factors as part of the symptoms. NOTE: Many investigators think it is possible to have simultaneous true organic pathology and a conversion component.
3. Symptoms that are *not* conscious or voluntary. The loss of functioning is usually in the voluntary nervous system, rarely autonomic.
4. Symptoms that defy anatomic explanation

---

*For the adolescent runaway two resources may be useful: Runaway Hotline ([800] 231-6946) and National Runaway Switchboard ([800] 621-4000).

usually have some symbolic significance that may reduce anxiety; they may become manifest at time of stress.
5. Associated findings
   a. "La belle indifference" and is probably of *no* value in verifying the diagnosis.
   b. Some symbolism may be involved in the development of the symptom (e.g., paralyzed arm prevents patient from hitting wife). The patient may try to emulate a relative's symptoms.
   c. A previous history of developing somatic symptoms is often present.
   d. Previous CNS pathology or trauma increases the risk for conversion disorder.
   e. Secondary gain is often present (i.e., the sick role is gratifying to the patient).

DIFFERENTIAL DIAGNOSIS

Conversion reactions should be differentiated from true organic pathology. Psychiatric disorders that must be excluded include:

1. Hypochondriasis: an unrealistic interpretation of normal body signs
2. Malingering: a conscious attempt to get attention through *voluntarily* feigned symptoms
3. Munchausen syndrome: an unconscious attempt to gain attention through voluntarily feigned symptoms
4. Depression: may occur with somatic symptoms without other signs of depression

MANAGEMENT

1. Conversion symptoms are often transient and disappear on their own. They may require hospitalization until they partially resolve.
2. *Psychotherapy is indicated in refractory cases.*
3. The patient may retrench and worsen if an attempt is made (especially initially) to prove that symptoms are mental.
4. Any other underlying psychopathology (e.g., schizophrenia) should be treated.
5. The prognosis is good, especially with acute

onset, short duration of symptom(s), adequate premorbid personality, and minimal secondary gain from symptom. It is crucial to focus on the reduction of stress.

Acute psychoses

These patients require immediate attention to their level of self-destructiveness and potential for violence. If there is any doubt, the patient should be legally and physically restrained (with hospital guards, etc.) until these questions can be answered. Although psychiatrists disagree about subtypes of psychoses in childhood, several categories have merged as distinct diagnostic entities, which should be familiar to anyone involved in caring for pediatric emergencies. A child with an acute psychosis often seems "off" or detached. Accurate diagnosis and disposition are paramount because such children, when they arrive at an emergency setting, often have come from isolated, suspicious families that rarely frequent hospitals.

INFANTILE AUTISM
Etiology

1. Unknown but former theories of "refrigerator parents" and abnormal rearing are being discarded in favor of a more dynamic etiology involving organic factors (in the child) triggering aberrant parenting.
2. The illness is probably evenly distributed socioeconomically.

Diagnostic findings

1. Age of onset usually under 30 mo
2. Highly unusual responses to environment (need for sameness, stereotypes), with poor social relations
3. Gross deficits in language development. Abnormal speech patterns (echolalia, pronoun reversals)
4. Absence of delusions or hallucinations

5. Frequent associated findings:
   a. Congenital blindness
   b. Retardation (70% have IQ <70)
   c. Grand mal seizures before adolescence
   d. Pockets of normal or even precocious development (e.g., unusual memory or ability to calculate quickly)
   e. Abnormal auditory-evoked responses

Differential diagnosis

1. Mental retardation. Usually with uniform lags in development in all spheres (e.g., motor, social, language). Mentally retarded children ordinarily demonstrate some social relatedness.
2. Diffuse CNS disease (cytomegalovirus, phenylketonuria, hepatic encephalopathy)
3. Deafness. Audiogram will help differentiate.

Management

1. Multifaceted management (behavioral, structured educational program, psychotherapy) is indicated. Hospitalization should *always* be considered.
2. Neuroleptics may help symptoms of agitation, anxiety, and destructiveness (e.g., thioridazine [Mellaril] starting dose: 0.5-1 mg/kg/24 hr q 8-12 hr [adult: 25 mg q 8-12 hr PO]). Titrate response.

The prognosis is very guarded and is best for children with high IQ and good language development.

SCHIZOPHRENIA
Etiology

There are multiple causative theories, ranging from abnormal family patterns to faulty neurotransmitter mechanism (dopamine hypothesis). Schizophrenia has a strong familial predilection.

Diagnostic findings

1. Usual onset in late adolescence but may occur in earlier childhood
2. Lengthy prodrome of at least 6 mo during which patients exhibit gradual withdrawal

from previous relationships and functioning
3. Delusions
4. Hallucinations (usually auditory)
5. Abnormal content of speech (loosening of associations)
6. Altered affect, which often is *inappropriate* to the content of speech (e.g., laughing while describing death of relative), but not predominantly euphoric or depressed
7. Associated findings
   a. Catatonia with either excitement or motoric rigidity
   b. Excitation can be life threatening. Poor impulse control or paranoia can make these patients very dangerous.

Differential diagnosis

1. Other nonorganic psychoses (manic-depression, which shows predominant mood problem)
2. Organic psychoses. Patient usually shows faulty cognition, which can be demonstrated with tests of memory (remembering three unrelated objects at 3 min) and orientation (to person, place, and time; disorientation to time is the first of these to be affected). Causes are multiple but, in the pediatric population, most frequently are ingestions (hallucinogens, etc.).
3. Reactive psychoses (also called schizophreniform psychoses). More acute and short-lived
4. Acute grief reaction

Management

The patient should be hospitalized for self-protection.

Neuroleptics

Neuroleptics usually should be administered after 1-2 days of hospitalization to see how well the patient will respond to a safe environment, unless patient is agitated, combative, or in need of seclusion.

- Thiothixene (Navane) 10-30 mg/24 hr or thioridazine (Mellaril) 200-800 mg/24 hr, reflecting the patient's age, size, and response to therapy

Side effects are important and must be considered (p. 299):

1. Acute dystonias, especially with high-potency neuroleptics (e.g., haloperidol [Haldol]). Treat with an anticholinergic agent (e.g., benztropine [Cogentin] 1-2 mg PO or IM q 12 hr).
2. Parkinsonian side effects. Treat with an anticholinergic agent (Cogentin as in *1*).
3. Akathisias (motor restlessness). Difficult to treat and often requires adjusting dosage of neuroleptic
4. Anticholinergic signs and symptoms, especially with low-potency neuroleptics (e.g., chlorpromazine, thioridazine [Mellaril])
5. Tardive dyskinesias. Incidence increases with duration of treatment. May be "unmasked" when dosage of neuroleptic is lowered. No effective treatment at this time
6. Rash, cholestatic jaundice

Other considerations

1. Electroconvulsive therapy only if all else fails or patient is in acute danger (e.g., agitated catatonia or acutely suicidal)
2. Family and individual psychotherapy
3. Discharge planning and follow-up: crucial in preventing relapse
4. Prognosis: guarded

ORGANIC PSYCHOSES
Diagnostic findings

1. Evidence for an organic etiology: ingestion (hallucinogens, cocaine, amphetamines, over-the-counter anticholinergics); systemic illness; endocrine disorder (adrenal, thyroid); renal, cardiac, and liver failures; sensory deprivation (ICU "psychosis")
2. Cognitive impairment (memory and disorientation)
3. Predominantly visual hallucinations (if any) vs. auditory hallucinations in schizophrenia

Management

1. Treatment of underlying disorder
2. Occasionally, seclusion, restraint, or neuro-

leptics (neuroleptics have sedative and anticholinergic properties and may be contraindicated)

MANIC-DEPRESSIVE PSYCHOSIS
Diagnostic findings

Manic-depressive psychosis is rare in childhood and principally involves:
1. Increased motor activity
2. Flight of ideas
3. Euphoric or dysphoric mood change
4. Associated findings: spending binges, decreased need for sleep, grandiosity, delusions, hallucinations, increased sexual activity.

Differential diagnosis

Adolescents who have taken stimulants or PCP or who have sustained brain damage may have some of these findings.

Management

Patients should be hospitalized and given some combination of neuroleptic and lithium treatment.

DEPRESSION
Diagnostic findings

Children may demonstrate signs and symptoms of depression, requiring recognition and intervention. Typically, patients have a variable appetite and some weight loss because of poor intake, whereas others gain weight secondary to an increased appetite. Insomnia or hypersomnia is common, with a loss of interest and pleasure in usual activities. Depressed individuals have thoughts of worthlessness and self-reproach and suicidal ideation.

Management

Of primary importance is to recognize the depressed state of the patient and make referral for both short-term evaluation and long-term therapy. The urgency of such counseling must reflect the severity of the depression and ensure that there is no immediate danger to the patient from self-injury.

Psychophysiologic presentations

A psychophysiologic illness has three components. The patient must (1) have an underlying biologic or genetic disposition to get a disease, (2) must have a characteristic personality style, and (3) must be in a stressful situation. Peptic ulcer disease and thyrotoxicosis are examples of such illnesses. Various illnesses are considered psychosomatic in that psychologic factors are seen as contributing to the actual disease process, but personality profiles and biologic markers and processes have yet to be delineated. The symptoms often are used to avoid undesirable activities, such as school phobias. The following are perhaps the most common presentations:
1. Rumination. An infant regurgitates and may have low weight, and symptoms worsen during separation from the mother.
2. Cyclic vomiting. In response to a subtle stress, a child vomits for several days and then is well for days to weeks.
3. Abdominal pain. This may result from a variety of physical conditions but also may be caused by a psychophysiologic illness (peptic ulcer, ulcerative colitis) or, possibly, anorexia nervosa. When no etiology is found, abdominal pain may be a conversion symptom.
4. Headache. This very common symptom is usually transient in anxiety states but may be disabling when it is secondary to repressed anger, sexual wishes, etc.
5. Anorexia nervosa. Nonorganic extreme weight loss in the preadolescent or adolescent female; initially associated with voluntary dieting and a preoccupation with food. The patient develops amenorrhea, withdrawal, depression, and an intense interest in physical activity that may lead to bradycardia and hypotension.

Differential considerations include hypopituitarism, ovarian dysfunction, malabsorption, or malignancy.

Behavioral modification with positive reinforcement is the basis for management to create a weight gain. The patient must be allowed to gain autonomy, effectiveness, and self-esteem, often requiring hospitalization for both psychiatric and medical therapy initially.

Suicide attempts

The incidence of suicide and suicide attempts in childhood is increasing. Any seemingly innocent ingestion or accident should raise the question of a suicide attempt. Furthermore, any child who appears depressed should be asked about suicidal ideation, since suicide occurs most frequently in depressed individuals. Studies of suicidal individuals reveal that the risk of attempting or reattempting suicide is usually limited to a short crisis period. Therefore safeguarding the patient with hospitalization or well-established supports is paramount in suicide management.

DIAGNOSTIC FINDINGS

Evaluation of the patient who has attempted or is threatening suicide should include:
1. Discovering the precipitant. Usually a loss or reminder of a loss (anniversary reaction) is causative, but simply an argument with parents can trigger an attempt.
2. Assessment of risk factors
   a. Girls attempt suicide more often than boys, but boys are more successful.
   b. A chronic illness in the patient increases the risk.
   c. A family history of suicide is often found.
   d. A personal history of previous suicide attempt is an ominous sign.
   e. An intoxicated patient is at greater risk.
   f. Depression in the patient increases the risk.

g. Estrangement from a loved one is also a risk factor.
3. A careful evaluation of the present illness and suicidal behavior
   a. How *lethal* was the method of suicide (gun or hanging vs. ingestion of a few Valium)? Always ask about suicidal intent and plan.
   b. Was suicide attempted in complete isolation, or had the patient considered that he or she might be found before dying?
   c. Does any suicide note or afterthought explain a motivation?
   d. Is the patient depressed or schizophrenic or taking drugs?
   e. Would he or she try again if discharged?
Common pitfalls in evaluation include the following.
1. No one asks the patient about suicidal ideation or plan. Plan: ask the patient directly.
2. On recovering from an overdose, the patient disappears. Plan: always have patients guarded or in a locked unit until their freedom would not jeopardize them.
3. The physician/staff treats the patient roughly or unempathically. Plan: treat suicidal behavior medically, *not* judgmentally.

MANAGEMENT

1. Treat the medical or surgical sequelae of the suicide attempt.
2. Protect the patient if necessary with hospitalization or sheltered environment.
3. Always include a psychiatrist in management.
4. Try to shore up family and other sources of emotional support.
5. Remove all sources of potential self-injury if patient is to return home.
6. Treat the underlying psychiatric illness:
   a. Depression—antidepressants, psychotherapy
   Warning: remember that the lethal-dose ratio of tricyclic antidepressants is very low; dispense with caution.
   b. Schizophrenia—neuroleptics and hospitalization are usually needed

  c. Intoxication or ingestion—do serial suicide evaluations and mental status examinations until return to baseline. Reevaluation when patient is sober

7. At discharge, carefully evaluate your alliance with patient (i.e., will he or she call you prn and *before* next attempt?).

REFERENCES

American Psychiatric Association: Diagnostic and statistical manual of the mental disorders, ed. 3, Washington, D.C., 1980, The Association.

Aylward, G.P.: Understanding and treatment of childhood depression, J. Pediatr. **107**:1, 1985.

Farley, G.K., Eckhardt, L.O., and Hebert, F.B.: Handbook of child and adolescent psychiatric emergencies, Garden City, N.Y., 1979, Medical Examination Publishing Co., Inc.

Kaplan, H.I., Freedman, A.M., and Sadock, B.J.: Comprehensive textbook of psychiatry, vol. 3, Baltimore, 1980, Williams & Wilkins.

84 Pulmonary disorders

Asthma

ALERT: All wheezing is not caused by asthma. All patients require oxygen. The asthmatic patient in severe respiratory distress may not wheeze.

Bronchoconstriction results from intrinsic mechanisms related to autonomic dysfunction or extrinsic sensitizing agents. A number of factors precipitate airway reactivity leading to hypoxia (Fig. 84-1).

ETIOLOGY: PRECIPITATING FACTORS

1. Infection: viral
2. Allergic/irritants: pollens, foods, drugs (salicylates), pollutants, gases (chlorine, ammonia), exercise
3. Intrapsychic: emotional stress, phobias
4. Intoxication: bronchoconstrictors (propranolol and other beta-blockers)

DIAGNOSTIC FINDINGS

A precipitating factor must be sought by determining the history of the patient's asthma, medications (type, dose, and time of last dose), duration of symptoms with the current episode, associated illness, and history of aspiration. Additionally, it is important to estimate fluid intake and determine the pattern of response to previous episodes and medication. Prior hospitalizations and ventilatory support should be assessed.

1. Labored respirations with retractions, nasal flaring, tachypnea, and tachycardia are present. Pulsus paradoxus (diminished amplitude of blood pressure with inspiration $\geq$15 mm

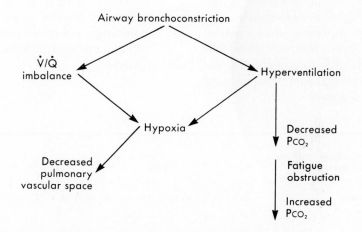

Fig. 84-1. Physiologic effect of bronchoconstriction.

Hg) may be present and, when combined with the degree of retractions, correlates with forced expiratory volume at 1 sec. (FEV_1). These are good indications of the severity of airway obstruction.

  a. Diffuse inspiratory and expiratory wheezing is noted with a prolonged expiratory phase. The patient with respiratory distress and without wheezing may not be moving enough air to generate air movement and may have a silent chest.

  b. Rales and rhonchi may be present.

  c. Pulsus paradoxus may accompany severe asthma, pericardial tamponade, and pneumothorax. Its presence is determined by having the patient breathe quietly while the physician lowers the blood pressure cuff toward the systolic level. The pressure when the first sound is heard is noted. The pressure is further dropped until sounds can be heard throughout the respiratory cycle. A difference of ≥ 10 mm Hg indicates the presence of paradoxic pulse.

2. Patients may have cyanosis, diminished blood-pressure, and fever as late findings.

3. Diaphoresis, agitation, somnolence, or confusion may result from hypoxia, hypercapnia, exhaustion, or drug intoxication, and the patient requires emergent intervention because of impending respiratory failure.

4. Status asthmaticus is present when a patient has moderate to severe obstruction and fails to respond significantly to epinephrine and other rapid beta-agonists administered in the initial treatment regimen.

5. Chronic cough may occasionally be the only presentation for reactive airway disease. The chest may sound clear, but wheezing can be induced by having the patient exercise. The condition requires a therapeutic trial of oral or inhaled bronchodilators.

Complications

1. Pneumothorax or pneumomediastinum
2. Pneumonia
3. Respiratory failure with $PaO_2 < 50$ mm Hg and $PaCO_2 > 50$ mm Hg at room air, sea level. These parameters may be useful, as will the pattern of progression of disease. Patients often develop significant retractions, decreased or absent breath sounds, impaired mental status and agitation, decreased response to pain, and labored speech.
4. Dehydration
5. Inappropriate ADH secretion
6. Theophylline overdose (p. 301)
7. Death secondary to respiratory failure with cardiac decompensation or dysrhythmias

Ancillary data

1. ABG is indicated for all patients with moderate or severe asthma and for those failing to respond to epinephrine. Severe airway obstruction is associated with increasing acidosis and hypercarbia and hypoxemia.
2. Pulmonary function tests (PFT) are useful in monitoring asthmatic patients and provide important prognostic information for an acute episode

	Severity of airway obstruction	PaO_2	$PaCO_2$	pH	Base excess
	Mild	WNL	↓	↑	Respiratory alkalosis
Status asthmaticus {	Moderate	↓↓	WNL or ↓	WNL or ↑	Normal
	Severe	↓↓↓	↑	↓	Metabolic acidosis Respiratory acidosis

a. The peak expiratory flow rate (PEFR) and the FEV_1 have been proved useful for adults as predictors of the severity of an attack, but this has not been shown in children. Furthermore, the difficulty in obtaining cooperation to take a full inspiration and then to expire through a peak flowmeter or spirometer makes the data less reliable.

b. For older children the initial values and those after treatment may be useful.

3. Chest roentgenogram classically demonstrates hyperinflation and, rarely, an infiltrate. It may be useful in children who are unresponsive to beta-adrenergic agents with continuing localized rales or wheezes, tachypnea, and tachycardia after therapy. It rarely is indicated in children who have a good response to initial bronchodilator therapy. If other diagnostic considerations are possible such as a foreign body aspiration or pneumonia, the chest x-ray study may be useful.

4. Serum theophylline level is crucial in managing patients with an acute episode who were previously taking "therapeutic" doses of theophylline. Therapeutic levels are in the range of 10-20 µg/ml. Rapid assays of serum theophylline levels may facilitate this process.

5. CBC may be useful in children who have been febrile. Optimally, it should be obtained before administration of beta-adrenergic agents.

6. Electrolytes should periodically be monitored in the severely ill patient who is hospitalized to exclude inappropriate ADH secretion.

DIFFERENTIAL DIAGNOSIS (Chapter 20)

The differential considerations in the child with wheezing vary with the age of the child. In the infant, bronchiolitis, asthma, and upper airway congestion or obstruction must be excluded. Older children may have asthma, foreign body aspiration, or pneumonia. Cystic fibrosis and other chronic lung diseases also should be considered past infancy. Other diagnostic entities include:

1. Infection/inflammation
   a. Pneumonia (p. 601)
   b. Bronchiolitis (p. 588)
   c. Aspiration
2. Trauma (Chapter 62)
   a. Pneumothorax (may be spontaneous)
   b. Foreign body (p. 599)
3. Vascular disorder
   a. Compression of trachea by vascular anomaly
   b. Pulmonary edema (Chapter 19)
   c. Pulmonary embolism (p. 428)
   d. Congestive heart failure (Chapter 16)
4. Congenital disease
   a. Cystic fibrosis
   b. Tracheoesophageal fistula or tracheal anomaly
5. Hyperventilation
6. Intoxication: metabolic acidosis (may cause tachypnea) (p. 269), toxic inhalation
7. Neoplasm: mediastinal or pulmonary

MANAGEMENT

The patient is often the best indicator of both the severity of the attack and the most effective therapeutic regimen. If the history or physical examination suggests that asthma is not the most likely etiology, an appropriate work-up (inspiratory and forced expiratory film, cardiac examination, fluoroscopy, etc.) should be initiated following stabilization of the patient's respiratory status.

1. When appropriate, blood pressure should be stabilized and correction of acid-base abnormalities initiated. Oxygen, IV fluids, and, occasionally, sodium bicarbonate are required.
2. Humidified oxygen should be administered by nasal cannula or face mask at 3-6 L/min (30%-40%) to all patients with significant wheezing.
3. Cardiac monitoring is important when ad-

ministering adrenergic agents and theophylline, particularly in patients with moderate or severe disease (status asthmaticus).

Adrenergic agents

Initially, a potent, rapid-acting beta-agonist bronchodilator is administered parenterally or by inhalation. The choice of agent should reflect the severity of disease, experience of the clinician, the age and level of cooperation of the child, and the past experience of the child with the therapeutic alternatives.

Parenteral agents are useful in the child with severe disease and poor air movement and in cases where cooperation is minimal, often because of the child's young age.

1. Epinephrine (Adrenalin) $(1:1,000):0.01$ ml (0.01 mg)/kg/dose (maximum: 0.35 ml/dose SQ q 20 min prn). Dosage may be repeated for a total of three administrations if the response is partial or absent. It should not be administered if the heart rate is >180/min.
2. Terbutaline (Brethine) (1 mg/ml):0.01 ml (0.01 mg)/kg/dose (maximum: 0.25 ml/dose SQ). May be repeated once in 20-30 min if initial response is partial or absent. May have a more prolonged effect than epinephrine.

Nebulized administration is useful in the cooperative child and is generally more effective than parenteral therapy.

1. Isoetharine 1% (Bronkosol): 0.25-0.5 ml (0.01 ml/kg) in 2-2.5 ml of saline administered by powered nebulizer or IPPB. It should not normally be repeated more often than every 20 min or within 20 min of administering a parenteral agent. Sulfites are present.
2. Metaproterenol 5% (Alupent): 0.1 ml for children 2 yr or younger; 0.2 ml for children 3-7 yr; 0.3 ml for children older than 7 yr; 0.01-0.02 ml/kg/dose mixed in 2-2.5 ml of saline and administered by powered nebulizer or IPPB. May be repeated once in 20 min or routinely q 4 hr, but should not exceed 12 inhalations in 24 hr.
3. Atropine decreases bronchoconstriction and

often is combined with other inhalation agents for prolonged effect. Dose: 0.01-0.02 mg/kg/dose (adult: 1-1.5 mg/dose) in solution q 3-4 hr.
4. Terbutaline may be an effective bronchodilator when given by nebulizer with a persistent action. The aerosol dose in children is 0.03-0.05 mg (0.03-0.05 ml)/kg mixed in 1-2.5 ml saline administered q 4 hr. The dose in adults is 0.5 mg (0.5 ml) diluted in 2.5 ml saline q 4 hr. Terbutaline comes as a solution of 1 mg/ml.
5. Albuterol is now available in nebulized form (0.5% solution). Adult dose is 0.5 ml diluted in 3 ml of 0.9% NS.

If there has been an excellent response from epinephrine, with total clearing and resolution of signs and symptoms after 1-2 doses, many clinicians elect to administer Sus-Phrine (1:200) 0.005 ml/kg/dose (maximum: 0.15 ml/dose) SQ. Optimally, the single vial ampule should be used to ensure consistency of dosage. This agent may give a prolonged bronchodilator effect when a therapeutic level of theophylline is being obtained in the minimally ill child.

Status asthmaticus exists when the initial response to 2-3 doses of beta-adrenergic agents is poor. Hypoxia, acidosis, and hypotension must be rapidly corrected and other causes of wheezing considered. The absence of improvement often is caused by airway obstruction from a prolonged inflammatory process, suggesting that steroid therapy may be useful in such patients.

Children who are taking theophylline preparations and have intermittent problems with wheezing and children with only very rare episodes may benefit from inhalers with a beta-agonist such as isoetharine or metaproterenol. It is imperative that such patients be advised not to abuse the inhaler on a chronic basis.

Theophylline

Theophylline should be initiated immediately following initial attempts at bronchodilation.

Parenteral, oral, and rectal preparations are available but require appropriate loading before placing the patient on maintenance therapy.

It is imperative that if the patient is taking theophylline at the time of the encounter, a determination be made regarding the amount and time of the last dose and the duraton of therapy to decide if a loading dose is necessary.

1. If the patient is taking a subtherapeutic dose, half the loading dose may be given pending determination of the theophylline level.
2. Therapeutic theophylline is 10-20 μg/ml. 1 mg/kg of theophylline will raise the theophylline concentration by about 2 μg/ml.
3. Dosage of theophylline must be adjusted to reflect changes in clearance. Alter the dose as indicated for the following conditions:

Increase dose	Decrease dose
Drugs: Phenobarbital, phenytoin (Dilantin), marijuana	Drugs: cimetidine, erythromycin
	Illness: viral infections, fever, congestive heart failure, abnormal liver function, renal failure
Smokers	
Diet: High-protein, low-carbohydrate, charcoal broiled meat	Other: infants younger than 3 mo; pregnancy, especially third trimester

4. Dosage determination is based on lean body weight and must reflect serum theophylline levels. Aminophylline is about 85% theophylline.
5. Half-life of intravenous theophylline in children is approximately 2.5 hr, while in adults it is 4.6 hr.

Parenteral theophylline

This is indicated for moderate or severe obstructive disease unresponsive to adrenergic agents (status asthmaticus). A loading dose is normally given over 20 min followed by an IV infusion of maintenance theophylline. Maintenance infusion may be mixed with aminophylline 100 mg in 100 ml 0.9%NS (1 mg/ml) and can be calculated from the daily oral theophylline dosage (divided by 24) with alterations for factors modifying clearance.

The following doses of aminophylline (theophylline) are for patients not previously receiving theophylline products:

Age-group	Loading dose* (mg/kg)	Maintenance dose* (mg/kg/hr)
<12 mo	6-7 (5-6)	See discussion below
1-9 yr	6-7 (5-6)	1.2 (0.9)
10 yr and up	6-7 (5-6)	0.8 (0.6)

*Aminophylline dose (theophylline equivalent).

Dosing of theophylline in infants *under 1 year* of age requires careful monitoring of theophylline levels because of the variability in pharmacokinetics. Suggested guidelines follow:

1. Preterm infants up to 40 weeks postconception (postconception age = gestational age at birth + postnatal age): 1 mg/kg q 12 hr
2. Term infants either at birth or 40 weeks postconception:
   a. Up to 4 weeks postnatal: 1-2 mg/kg q 12 hr
   b. From 4-8 weeks: 1-2 mg/kg q 8 hr
   c. Beyond 8 weeks: 1-3 mg/kg q 6 hr

Children under 1 year of age and those with moderate to severe or recurrent disease should have levels measured within 24 hr of loading and then periodically. New tests done on fingerstick samples in 15 min should make theophylline levels more readily available in the office or ED.

Oral therapy

This may be used with mild disease. Loading dose of theophylline 6-7 mg/kg/dose as a single dose is followed in 6 hr with a maintenance dose of 4-5 mg/kg/dose q 6 hr PO. The dose in children under 1 year of age should be reduced.

In the stable patient with good response to initial beta-adrenergic therapy, many clinicians prefer to begin sustained-release preparations after initial loading with a short-acting theophylline (Table 84-1). The daily dosage of sustained release drugs should reflect the age of the child. This approach may improve compliance.

Long-term therapy

Long-term therapy with oral theophylline preparations must reflect the therapeutic response and side effects. Once a patient is stabilized following an acute episode, an oral dos-

TABLE 84-1. Selected xanthine preparations

Preparation	Dosage form (theophylline)*	Frequency of dose (hr)
LIQUIDS		
Somophyllin	105 mg (90 mg theophylline)/5 ml	4-6
Slo-Phyllin	80 mg/15 ml	4-6
Choledyl	100 mg (64 mg theophylline)/5 ml	4-6
TABLETS		
Somophyllin	100, 200, 250 mg	4-6
Slo-Phyllin	100, 200 mg	4-6
Theophyl	100 mg (chewable), 225 mg	4-6
Choledyl	100, 200 mg (64, 128 mg theophylline)	4-6
Theolair	125, 250 mg	4-6
Aminophylline	100 mg (85 mg theophylline)	4-6
	200 mg (170 mg theophylline)	4-6
SUSTAINED RELEASE		
Slo-bid Gyrocap	50, 100, 200, 300 mg	8-12
Slo-Phyllin Gyrocap	60, 125, 250 mg	8
Theophyl-SR	125, 250 mg	8
Theo-Dur Sprinkle	50, 75, 125, 200 mg	12
Theo-Dur	100, 200, 300 mg	12
RECTAL		
Somophyllin	60 mg (51 mg theophylline)/ml	4-6

*If preparation is not pure theophylline, theophylline equivalent is indicated in parentheses.

age of 16 mg/kg/24 hr of theophylline is usually adequate but may be increased up to 24 mg/kg/24 hr for children under 9 yr of age. 20 mg/kg/24 hr for 9- to 12-year-olds, and 18 mg/kg/24 hr for 12- to 16-year-olds. These are administered every 6 hr orally. The serum concentration should be maintained at 10-20 μg/ml and is the best measure of the appropriate dosage. On occasion, patients will do well with lower levels, whereas some will require over 20 μg/ml. Serious toxicity usually is not noted until a level of 30 μg/ml is reached. Often sustained release formulations are used to maximize compliance (Table 84-1).

Other considerations: theophylline

1. Combination drugs (often with ephedrine) have no advantages and are not recommended. Avoid preparations with alcohol.
2. Solutions for rectal administration are available but may have a less consistent absorption pattern. Suppositories are very unreliable and are not recommended. Rectal solutions may be useful on a short-term basis for patients who are vomiting from an intercurrent illness. Oral and rectal dosages are identical (Table 84-1).

   NOTE: It is important to ascertain that the GI symptoms are not signs of toxicity.
3. Theophylline toxicity results in tachycardia, dysrhythmias, irritability, and seizures, as well as nausea, vomiting, and abdominal pain (p. 301).

Steroids

1. All patients with moderate or severe asthma (status asthmaticus) should receive a minimum of 3-4 days of steroid therapy, and many prefer to treat for 7-10 days.

a. Methylprednisolone (Solu-Medrol) 1-2 mg/kg/dose q 6 hr IV **or**

b. Hydrocortisone (Solu-Cortef) 4-5 mg/kg/dose q 6 hr IV

2. In the rare patient who responds initially to epinephrine with clearing but returns with significant wheezing within 12 hr and clears again, steroids may decrease the risk of recurrence. Begin prednisone 1-2 mg/kg/24 hr q 6-12 hr PO for 3 days.

3. Patients who have been taking steroids within 12 mo (including patients using steroids administered by inhalation) or who have a previous history of respiratory failure associated with asthma should have steroids initiated for an acute exacerbation.

4. Patients with severe asthma, particularly those with severe exacerbations, may benefit from long-term steroid therapy. Systemic steroids (prednisone 1-2 mg/kg/24 hr q 6-12 hr PO) commonly are used initially for chronic therapy. Many patients requiring 20 mg or less of prednisone may be converted to inhalation administration with maintenance of good respiratory function and reduction of adverse reactions. Beclomethasone (Vanceril, Beclovent) is provided in a metered dose inhaler delivering 42-50 μg/puff. Children 6-12 yr receive 1-2 puffs q 6-8 hr (maximum: 10 puffs/24 hr), whereas older children and adults take 2 puffs q 6-8 hr (maximum: 20 puffs/24 hr). The mouth should be rinsed after inhalation. Consultation with an allergist should be obtained.

Other considerations

1. IV isoproterenol infusions have been used successfully in children with severe asthma and impending respiratory failure. They are administered with an initial dose of 0.1 μg/kg/min by continuous infusion, with increments of 0.05 μg/kg/min q 15-20 min until clinical improvement, cardiotoxicity, or treatment failure ($Pco_2 > 65$-70 mm Hg). Patients require intensive pulmonary and cardiac monitoring in a critical care center be-

fore initiation of therapy. This approach is effective in as many as 75% of children but should be initiated only after consultation is obtained. Theophylline levels should be monitored since the clearance is increased.

2. Intubation and mechanical ventilation rarely are needed except in the occasional patient with respiratory failure who does not respond to pharmacologic therapy (including continuous isoproterenol) or who has either disease that is rapidly progressive or life-threatening respiratory failure.

a. Volume-controlled ventilators are preferred, often requiring large tidal volumes resulting in high peak pressures. Low PEEP may be required.

b. Sedation or neuromuscular blockade may be necessary.

c. Complications: pneumomediastinum (50%), pneumothorax, massive atelectasis, and dysrhythmias.

3. Postural drainage, if tolerated, is a useful adjunctive therapy, either at home or in the hospital.

4. Antibiotics are indicated if pneumonia is present and a bacterial process is suspected.

5. Cromolyn (Intal) may be useful in children with chronic, intractable asthma. The drug is administered by inhalation and should be initiated only in consultation with an allergist.

DISPOSITION

1. Patients with moderate or severe asthma in status asthmaticus require immediate hospitalization and continuation of therapy initiated in the ED.

a. Although parameters predictive of admission are indecisive, the presence of symptoms for >24 hr, marked retractions, respiratory obstruction (PEFR ≤ 10% of expected), and poor response to the first epinephrine (PEFR ≤ 40% of expected) are associated with high admission rates. Children who have had partial or absent response to two treatments of epinephrine (SQ) or inhaled beta-agonist need to be admitted in the first hour of their encounter.

    b. Patients with a history of poor compliance, multiple visits, evidence of fatigue, abnormal ABG, chronic or intermittent steroid therapy, or severe asthma also should be admitted.

2. The patient who has mild disease and clears may be discharged with adequate oral therapy after appropriate loading before discharge. Sustained-release preparations may be useful. Frequent phone calls and visits are necessary.

3. Good follow-up (including monitoring theophylline levels and noting clinical response and frequency of exacerbations) is essential for all patients with asthma. Often psychiatric intervention is required because of the emotional component of asthma in many children.

Parental education

1. Give all doses of medication.
2. Push clear liquids. Warm fluids are particularly helpful.
3. Try to keep your child calm.
4. Try to identify substances that precipitate attacks, and avoid them.
5. Many patients will develop reactive airway disease in response to an infection. Such children should take bronchodilator therapy (asthma medicine) at the first sign of a cough of respiratory infection if they do not take the medication every day.
   - Parents should give 1½ times the normal dose when initiating the theophylline medication and then continue it at the regular dose for 3-4 days after the resolution of major cold symptoms.
6. Call physician immediately if
   a. Breathing difficulty recurs or worsens, color changes, restlessness develops, or fluid intake decreases, or if child has difficulty speaking because of respiratory distress

    b. Nausea, vomiting, or irritability develops because of the theophylline medicine or child is unable to take medication

    c. Cough or wheezing persist or fever or chest pain develops

REFERENCES

Abramowicz, M.: Drugs in asthma, Med. Lett. Drugs Ther. **24:**83, 1982.

Carrier, J.A., Shaw, R.A., Porter, R.S., et al.: Comparison of intravenous and oral routes of theophylline loading in acute asthma, Ann. Emerg. Med. **14:**1145, 1985.

Fireman, P.: The wheezing infant, Pediatr. Rev. **7:**247, 1986.

Gershel, J.C., Holdman, H.S., Stein, R.E.K., et al.: The usefulness of chest radiographs in the first asthma attack, N. Engl. J. Med. **309:**336, 1983.

Lee, H., and Evans, H.E.: Aerosol bag for administration of bronchodilators to young asthmatic children, Pediatrics **73:**230, 1984.

Leffert, F.: The management of acute severe asthma, J. Pediatr. **96:**1, 1980.

Littenberg, B., and Gluck, E.H.: A controlled trial of methylpredisolone in the emergency treatment of acute asthma, N. Engl. J. Med. **314:**150, 1986.

Lulla, S., and Newcomb, R.W.: Emergency management of asthma in children, J. Pediatr. **97:**346, 1980.

Ownby, D.R., Abarzua, J., and Anderson, J.A.: Attempting to prevent hospital admission in acute asthma, Am. J. Dis. Child. **138:**1062, 1984.

Reinecke, T., Seger, D., and Wears, R.: Rapid assay of serum theophylline levels, Ann. Emerg. Med. **15:**147, 1986.

Weinberger, M., Hendeles, L., and Ahrens, R.: Clinical pharmacology of drugs used in asthma, Pediatr. Clin. North Am. **28:**47, 1981.

Willert, C., Davis, A.T., Harmon, J.J., et al.: Short-term holding room treatment of asthmatic children, J. Pediatr. **106:**707, 1985.

Bronchiolitis

ALERT: Patients with marked tachypnea, retractions, cyanosis, or decreased air exchange require immediate attention and hospitalization. Hydration status must be assessed.

Bronchiolitis is an acute lower respiratory infection producing inflammatory obstruction of the small airways and reactive airway disease. It commonly occurs in children under 2 yr of age, with the highest incidence in those under 6 mo. The relationship of bronchiolitis to asthma and later reactive airway disease is unclear at the present time. In contrast to asthma, which primarily has bronchoconstriction with secondary inflammation, bronchiolitis is primarily an inflammatory process with a bronchoconstrictive component that is variably present.

ETIOLOGY

Viral infection caused by respiratory syncytial virus (RSV) accounts for 90% of isolates. Parainfluenza, adenovirus, and influenza are less common.

DIAGNOSTIC FINDINGS

1. The majority of patients have a preceding respiratory tract infection followed by the onset of marked tachypnea (often >60/min) and diffuse wheezing.
   a. Most children appear well and are attentive, alert and, in no distress despite the tachypnea.
   b. Many have an accompanying otitis media and viral pneumonia.
2. Patients with respiratory distress have marked retractions, nasal flaring, and cyanosis. With the progression of inflammation, air movement may decrease, with disappearance of audible wheezing. Vital signs may be altered.
3. Restless, apprehensive behavior may appear if hypoxia or fatigue is present.

Complications

1. Apnea is most commonly found in children under 6 mo of age who were born prematurely.
2. Dehydration may be exacerbated by the abnormal insensible losses from the rapid respiratory rate. Intake may be decreased because of the increased respiratory effort.
3. Bacterial pneumonia may result from secondary infection.

4. Pneumothorax may occur with severe obstructive disease.
5. Residual parenchymal and airway disease may result from any acute episode of bronchiolitis, causing long-term abnormalities in pulmonary function. The relationship to asthma and later pulmonary and allergic disorders is uncertain.
6. Bronchiolitis fibrosa obliterans results from progressive fibrotic reaction, which obliterates the bronchioles.
7. Death in 1%-2% of patients is secondary to respiratory failure.

Ancillary data

1. ABG is useful in assessing hypoxia and hypercapnia when the clinical examination is not conclusive.
2. Chest x-ray films demonstrates hyperinflation, often associated with a diffuse, patchy infiltrate.

DIFFERENTIAL DIAGNOSIS (Chapter 20)

The most common considerations are asthma, pneumonia, and foreign bodies.
1. Asthma usually occurs in children over 1 yr of age (children with asthma generally experience more respiratory distress). Asthma is primarily caused by bronchoconstrictive disease, whereas bronchiolitis is primarily an inflammatory process.
2. Pneumonia may produce wheezing and asymmetric breath sounds. A chest x-ray film may be useful. Viral pneumonia often accompanies bronchiolitis.
3. Foreign bodies may be excluded by a negative history and normal inspiratory and expiratory films.
4. Other entities that should be excluded include congestive heart failure, cystic fibrosis, vascular ring, neoplasm, and toxic or smoke inhalation.

MANAGEMENT (Fig. 84-2)

1. The initial assessment should determine if acute stabilization is required. Oxygen, air-

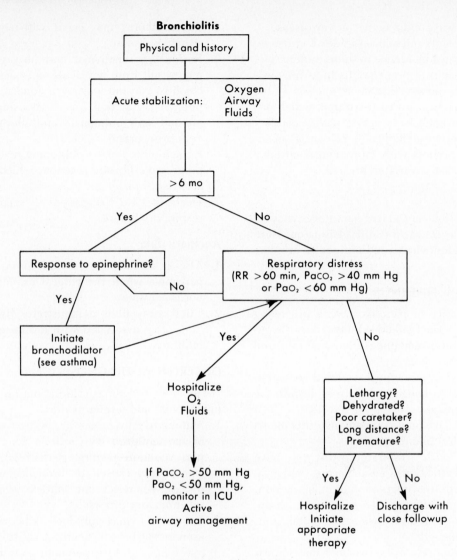

Fig. 84-2. Bronchiolitis.

way intervention, and fluids may be initiated.
2. If the child is over 6 mo of age, a trial of epinephrine (1:1,000) 0.01 mg/kg/dose (maximum: 0.35 ml/dose) SQ may be tried if there is moderate or severe distress. Repeat doses every 20 min. Up to a total of three doses may be given if there is a partial response to the initial administration and the heart rate is <180/min.

a. If there is a response to the epinephrine, bronchodilator therapy should be initiated (see the discussion on asthma on p. 585)
b. Patients under 6 mo of age rarely respond to epinephrine because of the relative scarcity of smooth muscles in the bronchioles. The use of bronchodilators in old-

er children is controversial, and efficacy has not been demonstrated.

3. Whatever the response to epinephrine, the patient requires evaluation for signs of respiratory distress.

   a. The patient who has a respiratory rate >60/min or any evidence of hypoxia, hypercapnia, fatigue, or progression should be hospitalized for humidified oxygen therapy, fluids, and monitoring.

   b. If respiratory failure is present or imminent (PaO_2 <50 mm Hg and $PaCO_2$ >50 mm Hg), the patient should be in an ICU and active airway intervention initiated. Continuous positive airway pressure (CPAP) should be instituted if there is a rising respiratory rate or pulse, decreased responsiveness, decreasing PaO_2, or increasing $PaCO_2$. Oxygen at 30%-40% with 5 cm H_2O pressure may be used. Mechanical ventilation with intubation is necessary if CPAP fails or apneic spells are frequent.

4. Aerosolized ribavirin speeds up improvement of illness in children with severe RSV lower respiratory tract disease, usually following documentation of the cause. Severe disease should be considered for such intervention if a prolonged (3 days) hospitalization is anticipated or there is underlying cardiopulmonary pathology. Special precautions are required for children who need mechanical ventilation.

DISPOSITION

1. Patients should be hospitalized if there is any evidence of apnea, lethargy, or dehydration or if the patient has unreliable caretakers, lives a long distance from a health care facility, or is premature.

2. Patients without respiratory distress or other modifying factors may be discharged with close follow-up.

   Parental education

1. Give all prescribed medications.

2. Push clear liquids. Do not worry about solids.

3. Humidified air may decrease congestion.

4. Call physician if

   a. Breathing effort or retractions increase

   b. Cyanosis or apnea are noted

   c. Fluid intake decreases

   d. Child develops an increasing fever, toxicity, or fatigue

REFERENCES

Hall, C.B., and McBride, J.T.: Vapors, viruses, and views: ribavirin and respiratory syncytial virus, Am. J. Dis. Child. 140:331, 1986.

Hall, C.B., McBride, J.T., Gala, C.L., et al.: Ribavirin treatment of respiratory syncytial viral infection in infants with underlying cardiopulmonary disease, JAMA 254:3047, 1985.

McConnochie, K.M., and Roghmann, K.J.: Bronchiolitis as a possible cause of wheezing in childhood: new evidence, Pediatrics 74:1, 1984.

Outwater, K.M., and Crone, R.K.: Management of respiratory failure in infants with acute viral bronchiolitis, Am. J. Dis. Child. 138:1071, 1984.

Tercier, J.A.: Bronchiolitis: a clinical review, J. Emerg. Med. 1:119, 1983.

Croup and epiglottitis

ALERT: Ensure adequate airway. Differentiate croup from epiglottitis. Epiglottitis requires that the patient be intubated. Always consider foreign body and allergic croup in the different diagnosis. A clinician skilled in airway management must accompany the patient until diagnosis and stabilization are complete.

Infections of the supraglottic area result in swelling of the laryngeal and epiglottic structures and may additionally involve the trachea as in croup (laryngotracheobronchitis).

ETIOLOGY

1. Infection

   a. Croup is viral, and the agents include parainfluenza, RSV, and influenza.

   b. Epiglotittis is caused by *Haemophilus influenzae;* rarely, other bacteria

2. Allergy. Allergic croup is a rapid supraglottic

TABLE 84-2. Comparison of croup and epiglottitis

	Croup	Epiglottitis
Age	6 mo-3 yr	Any age (peak: 2-5 yr)
Seasonal occurrence	Fall/winter	None
Worst time of day	Night/early AM	Throughout day
Etiology	Viral	*H. influenzae*
Clinical signs/symptoms		
Onset	Insidious	Rapid
Preceding URI	Yes	Rare
Fever	<39.50° C (103° F)	High
Toxic	No	Yes
Sore throat	Variable	Yes
Voice	Hoarse	Muffled
Drooling	None	Yes
Dysphagia	None	Yes
Cough	"Barking seal"	None
Preferred position	Variable	Prefers sitting
Stridor	Inspir/expir	Inspir
Epiglottis	WNL	"Cherry red"
Ancillary data		
WBC	WNL	High
Blood culture	Negative	Positive
ABG	Variable	Variable
X-ray, lateral neck (Fig. 84-4)	WNL	Enlarged epiglottis

swelling resulting from exposure to a precipitating or sensitizing agent.

DIAGNOSTIC FINDINGS (Table 84-2)

1. Respiratory failure may occur with both croup and epiglottitis; may have accompanying pulmonary edema
2. Spasmodic or allergic croup has a rapid onset of croup syndrome following exposure to a precipitating factor and without a preceding viral respiratory infection as in infectious croup.
3. Other conditions resulting in upper airway obstruction and dyspnea must be considered in the history and physical examination.
4. Extraepiglottic foci commonly are associated with epiglottitis. Pneumonia, lymphadenitis, and otitis media are most common. Pulmonary edema occurs, not uncommonly, following relief of the obstruction.

DIFFERENTIAL DIAGNOSIS (Chapter 20)

Stridor indicates that there is some degree of upper airway obstruction. Inspiratory stridor usually indicates a supraglottic lesion, whereas expiratory stridor usually emanates from a lower airway involvement. Common entities to consider include the following:

1. Supraglottic
   a. Viral infection
   b. Bacterial infection: group A streptococcus, *Staphylococcus aureus*, anaerobes of the mouth (*Peptococcus, Bacteroides*), *Corynebacterium diphtheriae*
   c. Epiglottitis: *H. influenzae*
   d. Noninfectious: foreign body, trauma, caustic ingestion, neoplasm, angioneurotic edema
2. *Infraglottic* or subglottic (laryngitis, laryngotracheitis, laryngotracheobronchitis
   a. Viral: parainfluenza, influenza A and B, measles, adenovirus, RSV

  b. *Mycoplasma pneumoniae*
  c. Of bacterial infections, which are usually secondary, the most important entity is **bacterial tracheitis**. This is secondary to superinfection of damaged trachea from an antecedent viral infection. It is commonly caused by *S. aureus* or *H. influenzae* with accumulation of pus in the trachea causing a thick plug and ultimately leading to obstruction. It often is associated with pneumonia and appears clinically as a crouplike syndrome with toxicity and rapid progression. Active airway intervention often is required, combined with aggressive pulmonary drainage and toilet and appropriate antibiotics for potential pathogens.

MANAGEMENT (see box on pp. 595-596 and Fig. 84-3)

1. The patient with upper airway obstruction from croup or epiglottitis requires urgent attention to:
   a. Ensure adequate airway
   b. Differentiate croup from epiglottitis
   c. Provide ongoing management and airway stabilization
2. Respiratory failure caused by upper airway obstruction may occur. Airway intervention is indicated if hypoxia (PaO_2 <50 mm Hg with supplemental O_2) or hypercapnia ($PaCO_2$ >50 mm Hg) is present, if the patient demonstrates evidence of fatigue, or if there is progressive anxiety or severe obstruction. Patients with epiglottitis (see following discussion) usually require intubation on a prophylactic basis. All patients requiring intubation should have the procedure performed with extreme care and maximal support, usually under controlled conditons in the operating room with equipment and personnel mobilized (see box, pp. 595-596, and Fig. 84-3). Often a smaller tube size is used to minimize the risk of subglottic stenosis. Tube should be well immobilized. There may be some contribution of bacterial tracheitis in children with severe disease, particularly in those with croup who require intubation.
3. Following evaluation for respiratory failure, the epiglottis should be visualized to determine its configuration, size, and color. The epiglottis in the child is somewhat easier to see because it is at the level of C2-C3 rather than the C5-C6 level found in adults.
   a. If there is evidence of obstruction or the clinical signs and symptoms are consistent with epiglottitis, visualization is optimally done in the operating room with clinicians experienced in surgical airway management (anesthesiologist, otolaryngologist, and surgeon) present. Patients should be preoxygenated and initially allowed to sit in their most comfortable position. Children are usually more comfortable sitting; a supine position may lead to acute obstruction. Minimize agitation. At the time of visualization, the patient care team must be prepared to intubate the child if obstruction occurs or epiglottitis is diagnosed (see box pp. 595-596, and Fig. 84-3).
   b. Some clinicians prefer to use a lateral neck x-ray film before visualization because of the potential risk of exacerbating the disease if the posterior pharynx is further inflamed. This technique may be useful if the child is not in severe respiratory distress and no evidence of obstruction exists, but direct controlled visualization is usually more desirable. *A clinician capable of intubating the patient must accompany the patient at all times*. Portable films should be considered. Classic findings of croup on lateral radiograph include ballooning of the hypopharynx with narrowing of the cervical trachea on inspiration and ballooning of the cervical trachea on expiration (Fig. 84-4).

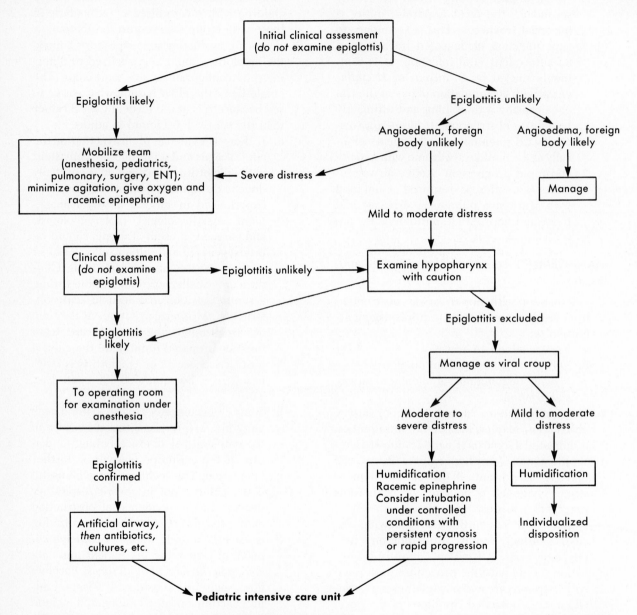

Fig. 84-3. Optimal assessment and management of epiglottitis and severe croup. Care must be individualized to reflect resources and logistic issues within a given institution.

SUGGESTED PROTOCOL FOR MANAGEMENT OF UPPER AIRWAY OBSTRUCTION DUE TO INFECTION IN CHILDREN

OVERVIEW

Children with evidence of upper airway obstruction commonly have stridor, most commonly inspiratory if the pathology is supraglottic, whereas expiratory stridor emanates from the trachea. For children with stridor or any evidence of upper airway obstruction it is imperative to rapidly evaluate the degree of respiratory distress and intervene in an appropriate fashion, considering the degree of compromise, the diagnostic considerations, and the personnel, equipment, and facilities available.

Obviously, the management described below of the child with severe croup or epiglottitis as the underlying pathology requires a markedly different intervention than does the child with a suspected or proved foreign body. Furthermore, mild croup unassociated with significant respiratory distress often can be managed after a careful evaluation with humidification at home and parental education regarding the danger signals indicating progression of disease.

MANAGEMENT

1. When the diagnosis of upper airway obstruction with respiratory compromise is suspected, secondary to an infectious process, a designated senior physician (attending or fellow) experienced in airway management should be called and should remain in constant attendance to coordinate and facilitate the patient's care. The senior physician should be responsible for activating this protocol.
2. The child should be kept in the company of parents, given humidified oxygen by mask, monitored for cardiac and respiratory function, and allowed to remain in the most comfortable position. Keep the child calm, reducing anxiety whenever possible.
3. Following rapid assessment of the severity and pattern of progression of the respiratory obstruction, the senior physician should call the pediatric pulmonary and surgery fellows and the attending anesthesiologist.
4. If significant obstruction appears to be present, the operating room personnel should be alerted to prepare for direct laryngoscopy and possible intubation. Preparations also should be made for rigid bronchoscopy and tracheostomy.
5. Should the operating room be unable to accommodate the patient immediately, transfer the patient to the PACU (recovery room). The third line of transfer is the pediatric intensive care unit.
6. For children who have possible severe croup and there is a delay in achieving definitive visualization, a trial of nebulized racemic epinephrine (dilute 0.25-0.50 ml in 2.5 ml sterile water or saline and administer by nebulizer) may be of value. This should be done only in *stable, cooperative* patients under constant supervision who are not progressing rapidly and have no evidence of impending total obstruction.
7. Do not agitate the child while obtaining bloods, starting IVs, x-ray studies, or separation from parents. Do not leave the child unattended or send the patient for any diagnostic studies.
8. *Do not* attempt laryngoscopy in the ED unless other options do not exist. The etiology of progressive airway obstruction is best delineated under optimal conditions in the operating room where the patient can be given inhalation anesthesia and the epiglottis visualized under total control. If the diagnosis of epiglottitis is confirmed, the patient will be intubated with a tube 0.5-1.0 mm smaller than would normally be used.

NOTE: This protocol should be modified to reflect the availability of personnel, equipment, and facilities, as well as the service and educational focus, in a given institution.   *Continued.*

SUGGESTED PROTOCOL FOR MANAGEMENT OF UPPER AIRWAY OBSTRUCTION DUE TO INFECTION IN CHILDREN—cont'd

9. In the event of an acute obstructive event in the ED, ventilation usually can be achieved using positive pressure ventilation and a self-inflating bag with 100% oxygen until definitive stabilization is achieved with available resources.

10. After satisfactory establishment of the airway, diagnostic studies can be obtained, pharmacologic therapy initiated, and transfer to the pediatric intensive care unit accomplished.

11. Management of croup with stridor at rest in the ED. Stridor at rest is an indication for hospital admission. Visualization of the epiglottis should be performed in the ED before admission to the ward or ICU if there is *no* evidence of obstruction and epiglottitis is not considered to be the likely diagnosis. The attending ED physician should be notified of the presence of such patients and involved with the procedure. At the time of visualization, the child should have been preoxygenated and a nurse and attending physician should be present. Equipment necessary for airway management, including self-inflating bag, appropriate ET tube size (with stylet), oxygen, suction, and laryngoscope, must be immediately available.

   Frequently, nebulized racemic epinephrine (see 6) may be administered to the cooperative patient. Steroids, although controversial, often are given to patients who require nebulized racemic epinephrine.

Epiglottitis (see box on pp. 595-596 and Fig. 84-3)

Immediate intervention is required. Initially 100% oxygen should be given. The patient who is already obstructed may be ventilated by bag-mask positive pressure with a nonrebreathing 100% oxygen bag. The patient should be intubated with an endotracheal or nasotracheal tube one to two sizes smaller than would normally be indicated. Topical 4% cocaine or topical epinephrine may be useful as may atropine (0.01-0.02 mg/kg IV), the latter decreasing the vagal response. After intubation, most patients are allowed to breath spontaneously with 4-6 mm Hg of CPAP and 40% FIO_2 (humidified). The CPAP helps to stabilize the lungs following relief of the obstruction.

1. If time and clinical status permit, the optimal place to perform intubation (and visualize the epiglottis) is in the operating room with appropriate relaxation and with the assistance of an anesthesiologist and others experienced in airway management.

2. An otolaryngologist or surgeon should be available to assist if a surgical airway is required.

3. If personnel resources are limited, intubation, if necessary, can usually be achieved by a clinician skilled in pediatric airway management. The older child often can be intubated in the position of greatest comfort (usually sitting up and leaning forward). This means that in this circumstance clinicians have been successful in blindly intubating the child with the intubator behind the child (usually on stretcher with child). To be successful, this approach usually requires that the child (over 5 yr) be able to tolerate a 6 mm tube.

4. Following intubation, patients are monitored in an intensive care unit. Blood cultures and other studies may be done and antibiotics initiated. Patients usually remain intubated for 36 ± 14 (1 SD) hr. Direct visualization, often using fiberoptic laryngoscopy, should serve as a guide to the timing of elective extubation.

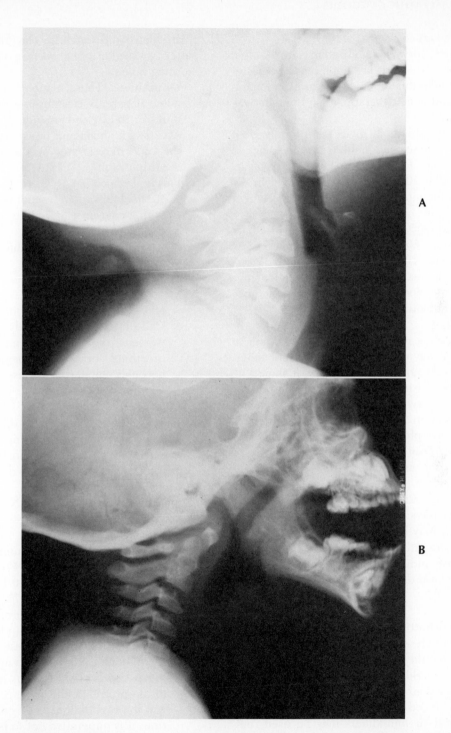

Fig. 84-4. Soft tissue lateral neck films. **A,** Normal. **B,** Markedly swollen epiglottis. Patients with epiglottitis have narrow valleculae and thick mass of tissue ("thumb" sign) extending from the valleculae to the arytenoids. (Courtesy Dr. S.Z. Barkin, Denver, Colo.)

Intravenous line

Following airway stabilization, an IV line should be started if it has not already been initiated. Fluid status should be assessed and maintenance and deficit therapy (if any) initiated.

Antibiotics

Antibiotics should be given parenterally for at least 5 days (at which time they may be changed to oral therapy for a total course of 10 days):

1. Ampicillin 100-200 mg/kg/24 hr q 4 hr IV *and* chloramphenicol 75-100 mg/kg/24 hr q 6 hr IV; **or**
2. Cefotaxime 50-150 mg/kg/24 hr q 6 hr IV; **or** ceftriaxone 50-75 mg/kg/24 hr q 12 hr IV; **or** cefuroxime 100 mg/kg/24 hr q 6-8 hr IV

Antibiotics may be altered to reflect sensitivity data from blood cultures obtained before beginning antibiotics.

Disposition

1. All patients require emergent admission to an ICU for airway management and monitoring. If transport is necessary, it should be arranged, using an ambulance equipped for airway intervention, ventilatory support, and resuscitation. Trained personnel and an experienced physician should accompany the patient. *Transport without means to control the airway and ventilate the patient is inappropriate.* Ongoing involvement by an anesthesiologist, otolaryngologist, and critical care physician is helpful.
2. Patients may be extubated under controlled conditions after an average of 36 hr if clinical response indicates, and they may be discharged 4-6 days after admission.

Croup

If the epiglottis is normal and other entities within the differential are excluded, treatment for croup should be initiated.

Absence of stridor at rest

Humidified air is the mainstay of therapy and may be achieved by a variety of cool air vaporizers. Warm air humidifiers may be used, but they have the potential disadvantage of causing burns.

Parents should watch for changing breathing patterns. Stridor often worsens in the early morning hours.

1. **Disposition.** These patients may be sent home if parents can observe the child, administer fluids, and provide humidified air. Access to a phone and transportation in case the child deteriorates may serve to modify the disposition.
2. **Parental education**
   a. Keep child's room humidified, preferably with a cold-mist humidifier.
   b. Push clear liquids.
   c. Control fever to make child more comfortable.
   d. Take the child who awakens with stridor outside for 5 min. If the stridor persists, take the child to the hospital.
   e. Call physician immediately if the stridor worsens or child has more difficulty breathing, turns blue, begins drooling, becomes agitated or listless, has poor intake, or does not improve in 4-5 days.

Stridor at rest

1. These patients should be hospitalized. Humidified air remains the mainstay of therapy and may be achieved by vaporized rooms or mist tents. The latter has the disadvantage of decreasing patient visibility.
2. Racemic epinephrine (MicroNefrin) is useful for patients with stridor at rest and respiratory distress.
   a. Racemic epinephrine is administered by diluting the solution (2.25%) (<20 kg: 0.25 ml in 2.5 ml saline; 20-40 kg: 0.5 ml in 2.5 ml saline; >40 kg: 0.75 ml in 2.5 ml saline), which is administered by nebulizer with or without IPPB up to every 2 hr for increasing stridor at rest.
   b. The therapeutic effect lasts up to 4 hr, and the patient's clinical status often returns to the pretreatment level. Since patients will improve following racemic epinephrine, it is imperative not to be lulled into early discharge on the basis of clinical improvement.

3. Steroids may reduce the severity of disease, and they are indicated for patients requiring racemic epinephrine because of stridor at rest and respiratory distress. Their use is controversial.
   • Dexamethasone (Decadron) 0.25-0.5 mg/kg/dose q 6 hr IV or IM is given for 24-36 hr.
4. Hydration must be maintained by oral or parenteral therapy. Antipyretics are often useful.
5. Oxygen without intubation rarely is indicated since hypoxia is usually an indication for airway intervention. Oxygen, when administered, should be given only in an ICU where intensive monitoring and observation are possible. On occasion, intubation is required because of respiratory failure.
6. **Disposition.** Most patients with stridor at rest should be admitted for observation and therapy to a unit that provides close supervision and access to airway intervention should it become necessary.

Spasmodic or allergic croup

This is rapid in onset and usually treated very effectively with nebulized racemic epinephrine (0.25-0.50 ml [adult: 0.75 ml] diluted in 2.5 ml of saline). Patients respond dramatically but may require additional treatments in the ensuing 24 hr.

Patients with allergic croup should be hospitalized for observation, humidified air, and additional racemic epinephrine treatments.

REFERENCES

Battaglia, J.D.: Severe croup: the child with fever and upper airway obstruction, Pediatr. Rev. **7**:227, 1986.

Fried, M.P.: Controversies in the management of supraglottitis and croup, Pediatr. Clin. North Am. **28**:931, 1979.

Goldhagen, J.L.: Croup: pathogenesis and management, J. Emerg. Med. **1**:3, 1984.

Liston, S.L., Gehrz, R.C., Siegel, L.G., and Tilelli, J.: Bacterial tracheitis, Am. J. Dis. Child. **137**:764, 1983.

Molteni, R.A.: Epiglottitis: incidence of extraepiglottic infection: report of 72 cases and review of the literature, Pediatrics **58**:526, 1976.

Rothstein, P., and Lister, G.: Epiglottitis: duration of intubation and fever, Anesth. Analg. **62**:785, 1983.

Westley, C.R., Cotton, E.K., and Brooks, J.G.: Nebulized-racemic epinephrine by IPPB for the treatment of croup, Am. J. Dis. Child. **132**:484, 1978.

Willis, R.J., and Rowland, T.W.: The early management of acute epiglottitis: a survey of current practice, J. Emerg. Med. **2**:13, 1984.

Foreign body in airway

ALERT: Laryngotracheal foreign bodies require immediate airway stabilization, either by removal of the material or surgical intervention. Foreign bodies may cause wheezing.

The clinical presentation of an airway foreign body will reflect the acuteness and location of the obstruction. Laryngotracheal foreign bodies typically produce an acute obstruction, whereas bronchial foreign bodies produce a more subacute course. Bronchial obstruction may result from a variety of mechanisms:
1. Check valve in which air is inhaled but not expelled leading to emphysema
2. Stop valve, which allows no inhaled air to pass, resulting in distal atelectasis
3. Ball valve in which the foreign body is dislodged during expiration but reimpacts on inspiration, resulting in atelectasis
4. Bypass valve producing a partial obstruction to inflow and outflow with decreased aeration on the affected side

Food and vegetable matter (nuts, seeds, raisins, hard candy, sausage-shaped meat, or raw carrots) are most commonly aspirated by children. Objects are usually ≤32 mm, with round objects being more likely to plug the airway completely. The highest risk period is from birth to 48 mo; the peak age-group is between 1 and 2 yr.

DIAGNOSTIC FINDINGS

1. Although a history of aspiration is useful, the absence of a positive history does not exclude a foreign body.
2. Acute airway obstruction secondary to ma-

terial in the laryngotracheal area results in acute, life-threatening respiratory distress. Cyanosis, apnea, stridor, wheezing, cough, and dysphonia may be present. Facial petechiae may appear secondary to increased intrathoracic pressure.

3. Subacute obstruction occurs with bronchial foreign bodies and, rarely, partial obstruction of the laryngotracheal segment. Clinically, patients develop air trapping, wheezing, cyanosis, a muffled voice, and cough. Atelectasis is commonly present.

Complications

1. Specific pulmonary complications may include atelectasis, pneumonia, erosion through trachea and bronchus, and abscess.
2. Respiratory arrest occurs with any delay in clearing an acute obstruction. Attempts at removal of bronchial foreign bodies may produce total obstruction.
3. Dysrhythmias and other complications of hypoxia may develop, including a full cardiac arrest.
4. Pulmonary edema is uncommonly reported secondary to obstruction and increased intrathoracic pressure.

Ancillary data

Relief of the obstruction should not be delayed awaiting results of ancillary data. Immediate intervention may be necessary. However, if obstruction is only partial, a number of ancillary diagnostic tests may be useful in defining the location of the foreign body and in considering other diagnostic entities.

1. ABG to determine hypoxia and ventilatory status
2. Chest x-ray films, inspiratory and expiratory, to determine if a bronchial foreign body is likely to be present. It is often important to distinguish a foreign body in the trachea from one in the esophagus. Foreign bodies lie in the plane of least resistance. Flat foreign bodies like coins in the esophagus lie in the frontal plane, appearing as a full circle on the PA view, whereas those in the trachea rest in the sagittal plane and will appear end-on in the PA chest x-ray film and flat on a lateral view.
3. Soft tissue lateral neck
4. Laryngoscopy. May be both diagnostic and therapeutic. Magill forceps or Kelly clamps can remove the foreign body under direct visualization of the laryngotracheal area.
5. Fluoroscopy may be useful. Tracheal foreign bodies may have a paradoxic movement.
6. Bronchoscopy is the definitive therapy but is also useful as a diagnostic tool. The procedure is rapidly and safely performed with fiberoptic equipment used by a physician experienced in this procedure.

DIFFERENTIAL DIAGNOSIS (Chapter 20)
MANAGEMENT

1. The initial stabilization of the patient with a foreign body involves attention to the airway while managing shock, respiratory, or cardiac arrest and the complications of hypoxia the patient has experienced. Concurrent with immediate resuscitation, other considerations in the differential diagnosis must be considered.
2. Efforts should be initiated on the first contact to relieve airway obstruction according to the guidelines of the American Heart Association. Attempts at clearing the airway followed by back blows and manual thrusts should be considered as an essential part of prehospital care and will, ultimately, determine the patient's prognosis.
3. If the patient is not acutely obstructed and can cough and phonate, coughing should be encouraged.
   a. Although there are no controlled studies, the bulk of the literature suggests that a combination of maneuvers may be more effective than any single method used alone. These recommendations are under constant reevaluation.

b. In the infant under 12 months, the rapid increase in pressure resulting from four back blows may expel or loosen a foreign body since many of these lodge high in the throat. If the material is not expelled by the patient, manual chest thrusts should be done immediately to provide a more sustained increase in pressure and airflow.

c. Older children should be handled by doing a manual abdominal (Heimlich) or chest thrust as the primary technique, whereas in the adolescent or adult, a manual abdominal thrust is recommended, because of the relative decrease in chest wall compliance.

4. If the above procedures are not *rapidly* successful, an attempt may be made to remove the foreign body with laryngoscopy and a Magill forceps or Kelly clamp.

5. Bronchoscopy is the definitive therapy and must be performed rapidly in all patients with unrelieved respiratory obstruction or in those with a bronchial foreign body present for > 24 hr.

6. If these procedures are not available or immediately successful at relieving the obstruction, surgical intervention by cricothyroidotomy may be appropriate.

7. Postural drainage in an ICU, in combination with inhaled bronchodilators, is useful in removing non vegetable matter foreign bodies that have been present in the tracheobronchial tract for <24 hr and that are not associated with respiratory distress. Bronchoscopy may, of course, be used instead.

DISPOSITION

1. Patients who have experienced significant hypoxia or any other complications of an upper airway foreign body should be hospitalized for monitoring if definitive therapy has been rendered either before arrival at the hospital or in the ED.

2. Patients with ongoing obstruction need emergent airway stabilization and critical care facilities.

3. The patient who has experienced a very transient episode of obstruction or choking and is free of distress or signs and symptoms referable to the incident may be followed closely as an ambulatory patient.

Parental education

Small, hard foods such as nuts, seeds, raisins, hard candy, sausage-shaped meat and raw carrots should not be given to small children unless cut into very small pieces. Parents should be taught the techniques of back blow and manual chest thrust.

REFERENCES

Abman, S.H., Fan, L.L. and Cotton, E.K.: Emergency treatment of foreign body obstruction of the upper airway in children, J. Emerg. Med. **2**:7, 1984.

American Heart Association: Standards and guidelines for cardiopulmonary resuscitation (CPR) and emergency cardiac care (ECC), JAMA **255**:2954, 1986.

Blazer, S., Naveh, Y., and Friedman, A.: Foreign body in the airway, Am. J. Dis. Child. **134**:68, 1980.

Fulkerson, W.J.: Fiberoptic bronchoscopy, N. Engl. J. Med. **311**:511, 1984.

Greensher, J., and Mofenson, H.C.: Emergency treatment of the choking child, Pediatrics **70**:110, 1982.

Harris, C.S., Baker, S.P., Smith, G.A., and Harris, R.M.: Childhood asphyxia by food: anatomical survey and overview, JAMA **251**:2231, 1984.

Kosloske, A.M.: Bronchoscopic extraction of aspirated foreign bodies in children, Am. J. Dis. Child. **136**:924, 1982.

Pneumonia

Pneumonia is an acute infection of the lung parenchyma presenting as an interstitial process involving either the alveolar walls or the alveoli.

ETIOLOGY AND DIAGNOSTIC FINDINGS: INFECTION (Table 84-3)

1. Bacterial infection (Table 84-4)
   a. Common organisms: *Streptococcus pneumoniae, Haemophilus influenzae,* group A

TABLE 84-3. Differentiating features of pneumonia

	Bacterial	Viral	Mycoplasmal
Age	Any	Under 5 yr	5-15 yr
Season	Any	Epidemic	Any
Onset	Rapid	Gradual	Gradual
Toxicity	Severe	Mild/moderate	Mild
Fever	High	Moderate	Low
Chills	Common	Rare	Rare
Tachypnea	Moderate/severe	Mild/moderate	Mild/moderate
Cough	Productive, variable	Dry, variable	Dry, prominent
Myalgia/headache	None	Common	Headache, pharyngitis
Auscultation	↓ breath sounds, rales, rhonchi	Rare wheezes, rare rales	Very rare rales
Pleural effusion	Common	Very rare	Rare
Segmental consolidation	Common	Rare	Variable
Chest x-ray	Lobar consolidation	Interstitial, delayed resolution	Interstitial (more than physical exam would indicate)
WBC (cells/mm³)	>10,000	Normal	Normal
Diagnostic procedures	Positive blood culture; rarely: lung tap or thoracentesis	Viral culture, serology	Cold agglutinin, complement-fixation
Primary antibiotics	Ampicillin/amoxicillin: 8 yr or under Penicillin or erythromycin: 9 yr or older	None	Erythromycin

TABLE 84-4. Bacterial pneumonias: diagnostic findings

	Streptococcus pneumoniae	*Haemophilus influenzae*	Group A streptococci	*Staphylococcus aureus*
Age	4 yr or under	8 yr or under	Over 10 yr	Under 1 yr
Onset	Rapid	Gradual	Gradual	Rapid
Diagnostic features	Infant: poor feeding, cough, irritable; child: fever, cough, toxic, abdominal pain	Fever, cough, toxic, otitis media (variable)	Fever, tachypnea, chill, pleuritic pain, hemoptysis	High fever, respiratory distress, nausea, vomiting
Complications	Bacteremia Empyema Effusion	Bacteremia Meningitis Empyema Lung abscess Bronchiectasis	Empyema (serosanguineous)	Pneumatocele Empyema Pneumothorax Pyopneumothorax
Chest x-ray film	Lobar consolidation Patchy bronchopneumonia	Unilateral lobar consolidation	Infiltrate	Segmental, lobar infiltrate

streptococci, and *Staphylococcus aureus*
  b. Unusual organisms
     (1) Pertussis: catarrhal stage followed by staccato, paroxysmal cough (p. 168*t*)
     (2) *Pseudomonas aeruginosa:* usually in debilitated or immunocompromised patients, especially those with cystic fibrosis. May involve pulmonary tract, ear, sinus, or meninges
     (3) *Klebsiella pneumoniae:* usually in infants, alcoholics, or those who are immunocompromised. Explosive pulmonary symptoms with gastroenteritis and neurologic findings. Chest roentgenogram shows bulging fissures.
     (4) Anaerobes such as *Peptostreptococcus* organisms, often as secondary infection or abscess
2. Viral infections: RSV and parinfluenza predominant in children under 2 yr; influenza A and B in older children; other agents: adenovirus, measles, and chickenpox
3. *Mycoplasma pneumoniae:* frequent in children over 5 yr
4. *Chlamydia trachomatis*
  a. Tachypnea, staccato cough, conjunctivitis, rarely toxic; fairly common in the second to sixth weeks of life
  b. Chest x-ray film; hyperexpansion; CBC; eosinophilia
5. *Mycobacterium tuberculosis*
  a. History of exposure; fever, anorexia, cough
  b. Chest x-ray film with hilar adenopathy and apical findings; sputum and gastric aspirates may be helpful. PPD skin test on patient and family should be done.
6. Parasitic infection: *Pneumocystis carinii*
  a. Fever, tachypnea, cough, dyspnea, cyanosis; occurs in immunosuppressed or malnourished patients
  b. Chest x-ray film: diffuse interstitial pneumonitis; ABG; hypoxia, usually greater than would be indicated by chest x-ray study; lung aspirate or biopsy using methenamine-silver nitrate stain

7. Fungal infection
  a. Coccidiomycosis
     (1) Fever, pleuritis, productive cough with weight loss, anorexia, myalgias, headache, and rash
     (2) Chest x-ray study; pneumonia (interstitial), effusions, granuloma, cavitation
     (3) Skin test and complement-fixation test
  b. Histoplasmosis
     (1) Pulmonary cavitation, hemoptysis, variable hepatosplenomegaly, variable weight loss, lymphadenopathy
     (2) Chest x-ray film; pulmonary calcification; CBC; anemia
8. Rickettsial infection: Q fever
  a. Fever, chest pain, headache, sore throat, chills, and respiratory symptoms; self-limited disease of 3 wk
  b. Complement fixation

Ancillary data

Laboratory studies must be individualized for the specific patient and the presenting clinical complex.
1. Chest roentgenogram: PA and lateral
  a. Inspiratory and expiratory views may be useful in excluding a foreign body, if in doubt.
  b. Lateral decubitus can define an effusion.
2. CBC with differential
3. ABG. For all patients with cyanosis, apnea, dyspnea, or respiratory distress
4. Blood cultures. Positive in 10%-20% of bacterial pneumonias and should be obtained on all patients requiring hospitalization (e.g., toxic, respiratory distress)
5. Counterimmuno electrophoresis may be useful in hospitalized patients with negative cultures.
Pulmonary cultures
Invasive procedures are indicated for patients with severe toxicity and life threatening infection, for those failing to respond to appropriate antibiotic therapy, and for those who are immunosuppressed.

Nasopharyngeal (NP) or throat cultures are of no value except for pertussis (NP swab) and viral cultures.

1. Sputum. Usually difficult to obtain in children and contaminated with mouth flora. Reliable only with productive cough and if single organism is recovered
2. Tracheal suctioning via direct laryngoscopy. Fairly reliable but patient may have upper airway contamination
3. Transtracheal aspiration. Difficult to do in children and usually should be avoided. Absolute contraindication is a bleeding diathesis or an uncooperative, young child.
4. Bronchoscopy with direct aspiration and brush border biopsy. Excellent approach yielding direct visualization with aspiration of good culture material. Requires equipment and experience, which are rarely available emergently
5. Direct needle aspiration of the lung (useful in critically ill and immunocompromised children)
   a. Unless the infiltrate is in the upper lobes, the patient is placed in a sitting position and is told to take a deep breath and hold in expiration if old enough to cooperate. A needle (18-20 gauge, 1-1½ in) is inserted rapidly under negative pressure, along the top of the rib, with an attached syringe containing nonbacteriostatic saline. Patient requires hospitalization for observation after procedure.
   b. Aspirate is excellent specimen for Gram's stain and culture.
   c. Contraindications include hyperexpansion with air trapping, pneumothorax, bleeding diathesis, pulmonary hypertension, uncontrolled coughing or seizures, poor cooperation, and lack of facility to observe the patient after the procedure.

Thoracentesis (Appendix A-8)

This is indicated for the removal of pleural fluid for either diagnostic or therapeutic purposes.

1. Patient is maintained in an upright position and the site for thoracentesis is defined by x-ray film and physical examination.
2. Needle (18-20 gauge) with a 20 ml syringe is attached to a three-way stopcock. Using negative pressure, it is passed along the top of the ribs and fluid is withdrawn. The amount removed should reflect the degree of respiratory distress and that required for diagnosis. Patient must be hospitalized for observation after procedure.

Evaluation of the fluid should include Gram's stain and culture, cell count and differential, protein, LDH, and glucose.

DIFFERENTIAL DIAGNOSIS (Chapter 20)

1. Allergy: asthma (p. 581)
2. Trauma
   a. Foreign body (p. 599)
   b. Drowning (Chapter 47)
3. Atelectasis
4. Vascular disease
   a. Congestive heart failure and pulmonary edema (Chapters 16 and 19)
   b. Pulmonary embolism (p. 428)
5. Intoxication: hydrocarbon (p. 292)
6. Recurrent aspiration (gastroesophageal reflux, vascular ring, pharyngeal incoordination, H type tracheoesophageal fistula)
7. Congenital absence of lung, hemangioma, etc.
8. Neoplasm: primary or metastatic

MANAGEMENT

1. The majority of patients with pneumonia have only mild disease and require no immediate stabilization or airway support. However, if respiratory distress is present, stabilization of the airway is of the highest priority.
   a. Oxygen, optimally with humidification, should be initiated if respiratory distress is present.
   b. Intubation, may be indicated if respiratory failure (PaO_2 <50 mm Hg and $PaCO_2$ >50 mm Hg) is present.

c. ABG is indicated for moderately ill patient.

d. Suctioning and postural drainage are useful adjunctive measures.

2. Antibiotics should be initiated with all cases of pneumonia in which bacteria or mycoplasmas are the suspected pathogens (Table 84-5).

a. If appropriate, cultures (blood and rarely lung tap) should be obtained before initiating medication.

b. Viral infections do not require antibiotics although if the patient is toxic or having respiratory distress, antibiotics are indicated until culture results are available.

c. The majority of patients may be treated with oral medications as outpatients.

d. The initial choice must reflect common etiologies for the patient's age, allergies, signs and symptoms, and known bacterial sensitivity patterns.

e. Antibiotic failures commonly result from resistant organisms (particularly *H. influenzae*), viral infections or poor compliance.

f. Organisms, such as tuberculosis, and *Pneumocytis* carinii, require alternative therapy.

3. Bronchodilators are indicated if wheezing or reactive airway disease is present (p. 584).

4. Special considerations must be recognized in the management of the newborn (Chapter 11).

DISPOSITION

Hospitalization rarely is necessary but is indicated if any of the following exist:

1. Significant toxicity with high fever, dyspnea, apnea, cyanosis, or fatigue

2. Any evidence of potential respiratory failure or progression

3. Age of less than 2-3 mo

TABLE 84-5. Antibiotic therapy for bacterial pneumonia

Age-group	Major etiologies	Antibiotic therapy	
		PO	IV
Under 2 mo*	E. coli Group B streptococci S. aureus C. trachomatis	Rarely given	Ampicillin 100-200 mg/kg/24 hr q 6-12 hr **and** gentamicin 5-7.5 mg/kg/24 hr q 8-12 hr
2 mo to 8 yr	Virus S. pneumoniae H. influenzae S. aureus (rare)	Amoxicillin 30-50 mg/kg/24 hr q 8 hr **or** Augmentin	Ampicillin 200 mg/kg/24 hr q 4 hr; **or** cefotaxime 50-150 mg/kg/24 hr q 6 hr IV.† **If poor response, add** nafcillin (or equiv) 100 mg/kg/24 hr q 4 hr
9 yr or over	Virus S. pneumoniae Mycoplasma S. aureus (rare) Group A streptococci (rare) H. influenzae (rare)	Erythromycin 30-50 mg/kg/24 hr q 6 hr	Ampicillin 200 mg/kg/24 hr q 4 hr; if poor response, consider erythromycin (PO) or nafcillin

*If *C. trachomatis* is suspected, **add** erythromycin 30-50 mg/kg/24 hr q 6 hr PO.

†Other alternatives include ceftriaxone 50-75 mg/kg/24 hr q 12 hr IV or cefuroxime 100 mg/kg/24 hr q 6-8 hr IV.

4. Immunocompromised host: underlying disease (e.g., leukemia), drugs (steroids or other immunosuppressive agents), or sickle cell disease

   NOTE: Patients with cystic fibrosis or other chronic pulmonary disease should be hospitalized for acute deterioration and distress with the aim of controlling the infection and instituting aggressive pulmonary toilet.
5. Pleural effusion or after lung aspiration or thoracentesis.
6. Unreliable home environment or questionable compliance

   Most patients may be discharged with appropriate medications.
1. Close follow-up must be ensured to assess the patient's condition after 24 and 48 hr to ensure that resolution has occurred.
2. A repeat chest x-ray film should be obtained 4-6 wk after the initial diagnosis in patients who have segmental or lobar infiltrates.

Parental education

1. Give medication for entire treatment course.
2. Call or bring your child to the primary care physician in 24 hr to assess the response to treatment.
3. Perform postural drainage, if suggested.
4. Call physician if
   a. Your child is having more difficulty breathing or develops a high fever, more rapid breathing, increased retractions, cyanosis, or apnea
   b. Your child has trouble taking medications or fluids
   c. Your child is not afebrile and much improved in 48 hr

REFERENCES

Asmar, B.I., Slovis, T.L., et al.: Hemophilus influenzae type b pneumonia in 43 children, J. Pediatr. **93**:389, 1978.

Glezen, W.P., and Denny, F.W.: Epidemiology of acute lower respiratory disease in children, N. Engl. J. Med. **288**:498, 1973.

Paisley, J.W., Lauer, B.A., McIntosh, K., et al.: Pathogens associated with acute lower respiratory tract infection in young children, Pediatr. Inf. Dis. **3**:14, 1984.

85 Renal disorders

Acute glomerulonephritis

AILEEN B. SEDMAN

Although glomerulonephritis is a histopathologic diagnosis, the term *acute glomerulonephritis* is commonly used to define the clinical presentation of hematuria, edema, and hypertension. The disease most frequently occurs between ages 3-7 and rarely under 2 yr.

Commonly, acute glomerulonephritis occurs as a sequela of a group A beta-hemolytic streptococcal infection of either the pharynx or skin. The pathogenesis is poorly understood but probably results from the deposition of circulating immune complexes in the kidney. Although the disease is self-limited with careful clinical management, strict attention must be given to the initial evaluation, differential diagnosis, and recognition of complications.

DIAGNOSTIC FINDINGS

1. There is usually a preceding streptococcal infection or exposure 1-2 wk (average: 10 days) before the onset of glomerulonephritis. An interval <4 days is associated with an exacerbation of preexisting disease rather than an initial attack.
2. Patients commonly have hematuria (90%), fluid retention and edema (100%), hypertension (60%-70%), and oliguria (80%). Fever, malaise, and abdominal pain are frequently reported.

Complications

1. Circulatory congestion is frequently noted with dyspnea, cough, pallor, and pulmonary edema.
2. Hypertensive encephalopathy with confusion, headaches, somnolence, and seizures evolves.
3. Anuria and renal failure occur in 2% of patients.

Ancillary data

1. Urinalysis
   a. Hematuria may be microscopic or gross. Erythrocyte casts are present in 60%-85% of hospitalized children.
   b. Leukocyturia and hyaline and granular casts are common.
   c. Proteinuria is usually <2 g/m²/24 hr.
   d. Urinary concentrating ability is preserved.
2. Fractional excretion of sodium (p. 616) may be reduced.
3. Streptozyme (p. 427) is elevated.
4. Total serum complement and specifically C3 is depressed in 90%-100% of patients during the first 2 wk of illness, returning to normal within 3-4 wk. Persistently low levels suggest that a chronic renal disease may exist.
5. Immunoglobulin G levels are elevated, often associated with rheumatoid factor titers >1:32.
6. Anemia is present, possibly because of dilution. Thrombocytopenia is reported, and fibrinogen, factor VIII, and plasma activity may be acutely elevated.
7. BUN is elevated disproportionately to the se-

rum creatinine. Hyponatremia and hyperkalemia may be present, specifically related to the degree of oliguria.

8. Chest roentgenogram may show cardiomegaly and pulmonary congestion.

DIFFERENTIAL DIAGNOSIS (Chapter 37)

The diagnosis of poststreptococcal acute glomerulonephritis is established by the acute onset of edema, hypertension, and gross or microscopic hematuria with erythrocyte casts and proteinuria. There is evidence of an antecedent streptococcal infection, decreased complement, and spontaneous improvement in the renal disease and its complications. Other diagnoses should be considered when the clinical syndrome is aberrant, the renal failure is severe, the individual's age does not fall within the predicted range, or resolution is prolonged.

MANAGEMENT

The initial focus must be on management of complications and evaluation of the extent of renal injury.

Fluid overload

1. Fluid and salt are restricted to maintain normal intravascular volume.
2. Diuretics may be required.

Hypertension (Chapter 18)

1. Although a wide variety of drugs may be useful, the following are consistently effective:
   a. Diazoxide 1-3 mg/kg/dose q 6 hr IV (potent vasodilator)
   b. Furosemide (Lasix) 1-2 mg/kg/dose IV (diuretic)
2. For prolonged therapy, the following are given:
   a. Propranolol 1 mg/kg/dose q 6 hr PO
   b. Hydralazine 1-3 mg/kg/24 hr q 6 hr PO

DISPOSITION

1. All patients who have evidence of uncontrolled hypertension, congestive heart failure, or azotemia should be hospitalized. Children without any of these problems can be followed at home but must have adequate medical care available, including frequent blood pressure measurements.
2. A nephrologist should be involved in the child's care.

REFERENCE

Baldwin, D.S.: Poststreptococcal glomerulonephritis: a progressive disease? Am. J. Med. **62**:1, 1977.

Hemolytic-uremic syndrome

Hemolytic-uremic syndrome (HUS) normally is accompanied by nephropathy, microangiopathic hemolytic anemia, and thrombocytopenia following an episode of gastroenteritis or respiratory infection. It is primarily a disease of children, usually occurring before 5 yr of age. Although it rarely occurs in adults, it has been reported in women taking oral contraceptives and during the postpartum period. There is a familial predilection.

HUS results from localized intravascular coagulation and endothelial injury within the kidney. The prostacyclin/thromboxame (coagulation/anticoagulation) equilibrium is disturbed.

ETIOLOGY-INFECTION

1. Bacteria: *Shigella* and *Salmonella* organisms and group A streptococci
2. Virus: coxsackievirus, influenza, and respiratory syncytial virus (RSV)
3. Many other unspecified infections may trigger the disorder.

DIAGNOSTIC FINDINGS

1. Patients have a history of gastroenteritis with vomiting, bloody diarrhea, and crampy abdominal pain up to 2 wk preceding the onset of HUS. The absence of a gastrointestinal prodrome is associated with a poor prognosis. Some patients experience respiratory infections before the illness.

2. The spectrum of clinical disease is highly variable, ranging from mild elevation of BUN without anemia to severe, total anuria with marked anemia and thrombocytopenia.
3. Patients may have marked hypertension, pallor, petechiae and easy bruising, hepatosplenomegaly, and edema.
4. CNS findings are variably noted, including irritability and lethargy progressing to coma, seizures, and hemiparesis.

Complications

1. Recurrence, often without prodrome, and mortality rate of 30%
2. Renal failure, rarely progressing to end-stage renal disease
3. Bowel perforation or necrosis
4. Severe CNS findings including drowsiness, personality changes, and hemiparesis, progressing to cerebral infarction, seizures, and coma
5. High output cardiac failure from volume overload. Rare myocarditis

Ancillary data

1. Assessment of renal function (p. 616)
   a. Electrolytes (elevated K and acidosis may be present), BUN, creatinine, calcium (often low), and phosphorus (usually elevated)
   b. Urinalysis demonstrating hematuria and proteinuria
   c. In dehydration the BUN is often elevated and should decrease by 50% over the first 24 hr of appropriate rehydration. If fall does not occur, HUS should be considered.
2. Hematologic findings
   a. A low hemoglobin (Hb) is usually present with RBC demonstrating a microangiopathic hemolytic anemia with burr cells and fragments on peripheral smear.
   b. The WBC count usually is elevated.
   c. Platelets are often decreased below 50,000/mm^3.

d. Coagulation studies are normal. Minimal evidence for DIC with fibrin split products is rarely found.
3. ABG for evaluation of acidosis and potential hypoxia
4. Bacterial and viral cultures, when appropriate

DIFFERENTIAL DIAGNOSIS

1. Inflammation and infection
   a. Ulcerative colitis is accompanied by bloody diarrhea and anemia. The length of illness may provide information.
   b. Surgical abdomen secondary to infection, perforation, or necrosis may be difficult to distinguish.
   c. An acutely dehydrated patient with acute tubular necrosis may have some parallel characteristics.
2. Trauma may be associated with hematuria and anemia secondary to an acute blood loss.
3. Other causes of acquired hemolytic anemia (p. 152)

MANAGEMENT

1. The initial management, after establishing the diagnosis, should involve careful monitoring, assessing, and treating the volume status of the patient. Many patients develop volume overload associated with electrolyte abnormalities, hypertension, and high output failure.
2. Renal failure requires attention to fluids and, when appropriate, to treatment of hypertension, volume overload, hyperkalemia, acidosis, hypocalcemia, hyperphosphatemia, and other metabolic abnormalities (p. 615). Consultation should be obtained.
   • If a routine medical management is ineffective, peritoneal dialysis usually is done when there is hypervolemia with oliguria or anuria, >24 hr of anuria, unresponsive electrolyte abnormalities, and life-threatening hyperkalemia in a patient in whom more conservative management is contraindicated.

3. Hb <5-6 g/ml or an Hct <20% requires intervention, particularly if there is evidence of high output failure or hypoxia associated with the anemia. It is crucial to initially transfuse only a small amount of blood slowly (5 ml/kg over 4 hr) to minimize volume overload. Transfusion should not be given, if the patient is hyperkalemic, until dialysis is established. Blood should be as fresh as possible.

4. Platelets have a shortened survival time, and transfused platelets may contribute to platelet plugging in the renal microvasculature. Transfuse only if count is <10,000/mm^3 and evidence of life-threatening bleeding or peritoneal dialysis occurs.

5. Seizures are controlled with diazepam (Valium) 0.2-0.3 mg/kg/dose IV, repeated in 10 min as required if seizures continue. Phenobarbital or phenytoin should be initiated for maintenance therapy (Chapter 21).

6. Since the etiology of HUS may involve prostacyclin deficiency, infusion of fresh frozen plasma may be beneficial.

DISPOSITION

1. Patients normally should be hospitalized for evaluation and treatment.

2. Rarely, patients may be discharged home if there is no clinical evidence of disease (normal BP, CNS status, and volume) and there are only minimal laboratory abnormalities (mildly hemolytic smear and normal Hb, Hct, platelet count, BUN, and creatinine). If the patient is discharged, it is imperative to follow the patient (including laboratory parameters) to ensure that there is no progression of disease.

3. Given that siblings may get the disease, it is important that other household members be monitored as outpatients.

4. Long-term follow-up (1-2 yr) is indicated because of the possibility of delayed onset of renal failure and hypertension.

REFERENCES

Dolishager, D., and Tune, B.: The hemolytic uremic syndrome, Am. J. Dis. Child **132**:55, 1978.

Misiani, R.: Haemolytic uremic syndrome: therapeutic effect of plasma infusion, Br. Med. J. **285**:1304, 1982.

Henoch-Schönlein purpura

Henoch-Schönlein purpura (HSP) is an acute vasculitis of unknown etiology but associated with group A streptococcal, *Mycoplasma,* and viral (e.g., varicella, EB virus) infections; drugs (penicillin, tetracycline, aspirin, sulfonamides, and erythromycin); and allergens (insect bites, chocolate, milk, and wheat). It most commonly occurs in the winter months. A male predominance has been noted.

Multisystem involvement occurs primarily in children 2-11 yr of age with progression of renal disease occurring more commonly in older children and adults (children: 5%; adults: 13%-14%). Children under 3 mo commonly have only skin manifestations without gastrointestinal or renal involvement.

DIAGNOSTIC FINDINGS

1. Skin lesions are pathognomonic, beginning on the gravity-dependent areas of the legs and buttocks and the extensor surfaces of the arms. They begin as erythematous, maculopapular lesions that blanch and progress to become petechial and purpuric, at which time they are often palpable. They may be discrete, confluent, clustered, or individual. The entire body may be involved, although the lower extremities usually demonstrate the greatest eruption. A rash is the presenting symptom in 50% of patients. It may recur in 40% of patients within 6 wk, often without systemic signs.

2. Colicky abdominal pain with diarrhea, often bloody, is commonly present. Approximately 60%-85% of patients have melena or hematemesis. Intussusception or perforation must be considered.

3. Nephritis associated with hematuria, proteinuria, and other nephrosis may develop. Renal involvement may begin after other symptoms and requires ongoing follow-up.
4. Migratory polyarthritis, often transient, is present with greatest tenderness of ankles, knees, and wrist.
5. Other findings include soft tissue edema (scalp, ear, face, and dorsum of hands and feet), testicular pain, and parotitis.

Complications

1. Intussusception and abdominal distension
2. Severe renal involvement progressing to nephritis. Renal involvement is the ultimate determinant of outcome and long-term sequelae and increases with advancing age.
3. CNS presentations include mental status change, hemiparesis, seizures, and intracranial hemorrhage.

Ancillary data

1. CBC is variably elevated with left shift. Anemia may be present. Bleeding screen and platelet count are normal; ESR is elevated.
2. Urinalysis reflects the degree of renal involvement. Hematuria, proteinuria, leukocytosis, and cylinduria may be noted. If urinalysis is abnormal, other assessments of renal function are indicated.
3. Throat cultures for group A streptococci.
4. Blood cultures if bacteremia is diagnostic consideration.
5. Serum complement is normal.
6. Barium enema may be indicated to exclude intussusception if there is acute abdominal pain without evidence of perforation.
7. Renal biopsy is done in patients with severe nephropathy, following the acute phase of the illness.

DIFFERENTIAL DIAGNOSIS

1. Infections, particularly those associated with petechial and purpuric eruption (e.g., meningococcemia, Rocky Mountain spotted fever) (Table 42-1)

2. Thrombocytopenic purpura (platelet count should differentiate)
3. Nonthrombocytopenic purpura: Ehlers-Danlos syndrome, scurvy, massive steroid therapy, vasculitis
4. Glomerulonephritis (p. 607)
5. Intraabdominal pathology: intussusception, trauma, appendicitis (p. 494)

MANAGEMENT

1. Supportive care. If there is evidence of GI hemorrhage or hypovolemia, fluids and stabilization should be initiated.
   a. Management of renal disease if there is abnormal function
   b. Evaluation for intussusception with severe abdominal pain (p. 498)
   c. Exclusion of septicemic process
2. With significant GI pain and symptoms (once an acute abdomen is excluded), steroids may be useful: prednisone 1-2 mg/kg/24 hr q 12 hr PO for 1 wk. There is suggestive evidence that steroids play a beneficial role in soft tissue and joint swelling and glomerulonephritis, the latter requiring high-dose, pulsed therapy.
3. If acute renal failure or nephrosis is present, a nephrologist should be consulted. Specific attention must be given to the control of blood pressure and intake and output (p. 113).

DISPOSITION

The patient should be hospitalized for observation and treatment unless skin manifestations are the only problem and close outpatient follow-up is possible. A poor prognosis is associated with children under 6 yr, as well as the presence of nephrotic syndrome or crescent formation in the glomeruli.

REFERENCE

Hurley, R.M., and Drummond, K.N.: Anaphylactoid purpura nephritis: clinicopathological correlations, J. Pediatr. **81**:904, 1972.

Nephrotic syndrome

AILEEN B. SEDMAN

Massive proteinuria occurs secondary to increased glomerular permeability in nephrotic syndrome. Most commonly affecting children under 6 yr of age, it is marked by massive proteinuria, edema, hypoalbuminemia, and hyperlipidemia.

ETIOLOGY

1. Renal disorders
   a. Idiopathic or NIL disease
   b. Glomerular lesions (membranous glomerulopathy, focal glomerulosclerosis, membranoproliferative glomerulonephritis)
2. Intoxication: heroin, mercury, probenecid, silver
3. Allergic reactions
   a. Poison ivy or oak, pollens
   b. Bee sting
   c. Snake venom
   d. DPT immunization
4. Infection
   a. Bacterial
   b. Viral: hepatitis, cytomegalovirus, EB virus (infectious mononucleosis)
   c. Protozoa: malaria, toxoplasmosis
5. Neoplasm: Hodgkin's disease, Wilms' tumor etc.
6. Autoimmune disorders: Henoch-Schönlein purpura, systemic lupus erythematosus
7. Metabolic disorder: diabetes mellitus
8. Vascular disorders: congenital heart disease and congestive heart failure, pericarditis

DIAGNOSTIC FINDINGS

1. Patients often report flu-like syndrome and subsequent development of edema. Since infection often exacerbates nephrotic syndrome, the physician should always look for an infection in initial diagnosis or with patients who become unresponsive to steroids.
2. Blood pressure may be decreased if there is depletion of intravascular volume, or it may be increased with renal disease. Hypertension is usually mild and transient.
3. Patients have generalized peripheral edema and may have ascites with hepatomegaly.
4. Respiratory and cardiovascular status will reflect the extent of edema. Pleural effusion, pericardial effusion, pulmonary edema, and congestive heart failure may be present.

Complications

1. Infection. Patients are at increased risk of peritonitis and, if immunosuppressed, are susceptible to systemic infection. Septicemia, cellulitis, peritonitis, and pneumonitis are commonly caused by *S. pneumoniae*. They also are caused by *E. coli*, pseudomonas, and *H. influenzae*.
2. Renal failure
3. Protein malnutrition
4. Thromboembolism. Patients are hypercoagulable.
5. Relapse

Ancillary data (Figure 85-1)

1. WBC to evaluate for infection
2. Electrolytes, BUN, creatinine, calcium, and phosphorus. BUN and creatinine are elevated in 25% of children with minimal change nephrotic syndrome.
3. Triglycerides and cholesterol. Plasma cholesterol carriers (low-density lipoprotein [LDL] and very low-density lipoprotein) are increased. Elevated lipids result from increased synthesis, as well as defect in catabolism of phospholipid.
4. Hypoalbuminemia
5. Protein in 24 hr urine collection >3.5 g protein/1.73 m^2/24 hr. Creatinine clearance is normal. Spot protein/creatinine ratio >3.0
6. Serum complement (C_3) decreased
7. Tests to evaluate potential etiology. Include ASO titer
8. IVP or ultrasound to exclude renal anatomic abnormalities (with abnormal laboratory val-

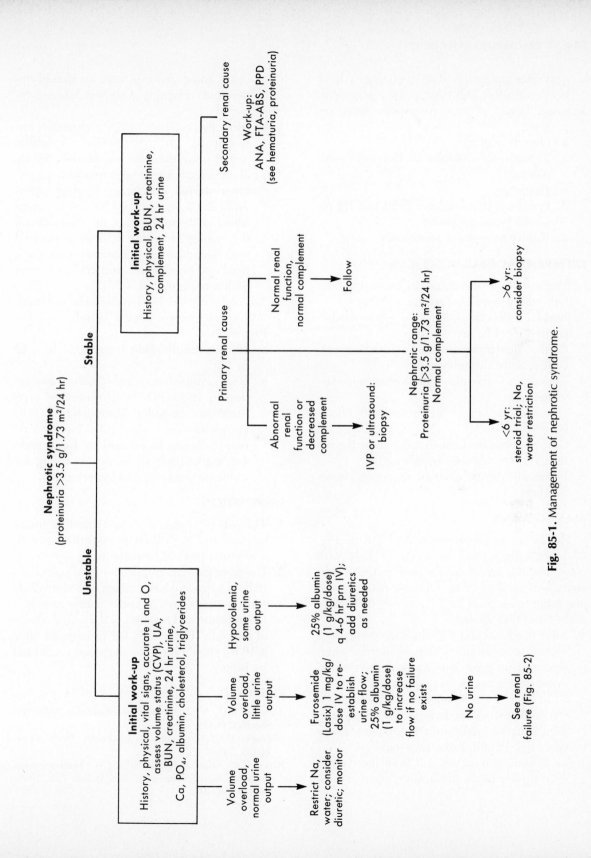

Fig. 85-1. Management of nephrotic syndrome.

ues) once patient is stable, etiologies have been evaluated, and volume status is normal.
9. Renal biopsy if poor prognostic signs are present:
   a. Over 6 yr of age
   b. Evidence of azotemia or decreased complement
   c. Hematuria
   d. Persistent hypertension (>90 mm Hg diastolic blood pressure)
   e. Failure to respond to steroids

DIFFERENTIAL DIAGNOSIS (Chapter 37)

Diagnostic considerations in evaluating the patient with generalized *edema* include:
1. Renal: nephrotic syndrome, glomerulonephritis, renal failure
2. Cardiovascular: congestive heart failure, vasculitis, acute thrombosis
3. Endocrine/metabolic: hypothyroidism, starvation
4. Hematologic: hemolytic disease of the newborn
5. Gastrointestinal: cirrhosis, protein-losing enteritis, cystic fibrosis, lymphangitis
6. Iatrogenic: drugs (steroids, diuretics), water overload

MANAGEMENT

The initial management is outlined in Fig. 85-1. Patients should be weighed daily with close monitoring of intake and output, vital signs, and renal function. Of those patients who are going to respond 73% do so within 14 days and 94% within 28 days.
1. After diagnosis and stabilization, the patient without complications (1-6 yr, normal complement, no gross hematuria, large protein urine loss) is begun on prednisone: 2 mg/kg/24 hr (maximum: 80 mg/24 hr) q 24 hr in AM PO until protein has disappeared from urine, then 2 mg/kg (maximum: 80 mg/dose) every other day PO for 2 mo, then tapered.
   a. If remission occurs and then the patient relapses, begin prednisone again and bi-

opsy. Some children may be steroid dependent, relapsing as steroid dosage is tapered.
   b. After two relapses or if the patient is unresponsive to prednisone, cytotoxic agents may then be considered. Subtle acute infection may be responsible for relative steroid resistance. Cyclophosphamide 2-2.5 mg/kg/24 hr for 2-4 mo combined with prednisone; or chlorambucil 0.2 mg/kg/24 hr for 5-15 wk combined with low-dose prednisone currently are used and may be initiated in consultation with a nephrologist.
2. Salt and water restriction should be initiated. Additional therapy usually is indicated (see Fig. 85-1):
   a. Hydrochlorothiazide 1 mg/kg/24 hr q 12 hr PO
   b. If no results: furosemide (Lasix) 1 mg/kg/dose q 12 hr PO. With continued poor response, consider administering salt-poor human albumin 1 g/kg/dose over 60 min, followed in 30 min by furosemide 1-2 mg/kg/dose IV while observing for pulmonary edema and hypertension.

DISPOSITION

1. The patient should be hospitalized for initial workup and evaluation in consultation with a nephrologist. Most patients do very well.
2. Unstable patients require hospitalization until fluid balance is determined and controlled.
3. Most patients have minimal-change nephrotic syndrome and respond to the initial course of steroids. Those who fail to respond after 4-10 wk should have the diagnosis confirmed by biopsy.

REFERENCES

Adelman, R.D.: Nephrotic syndrome, Contemp. Issues Nephrology **12**:191, 1984.
Glassock, B.J.: The nephrotic syndrome, Hosp. Pract. **14**:105, 1979.
Rance, C.P., Arbus, G.S., and Balfe, J.W.: Management of the nephrotic syndrome in children, Pediatr. Clin. North Am. **23**:735, 1976.

Acute renal failure

AILEEN B. SEDMAN

Acute renal failure occurs when there is a sudden impairment of the kidneys' ability to regulate urine volume and composition to maintain homeostasis. Once diagnosed, it is imperative that the cause be delineated rapidly to facilitate implementation of appropriate therapeutic steps. It may be prerenal (decreased perfusion of the kidney), intrarenal (damage to the actual nephron), or postrenal (downstream obstruction of the urinary tract).

ETIOLOGY

See Table 85-1.

DIAGNOSTIC FINDINGS

1. The history can provide some clue regarding the etiology of renal failure.
   a. Prerenal patients have a history of decreased perfusion of the kidney. This may include dehydration from vomiting, diarrhea, diabetic ketoacidosis, decreased intravascular volume secondary to nephrotic syndrome, burns, or shock resulting from hemorrhage, sepsis, cardiac failure, or anaphylaxis.
   b. Intrarenal failure results from direct nephron damage occurring in glomerulonephritis (hematuria, proteinuria, edema, and hypertension), HUS (anemia, uremia, and thrombocytopenia), nephro-

TABLE 85-1. Common causes of acute renal failure

Prerenal (decreased perfusion of an intact nephron)	Intrarenal (damage to the actual nephron)	Postrenal (downstream obstruction with initially intact nephron*)

Shock: hypovolemic
  Dehydration
  Hemorrhagic
  Diabetic ketoacidosis
  Burn
Shock: distributive
  Septic
  Anaphylactic
Shock: cardiogenic
Nephrotic syndrome with intravascular volume depletion from decreased oncotic pressure
Renal vessel injury of obstruction
	Glomerulonephritis
	  Acute postinfectious (including bacterial, viral, secondary endocarditis or shunt infections)
	  Hemolytic-uremic syndrome
	  Membranoproliferative
	  Henoch-Schönlein purpura
	  Goodpasture's syndrome (anti–glomerular basement membrane)
	  Lupus erythematosus
	Acute tubular necrosis caused by prolonged decreased perfusion
	Nephrotoxins: aminoglycosides, cephalosporins, methicillin, phenytoin, radiocontrast materials, heavy metals
	Rhabdomyolysis: pigment damage to nephron
	Neoplasms
		Posterior urethral valves
		Ureteropelvic junction abnormality
		Stones
		Crystals
		  Sulfonamides
		  Uric acid
		Retroperitoneal fibrosis or tumor
		Trauma to collecting system
		Ureterocele

*Prolonged obstruction eventually leads to irreversible nephron damage.

toxic exposures, massive crush injuries, overwhelming infection, or DIC.

   c. Obstruction leads to postrenal failure and may be accompanied by abdominal and flank pain, although the blockage may be insidious without symptoms.

2. Physical examination can reflect the underlying renal and fluid abnormality:

   a. Hypovolemia (hypotension or orthostatic changes and tachycardia)

   b. Volume overload (increased blood pressure, edema, congestive heart failure)

   c. Obstruction (increased kidney size or large bladder)

3. Patients may be oliguric (urine output <1 ml/kg/hr) or nonoliguric with a volume inappropriate to maintain hemostasis. Azotemia (increase in plasma concentration of nitrogenous waste products, i.e., BUN and creatinine) is present.

Complications

1. Fluid overload with associated congestive heart failure
2. Hypertension from fluid overload or inappropriate renin production
3. Azotemia with elevated potassium, BUN, and creatinine

4. Dysrrhythmias
5. Hypocalcemia and high phosphorus, leading to cardiac dysrhythmias, tetany, and altered mental status
6. Acidosis from diminished H^+ secretion by kidney
7. Hyperphosphatemia and high $Ca^{++} \times PO_4^{--}$ product (>70 when Ca^{++} mg/dl $\times$ PO_4^{--} mg/dl) can produce calcification in soft tissues and reciprocal hypocalcemia.
8. Altered level of consciousness, seizures, and coma from metabolic derangements (e.g., elevated BUN and potassium and decreased Ca^{++}), cerebral edema, and hypertension
9. Bleeding secondary to platelet dysfunction associated with uremia. Anemia. Platelets low in HUS

Ancillary data

1. Electrolytes, Ca^{++}, PO_4^{--}, BUN and creatinine, CBC, and platelets
2. ECG and cardiac monitor
3. Combining data from serum, urine, and ultrasonography: best method for differentiating among prerenal, intrarenal, and postrenal failure:

Prerenal	Intrarenal	Postrenal
Ultrasound: normal	Ultrasound: can have increased renal density or slight swelling	Ultrasound: dilated bladder or kidney
Serum BUN to creatinine ratio >15:1		History and exam may be diagnostic
Urine Na^+ <15 mEq/L	Urine Na^+ >20 mEq/L	Indexes not helpful
Urine osmolality >400 mOsm	Urine osmolality <350 mOsm	
Urine to plasma creatinine ratio >14:1	Urine to plasma creatinine ratio <14:1 (often <5:1)	
Fractional excretion of Na^+ <1 (<2.5 in neonates)	Fractional excretion of Na^+ >3 (>2.5 in neonates)	

$$\text{Fractional excretion of } Na^+ = \frac{\text{Urine } Na^+ \text{ mEq/L}}{\text{Plasma } Na^+ \text{ mEq/L}} \times \frac{\text{Plasma creatinine mg/dl}}{\text{Urine creatinine mg/dl}} \times 100$$

4. Creatinine clearance. A good measure of glomerular filtration rate and particularly helpful in monitoring children with renal disease. A 24 hr urine collection is needed.

$$\text{Creatinine clearance (ml/min/1.73 m}^2) = \frac{UV}{P} \times \frac{1.73}{SA}$$

where

U = Urinary concentration of creatinine (mg/dl)

V = Volume of urine divided by the number of minutes in collection period (24 hr = 1440 min) (ml/min)

P = Plasma concentration of creatinine (mg/dl)

SA = Surface area (m²)

a. Normal newborn and premature: 40-65 ml/min/1.73 m²

b. Normal child: 109 ml (female) or 124 ml (male)/min/1.73 m²

c. Adult: 95 ml (female) or 105 ml (male)/min/1.73 m²

5. Single voided urine samples in adults have been of some use in assessing renal function. In patients with stable renal function, a spot protein/creatinine ratio of >3.0 can represent nephrotic range proteinuria; a ratio of <0.2 is normal. This may be particularly useful in monitoring patients; however diagnostic confirmation should be done by the traditional methods outlined in 4.

MANAGEMENT

Initial stabilization must focus on determining the etiology and classification of the acute renal failure to permit appropriate therapeutic intervention. The initial approach is outlined in Fig. 85-2. Intake and urine output must be measured closely. A catheter (6 mo: 8 Fr; 1-2 yr: 10 Fr; 5 yr: 10-12 Fr; 8-10 yr: 12 Fr) is usually necessary.

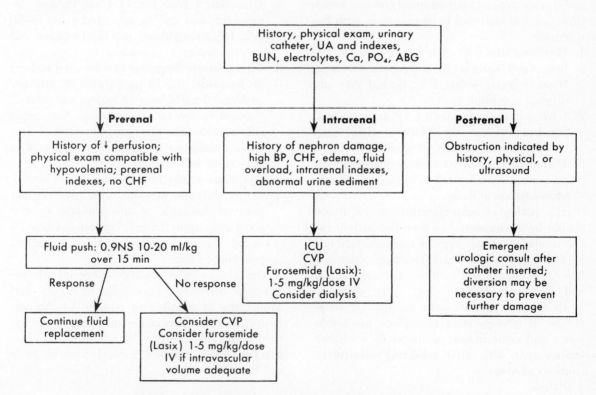

Fig. 85-2. Acute renal failure: initial assessment and treatment.

Fluid balance

Furosemide

Furosemide (Lasix) is the most potent diuretic available and should be given if the intravascular volume is adequate or overloaded according to CVP measurements.

1. Give 1-6 mg/kg/dose q 2-6 hr IV (high dose to be used if creatinine is >2 mg/dl)
2. If there is no response after two doses at maximum amount, do not continue because of potential nephrotoxicity and ototoxicity.
3. Do not give if there is evidence of obstruction.
4. A good response to diuretics is the formation of 6-10 ml/kg of urine over the subsequent 1-3 hr.

Mannitol

Mannitol may be useful if there is no response to furosemide in patients with prerenal failure and if response can be monitored closely. Some clinicians use mannitol in combination with furosemide.

1. Give mannitol 0.75 g/kg/dose q 6 hr IV. Infuse over 3-5 min at rate of ≤5 g/min. If there is no response within 2 hr, do not give additional mannitol.
2. Give only to patient with CVP line in place, because of risk of severe fluid overload, pulmonary edema, and hyperosmolality.
3. Do not give if there is evidence of obstruction or acute renal failure of an intrarenal nature.

Administration of fluids

If the patient remains oliguric or anuric, fluids should be administered to keep the patient intravascularly normal. Replace insensible (30 ml/kg/24 hr) and extraordinary (vomiting, diarrhea, fever, etc.) losses and maintain normoglycemia and metabolic balance (e.g., give calcium, $NaHCO_3$). In patients with nonoliguric renal failure, it is imperative to replace insensible losses and urine output (milliliter for milliliter replacement with fluid reflecting electrolyte contents of urine).

Dialysis

Rapid referral for dialysis is mandatory for those patients with severe fluid overload or metabolic derangement who do not respond to diuretic therapy.

Hypertension (Chapter 18)

Hypertension may be caused by fluid overload or high renin secretion. Any child having acute hypertension with a diastolic pressure >100 mm Hg should be treated parenterally because of the risk of seizures, encephalopathy, and other sequelae of hypertension. Only a mild reduction in pressure is needed in an acute situation, often to the range of 90-100 mm Hg.

Parenteral therapy

Parenteral therapy should be given sequentially, with observation for a response.

1. Furosemide (Lasix) 1 mg/kg/dose q 2-6 hr IV facilitates action of vasodilators by volume contraction.
2. Diazoxide (Hyperstat) 1-3 mg/kg/dose by rapid infusion may be repeated every 30-60 min. It is a vasodilator, and fluid infusion will reverse severe hypotension.
3. Nitroprusside (Nipride) may be used instead of diazoxide: 0.5-10 µg/kg/min IV infusion (average: 3 µg/kg/min). A potent vasodilator, it requires constant monitoring. Nitroprusside provides the most exact method of controlling malignant hypertension because of its very short half-life.
4. Hydralazine may be used if a slower acting, longer duration vasodilator is preferred in place of diazoxide or nitroprusside: 0.1-0.2 mg (rarely up to 0.5 mg)/kg/dose q 4-6 hr IV or IM. Use in combination with diazoxide to potentiate effect.

The choice of medication depends on urgency of treatment, knowledge of agents, and availability of monitoring equipment. Vasodilators may eventually cause compensatory tachycardia and may require the addition of a beta-blocker like propranolol (Inderal) 1 mg/kg/24 hr q 6 hr PO.

Hyperkalemia

Hyperkalemia causes membrane excitability with possible cardiac dysrhythmias. K^+ >6.5 mEq/L can cause ECG changes consisting of peaked T waves and, eventually, widened QRS complex. Cardiac toxicity is enhanced by hypocalcemia, hyponatremia, acidosis, or rapid change.

Potassium

Potassium >7.0 mEq/L requires rapid intervention in the following sequence:

1. Calcium chloride 10% 0.2-0.3 ml (20-30 mg)/kg/dose (maximum: 5 ml or 500 mg/dose) IV slowly over 5-10 min monitoring for bradycardia
   a. It changes the cell-action potential protecting the heart from dysrhythmias.
   b. It can be repeated up to four times or until serum calcium increases.
   c. Its effect lasts about 30 min.
2. $NaHCO_3$
   a. Alkalosis helps to exchange H^+ for K^+, thereby moving potassium intracellularly and normalizing membrane potential.
   b. $NaHCO_3$ 1-2 mEq/kg/dose IV push q 2-4 hr or as required by pH is useful in emergent situations (as well as in combination with kayexalate for asymptomatic hyperkalemia ([K^+ <6.5 mEq/L]).
3. Glucose and insulin (to move K^+ intracellularly)
   a. Give glucose 0.5-1.0 g/kg followed by 1 unit of insulin IV for every 4 g of glucose infused; may repeat q 10-30 min.
   b. Monitor Dextrostix/Chemstrip tests and glucose carefully. The effect lasts 1-3 hr.
4. Kayexalate (an ion exchange resin). Give 1 g resin/kg/dose q 4-6 hr preferably mixed with 70% sorbitol PO (may use NG tube) or PR. For newborn give 1 g/kg/dose with kayexalate dissolved in 10% dextrose to make 25% solution.
   a. It is useful in combination with $NaHCO_3$ for K^+ <6.5 mEq/L.
   b. It may cause hypocalcemia and hypomagnesemia, gastric irritation, and diarrhea.

Metabolic acidosis

Give $NaHCO_3$ 1-2 mEq/kg/dose q ½-6 hr IV push as indicated by ABG, exercising care to avoid fluid overload. Substitute $NaHCO_3$ for NaCl in IV fluids.

NOTE: If severe acidosis and fluid overload are present, rapid dialysis is mandatory.

Hyponatremia

Hyponatremia usually is secondary to water overload. Water intake should be restricted to insensible plus extraordinary losses.

Hyperphosphatemia

Aluminum hydroxide antacids (Amphojel or Basaljel) 10-30 ml q 1-4 hr PO or NG should be given. Aluminum is potentially toxic and should be used only for short-term therapy.

Rapid dialysis (peritoneal or hemodialysis)

Indications are:
1. Fluid overload with congestive heart failure
2. Severe hyperkalemia
3. Severe hyponatremia or hypernatremia
4. Unresponsive metabolic acidosis, particularly with fluid overload
5. BUN >80-100 mg/dl
6. Uremia producing alteration in consciousness or seizures

Technology has made dialysis possible for even the smallest child.

Other considerations

An intravenous pyelogram should not be done in an individual with renal failure because of the risk of nephrotoxicity from the dye. Ultrasound and renal scans are preferable for initial evaluation.

DISPOSITION

All patients require hospitalization and a nephrology consultation.

REFERENCES

Fine, R.N.: Peritoneal dialysis update, J. Pediatr. **100**:1, 1982.

Ginsberg, J.M., Chang, B.S., Matarese, R.A., et al.: Use of single voided urine samples to estimate quantitative proteinuria, N. Engl. J. Med. **309**:1543, 1983.

Gordillo-Paniqua, G., and Velasquez-Jones, L.: Acute renal failure, Pediatr. Clin. North Am. **23**:817, 1976.

Siegel, N.J.: Acute renal failure, Contemp. Issues Nephrology **17**:297, 1984.

Urinary tract infection

ALERT: Symptoms often are nonspecific. A high index of suspicion is required, combined with appropriate cultures, treatment, and follow-up.

Urinary tract infections (UTI) range from being asymptomatic to causing systemic disease associated with pyelonephritis.

ETIOLOGY: INFECTION

Bacteria causing the majority of infections are normal rectal and perineal flora, including *Escherichia coli*, *Klebsiella* organisms, enteric streptococci, and, rarely, *Staphylococcus aureus* or *epidermidis*.

Uncommonly, viral, fungal, and mycobacterial agents are causative.

DIAGNOSTIC FINDINGS

Predisposing factors include poor perineal hygiene, the short urethra of females, infrequent voiding, and sexual activity. Females have a higher incidence. Males with UTI have a high incidence of anatomic pathology.

Symptoms in younger children are often nonspecific.

1. Neonates may have fever or hypothermia, poor feeding, failure to thrive, jaundice, sepsis, or cyanosis.
2. Infants may experience vomiting, diarrhea, fever, and poor feeding.

3. Older children have the more classic signs and symptoms of fever, abdominal pain, vomiting, enuresis, and urinary frequency, dysuria, and urgency.

Systemic toxicity accompanied by high temperatures, chills, and variably, costovertebral angle (CVA) pain usually accompany upper urinary tract disease and *pyelonephritis*. Often there is increased warmth over the involved kidney.

Historically, it is important to ascertain if the patient has had previous episodes of infection. The physical examination should determine if there is evidence of genitourinary malformations, hypertension, or poor growth.

Complications

1. Chronic renal failure secondary to recurrent pyelonephritis
2. Bacteremia
3. Perinephric abscess
4. Sepsis

Ancillary data

Urine culture

Urine culture is the basis for making the diagnosis. In asymptomatic or minimally ill patients, a clean catch midstream specimen (CCMS) should be obtained after carefully cleaning the perineum and uretha. In patients who are toxic, specimens should be obtained by suprapubic aspiration (Appendix A-7) or a straight catheterization. In younger children the catheterization may be done by using a no. 5 Fr sterile feeding tube. The first 5 ml of urine is discarded and the remainder cultured. Bag urine is not satisfactory for adequate diagnosis.

1. The specimen must be cultured within 30 min or placed in a refrigerator. If not, the colony count may be elevated but is not reliable.
2. The interpretation of the culture varies with the method of collection.

Collection method	Colony forming units/ml		
	Uninfected	Uninterpretable	Infected
Suprapubic	<10		≥10
Straight catheter	<10^3		≥10^3
CCMS	<10^3	10^3-10^5	≥10^5
Bag	<10^3	10^3-10^5	≥10^5

Cultures that are uninterpretable need to be repeated. Dilution (e.g., specimens that are not first morning void) or improper medium may lower the colony count. Other causes of low colony counts include recent antimicrobial therapy, fastidious organisms, bacteriostatic agents in urine, and complete obstruction of the ureter.

Urinalysis

Urinalysis is a useful diagnostic tool but not definitive.

1. Pyuria (>5 WBC/HPF) is present in over half of patients with UTI.
2. Causes of pyuria besides UTI include chemical (bubble bath) or physical (masturbation) irritation, other irritation, dehydration, renal tuberculosis, trauma, acute glomerulonephritis, respiratory infections, appendicitis, other abdominal and pelvic infections, gastroenteritis, and administration of oral polio vaccine.

Radiologic studies

These rarely are emergently indicated unless there is severe toxicity or evidence of obstruction. Those children who require radiologic evaluation 4-6 wk after UTI include:

1. Children under 1 yr of age
2. Males (increased association with anomaly)
3. Clinical signs and symptoms consistent with pyelonephritis
4. Clinical evidence of renal disease (e.g., high blood pressure, BUN, or creatinine)
5. After the second documented lower tract UTI in females, although some authorities recommend that these patients should be studied after the first infection

The optimal approach to evaluation remains controversial. Traditionally, patients have had an IVP and voiding cystourethrography (VCU). More recently, ultrasonography has been used as the initial procedure, evaluating for size, location, and associated anomalies. If the sonogram is normal, a VCU is done to evaluate for vesicoureteral reflux. If the ultrasound is abnormal, an IVP and a VCU should be done.

Blood cultures

These are indicated in the febrile, toxic patient.

Blood creatinine and urea nitrogen

These should be obtained in patients with evidence of pyelonephritis, recurrent infections, or hypertension.

DIFFERENTIAL DIAGNOSIS

1. Trauma. Chemical (bubble bath) or physical (masturbation or perineal injury) irritation may cause discomfort.
2. Infection
   a. Viral, mycobacterial, and fungal agents may cause similar symptoms with associated pyuria. Culture techniques need to be specific for these organisms.
   b. Vaginitis may cause irritation with comparable symptoms.
   c. Pinworms may cause perineal pain secondary to both inflammation and itching.
   d. *Urethritis* caused by *Neisseria gonorrhoeae* or *Chlamydia trachomatis* often is associated with a discharge. It may cause dysuria, supra pubic discomfort, and, in the male, prostatic or rectal tenderness (p. 511).

MANAGEMENT

1. The first step in management is to have a high index of suspicion. When UTI is suspected, an appropriate urine culture should be obtained. Suprapubic or catheterized specimens are indicated for moderately ill patients. A CCMS specimen for the minimally ill individual is appropriate and, if abnormal, should be repeated.

2. A UA should be done. If normal, urine should be sent for culture. If pyuria or bacteriuria are found, the specimen should be sent for culture and the appropriate medication initiated.

3. A **lower urinary tract** infection (cystitis) commonly has associated urinary symptoms of urgency, frequency, and dysuria. Appropriate management is to push fluids initially and to begin antibiotics:
   a. Amoxicillin 30-50 mg/kg/24 hr q 8 hr PO **or**
   b. Sulfisoxazole (Gantrisin) 120-150 mg/kg/24 hr q 6 hr PO **or**
   c. Trimethoprim (TMP) with sulfamethoxazole (SMZ) 8 mg TMP and 40 mg SMZ/kg/24 q 12 hr PO **or**
   d. Cephalexin (Keflex) 25-50 mg/kg/24 hr q 6 hr PO
   NOTE: There is conflicting data about the efficacy of single-dose therapy, and it cannot at present be recommended without further substantiation of its efficacy in both short-term treatment and long-term recurrences.

4. **Pyelonephritis** has associated systemic toxicity (temperature, chills, CVA tenderness) and requires broader coverage antibiotics. Until cultures and sensitivities are available (24-48 hr), a combination of one of the drugs in 3 used in treating lower tract infection; **and** gentamicin *or* tobramycin 5.0-7.5 mg/kg/24 hr q 8-12 hr IM or IV should be given. For the patient with only moderate toxicity who is to be followed as an outpatient, administration of gentamicin 1.5-2.0 mg/kg/dose (maximum: 80 mg/dose) IM once, in combination with continuing oral therapy provides sufficient treatment pending isolation and determination of sensitivities in 24-48 hr. Those requiring hospitalization should be treated with standard parenteral daily doses.

5. If urinary dysuria, urgency, or frequency are predominant symptoms, temporary relief can be obtained with phenazopyridine (Pyridium), a urinary tract analgesic, at 12 mg/kg/24 hr orally in three doses q 8 hr up to 200 mg/dose. Urine will turn orange.

6. Follow-up should be ensured in 48 hr to determine if the patient is clinically improved and that the etiologic organism is sensitive to the medication. If there is any question, a repeat UA and urine culture should be obtained. Medication may need to be altered.

7. The patient should return in 14 days after a total course of antibiotics of 10 days for a repeat UA and culture. Close follow-up over the next year is appropriate because of the increased risk of recurrence. The greater the number of previous episodes, the more likely the infection will recur. In the first year the chance of recurrence is as high as 50%.

DISPOSITION

1. Patients who are toxic, pregnant, or compromised hosts; who are unable to maintain hydration or retain medications; or who have debilitating systemic disease sould be hospitalized. In addition, those with previous renal disease associated with impaired function, foreign bodies (catheter), or stones should be hospitalized. Other criteria that should be considered include the likelihood of resistant organisms, failure on previous outpatient therapy, prevous pyelonephritis within 30 days, and the reliability of the patient.

2. Most patients may be followed at home with appropriate antibiotic therapy. Compliance must be ensured and follow-up arranged in 1-2 days.
   a. High-risk patients should be evaluated radiologically.
   b. Patients with recurrent UTI should be referred to a urologist.

Parental education

1. Give all of the medication. Call physician if your child does not tolerate medication.

2. A urine culture has been obtained. In 2 days you should contact your care provider to be sure that your child is taking the correct medicine and feeling better.
3. Two weeks after your initial visit, your care giver will want to see your child again for another culture. Periodic checks will be made over the next year.
4. To help prevent repeat infections, particularly in girls, try the following.
   a. Teach her to wipe correctly from front to back.
   b. Do *not* use bubble baths or let the soap float around in the bath.
   c. Minimize constipation.
   d. Encourage frequent urination.
5. Call physician if
   a. Fever or pain with urination is not gone in 48 hr after beginning antibiotics.
   b. Your child gets worse or does not tolerate medication.

REFERENCES

Adelman, K.D.: Urinary tract infections in children, Contemp. Issues Nephrology **12**:155, 1984.

Bergstrom, T., Larson, H., Lincoln, K., et al.: Studies of urinary tract infections in infancy and childhood. XII. Eighty consecutive patients with neonatal infection, J. Pediatr. **80**:858, 1972.

Durbin, W.A., and Peter, G.: Management of urinary tract infections in infants and children, Pediatr. Inf. Dis. **3**:564, 1984.

Fine, J.S., and Jacobson, M.S.: Single-dose versus conventional therapy of urinary tract infections in female adolescents, Pediatrics **75**:916, 1985.

Ginsburg, C.M., and McCracken, G.H.: Urinary tract infections in young infants, Pediatrics **69**:409, 1982.

Margileth, A.M., Pedreira, F.A., Hirschman, G.H., et al.: Urinary tract infection, Pediatr. Clin. North Am. **23**:721, 1976.

Stahl, G.E., Topf, P., Fleisher, G.R., et al.: Single dose treatment of uncomplicated urinary tract infections in children, Ann. Emerg. Med. **13**:705, 1984.

Todd, J.K.: Urinary tract infections in children and adolescents, Postgrad. Med. **60**:225, 1976.

APPENDIX A Procedures

Several procedures are unique to the pediatric patient. Others are done infrequently and require some familiarity with the crucial landmarks. The descriptions included in this section are not meant to be inclusive but to serve as reminders of important aspects of techniques to those individuals who have had experience performing them in a supervised setting that included direct observation and instruction. The section is not intended to be a training manual for practitioners without previous experience in invasive procedures. Consents should be obtained when appropriate but should not delay life-saving procedures.

Preparing a child for a procedure may facilitate the process and must be related to the child's age, developmental status, and ability to understand. Initially determine what the parents know about the procedure and what they have told the child. When appropriate explain the procedure rather than offering choices, especially if there are no choices. Encourage the child to ask questions while presenting small amounts of information at a time. Describe the procedure in terms of what the child will feel, taste, see, or smell while making the child as comfortable as possible. Appeal to older toddlers (2-4 yr), who desire to please, by encouraging them to help or assist with the Band-Aid.

Appendix A-1: Arterial punctures

Arterial punctures are used routinely to obtain heparinized blood for ABG determinations. Most laboratories can make the determina-
tion with <1 ml of heparinized blood. A tuberculin syringe is filled with heparin that is then squirted out, allowing a small amount to remain in the hub. A 25-gauge needle is used in newborns and infants. The site is identified and prepared before puncture. After withdrawal of the needle, pressure should be applied to the site for at least 5 min.

1. The radial artery is the preferred site because of its stability and lack of an accompanying vein. It is entered tangentially with the artery being localized by placing fingers proximal and distal to the point of entry (Fig. A-1).
2. The brachial artery may be entered at its most superficial point at the median side of the antecubital fossa.
3. The superficial temporal artery is useful in the infant. The overlying hair is shaved, the area prepared, and the artery located and immobilized by one finger while the puncture is made, often with a scalp-vein needle in place of a straight needle.

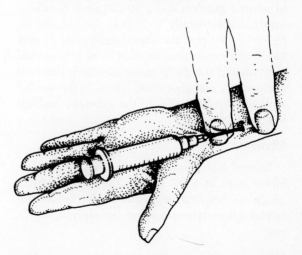

FIG. A-1. Localization of radial artery for puncture.

Other sites include:
1. The dorsalis pedis on the dorsum of the foot
2. The posterior tibial artery located between the medial malleolus and the Achilles tendon
3. The femoral artery, which should be used only in life-threatening situations

Appendix A-2: Arthrocentesis

Arthrocentesis is essential in excluding infection in a joint that is acutely swollen or painful or that has limited range of motion.

SITE AND POSITION
Knee

The patient is placed on his or her back with the knee fully extended. The needle (18-gauge) is passed laterally or medially beneath the midpoint of the patella so that it enters the knee joint midway between the patella and the patellar grove of the femur.

Ankle

The ankle is approached either medially or laterally, reflecting the area of maximal swelling. For those with lateral swelling, the foot is placed in neutral position and a 20-22 gauge needle is inserted horizontally 1 cm both medial and inferior to the tip of the lateral malleolus. Medial swelling also requires the foot to be in a neutral position and the 20-22 gauge needle is directed horizontally just above and lateral to the medial malleolus, just medial to the extensor hallucis longus tendon.

Elbow

Lateral aspiration is done by positioning the elbow joint at a 90° angle. The needle (20-22 gauge) is inserted perpendicularly, below the lateral epicondyle and above the olecranon process.

Hip

Arthrocentesis usually is done by an orthopedic consultant.

PROCEDURE

Aseptic technique is essential. The area should be shaved (if necessary) and the skin prepared with a povidine-iodine scrub followed by cleansing with an alcohol scrub. The procedure is not routinely done in the presence of overlying cellulitis or a coagulation disorder.

Anesthetic agents (1%-2% lidocaine) are infiltrated into the skin with a 23-25 gauge needle. A new bottle of anesthetic agent should be used to ensure sterility.

A large 18 gauge needle normally should be attached to a 5-10 ml syringe for aspiration of large joints (20-22 gauge for smaller joint). If large amounts of fluid are anticipated, the syringe may be attached to a stopcock and a larger syringe attached once free flow is established. Negative pressure usually is maintained.

COMPLICATIONS

Bleeding within the joint or in the subperiosteum may occur, as may infection. Strict aseptic technique must be maintained.

FLUID ANALYSIS (Table 82-1)

Fluid obtained by arthrocentesis should always be analyzed completely. This analysis should include:
1. Cell count
2. Gram's stain and culture, both aerobic and anaerobic
3. Protein and glucose
4. Examination for crystals (monosodium urate or calcium pyrophosphate dihydrate)
5. Mucin clot

Appendix A-3: Intravenous infusion

Obtaining venous access in the pediatric patient requires familiarity with potential sites and techniques, as well as expertise and patience. The choice of technique may require modification because of the nature of the injury or illness and the patient's condition, size, and fluid requirements.

PERIPHERAL VEIN PERCUTANEOUS PUNCTURE
Site

Peripherally, the preferred sites are the antecubital vein, veins on the dorsa of the hand and foot, and, in the child under 2 yr of age, the scalp. The external jugular (p. 629) or femoral vein also may be used.

Position

1. The patient is immobilized to the extent necessary. For smaller children a papoose board may be useful.
2. Extremities require careful immobilization with tape (Fig. A-3, *A*). Hands may be better positioned if a small amount of cotton or gauze is placed under the wrist when using veins on the dorsum of the hand.

Preparation

1. Cleanse the area to be entered.
2. Shave the area if necessary, e.g., the head.

Tourniquet

1. Apply a tourniquet proximal to the point of venous access.
2. On the head a rubber band may serve as the tourniquet. Place a small amount of tape at one point on the rubber band to facilitate removal of the tourniquet (Fig. A-3, *B*).

Needles and cannulas

The choice is based on personal preference.
1. *Scalp vein needle.* May be used in all areas except for veins overlying joints. The inherent problem is the lack of true stability of the needle after it is inserted.
   a. Before inserting the needle, flush with saline, leaving the syringe attached until the skin is punctured. Once the skin is entered, remove the syringe to permit a flashback on entering the vein.
   b. Insert the needle tangentially through the skin approximately 1 cm distal to the point of vein entry. Grasp the needle by the winged tabs. Advance the needle gently

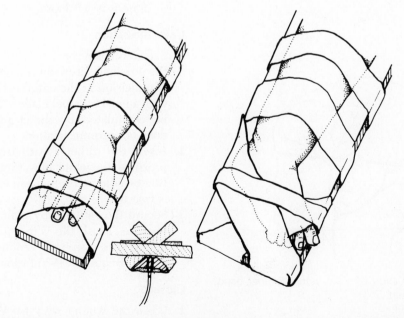

FIG. A-3, A. Immobilization of extremity for percutaneous venous puncture. Scalp-vein needle taping.

until the vein is entered and a flashback is visible. Unless the vein is large, do not thread the needle further.

   c. Place a 1 cm wide tape over the needle at the point of entry to provide initial stabilization, and loop a second piece around the winged tabs.

   d. Intermittently flush the needle to ensure patency and position.

   e. Tape the needle carefully to minimize movement. Placement of a half medicine cup with the edges taped provides additional protection.

2. *Over-the-needle or through-the-needle catheter.* Inserted according to manufacturer's directions. Remember that once a flashback is noted in the over-the-needle catheter, the needle should be inserted 1-3 mm more to ensure that it is well in the vein.

Intravenous infusion

An IV infusion set should be attached after the patient is stabilized. In children under 5 yr of age, there should always be a volume-limiting device such as a Buretrol in line to avoid excessive fluid administration.

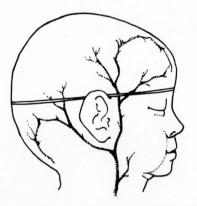

FIG. A-3, B. Location of scalp veins. Rubber band used for tourniquet.

VENOUS CUTDOWN
Site

The greater saphenous vein is located anterior to the medial malleolus and medial to the anterior tibial tendon.

Position

The foot is immobilized with careful visualization of the malleolus.

Procedure

1. After cleansing, draping, and infiltrating locally with 1% lidocaine, apply a tourniquet.
2. Make a l cm transverse incision perpendicular to the vein, usually one fingerbreadth above and one fingerbreadth anterior to the medial malleolus.
3. Bluntly dissect down to the tibia in the direction parallel to the vein and identify the vein. Free the vein, and place two 3-0 Vicryl or silk sutures loosely around it.
   a. The distal suture is ligated to control venous return.
   b. The proximal suture is tied after the venous catheter has been placed. At this time it is left loose.

Catheterization

1. Select the appropriate size catheter. Using the proximal suture for traction, make a small flap incision in the anterior third of the vein with a no. 11 scalpel blade. The vein also can be cannulated by direct puncture, which does not require ligation.
2. Insert the catheter with traction from the proximal tie while elevating the vein flap. Remove the tourniquet and ensure that there is free flow.
3. Secure the catheter by tightening the proximal tie. Flush the vein with 1-2 ml of 1% lidocaine to overcome venous spasm, if necessary. Begin the IV infusion.

Closure

1. Close the wound with 4-0 Vicryl or Dexon sutures (some prefer silk or nylon), and fur-

ther secure the catheter by looping the IV tubing around the patient's great toe.

2. Cover with sterile dressing.

EXTERNAL JUGULAR VEIN
Site

The external jugular vein is easily accessible in children whose necks are not unduly short or obese. The vein courses from the angle of the mandible to the middle of the clavicle over the sternocleidomastoid muscle. The vein may be used for venipuncture, as well as for establishing peripheral or central venous access.

Position

The child is restrained in a supine position on a firm table. The head is rotated to the side away from the procedure and held off the edge of the table with the shoulders firmly touching the table (Fig. A-3, *C*).

Although the vein may be visible without additional measure, distension may be increased by placing the child in modified Trendelenburg's position, by having the child cry, or by occluding the vein with a finger on the clavicle.

Catheterization

After the area is prepared and draped, the *catheter* is inserted.

1. If peripheral access is desired, the largest catheter that is easily inserted should be employed.
2. If central access is desired, a guide-wire technique normally is used as described on p. 631.
3. The IV infusion is attached and the catheter secured.

INTRAOSSEOUS INFUSIONS

These are indicated only when intravenous sites are not available and immediate access is required on a temporary basis for infusion of crystalloid. Other agents have been infused without apparent complications but without controlled follow-up. The safety of infusion of hypertonic or strongly alkaline solutions has not been established.

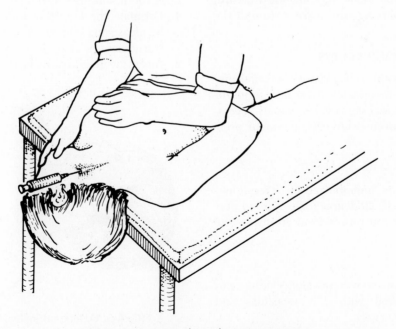

FIG. A-3, C. External jugular vein puncture.

Position

The patient is immobilized in the supine position. It is often helpful to position a small sandbag under the leg, immediately behind the operative site.

Needle

An 18-20 gauge spinal needle with stylet or a small bone marrow trephine needle is optimal.

Procedure

1. Strict aseptic technique must be maintained.
2. Local infiltration with lidocaine is desirable.
3. The needle is inserted perpendicular to the skin or at a 60 degree-inferior angle.
4. The needle is in the marrow when there is a lack of resistance after the needle passes through the cortex and stands upright without support, bone marrow is aspirated by the syringe, and the infusion flows smoothly.

Complications

The procedure is meant only as a temporizing measure. Complications may include fracture, osteomyelitis, abscess, and leakage around the needle.

CENTRAL VENOUS ACCESS

This involves the subclavian or internal jugular veins. The femoral vein also may be used. Central venous access provides venous access, as well as measurement of central venous pressure.

Position

The patient is immobilized in Trendelenburg's position (15-20 degrees) if condition permits, with the head turned away from the site of puncture.

Site and needle

The site is cleansed with povidone-iodine (Betadine), infiltrated with 1% lidocaine, and draped if time permits.

Internal jugular vein

The vein runs posterior to the sternocleidomastoid muscle between its two heads and behind the anterior portion of the clavicular head as it courses to meet the subclavian vein just above the medial end of the clavicle.

For the central or middle approach:
1. Landmarks are the triangle created by the sternal and clavicular heads of the sternocleidomastoid muscle and the clavicle at the base. The internal jugular vein is just behind the medial border of the clavicular head. The carotid artery is just medial to it.
2. The needle is inserted at the apex of the triangle at a 45-degree angle and aimed caudal and toward the ipsilateral nipple. The needle is inserted only 1-2 cm. If the vein is not entered, the needle is withdrawn and redirected slightly more laterally (Fig. A-3, *D*).

Subclavian vein

The vein crosses over the first rib and passes in front of the anterior scalene muscle and continues behind the medial third of the clavicle, where it unites with the internal jugular vein to form the innominate vein.
1. Estimate the length of the catheter needed by measuring from the site of insertion to the sternomanubrial angle.
2. Insert the needle infraclavicularly at the junc-

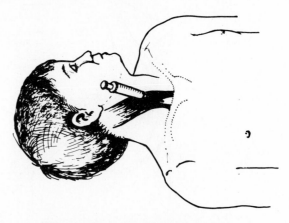

FIG. A-3, D. Internal jugular puncture.

ture of the middle and medial thirds of the clavicle parallel to the frontal plane. Direct it medially and slightly cephalad behind the clavicle toward the sternal notch.

NOTE: It is often useful to place a finger in the suprasternal notch for reference (Fig. A-3, *E*).

3. Insert the needle with the bevel upward. Once the lumen of the vessel is entered, rotate it so that the bevel is directed caudally.
4. Attach the needle to a syringe and insert under negative pressure until a free flow of blood back into the syringe is achieved. The syringe is then removed and a thumb placed over the needle hub to prevent air embolization.
5. A supraclavicular approach is preferred by some clinicians. The site of insertion is the angle and junction formed by the lateral border of the sternocleidomastoid muscle and the clavicle. The needle is inserted behind the sternocleidomastoid muscle and clavicle at an angle bisecting the angle formed by the landmarks and directed toward the contralateral nipple. The needle is advanced with the barrel of the syringe 5-10 degrees below the horizontal plane. The vein is entered 0.5-4.0 cm of depth. If unsuccessful, elevate the syringe 5 degrees above the horizontal plane.

The cannula

The *cannula* type determines the next step (Table A-3).

1. If the *catheter-through-the needle* technique is used, the catheter is slipped through the needle the appropriate distance and the needle is slid off the cannula once the cannula is in place. The catheter is never withdrawn through the needle because of the risk of shearing it.
2. If a *guide wire* is used, a wire guide is inserted through the needle and the needle is withdrawn. The dilator and overlying cath-

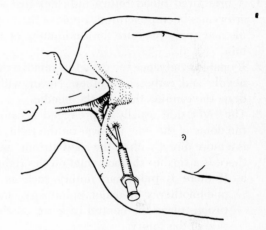

FIG. A-3, E. Subclavian vein puncture.

TABLE A-3. Suggested central venous catheters

Age	Catheter over wire (Seldinger)	Catheter through needle
Under 2 years	Steel needle: thin-walled, 21 gauge Guide wire: 0.018 in (0.46 mm), 20 cm Catheter: 4.0 Fr 7 cm Teflon or Silastic (5.0 Fr if >6 mo)	
2-10 years	Steel needle: thin-walled, 20 gauge Guide wire: 0.021 in (0.53 mm), 30 cm Catheter: ≥5.0 Fr, 12-cm Teflon or Silastic	Needle: 17 gauge, 4 cm Catheter: 19 gauge
Over 10 years	Steel needle: thin-walled, 18 gauge Guide wire: 0.035 in (0.89 mm), 40 cm Catheter: ≥6.0 Fr 15-cm Teflon or Silastic	Needle: 14 gauge, 4 cm Catheter: 16 gauge

There is tremendous variability among catheters, and these represent only guidelines. Before inserting, check to be certain that the needle, guide wire, and catheter are compatible. Prepackaged kits are available with all materials necessary for catheter insertion.

eter are then fed over the wire and, once in place, the wire and dilator are removed.

Procedure

1. The IV infusion is attached with an inline manometer to measure central venous pressure (CVP).
2. The catheter is secured with suture through the skin and wrapped around the catheter. A sterile dressing is applied.
3. CVP is determined.

Cautions

1. A bright-red blood return indicates that an artery has been punctured. Remove the needle and apply pressure for a minimum of 10 min.
2. If unable to advance the catheter, remove the needle and catheter together. Never withdraw the cannula through the needle.
3. The right side usually is preferred because the dome of the lung is lower on the right, it is a more direct path to the right atrium, and there is a smaller thoracic duct on the right.
   a. If there is pulmonary injury such as a pneumothorax or major pulmonary contusion, place the central catheter on the side of the injury.
   b. If there is potential vascular injury to the subclavian, internal jugular, or innominate veins, place the catheter on the other side.
4. Following insertion, a chest roentgenogram (AP or PA and lateral) should be obtained for defining placement, as well as excluding immediate complications.
   NOTE: Many believe that the external jugular is the safest approach, followed by the internal jugular technique.

Complications

These include pneumothorax, hemothorax, hydrothorax, air or catheter embolization, and brachial plexus injury. Preparations always should be made to treat them. Cervical hematomas are common, and while bleeding is usu-

ally trivial, it can produce occlusion of the airway. A common error, if a pneumothorax occurs, is to try to reverse it with too small an intrathoracic catheter. A thoracostomy should be performed with underwater drainage and, at times, additional suction.

UMBILICAL ARTERY AND VEIN

This is useful in the newborn (Chapter 9).

Appendix A-4: Lumbar puncture

Lumbar punctures (LP) commonly are performed to exclude CNS infection. It is important to exclude potential increased intracranial pressure on the basis of history and physical examination before performing the LP. If there is any question, a CT scan should be obtained before the LP.

POSITION

The patient's position is crucial. The patient should be placed at the edge of a firm examination table and maintained in a position with the neck flexed and the knee drawn upward (fetal position). *The key to performing an LP is to properly position the child* (Fig. A-4).
1. The shoulders and back of the patient should be perpendicular to the table.
2. An alternative position for the small infant is to have the patient sitting, flexing the thighs up to the abdomen. This is recommended only if the holder and clinician are experienced with this approach.
3. In the preterm infant, the optimal position is either the lateral recumbent one with the hips flexed and partial neck extension or the upright position. Full flexion of the neck may cause hypoventilation.

PROCEDURE

1. The patient's back is cleansed with a surgical scrub—using povidone-iodine (Betadine)—and then draped. Steri-drapes are particularly useful because they are adherent and do not obscure the landmarks.

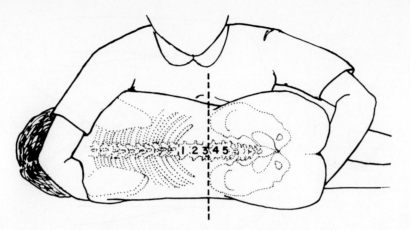

FIG. A-4. Position for lumbar puncture.

2. Meticulous sterile technique is used.
3. Local anesthetic is used for children over 5 yr of age who will cooperate more easily if the pain is minimized.

Site

The puncture is at the intersection of the line joining the superior portion of the iliac crest with the spine. This point is the spinous process of L4. The needle is optimally inserted at L3-L4 but may be inserted one space above or below.

Spinal needle

This is a 22-gauge, 1½-inch needle for children under 5 yr, increased to 3 inches long in the adult.

Insertion

The needle is inserted into the designated spot with the stylet in place.
1. The needle should be inserted perpendicular to the back and aimed toward the umbilicus.
2. In the younger child it is advisable to puncture the skin and allow the child to calm down and then to reassess the position before proceeding.
3. Younger children will not demonstrate the increasing resistance and "pop" noted in older children. It is advisable to frequently remove the stylet and examine the needle hub for fluid as the needle with stylet is advanced.

Manometry

This can be performed in cooperative children over 5 yr when it is important. A three-way stopcock and manometer are attached to the spinal needle and the pressure determined. Normal relaxed pressure is 5-15 cm of water.

Fluid analysis

Analysis of the cerebrospinal fluid (CSF) must be done expeditiously.
1. Tube no. 1: culture and Gram's stain. If Gram's stain is negative: methylene blue. Cultures beyond routine bacterial ones should be specified.
2. Tube no. 2: protein and glucose. (Serum glucose should be obtained before performing the LP.)
3. Tube no. 3: cell count. If bloody, it may be desirable to compare tube no. 1 and tube no. 3 cell count to determine if the tap was traumatic.
4. Analysis is outlined in detail on p. 552.

COMPLICATIONS

1. Cardiac respiratory arrest may result from the child being held too tightly, with subsequent respiratory arrest and impaired venous return.

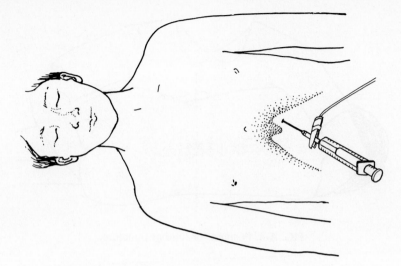

FIG. A-5. Position of needle for pericardiocentesis.

2. Infection secondary to introduction of pathogens during the procedure may occur. Controversy exists as to the risk of performing an LP in the child with bacteremia. The risk is not substantiated, and this question should not serve to inhibit clinicians from doing necessary studies.
3. Herniation through the foramen magnum may occur because of antecedent increased intracranial pressure. If increased pressure is noted at the time of the procedures, only a small amount of fluid should be withdrawn and the needle quickly removed. The patient obviously requires immediate evaluation and treatment. Optimally an LP is avoided with such patients.
4. Headaches are more common in adults.
5. Intraspinal dermoids are avoided by using only needles with stylets.
6. Penetration of a nerve causes pain. In this case the needle is withdrawn and redirected.
7. Spinal cord hematoma occurs, particularly in patients with thrombocytopenia or coagulation defects.

Appendix A-5: Pericardiocentesis

Fluid collection in the pericardial sac, whether it results from effusion, infection, or hemorrhage, may be removed in the acute situation for both diagnostic and therapeutic reasons by pericardiocentesis. An echocardiogram may be an important diagnostic tool in the stable patient to establish the presence of an effusion. Following this life-saving procedure, definitive surgical care is immediately indicated.

POSITION

The patient is supine, leaning backward at a 45-degree angle, supported by the bed or pillows (reverse Trendelenburg's position).

SITE

The left subxiphoid is used, with the needle aimed cephalad and backward toward the tip of the left scapula (Fig. A-5). Some clinicians recommend aiming the needle toward the right scapula.

NEEDLE

An 18- or 20-gauge metal spinal needle (3 inch) is attached to a three-way stopcock and 20 ml syringe. One end of an alligator clip is attached to the needle's base and the other end to the V lead on an ECG. (Limb leads should be attached as usual.)

PROCEDURE

1. After preparing, cleaning, and draping the patient, the needle is inserted slowly under negative pressure through the puncture site, penetrating the diaphragm. As the pericardium is entered, there is a distinct "pop." A current of injury with ST-T wave changes will be noted if the epicardium is entered, and the needle should be withdrawn slightly.
2. Aspiration is performed. As little as 2 ml may be temporarily effective at relieving tamponade and improving cardiac output.
3. Vital signs should be monitored throughout the procedure.

COMPLICATIONS

1. Pneumothorax
2. Coronary artery injury or myocardial laceration
3. Dysrhythmias
4. Bleeding. In the stable patient, PT, PTT, and platelet count may be obtained before the procedure.

Appendix A-6: Subdural tap

The subdural space is a noncommunicating space between the dura matter and the arachnoid membrane. Although a CT scan can delineate the presence of fluid in the subdural space, the tap is done to define the nature of the collection: hematoma, effusion, or empyema.

SITE

The *puncture site* is the lateral corner of the anterior fontanel or further lateral along the su-

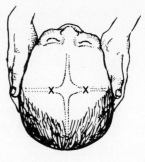

FIG. A-6. Puncture site for subdural tap.

ture. Optimally, this is at least 5 cm from the midline or 1-2 cm lateral to the edge of the anterior fontanel (Fig. A-6). If the fontanel is not open (usually over 12 mo), a neurosurgeon should be consulted.

POSITION

The patient is in the supine position with the head at the edge of an examining table. An assistant should immobilize the patient with the help of a papoose board.

NEEDLE

A *subdural needle* (short bevel) is used. If one is unavailable, a short spinal needle with a short bevel may be substituted. It is often advisable with this needle to place a hemostat on the needle at the point of entry to prevent excessive penetration.

PROCEDURE

1. The anterior two thirds of the scalp are shaved and surgically scrubbed with povidone-iodine (Betadine). Meticulous surgical technique is essential. The needle is inserted slowly at right angle to the skin surface with total finger control. It is advanced slowly with the stylet in place until there is a sudden decrease in resistance, usually associated with a "pop," representing penetration of the dura.
2. The stylet is removed, and up to 15-20 ml of fluid is allowed to drain by gravity, avoiding

aspiration. Normally there are only a few drops in this space. Sometimes none is obtained.

3. In most cases the procedure is repeated on the other side.
4. If excessive fluid is present or reaccumulates, repeat taps may be necessary over a period of time. A neurosurgeon should be consulted.

ANALYSIS OF THE FLUID

This should parallel the studies performed on specimens obtained by LP: culture, Gram's stain, glucose, protein, and cell count (p. 552). A subdural effusion usually is associated with grossly xanthochromic or bloody fluid.

COMPLICATIONS

1. Infection secondary to introduction of pathogens during the procedure
2. Bleeding from small vessels (lateral position of puncture site should be maintained to avoid superior sagittal sinus).
3. Removal of >20 ml/tap can produce CNS sequelae. If >20 ml is present, a neurosurgeon should be consulted.
4. Injury to the cerebral cortex if needle is inserted too deeply

Appendix A-7: Suprapubic aspiration

Suprapubic aspiration is a safe method to obtain urine from the newborn and infants under 2 yr of age, because the distended bladder in this age-group is primarily intraabdominal.

The infant's bladder must be full. Determining that the diaper has been dry for 45 min is good evidence of a full bladder.

POSITION

The patient is restrained in the supine position.

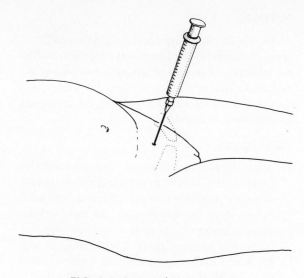

FIG. A-7. Suprapubic aspiration.

SITE

The site is 2 cm (a fingerbreadth) above the symphysis.

PROCEDURE

1. Surgically cleanse the suprapubic area with povidone-iodine (Betadine).
2. Identify the pubic bone without contaminating the area of puncture.
3. Insert a 1½ inch, 22-gauge needle attached to a 5 ml syringe at midline, angling the needle 10-20 degrees cephalad and advancing it through the skin under negative pressure at all times (Fig. A-7).

Entry into the bladder is indicated by return of urine. If no urine is obtained:

1. Angle the needle perpendicular to the frontal plane and try once more.
2. Avoid excessive probing or manipulation of the needle.
3. If no urine is obtained, try again in 15 min, or use a different technique such as catheterization (an infant can be catheterized with a 3.5 or 5.0 Fr feeding tube).

COMPLICATIONS

These include gross hematuria (some hematuria usually will follow the procedure), anterior abdominal wall abscess, and bowel puncture. Peritonitis is uncommon.

Appendix A-8: Thoracentesis

Thoracentesis is indicated to remove pleural fluid for diagnostic or therapeutic reasons or in the emergency treatment of a pneumothorax pending placement of a chest tube.

POSITION

For posterior or posterior-lateral approaches to fluid removal the patient sits in a flexed position, leaning forward against a bed stand or chair back. A small infant may be held in the "burping" position.
1. If the patient is too ill to sit, the procedure may be performed with the patient lying on the involved side on a firm surface with a portion of the lateral chest wall extending over the edge of the bed. An alternative for gaining access to the lateral chest wall is for the patient to lie across two beds or examination tables with the involved side down.
2. If a pneumothorax is to be decompressed the patient should be lying supine.

SITE

The *site* of puncture is dependent on the location of the pleural fluid. If a pneumothorax is being decompressed before placing chest tube (A-9), venting is done at the second or third intercostal space at the midclavicular line.

NEEDLE

An 18- or 19-gauge needle with a short bevel attached to a three-way stopcock and 10 ml syringe is used. If fluid is expected, plastic tubing is attached to the sidearm of the stopcock to facilitate removal of fluids.

Flexible cannulas over needle also are useful and may replace the needle. They decrease the risk of lung puncture and are particularly valuable for emergency relief of the patient.

PROCEDURE

1. The patient is prepared and draped, and 1% lidocaine is infiltrated locally.
2. With sterile technique the needle or catheter over needle is inserted, passing over the superior edge of the rib under negative pressure, and advanced slowly. There is a sudden decrease in resistance once the pleural space is reached. A hemostat should be placed on the needle at the skin to prevent further penetration once the pleural space is entered.
3. Fluid is aspirated, the volume reflecting cardiopulmonary status and the therapeutic goals of the procedures.

ANALYSIS OF THE FLUID

This should include a culture, Gram's stain, protein, glucose, LDH, cell count, and a check for chyle (see below).

The distinction between transudate and exu-

	Transudate	Exudate
Etiology	CHF, cirrhosis	Infection: bacterial, mycobacterial; infarction, neoplasm, pancreatitis
Protein	<3.0 g/dl (PF/S* <0.5)	>3.0 g/dl (PF/S >0.5)
LDH	Low (<200 IU/L) (PF/S <0.6)	High (>200 IU/L) (PF/S >0.6)
Glucose	Same as blood	Variable (infection: low)
RBC	<10,000/mm^3	Variable (if >100,000/mm^3, consider infarction, trauma, neoplasm)
WBC	<1,000/mm^3	>1,000/mm^3 (infection)

*PF, Pleural fluid; S, serum.

date may be useful in differentiating the causes of pleural effusion. Transudates usually are associated with congestive heart failure, cirrhosis, nephrotic syndrome, acute glomerulonephritis, myxedema, and peritoneal dialysis. Exudates with proteins over 3 g/dl occur with pulmonary infarction, neoplasms, infection (viral or bacterial such as *S. aureus, H. influenzae,* or streptococcus; tuberculosis; fungus; or parasites), collagen vascular disease, subphrenic abscess, trauma, and lymphatic abnormalities.

COMPLICATIONS

These include introduction of infection, pneumothorax, hemothorax, or pulmonary laceration. Hospitalize patient to observe after procedure.

Appendix A-9: Thoracostomy

Chest tubes are used for the treatment for pneumothorax or hemothorax, often before making a definitive radiologic diagnosis (Chapter 62). Management in newborns is discussed in Chapter 11.

INDICATIONS

1. Tension pneumothorax
2. Traumatic moderate to large pneumothorax. A small (<10% simple) pneumothorax in a symptom-free patient (with no increase on repeat roentgenogram) may be observed in the hospital if general anesthesia or mechanical ventilation is not required for other injuries.
3. Any pneumothorax with respiratory symptoms
4. Increasing pneumothorax after initial conservative therapy
5. Pneumothorax in a patient who needs mechanical ventilation or general anesthesia
6. Associated hemothorax
7. Bilateral pneumothorax

POSITION

The *position* of the patient is supine with appropriate immobilization.

SITE

The *site* for insertion is at the fourth or fifth intercostal space in the midaxillary line.

TUBE SIZE

The *tube* should be the largest one that can be inserted. This is particularly important if a hemothorax is present.
1. The following are estimates of appropriate size:
   a. Newborn 8-12 Fr
   b. Infant 14-20 Fr
   c. Children 20-28 Fr
   d. Adolescent 28-42 Fr
2. Length of the tube should be approximated before insertion. All holes in the tube must be within the pleural cavity.

PROCEDURE

1. The area is prepared, draped, and locally infiltrated with 1% lidocaine down to the rib and along the subcutaneous tissue to be tunneled.
2. The skin is incised with a scalpel parallel to the long axis of the rib. The incision should be adequate to permit manipulation of the tube (3-5 cm).
3. The area is bluntly dissected down to the rib with a clamp or scissors. If tunneling is desired, the dissection is continued across the intercostal space above the incision site and over the next rib. A clamp is then curved over the superior edge of the rib, dividing the intercostal muscles down to the parietal pleura, which is penetrated. The opening is enlarged by blunt dissection.
4. In older infants and children, a finger is inserted to ensure that there are no adhesions of the lung and that the tube will be inserted into the chest and not subdiaphragmatically.

5. The thoracostomy tube is grasped at the tip by a curved clamp and advanced through the tunnel and intercostal space into the chest. It is directed posteriorly and apically. The interspace is entered superior to the rib to avoid injuring the neurovascular bundle (Fig. A-9). All holes must be within the pleural cavity.
6. The tube is attached to an underwater seal. If there is a continuous air leak or an associated hemothorax, additional pleural suction may be needed up to 15-25 cm water.
7. The tube is sutured in place and dressed with a sterile covering, often including a petrolatum-soaked gauze as an air seal.

8. A chest x-ray film should be obtained following the procedure.

COMPLICATIONS

1. Inserting the tube too low, causing penetration of the diaphragm and injury to the liver or spleen
2. Injury to the neurovascular bundle, causing persistent hemorrhage
3. Injury to the underlying lung
4. Air leak if the tube is not placed far enough to include all the holes in the pleural cavity, causing extensive subcutaneous emphysema and failure to reexpand the collapsed lung
5. Empyema

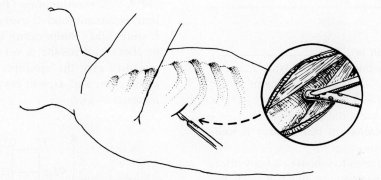

FIG. A-9. Placement of chest tube. (Modified from Rosen, P., and Sternbach, G.: Atlas of emergency medicine, Baltimore, 1983, The Williams & Wilkins Co.)

Parent instruction sheets for common pediatric illnesses

This section consists of material designed for reproduction and distribution. It is also useful for telephone triage and advice.

Appendix B-1: General information for parents

MEDICATION

1. Your medication is _____ .
   Give _____ teaspoon/tablet/capsule _____ times per day. Give every dose, even if your child begins to feel better.
   a. If a liquid, use a measuring spoon.
   b. Store medication in refrigerator if indicated.
   c. If your child goes to school or a babysitter, arrange for someone to give the medicine if necessary.
2. Call physician if your child refuses to take the medicine or you think your child is having a reaction to the medicine.

FEVER

1. For children over 3 months of age, give fever medicine if the temperature is over 101.5° F (38.6° C), if child is very uncomfortable, or if any fever is present at bedtime. If your child is acting normally, fever medicines may be delayed until the temperature is 102.2° F (39° C). Acetaminophen (Tylenol or equivalent) is recommended every 4-6 hours.
2. If your child's temperature is 103° F (39.5° C) or above and he/she is very uncomfortable, you may give the appropriate dose of acetaminophen **and** aspirin every 5-6 hours (see material below).

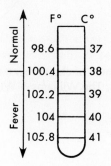

F°	C°
98.6	37
100.4	38
102.2	39
104	40
105.8	41

Dose of fever medicine

Brand	0-3 mo	4-11 mo	12-23 mo	2-3 yr	4-5 yr	6-8 yr	9-10 yr	11-12 yr
Acetaminophen drops (80 mg/0.8 ml)	0.4 ml	0.8 ml	1.2 ml	1.6 ml	2.4 ml			
Acetaminophen elixir (160 mg/tsp)		½ tsp	¾ tsp	1 tsp	1½ tsp	2 tsp	2½ tsp	
Chewable acetaminophen or aspirin (80 mg)			1½	2	3	4	5	6
Junior swallowable tablet (160 mg)				1	1½	2	2½	3
Adult tablet acetaminophen or aspirin (325 mg)						1		1½

3. If the temperature remains over 104° F (40° C) after medication, it may be helpful to sponge or partially submerge your undressed child in lukewarm water (96°-100° F) for 15-30 minutes. Some prefer laying the undressed child on a towel. Another towel soaked in lukewarm water is placed on the child. The towel is changed every 1-2 minutes for 15-30 minutes.
4. Dress child lightly. Push fluids.
5. Do **not** use aspirin if your child has chickenpox or an influenza-like illness.
6. Call physician if
   a. Fever goes above 105° F (40.5° C)
   b. Fever lasts beyond 48-72 hours
   c. Child is under 3 months and has a fever over 100.4° F (38° C)
   d. Child has a seizure (convulsion); develops abnormal movements of face, arms, or leg; stiff neck; fullness of soft spot, purple spots, difficulty breathing, burning on urination, decreased urination, or abdominal pain; marked change in behavior, level of consciousness, or level of activity; looks sicker than expected.

CULTURES

Throat: _____
Other: _____

A culture has been obtained. The results will be available in 24-48 hours. Call your physician/Emergency Department (circle one) at that time.

X-RAY FILMS

An emergency reading has been made. A final reading will be made by the radiologist, and if there are any changes in diagnosis or instructions, you or your physician will be notified.

FOLLOW-UP

1. Call your physician or the Emergency Department if your child develops any problems that concern you.
2. Call physician to arrange to see _____

in the office in _____ days. The phone number is _____ .

OTHER INSTRUCTIONS

_____

Appendix B-2: Respiratory tract problems

EAR INFECTION

1. Fever medicines may make your child feel better.
2. A return appointment in 2-3 weeks should be made to be certain the infection has cleared up and more treatment is not necessary.
3. Your child can return to school or day care when feeling better and the fever is down. Swimming is permitted if there is no hole in the eardrum.
4. Call physician if
   a. There is no improvement in 36 hours
   b. Fever is not gone in 72 hours
   c. Child is increasingly irritable or listless
   d. Child develops vomiting or diarrhea

SORE THROAT

1. Gargle with warm salt water (1 tsp salt in 8-ounce glass) or suck hard candies.
2. Fever medicines may make your child feel better.
3. Call physician if
   a. Child develops severe pain or drooling
   b. Swallowing or breathing becomes difficult
   c. Child develops big swollen lymph nodes (glands) in the neck
   d. Fever lasts over 48 hours.

STREP THROAT

1. See *Sore throat* and *Medication* instructions.

2. Your child may return to school or day-care 24 hours after beginning antibiotics.
3. Family members who are symptomatic with fever, sore throat, or other symptoms suggestive of a strep throat should have a throat culture.

COLD

1. Children with a dry or stuffy nose will benefit from placing 2-3 drops of water in each nostril. For the younger child use a soft rubber suction bulb to clear discharge. Have older children blow their nose.
2. Fever medicines may make your child feel better.
3. A humidifier may be useful in maximizing comfort.
4. Call physician if
   a. Fever lasts more than 24-48 hours
   b. Child has fever at less than 3 months of age or has underlying heart or lung problems
   c. Evidence of infection elsewhere is present such as red eye, ear pain, or breathing problems, including wheezing or croup
   d. Skin under nose becomes crusty

COUGH

1. Sucking on cough drops or hard candy may be useful. A good cough medicine can be made at home by mixing equal amounts of honey (corn syrup for child under 1 year of age), lemon concentrate, and liquor like Scotch or bourbon. You may omit the liquor for younger children.
2. Cough syrups rarely are useful. Stronger cough medicines containing dextromethorphan (DM) or codeine must be prescribed by a physician, and they have the danger of reducing the cough reflex that protects the lungs.
3. Call physician if
   a. Difficulty breathing, shortness of breath, or blue color of skin or around mouth develops

   b. Cough lasts over 2 weeks
   c. Cough changes to croup ("barking seal" cough) or wheezing
   d. Child develops fever that lasts over 72 hours
   e. Coughing spasms occur that cause choking, passing out, or bluish lip color
   f. There is blood in the mucus
   g. Chest pain develops

EYE INFECTION (CONJUNCTIVITIS)

1. Before using topical medicine, clean the eye by removing the yellow discharge and dried matter with a wet cotton ball and warm water.
2. Put 2 drops of medicine in each eye every 2 hours (or as often as possible) while the child is awake. Once the infection is improving, the drops may be given 4 times per day.
3. For younger children, you may receive only an ointment that may be used 4 times per day but stays in the eye longer. It is also useful for older children before bedtime.
4. Continue medication until your child has awakened for two mornings without a discharge in the eyes.
5. Your child may infect other people. Separate towels and washcloths; careful handwashing may be useful.
6. Call physician if
   a. Infection is not improved in 72 hours
   b. Eyelid is red, swollen, warm, tender, or painful
   c. Eyeball is cloudy or sores develop on it
   d. Vision if blurred
   e. Eye becomes painful or develops photophobia

NOSEBLEED

1. If bleeding occurs, apply pressure for a full 10 minutes, compressing the soft and bony parts of the nose, pressing downward toward the cheeks with the thumb and forefinger. Preceding this, blow the nose if possible.
2. Increase home humidity. Minimize nose trauma and picking.

3. Apply Vaseline daily to the interior nose for 4-5 days.
4. Call physician if
   a. Unexplained bruising occurs
   b. Large amounts of blood are lost
   c. Bleeding cannot be controlled by pressure

CROUP

1. Keep child's room humidified. A cold-mist humidifier is best.
2. Push fluids. Try to keep child calm.
3. Fever medicine may make your child feel better.
4. If child worsens and develops increased breathing difficulty:
   a. Take child outside in cold air for 5 minutes.
   b. Try to get child to relax
   c. Arrange to go to hospital
5. Call physician immediately if
   a. Child has great difficulty breathing
   b. Lips or skin turn blue
   c. Drooling or difficulty swallowing develops
   d. Child does not improve with cold air
   e. Agitation or listlessness develops
   f. Cough does not improve in 4-5 days

ASTHMA

1. Give all doses of medication. Continue until there has been no wheezing for 48 hours. If your child wheezes often, your care provider may want to give the medicine for a long period.
2. Push clear liquids. Warm fluids are particularly helpful. Keep your child quiet and calm.
3. Try to identify substances that trigger attacks and avoid them. Typically, animals, feather pillows, dust, and pollens are involved. Pollutants and smoke may contribute to the problem.
4. Many patients with asthma will develop wheezing in response to an infection. If this is a trigger in your child, you should start medicine at the first sign of a cold or cough.

- Give 1½ times the normal dose when beginning asthma medicine, and then continue the regular dose for 3-4 days after resolution of symptoms.
5. Call physician immediately
   a. Breathing difficulty recurs or worsens or child has difficulty speaking
   b. Lips or skin turn blue
   c. Restlessness or sleeplessness is present
   d. Fluid intake decreases
   e. Nausea, vomiting, or irritability develops because of medicine or inability to take medication
   f. Cough or wheezing persists or chest pain or fever develops

Appendix B-3: Trauma

HEAD INJURY

1. Limit activities and restrict to light diet. With recent injury, apply ice pack to swelling.
2. Waken child every 2 hours and observe.
3. Aspirin or acetaminophen may be given for pain.
4. Call physician immediately if
   a. Increasing sleepiness, drowsiness, or inability to awaken patient develops
   b. Change in equality of pupils (black center of eye) or blurred vision, peculiar movements of the eyes, or difficulty focusing develops
   c. Stumbling, unusual weakness, or problem using arms or legs develops
   d. Change in normal gait or crawl develops
   e. Seizures occur
   f. Change in personality or behavior occurs such as increasing irritability, confusion, unusual restlessness, or inability to concentrate
   g. Persistent vomiting (more than three times) occurs
   h. Drainage of blood or fluid from nose or ear occurs
   i. Severe headache occurs

CARE OF SUTURED WOUNDS

1. Mild bleeding and some discomfort may occur after suturing as the anesthesia wears off
2. Keep wound clean and dry for 2 days, then begin gentle cleaning of wound twice daily with soap and water.
3. Try to keep area elevated.
4. Call physician if
   a. Wound becomes red or swollen or drains pus, or if red streak appears
   b. Wound becomes more painful
5. Change dressing in _____ days.
6. Return in _____ days for suture removal or wound check.

SPRAINS AND FRACTURES

1. Elevate the injured limb to lessen swelling. Ice packs may be useful for 12-24 hours.
2. If child is wearing an elastic Ace bandage, rewrap it if too loose or tight.
3. If child has a *cast*, keep it dry.
4. Call physician immediately if
   a. Severe pain or pressure within the cast (if present) develops
   b. Increasing coldness or blueness of the fingers or toes occurs
   c. Excessive swelling or decreased motion of toes or fingers is present

BURNS

1. Keep the wound clean and dry.
2. Change the dressing in _____ days. Wash burn gently, apply cream, and dress as directed.
3. Call physicians if
   a. Increasing redness or discoloration of the normal tissue around the burn site develops
   b. Red streaks radiating from the burn area develop
   c. Fever or chills occur
   d. Swelling or progressive inability to use fingers and toes (if extremity) develops
   e. Shortness of breath or increased cough develops
   f. Blurred vision (if face is involved) develops
   g. Swallowing difficulty (if neck is involved) develops

ANIMAL BITES AND SCRATCHES

1. Take medication _____ for _____ days. Give every dose. Call physician if your child refuses medicine or appears to have a reaction.
2. Call physician if
   a. Wound becomes red or swollen, drains pus, becomes more painful, or if red streaks develop
   b. Tender lump appears in the groin or under the arm
   c. Fever or chills are present

Appendix B-4: Other pediatric problems

DIARRHEA

1. Give only clear liquids; give as much as your child wants. The following may be used during the first 24 hours:
   a. Pedialyte RS, Lytren, or Infalyte (requires mixing)
   b. Gatorade
   c. Jell-O water—one package strawberry per quart water (twice as much as usual)
   d. Defizzed, room-temperature soda for older children (over 2 years) if diarrhea is only mild
2. If child is vomiting, give clear liquids *slowly*. In younger children, start with a teaspoonful and slowly increase the amount. If vomiting occurs, let your child rest for a while and then try again. About 8 hours after vomiting has stopped, child can return gradually to a normal diet.
3. After 24 hours, your child's diet may be advanced if the diarrhea has improved. If child

is taking only formula, mix the formula with twice as much water to make up half-strength formula, which should be given over the next 24 hours. Applesauce, bananas, and strained carrots may be given if child is eating solids.

If this is tolerated, the child may be advanced to a regular diet over the next 2-3 days.

4. If child has had a prolonged course of diarrhea, it is helpful in the younger child to advance from clear liquids to a soy formula (Isomil, ProSobee, or Soyalac) for 1-2 weeks. Children over 1 year should not be given cow's milk products (milk, cheese, ice cream, or butter) for several days.

5. Do not use boiled milk. Kool-Aid and soda are not ideal liquids, particularly in younger infants, because they contain few electrolytes.

6. Call physician if
   a. The diarrhea or vomiting is increasing in frequency or amount.
   b. The diarrhea does not improve after 24 hours of clear liquids or resolve entirely after 3-4 days
   c. Vomiting continues for more than 24 hours
   d. The stool has blood or the vomited material contains blood or turns green
   e. Signs of dehydration develop, including decreased urination, less moisture in diapers, dry mouth, no tears, weight loss, lethargy, or irritability

VOMITING

1. Clear liquids only should be given slowly and may include defizzed soda pop (cola, ginger ale), Pedialyte, Lytren, Gatorade, etc. In younger children, start with a teaspoon and slowly advance the amount. If vomiting occurs, let your child rest for a while and then try again.

2. About 8 hours after your child has stopped vomiting, he/she gradually return to a normal diet. For older infants and children bland items (toast, crackers, clear soup) may be given slowly.

3. Call physician if
   a. Vomiting increases in frequency or amount
   b. Vomiting continues for more than 24 hours
   c. Child develops signs of dehydration including decreased urination, less moisture in diapers, mouth, no tears, weight loss, lethargy, or listlessness
   d. Child becomes sleepy, difficult to awaken, or irritable
   e. Vomited material has blood in it or turns green

URINARY TRACT INFECTIONS

1. A urine culture has been obtained.
2. Two days after your child begins antibiotics, you should contact your care provider about the urine culture to be sure that your child is taking the correct medicine and feeling better.
3. Two weeks after your initial visit, your physician will want to see your child again for another urine culture. Arrangements also will be made for periodic urine checks over the next year.
4. Several steps may assist in preventing repeat infections in the future, particularly in girls.
   a. Teach your child to wipe correctly from front to back.
   b. Do not use bubble bath or let the soap float around in the bath.
5. Call physician if
   a. Fever or pain with urination is not gone 48 hours after beginning antibiotics
   b. Your child gets worse or does not tolerate medication

Reference standards

Appendix C-1: Growth curves

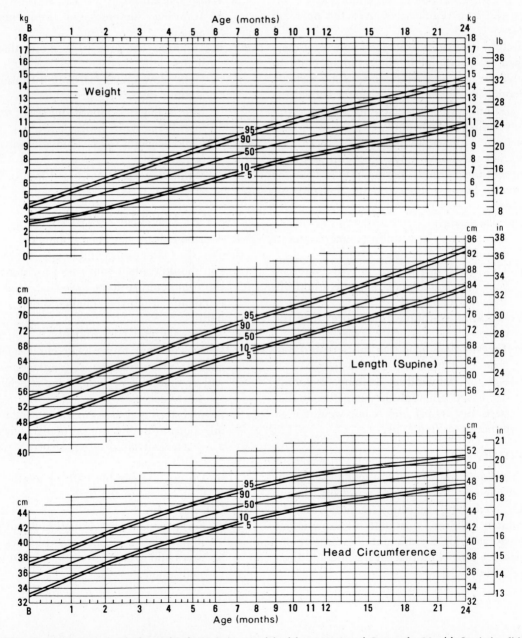

Percentile standards for growth: **boys (birth-24 mo).** (Modified from National Center for Health Statistics [NCHS] growth charts, 1976.)

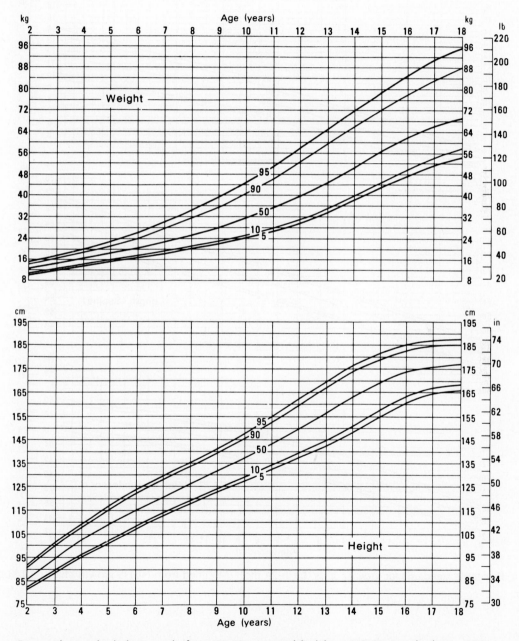

Percentile standards for growth: **boys (2-18 yr).** (Modified from NCHS growth charts, 1976.)

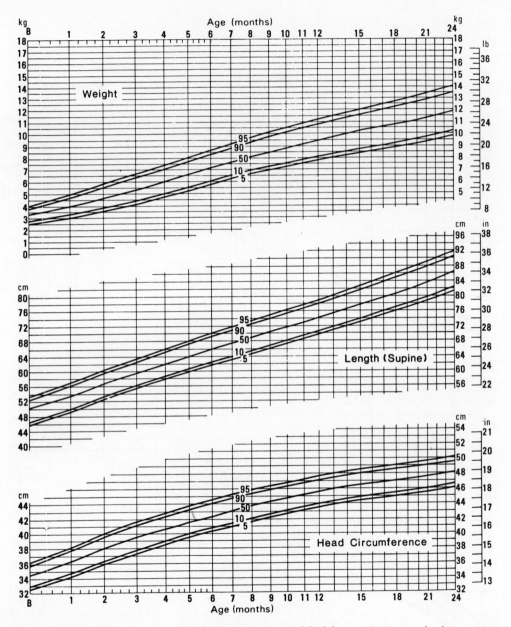

Percentile standards for growth: **girls (birth-24 mo).** (Modified from NCHS growth charts, 1976.)

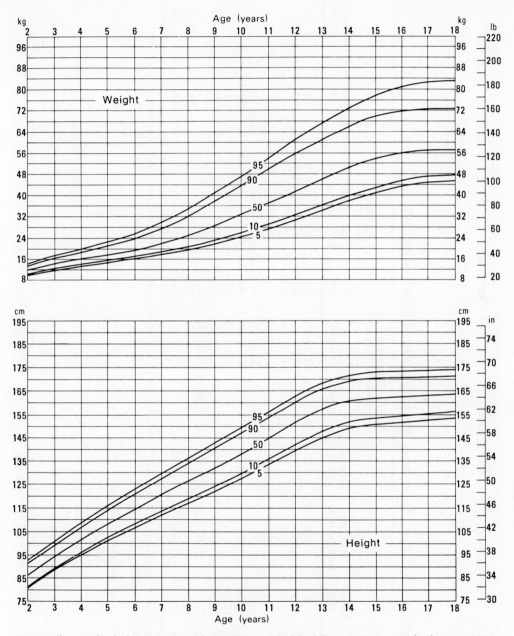

Percentile standards for growth: **girls (2-18 yr).** (Modified from NCHS growth charts, 1976.)

Appendix C-2: Vital signs and ancillary ventilatory support

| Age | Weight (kg) | Heart rate (average/min) | Respiratory rate | Blood pressure (mean ± 2 SD) | | ET tube | | | Chest tube (Fr) | Laryngoscopy blade |
				Systolic	Diastolic*	ID† (mm)	Length (cm)	Suction catheter (Fr)		
Premature	1	145	<40	42 ± 10	21 ± 8	2.5	10	6	8-10	0
Newborn	1-2	135		50 ± 10	28 ± 8	3.0	11	6-8	10-12	1
Newborn	2-3	125		60 ± 10	37 ± 8	3.0	12			
1 mo	4	120	24-35	80 ± 16	46 ± 16	3.5	13	8		
6 mo	7	130		89 ± 29	60 ± 10	3.5	14			
1 yr	10	125	20-30	96 ± 30	66 ± 25	4.0	15	8-10	16-20	1
2-3 yr	12-14	115		99 ± 25	64 ± 25	4.5	16	10		
4-5 yr	16-18	100		99 ± 20	65 ± 20	5.0-6.0	17		20-28	2
6-8 yr	20-26	100	12-25	See figure on p. 651		6.0-6.5	18			
10-12 yr	32-42	75				7.0	20	12	28-32	2-3
Over 14 yr	>50	70	12-18			7.5-8.5	24		32-42	3

Modified from Nadas, A: Pediatric cardiology, ed. 3, Philadelphia, 1976, W.B. Saunders Co.; Vesmond, H.T., et al.: Pediatrics **67**:607, 1981.

*Point of muffling (Nadas).

†Variability of 0.5 mm is common. Estimate: $\dfrac{16 + age\ (yr)}{4}$

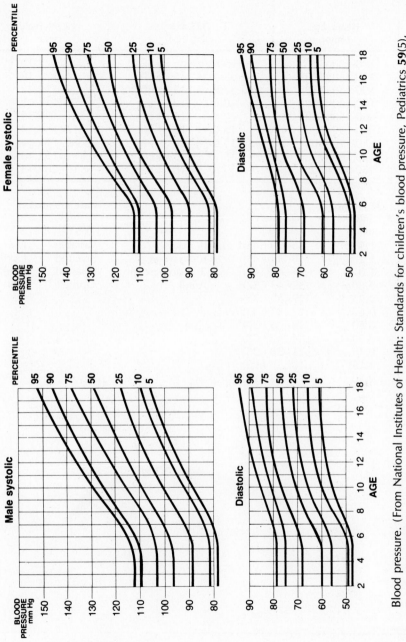

Blood pressure. (From National Institutes of Health: Standards for children's blood pressure, Pediatrics **59**(5), Part 2, May 1977.)

Appendix C-3: Electrocardiographic criteria

Age	Heart rate (/min)	QRS axis (degrees)	PR interval (sec)	QRS duration* (sec)
0-1 mo	100-180 (120)†	+75 to +180 (+120)	.08-.12 (.10)	.04-.08 (.06)
2-3 mo	110-180 (120)	+35 to +135 (+100)	.08-.12 (.10)	.04-.08 (.06)
4-12 mo	100-180 (150)	+30 to +135 (+60)	.09-.13 (.12)	.04-.08 (.06)
1-3 yr	100-180 (130)	0 to +110 (+60)	.10-.14 (.12)	.04-.08 (.06)
4-5 yr	60-150 (100)	0 to +110 (+60)	.11-.15 (.13)	.05-.09 (.07)
6-8 yr	60-130 (100)	−15 to +110 (+60)	.12-.16 (.14)	.05-.09 (.07)
9-11 yr	50-110 (80)	−15 to +110 (+60)	.12-.17 (.14)	.05-.09 (.07)
12-16 yr	50-100 (75)	−15 to +110 (+60)	.12-.17 (.15)	.05-.09 (.07)
Over 16 yr	50-90 (70)	−15 to +110 (+60)	.12-.20 (.15)	.05-.10 (.08)

Rate/min	QT interval R-R interval (sec)	QT interval (sec)	Age	T-wave orientation V1,V2	AVF	I,V5,V6
40	1.5	.38-.50 (.45)†	0-5 days	Variable	Upright	Upright
50	1.2	.36-.48 (.43)	6 days-2 yr	Inverted	Upright	Upright
60	1.0	.34-.46 (.41)	3 yr-adolescent	Inverted	Upright	Upright
70	0.86	.32-.43 (.37)	Adult	Upright	Upright	Upright
80	0.75	.29-.40 (.35)				
90	0.67	.27-.37 (.33)				
100	0.60	.26-.35 (.30)				
120	0.50	.24-.32 (.28)				
150	0.40	.21-.28 (.25)				
180	0.33	.19-.27 (.23)				
200	0.30	.18-.25 (.22)				

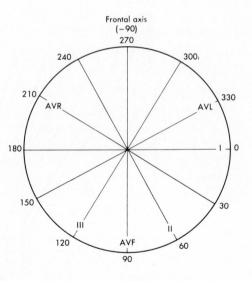

Frontal axis (−90)

Modified by permission of Garson, A., Jr., Gillette, P.C., and McNamara, D.G.: A guide to cardiac dysrhythmias in children, New York, 1980, Grune & Stratton, Inc.; Guntheroth, W.G.S.: Pediatric electrocardiography, Philadelphia, 1965, W.B. Saunders Co.

*If QRS duration is normal, add R + R′ and compare total (R + R′) with standards; R/S undefined because S can be equal to 0.

†Minimum-maximum (mean).

Lead V1			Lead V6			
R-wave amplitude (mm)	S-wave amplitude (mm)	R/S ratio	R-wave amplitude (mm)	S-wave amplitude (mm)	R/S ratio	Age
4-25 (15)	0-20 (10)	0.5 to ∞ (1.5)	1-21 (6)	0-12 (4)	0.1 to ∞ (2)	0-1 mo
2-20 (11)	1-18 (7)	0.3 to 10.0 (1.5)	3-20 (10)	0-6 (2)	1.5 to ∞ (4)	2-3 mo
3-20 (10)	1-16 (8)	0.3 to 4.0 (1.2)	6-20 (13)	0-4 (2)	2.0 to ∞ (6)	4-12 mo
1-18 (9)	1-27 (13)	0.5 to 1.5 (0.8)	3-24 (12)	0-4 (2)	3.0 to ∞ (20)	1-3 yr
1-18 (7)	1-30 (14)	0.1 to 1.5 (0.7)	4-24 (13)	0-4 (1)	2.0 to ∞ (20)	4-5 yr
1-18 (7)	1-30 (14)	0.1 to 1.5 (0.7)	4-24 (13)	0-4 (1)	2.0 to ∞ (20)	6-8 yr
1-16 (6)	1-26 (16)	0.1 to 1.0 (0.5)	4-24 (14)	0-4 (1)	4.0 to ∞ (20)	9-11 yr
1-16 (5)	1-23 (14)	0 to 1.0 (0.3)	4-22 (14)	0-5 (1)	2.0 to ∞ (9)	12-16 yr
1-14 (3)	1-23 (10)	0 to 1.0 (0.3)	4-21 (10)	0-6 (1)	2.0 to ∞ (9)	>16 yr

Chamber enlargement ("hypertrophy")

Right ventricular
1. RV1 >20 mm (>25 mm under 1 mo)
2. SV6 >6 mm (>12 mm under 1 mo)
3. Abnormal R/S ratio (V1 >2 after 6 mo)
4. Upright TV3R, RV1 after 5 days
5. QR pattern in V3R, V1

Left ventricular
1. RV6 >25 mm (>21 mm under 1 yr)
2. SV1 >30 mm (>20 mm under 1 yr)
3. RV6 + SV1 >60 mm (Use V5 if RV5 >RV6)
4. Abnormal R/S ratio
5. SV1 >2 × RV5

Combined
1. RVH and SV1 or RV6 exceed mean for age
2. LVH and RV1 or SV6 exceed mean for age

Right atrial
1. Peak P valve >3 mm (<6 mo), >2.5 mm (≥6 mo)

Left atrial
1. PII >0.09 sec
2. PV1 late negative deflection >0.04 sec and >1 mm

Maximal PR interval (sec)

Rate/min	<1 mo	1 mo-1 yr	1-3 yr	3-8 yr	8-12 yr	Adult
<60					0.18	0.21
60-80				0.17	0.17	0.21
80-100	0.12			0.16	0.16	0.20
100-120	0.12		0.16	0.16	0.15	0.19
120-140	0.11	0.14	0.14	0.15	0.15	0.18
140-160	0.11	0.13	0.14	0.14		0.17
>160	0.11	0.11				

Appendix C-4: Surface area nomograms

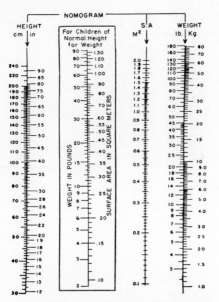

Nomogram for estimation of surface area. The surface area is indicated where a straight line which connects the height and weight levels intersects the surface area column; or the patient is roughly of average size, from the weight alone (enclosed area). (Nomogram modified from data of E. Boyd by C. D. West.)

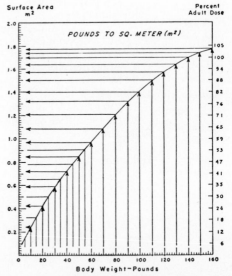

Relations between body weight in pounds, body surface area, and adult dosage. The surface area values correspond to those set forth by Crawford et al. (1950). Note that the 100 per cent adult dose is for a patient weighing about 140 pounds and having a surface area of about 1.7 square meters. (From Talbot, N. B., et al.: *Metabolic Homeostasis—A Syllabus for Those Concerned with the Care of Patients.* Cambridge, Harvard University Press, 1959.)

From Vaughan, V.C., McKay, R.J., and Behrman, R.E.: Nelson textbook of pediatrics, ed. 11, Philadelphia, 1979, p. 2055, W.B. Saunders Co.

Appendix C-5: Conversions and estimates

TEMPERATURE

To convert centigrade to Fahrenheit: ($\frac{9}{5}$ × temperature) + 32

To convert Fahrenheit to centigrade: (temperature − 32) × $\frac{5}{9}$

Centigrade (Celsius)	Fahrenheit	Centigrade (Celsius)	Fahrenheit
34.2	93.6	38.6	101.4
34.6	94.3	39.0	102.2
35.0	95.0	39.4	102.9
35.4	95.7	39.8	103.6
35.8	96.4	40.2	104.3
36.2	97.1	40.6	105.1
36.6	97.8	41.0	105.8
37.0	98.6	41.4	106.5
37.4	99.3	41.8	107.2
37.8	100.0	42.2	108.0
38.2	100.7	42.6	108.7

WEIGHT

To change pounds to grams, multiply by 454
To change kilograms to pounds, multiply by 2.2

Growth patterns

Birth weight (avg): 3.3 kg (7 lb 5 oz)
Newborn loses up to 10% of birthweight but should be up to birth weight again by 10 days
Infant gains 30 g (1 oz)/day for the first 1-2 mo
5 mo: birth weight should be doubled
12 mo: birth weight should be tripled
2 yr: birth weight should be quadrupled

Estimates of weight

4 to 8 year-old: 6 × Age + 12 = Weight (lb)
8 to 12 year-old: 7 × Age + 5 = Weight (lb)

Weight conversion table (pounds and ounces to grams)

Ounces	0 lb	1 lb	2 lb	3 lb	4 lb	5 lb	6 lb	7 lb	8 lb	9 lb
0		454	907	1361	1814	2268	2722	3175	3629	4082
1	28	482	936	1389	1843	2296	2750	3204	3657	4111
2	57	510	964	1418	1871	2325	2778	3232	3686	4139
3	85	539	992	1446	1899	2353	2807	3260	3714	4168
4	113	567	1020	1474	1928	2382	2835	3289	3742	4196
5	142	595	1049	1503	1956	2410	2863	3317	3771	4224
6	170	624	1077	1531	1984	2438	2892	3345	3799	4253
7	198	652	1106	1559	2013	2467	2920	3374	3827	4281
8	227	680	1134	1588	2041	2495	2948	3402	3855	4309
9	255	709	1162	1616	2070	2523	2977	3430	3884	4338
10	284	737	1191	1644	2098	2552	3005	3459	3912	4366
11	312	765	1219	1673	2126	2580	3034	3487	3940	4394
12	340	794	1247	1701	2155	2608	3062	3516	3969	4423
13	369	822	1276	1729	2183	2637	3090	3544	3997	4451
14	397	850	1304	1758	2211	2665	3119	3572	4026	4479
15	425	879	1332	1786	2240	2693	3147	3601	4054	4508

If patient weighs ≥10 lb, the following are used, adding the intermediate value in pounds and ounces to determine the final conversion:

10 lb	4.53 kg	110 lb	49.89 kg
20 lb	9.07 kg	120 lb	54.43 kg
30 lb	13.60 kg	130 lb	58.96 kg
40 lb	18.14 kg	140 lb	63.50 kg
50 lb	22.68 kg	150 lb	68.04 kg
60 lb	27.21 kg	160 lb	72.57 kg
70 lb	31.75 kg	170 lb	77.11 kg
80 lb	36.28 kg	180 lb	81.64 kg
90 lb	40.82 kg	190 lb	86.18 kg
100 lb	45.36 kg	200 lb	90.72 kg

LENGTH

To convert inches to centimeters, multiply by 2.54

To convert centimeters to inches, multiply by 0.394

Growth patterns

Birth length (avg): 50 cm (20 in)
12 mo: birth length should be doubled

HEAD CIRCUMFERENCE
Growth patterns

Birth head circumference (avg): 35 cm (14 in)
12 mo head circumference (avg): 47 cm (19 in)
Head circumference grows 1 cm/mo during first 9 mo

BLOOD PRESSURE (estimate)

Systolic BP (mm Hg) = $2 \times$ Age (yr) + 80
Diastolic BP (mm Hg) = $\frac{2}{3}$ systolic

Appendix C-6: Denver Developmental Screening Test

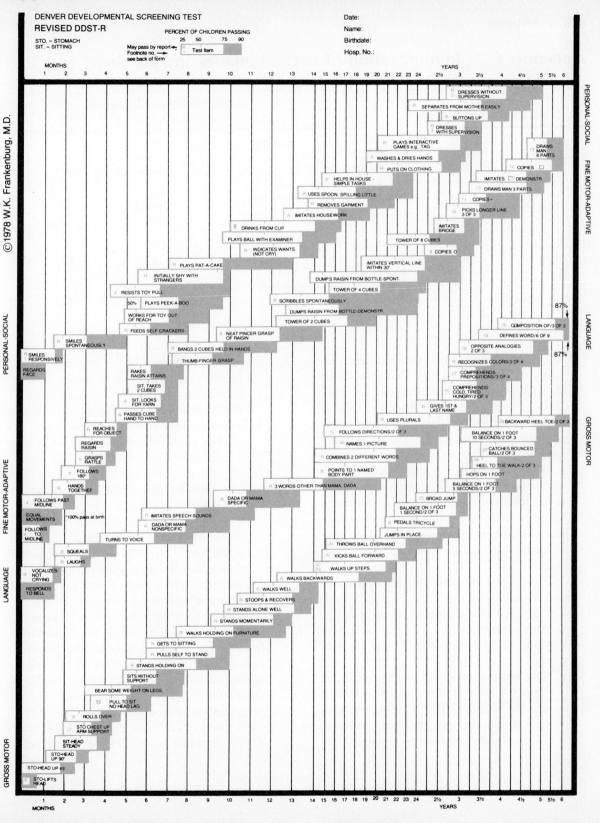

From Frankenburg, W.K., Fandal, A.W., and Sciarillo, W., et al.: J. Pediatr. **99**:998, 1981.

Appendix C-7: Immunization of normal infants and children

	Routine schedule		Schedule for children not immunized in infancy (Over 18 mo)		
2 mo	DTP	TOPV	First visit	DTP	TOPV
4 mo	DTP	TOPV		Tuberculin test	
6 mo	DTP	TOPV		Measles, mumps, rubella	
12 mo	Tuberculin test		2 mo later	DTP	TOPV
15 mo	Measles, mumps, rubella		4 mo later	DTP	TOPV
18 mo	DTP	TOPV	≥2 yr	H. influenzae	
2 yr	H. influenzae		10-16 mo later or preschool	DTP	TOPV
4-6 yr	DTP	TOPV			
14-16 yr	Td and thereafter every 10 yr		14-16 yr	Td and thereafter every 10 yr	

Modified Report of the Committee on Infectious Diseases, American Academy of Pediatrics, Evanston, Ill., 1982.

1. **DTP** (diphtheria, tetanus toxoid, and pertussis vaccine: 0.5 ml IM). Contraindicated if, with previous administration, seizures, CNS disorder, shock, or thrombocytopenia occurred or if patient experienced excessive somnolence, screaming, or temperature over 40.5° C. Generally not recommended in children with seizure disorders or evolving or progressive neurologic disease, or if monitoring patient for presence of fever in subsequent 24-48 hr. It is important to evaluate concurrent condition. (DT or Td may be given.) Do not give during an acute illness.

    Do not give to patients over 6 years of age. Prophylactic antipyretics are indicated. Do not give to children in whom it is important to monitor fevers over the ensuing 24-48 hr. Half doses of DTP may be adequate.

    a. **Td** (Tetanus and diphtheria toxoid, adult type: 0.5 ml IM). For those over 6 yr of age Td is given. This product contains less diphtheria antigen than pediatric DT and may be given to younger children if pediatric DT is unavailable. If primary immunization is begun after 6 yr of age, a series of only 3 Td immunizations is necessary.

    b. **Booster.** Td is recommended every 10 yr. For contaminated wounds, an additional booster dose is given if >5 yr has elapsed since the last dose. Human tetanus immune globulin (TIG) is indicated if the injured patient has had fewer than 2 previous immunizations of tetanus toxoid or has a serious wound that has been unattended for >24 hr. Prophylactic dose is 250-500 units/dose IM given concurrently with tetanus toxoid in separate sites and syringes (p. 546).

2. **TOPV** (trivalent oral polio virus vaccine: 2 drops PO). This recommendation is suitable for breast-fed as well as bottle-fed infants. Infants should not be fed for 30 min after administration to prevent spitting up. Vaccination at 6 mo of age is optional.

3. **Interruption of schedule.** Regardless of the time interval between doses of DTP and TOPV, continue where the patient left off.

4. **MMR** (measles, mumps, rubella vaccine: unit dose SQ). The combined vaccine (MMR) is equivalent to the protection achieved when the antigens are given separately. It is maximally effective when administered at 15 mo of age or older. It may be administered at the same time as DTP or TOPV, if necessary.

5. **Rubella vaccine.** Not to be administered to any female after the onset of menses without obtaining appropriate informed consent. The woman should be vaccinated only if she understands that it is imperative to avoid becoming pregnant in the subsequent 2 mo.

6. *H. influenzae vaccine. H. influenzae* type B vaccine is recommended for children 24 mo of age and older. High-risk children (attending day-care or having underlying disease that increases risk such as sickle cell anemia) may be immunized at 18 mo and will probably require reimmunization at a later date. Conjugate vaccines, currently under study, may be immunogenic in children as young as 6 mo of age.

7. *Influenzae vaccine* (inactivated). Recommended in high-risk patients including those with renal, metabolic, cardiac, or pulmonary disease, as well as immunocompromised hosts. The recommendation is reassessed annually but, in general, children 6-35 mo receive 0.25 ml (split virus) twice, those 3-12 yr receive 0.5 ml (split virus) twice, and children over 12 year should be given 0.5 ml (whole or split virus) once.

8. *Hepatitis B vaccine.* Administered to those with exposure to blood known to be HBsAg positive. Exposure may be percutaneous, ocular, or through mucosal membrane. A single dose of HBIG (0.06 ml/kg or 5.0 ml for adults) is given IM after exposure. HB vaccine 1 ml (children under 10 yr: 0.5 ml) should be given IM within 7 days of exposure, with a second and third dose at 1 mo and 6 mo after the first (p. 589).

9. **General contraindications for vaccinations:** (a) acute febrile illness, (b) immunodeficiency disorder, (c) immunosuppression therapy, (d) recent (within 8 wk) gamma globulin, plasma, or blood transfusion, (e) pregnancy, or (f) previous adverse or allergic reaction to vaccine. Children with evolving neurologic disease should avoid immunizations likely to cause fever or adverse neurologic reactions.

10. **Egg allergy.** Very rare anaphylactic reactions in children allergic to eggs have been reported from the administration of vaccines produced in chick or duck fibroblast tissues (measles, mumps, rubella). Patients with impressive histories for egg-white anaphylaxis should be skin tested with vaccine before administration.

11. **Tuberculin test.** A tuberculin test is optimally given before or simultaneously with the administration of measles (or MMR) vaccine. If there is a history of TB exposure or a high rate of endemicity, reactivity should be determined before administration of the measles vaccine. Routine skin testing on a biennial basis is recommended in high-risk populations.

12. **Immune serum globulin.** Indicated in individuals exposed to measles who are under 1 yr of age (0.25 ml/kg IM) or immunocompromised (0.5 ml/kg IM); viral hepatitis type A contact within 14 days of exposure (0.02 ml/kg IM); and selected immunodeficiency diseases. *Hepatitis B immune globulin (HBIG)* is used with significant exposure to HBsAG-positive blood within 24 hr and 1 mo later (0.06 ml/kg/dose, or 5 ml for adult, IM) (p. 590).

13. **Informed consent.** Parents and patients should be informed about the benefits and risks of immunizing procedures. Consent forms facilitate the presentation of this information and should state the benefits and risks, including adverse reactions.

Formulary

Appendix D-1: Common medications

Drugs	Dosages	Comments
Acetaminophen (Tylenol, Tempra)		
Drop: 80 mg/0.8 ml	10-15 mg/kg/dose q 4-6 hr PO	May give aspirin for synergistic
Elix: 160 mg/5 ml	(adult: 10 grains/dose); (max-	antipyretic effect
Tab: 80 (chew), 160 (junior) 325 mg	imum: 3.6 g/24 hr)	Tox: hepatic: overdose (Chapter
Supp: 120, 325 mg		55)
Acetazolamide (Diamox)		
Tab: 125, 250 mg	Diuretic: 5 mg/kg/24 hr q 6-24	Carbonic anhydrase inhibitor:
Cap (SR): 500 mg	hr PO, IV (adult: 250-375	IM painful; half-life: 4-10 hr;
Vial: 500 mg/5 ml	mg/24 hr)	Table 16-3
	Epilepsy: 8-30 mg/kg/24 hr q	Tox: hypokelemia, acidosis (long-
	6-8 hr PO, IM, IV (maxi-	term therapy), paresthesias
	mum: 1 g/24 hr)	
Acetylcysteine (Mucomyst)		
Sol'n: 10% (100 mg/ml)	Acetaminophen OD: load 140	Primary treatment for acetamin-
20% (200 mg/ml)	mg/kg PO, then 70 mg/kg q	ophen overdose (Chapter 55):
	4 hr PO × 17 doses	pulmonary mucolytic; also IV
	Nebulizer: 2-20 ml (10%) or	Tox: mucosal irritant, broncho-
	1-10 ml (20%) sol'n q 2-6 hr	spasm
Acyclovir (Zovirax)		
Cap: 200 mg	Herpes genitalis: 200 mg q 4	IV therapy indicated in immu-
Vial: 500 mg/10 ml	hr (5 doses/24 hr) PO × 10	nocompromised patient; may
Ointment: 5%	days	be effective in newborn; mod-
		ified dose for recurrent epi-
		sode
		Tox: diaphoresis, hematuria,
		phlebitis (IV)
Albumin		
25% salt-poor albumin (25 g/dl)	0.5-1 g/kg/dose IV repeated	Salt-poor albumin has 0.6 mEq
5% with 0.9%NS (5 g/dl)	prn	Na^+/g; caution with hypervo-
		lemia, CHF

Many oral drugs may be given 3-4 times per day with more flexibility than implied by the specific intervals noted. BR, Excreted in breast milk; NB, newborns under 7 days of age; Pen, penicillin; SR, sustained release; Tox, toxicity of drug.

Drugs	Dosages	Comments
Allopurinol (Zyloprim) Tab: 100, 300 mg	10 mg/kg/24 hr q 6 hr PO (<6-yr-old: 150 mg/24 hr: 6-10-yr-old: 300 mg/24 hr) (maximum: 600 mg/24 hr)	Titrate to serum uric acid level: reduce dose with renal failure Tox: rash, hepatic, cataract
Aluminum hydroxide (Amphogel) Tab: 300, 600 mg Susp: 320 mg/5 ml **Maalox** (also magnesium hydroxide) Tab: 200/200, 400/400 mg Susp: 225/200 mg/5 ml	Peptic ulcer: 5-15 ml (adult: 15-45 ml) 1 and 3 hr after meals and before bed PO Prophylaxis GI bleeding Infant: 2-5 ml/dose q 1-2 hr per NG tube Child: 5-15 ml/dose (adult: 30-60 ml) q 1-2 hr PO	Should be initiated early for prophylaxis. Alternative includes cimetidine
Amantidine (Symmetrel) Syr: 50 mg/5 ml Cap: 100 mg	4.4-8.8 mg/kg/24 hr q 12 hr PO (>9 yr and adult: 100 mg q 12 hr PO)	Continue for at least 10 days and longer in unprotected patient with ongoing exposure to influenza A in high risk patient; only children over 1 yr Tox: depression, CHF, psychosis, seizures
Amikacin (Amikin) Vial: 50, 250 mg/ml	15 mg/kg/24 hr q 8 hr IM, IV slowly over 30 min (maximum: 1.0 g/24 hr) (NB: 15 mg/kg/24 hr q 12 hr)	Therapeutic peak level: <35 μg/ml: caution in renal failure (reduce dose) Tox: renal, VIII nerve
Aminocaproic acid (Amicar) Syr: 250 mg/ml Tab: 500 mg	Load: 200 mg/kg PO (maximum: 6 g) Maint: 100 mg/kg/dose q 6 hr PO (maximum: 24 g/24 hr) for 2-5 days or until healing occurs	Useful for oral bleeding; Chapter 79 Tox: thrombosis, rash, hypotension
Aminophylline (Table 84-1)	Load: 7.5 mg/kg PO; maint: 5 mg/kg/dose q 6 hr PO Load: 6 mg/kg IV slowly, maint: 0.8-1.2 mg/kg/hr IV Neonatal apnea load: 5 mg/kg; then 2-3 mg/kg q 12 hr PO	85% theophylline: therapeutic level: 10-20 μg/ml; neonatal apnea (p. 76; Chapter 84) Tox: nausea, vomiting, irritability, seizures, dysrhythmias
Amoxicillin (Amoxil, Larotid) Susp: 125, 250 mg/5 ml Cap: 125, 250 mg	30-100 mg (avg: 50 mg)/kg/24 hr q 8 hr PO (adult: 250-500 mg q 8 hr)	Do not use for *Shigella* Tox: similar to ampicillin but less diarrhea: see Penicillin G

Drugs	Dosages	Comments
Amoxicillin (AMX)-clavulanic acid (CLA) (Augmentin) Susp: 125 mg AMX/ 31.25 CLA/ 5 ml 250 mg AMX/62.50 CLA/5 ml Tab: 250 mg AMX/125 CLA 500 mg AMX/125 CLA	30-50 mg AMX/kg/24 hr q 8 hr PO (adult: 250-500 mg AMX q 8 hr PO)	Dosage is based on amount of amoxicillin; 2 tab 250 mg are not equivalent to 500 mg tab; beta-lactamase inhibitor Tox: diarrhea, similar to amoxicillin
Ampicillin (Omnipen, Polycillin) Susp: 125, 250 mg/5 ml Cap: 250, 500 mg Vial: 250, 500, 1,000 mg	50-100 mg/kg/24 hr q 6 hr PO (adult: 250-500 mg/dose PO); 100-400 mg/kg/24 hr q 4-6 hr IV (NB: 50-100 mg/kg/24 hr q 12 hr IV) (adult: 4-12 g/24 hr IV)	Higher parenteral doses with severe infection: 3 mEq Na^+/g Tox: rash (esp. with infectious mononucleosis), diarrhea, superinfection: see Penicillin G
Aspirin (salicylate, ASA) Tab: 81 (chew), 325 mg Supp: 65, 130, 195, 325 mg	10-15 mg/kg/dose q 4-6 hr PO (adult: 10 grains/dose) Rheumatoid: 60-100 mg/kg/24 hr q 4-6 PO (maximum: 3.6 g/24 hr PO)	Synergistic antipyretic effect with acetaminophen; avoid with chickenpox or influenza-like illness Therapeutic level: 15-30 mg/dl Tox: GI irritation, tinnitus, platelet dysfunction; overdose (Chapter 55); BR
Atropine Vial: 0.1, 0.4, 1 mg/ml	0.01-0.03 mg/kg/dose IV (minimum: 0.1 mg/dose) (adult: 0.6-1.0 mg/dose; maximum total dose 2 mg) q 5 min prn; may also be given ET	Infants require higher dose (0.03 mg/kg); organophosphate poisoning (0.05 mg/kg) (Chapter 55) Tox: dysrhythmias, anticholinergic
Bicarbonate, sodium ($NaHCO_3$) Vial: 8.4% (50 mEq/50 ml) 7.5% (44 mEq/50 ml)	1 mEq/kg/dose q 10 min prn	Monitor ABG: dilute 1:1 with D5W or sterile water; incompatible with calcium, catecholamines Tox: alkalosis, hyperosmolality, hypernatremia
Bretylium (Bretylol) Vial: 50 mg/ml	5 mg/kg/dose IV followed prn by 10 mg/kg/dose q 15 min IV up to maximum total dose of 30 mg/kg	Table 6-3; limited experience in children Tox: nausea, vomiting, hypotension, bradycardia

Many oral drugs may be given 3-4 times per day with more flexibility than implied by the specific intervals noted. BR, Excreted in breast milk; NB, newborns under 7 days of age; Pen, penicillin; SR, sustained release; Tox, toxicity of drug.

Drugs	Dosages	Comments
Calcium chloride Vial: 10% (100 mg/ml-1.36 mEq Ca/ml)	20-30 mg/kg/dose (maximum: 500 mg/dose q 10 minimum IV [slow] prn); 250 mg/kg 24 hr q 6 hr PO (mix 2% solution)	Monitor heart, avoid extravasation; caution in digitalized patient; incompatible with $NaHCO_3$ Tox: bradycardia, hypotension
Calcium gluconate Vial: 10% (100 mg/ml-0.45 mEq Ca/ml) Tab: 1 g	100 mg/kg dose IV (slow) (maximum: 1 g/dose) q 10 min prn: 500 mg/kg/24 hr q 6 hr PO	See Calcium chloride
Captopril (Capoten) Tab: 12.5, 25, 50, 100 mg	1-6 mg/kg/24 hr q 8 hr PO (maximum: 450 mg/24 hr)	Table 18-2 Tox: renal, proteinuria, neutropenia, rash
Carbamazepine (Tegretol) Tab: 100 mg (chewable), 200 mg	15-30 mg/kg/24 hr q 8-12 hr PO (adult: 1600 mg/24 hr); begin 100-200 mg/dose q 12 hr PO with 100 mg/24 hr increments	Therapeutic level: 4-12 μg/ml: Table 81-6 Tox: hepatic, nystagmus, nausea, aplastic anemia
Carbenicillin (Geopen, Geocillin) Vial: 1, 2, 5, 10 g Tab: 382 mg	400-600 mg/kg/24 hr q 4-6 hr IV: 30-50 mg/kg/24 hr q 6 hr PO (NB: 200 mg/kg/24 hr q 12 hr IV) (adult: 40 g/24 hr IV; 2 g/24 hr PO)	Used in combination therapy with aminoglycoside; 5.2-6.5 mEq Na^+/g Tox: platelet dysfunction, rash; adjust dose with renal failure; see Penicillin G
Cefaclor (Ceclor) Susp: 125, 250 mg/5 ml Cap: 250, 500 mg	20-40 mg/kg/24 hr q 8 hr PO (adult: 250-500 mg q 8 hr)	Active against ampicillin-resistant *H. influenzae* Tox: renal, diarrhea, vaginitis; cross-reacts with pen
Cefamandole (Mandol) Vial: 0.5, 1, 2 g	50-150 mg/kg/24 hr q 4-6 hr IM, IV (adult: 4-12 g/24 hr)	Tox: bleeding, renal, hepatic, rash, neutropenia; cross-reacts with pen; adjust dose with renal failure
Cefazolin (Ancef, Kefzol) Vial: 0.25, 0.5, 1 g	25-100 mg/kg/24 hr q 6-8 hr IM, IV (NB: 40 mg/kg/24 hr q 12 hr) (adult 2-12 g/24 hr)	Tox: renal, hepatic, rash, phlebitis; cross-reacts with pen; adjust dose with renal failure
Cefoperazone (Cefobid) Vial: 1, 2 g	Adult: 2-12 g/24 hr q 6-12 hr IV slowly, IM	Little experience in children Tox: diarrhea, hypersensitivity

Drugs	Dosages	Comments
Cefotaxime (Claforan) Vial: 1, 2 g	50-150 mg/kg/24 hr q 4-6 hr IV, IM (neonatal meningitis: 100-150 mg/kg/24 hr q 8-12 hr) (adult: 1-2 g q 4-6 hr up to maximum 12 g/24 hr)	Third-generation cephalosporin; excellent broad-spectrum coverage; meningitis, UTI, bacteremia, pneumonia, skin infection Tox: hypersensitivity (cross-reacts with pen), phlebitis, pain (IM), diarrhea, colitis, renal, hepatic
Ceftriaxone (Rocephin) Vial: 0.25, 0.5, 1, 2 g	50-100 mg/kg/24 hr q 12-24 hr IV (adult: 1-2 g/dose q 12-24 hr IV)	Third-generation cephalosporin; less frequent administration; excellent broad-spectrum coverage Tox: diarrhea, abnormal liver function
Cefuroxime (Zinacef) Vial: 750, 1500 mg	50-240 mg/kg/24 hr q 6-8 hr IV (adult: 4.5-9.0 g/24 hr q 6-8 hr IV)	Second-generation cephalosporin; higher dose for meningitis; useful for *H. influenzae* disease; do not use for neonatal meningitis, sepsis
Cephalexin (Keflex) Susp: 125, 250 mg/5 ml Cap: 250, 500 mg	25-50 mg/kg/24 hr q 6 hr PO (adult: 250-500/mg/dose q 6 hr)	Tox: nausea, vomiting, renal, hepatic; cross-reacts with pen; adjust dose with renal failure
Cephalothin (Keflin) Vial: 1, 2, 4 g	75-125 mg/kg/24 hr q 4-6 hr IM, IV (NB: 40 mg/kg/24 hr q 12 hr) (adult: 4-12 g/24 hr)	Tox: renal, hepatic, phlebitis, neutropenia; cross-reacts with pen; adjust dose with renal failure
Cephradine (Anspor, Velosef) Susp: 125, 250/5 ml Cap: 250, 500 mg Vial: 0.25, 0.5, 1 g	25-50 mg/kg/24 hr q 6 hr PO; 50-100 mg/kg/24 hr q 6 hr IM (deep), IV	Tox: renal, hepatic, nausea, vomiting, neutropenia, vaginitis, phlebitis, cross-reacts with pen; adjust dose with renal failure
Chloral hydrate (Noctec) Syr: 500 mg/5 ml Cap: 250, 500 mg	Hypnotic: 50 mg/kg/24 hr q 6-8 hr PO, (maximum: 1 g/dose) Sedative: 1/2 hypnotic dose	Do not use with renal, hepatic disease
Chloramphenicol (Chloromycetin) Susp: 150 mg/5 ml Cap: 250 mg Vial: 1 g (100 mg/ml)	50-100 mg/kg/24 hr q 6 hr PO, IV (NB: 25 mg/kg/24 hr q 12 hr IV) (maximum 2-4 g/24 hr)	Tox: bone marrow suppression (reversible) and aplastic anemia; therapeutic level: 10-25 µg/ml: BR

Many oral drugs may be given 3-4 times per day with more flexibility than implied by the specific intervals noted. BR, Excreted in breast milk; NB, newborns under 7 days of age; Pen, penicillin; SR, sustained release; Tox, toxicity of drug.

Drugs	Dosages	Comments
Chlorothiazide (Diuril) Susp: 250 mg/5 ml Tab: 250, 500 mg	10-20 mg/kg/24 hr q 12 hr PO (NB: 30 mg/kg/24 hr PO) (adult: 250-500 mg q 12-24 hr PO)	Table 16-3 Tox: hyponatremia, hypokale- mia, alkalosis; reduce dose with renal failure
Chlorpheniramine (Chlor-Trimeton) Syr: 2 mg/5 ml Tab: 4 mg Tab/cap (SR): 8, 12 mg	0.35 mg/kg/24 hr q 6 hr PO (adult: 4 mg q 4-6 hr) Sustained release in children >12 yr: 16-24 mg/kg/24 hr q 8-12 hr PO	OTC antihistamine; Tox: drowsy, anticholinergic (Chapter 55), hypotension (IM)
Chlorpromazine (Thorazine) Syr: 10 mg/5 ml Tab: 10, 25, 50, 100 mg Cap (SR): 30, 75, 150 mg Supp: 25, 100 mg Vial: 25 mg/ml	0.5 mg/kg/dose q 6-8 hr PO, IM, IV prn (adult: 25-50 mg/dose) 1.0 mg/kg/dose q 6-8 hr PR prn (adult: 50-100 mg/dose PR)	Only children >6-mo-old Tox: phenothiazine-extrapyrami- dal, anticholinergic (Chapter 55); often mixed with meperi- dine and promethazine (see meperidine); BR
Cimetidine (Tagamet) Susp: 300 mg/5 ml Tab: 200, 300 mg Vial: 150 mg/ml	20-30 mg/kg/24 hr q 4-6 hr PO, IV (maximum: 2.4 g/24 hr) (adult: 300 mg/dose q 6 hr PO)	Tox: diarrhea, renal, neutrope- nia; reduce dose with renal failure
Clindamycin (Cleocin) Sol'n: 75 mg/5 ml Cap: 75, 150 mg Amp: 300, 600 mg	10-25 mg/kg/24 hr q 6 hr PO (adult: 600-1800 mg/24 hr PO) 15-40 mg/kg/24 hr q 6-8 hr IM, IV (NB: 15-20 mg/kg/24 hr q 6-8 hr IV) (maximum: 4.8 g/24 hr IV)	Caution in renal, hepatic disease Tox: colitis, rash, diarrhea, phle- bitis; only for child >1 mo
Clonazepam (Klonopin) Tab: 0.5, 1, 2 mg	0.01-0.2 mg/kg/24 hr q 8 hr PO; start at 0.01 mg/kg/24 and add 0.25-0.5 mg/24 hr q 3 days until control (maxi- mum: 20 mg/24 hr)	Therapeutic level: 0.013-0.072 µg/ml; caution in renal dis- ease; Table 81-6; previously Clonopin Tox: drowsy, ataxia, personality change
Clonidine (Catapres) Tab: 0.1, 0.2, 0.3 mg	0.005-0.01 mg/kg/24 hr q 8-12 hr PO (maximum: 0.9 mg/24 hr) (adult: 0.1 mg q 12 hr PO initially; increase 0.1-0.2 mg/24 hr up to 2.4 mg/24 hr PO)	Little experience in children; may be used acutely (p. 120) Tox: drowsiness, headache
Clotrimazole (Gyne-Lotrimin, Mycelex) Tab (vag): 100 mg Cream (vag): 1%	1 tablet or applicator-full vagi- nally nightly × 7-14 days	Tox: local irritation

Drugs	Dosages	Comments
Cloxacillin (Tegopen) Sol'n: 125 mg/5 ml Cap: 250, 500 mg	50-100 mg/kg/24 hr q 6 hr PO (maximum: 4 g/24 hr)	Administer on empty stomach Tox: GI irritant, see Penicillin G
Codeine Elix: 10 mg/5 ml (with antitussive) Tab: 15, 30, 60 mg Vial: 30, 60 mg/ml	Analgesic: 0.5 mg/kg/dose q 4-6 hr PO, IM (adult: 30-60 mg/dose) Antitussive: 1.0 mg/kg/24 hr q 4-6 hr PO (adult: 10-20 mg/ dose)	Also available combined with acetaminophen 120 mg with 12 mg codeine/5 ml and tab- lets Tox: dependence, CNS, and resp depression (Chapter 55); BR
Cortisone Tab: 5, 10, 25 mg Vial: 25, 50 mg/ml	Maintenance: 0.25 mg/kg/24 hr q 12-24 hr IM; 0.50-0.75 mg/kg/24 hr q 6-8 hr PO	Table 74-2
Deferoxamine (Desferal) Amp: 500 mg	If no shock: 90 mg/kg/dose q 8 hr IM If shock: 15 mg/kg/hr IV	Urine turns rose colored if SI >TIBC in iron overdose; Chapter 55 Tox: urticaria, hypotension
Dexamethasone (Decadron) Vial: 4, 24 mg	Croup: 0.25 mg/kg/dose q 6 hr IM, IV Cerebral edema: 0.25-0.5 mg/ kg/dose q 6 hr IM, IV Septic shock: 3 mg/kg/dose q 6 hr IV	Table 74-2; efficacy in cerebral edema controversial
Dextrose D50W (0.5 g/ml)	0.5-1.0 g (2-4 ml D25W)/kg/ dose IV	Dilute D50W 1:1 to avoid hy- pertonicity; draw glucose
Diazepam (Valium) Tab: 2, 5, 10 mg Vial: 5 mg/ml	Status epilepticus: 0.2-0.3 mg/ kg/dose IV (<1 mg/min) q 2-5 min prn (maximum total dose: child, 10 mg; adult, 30 mg) Sedation, muscle relaxation: 0.1-0.8 mg/kg/24 hr q 6-8 hr PO	If used for status epilepticus, must initiate additional drug (phenobarbital or phenytoin); respiratory depression (Chap- ter 21) Tox: drowsy, resp depression (increased with second drug); ?BR
Diazoxide (Hyperstat) Vial: 15 mg/ml	1-3 mg/kg/dose q 4-24 hr IV (fast); repeat in 30 min if no effect; may use intermittent smaller dose	Vasodilator: prompt (3-5 min) re- sponse (Table 18-2); also used to treat hyperinsulinemic hy- poglycemia

---

Many oral drugs may be given 3-4 times per day with more flexibility than implied by the specific intervals noted. BR, Excreted in breast milk; NB, newborns under 7 days of age; Pen, penicillin; SR, sustained release; Tox, toxicity of drug.

Drugs	Dosages	Comments
Dicloxacillin (Dynapen) Susp: 62.5 mg/5 ml Cap: 125, 250, 500 mg	25-100 mg/kg/24 hr q 6 hr PO (adult: 125-500 mg/dose)	Do not use for NB; although optimally given on empty stomach, may have to use open capsule mixed with food Tox: GI irritant, see Penicillin G
Digoxin	See Tables 6-3 and 16-2	
Diphenhydramine (Benadryl) Elix: 12.5 mg/5 ml Cap: 25, 50 mg Vial: 10, 50 mg/ml	5 mg/kg/24 hr q 6 hr PO, IM, IV (maximum: 300 mg/24 hr) Anaphylaxis or phenothiazine overdose: 1-2 mg/kg/dose q 6 hr PO, IM, IV	Antihistamine; OTC Tox: sedation, anticholinergic (Chapter 55)
Dobutamine (Dobutrex) Vial: 250 mg	1-15 µg/kg/min IV infusion (maximum: 40 µg/kg min IV) **Dilute:** 6 mg × weight (kg) in 100 ml D5W. Rate of infusion in µg/kg/min = ml/hr (1 ml/hr delivers 1 µg/kg/min); **or** 250 mg (1 vial) in 500 ml D5W = 500 µg/ml	Table 5-2
Dopamine (Intropin) Amp: 40 mg/ml Vial: 80 mg, 160 mg/ml	Low: 2-5 µg/kg/min IV drip Mod: 5-20 µg/kg/min IV drip High: >20 µg/kg/min IV drip **Dilute:** 6 mg × weight (kg) in 100 ml D5W. Rate of infusion in µg/kg/min = ml/hr (1 ml/hr delivers 1 µ/kg/min); **or** 200 mg (1 amp) in 500 ml D5W = 400 µg/ml	Table 5-2
Doxycycline (Vibramycin) Syr/susp: 25, 50 mg/5 ml Cap: 50, 100 mg Vial: 100, 200 mg	5 mg/kg/24 hr q 12 hr PO or IV slowly over 2-4 hr (adult: 100-200 mg/24 hr)	Do not use in children <9 yr of age Tox: GI irritant, hepatic, photosensitization, superinfection; adjust dose with renal failure; BR
Edrophonium (Tensilon) Vial: 10 mg/ml	Test for myasthenia gravis: 0.2 mg/kg/dose and if no response in 1 min, give 1 mg increments up to maximum total dose of 5-10 mg IV (NB: 1 mg single dose IV)	Have atropine available; may precipitate cholinergic crisis
Ephedrine Syr: 10, 20 mg/5 ml Tab/cap: 25, 50 mg	2-3 mg/kg/24 hr q 4-6 hr PO (adult: 25-50 mg q 4-6 hr PO)	Poor decongestant; potentiates side effects of theophylline without much therapeutic benefit (Chapter 84)

Drugs	Dosages	Comments
Epinephrine (Adrenalin) Vial (1:1000-1 mg/ml) (1:10,000-0.1 mg/ml) Sus-Phrine (1:200-5 mg/ml in oil)	Asthma: 0.01 ml (1:1000)/kg/dose (maximum: 0.35 ml/dose) q 15-20 min SQ prn × 3: Sus-Phrine 0.005 ml/kg/dose (maximum: 0.15 ml) × 1 Asystole: 0.1 ml (1:10,000)/kg/dose (maximum: 5 ml/dose) q 3-5 min IV, ET prn Shock: 0.05-0.5 μg/kg/min IV infusion **Dilute** (for infusion in *shock*): 0.6 mg × weight (kg) in 100 ml D5W. Rate of infusion in 0.1 μg/kg/min = ml/hr (1 ml/hr delivers 0.1 μg/kg/min); **or** 1 mg in 500 ml D5W = 2 μg/ml	Alpha- and beta-agonist first-line drug for asthma; Sus-Phrine unreliable in dosing unless using single dose vial; use in shock only after isoproterenol and dopamine are ineffective; not effective with acidotic patient; Table 5-2 Tox: tachycardia, dysrhythma, tremor, hypertension
Epinephrine, Racemic (Micro-NEF-RIN) Sol'n: 2.25%	0.25-0.5 ml in 2.5 ml of sterile water or saline administered by nebulizer	Rebounds, always admit patient; may use IPPB to administer
Erythromycin (Pediamycin, E.E.S., Erythrocin, E-Mycin ERYC) Susp: 200, 400 mg/5 ml Tab: 200 (chew), 250, 400, 500 mg	20-50 mg/kg/24 hr q 6 hr PO (adult: 250-1,000 mg/dose)	Also available as combination: erythromycin 200 mg + sulfisoxazole 600 mg/5 ml (Pediazole) Tox: GI irritant, rash; BR
Ethanol 100% (1 ml = 790 mg)	Methanol, ethylene glycol overdose: 1 ml/kg over 15 min, then 0.16 ml (125 mg)/kg/hr IV	Maintain ethanol level at ≥100 mg/dl; Table 54-5; BR
Ethosuximide (Zarontin) Syr: 250 mg/5 ml Cap: 250 mg	20-30 mg/kg/24 hr q 24 hr PO; begin 250 mg q 24 hr (3-6 yr old) and increase 250 mg/24 hr at 4-7 day interval; maximum: 1 g/24 hr	Therapeutic level: 40-100 μg/ml; Table 81-6 Tox: GI irritant, neutropenia, drowsy, dizzy, headache
Factor VIII, IX	Tables 79-2 and 79-3	
Fentanyl (Sublimaze) Amp: 50 μg/ml	2-3 μg/kg/dose IV slowly (adult: 50-100 μg/dose)	Narcotic-half-life: 20 min

Many oral drugs may be given 3-4 times per day with more flexibility than implied by the specific intervals noted. BR, Excreted in breast milk; NB, newborns under 7 days of age; Pen, penicillin; SR, sustained release; Tox, toxicity of drug.

Drugs	Dosages	Comments
Furazolidone (Furoxone) Liq: 50 mg/15 ml Tab: 100 mg	*Giardia:* 6 mg/kg/24 hr q 6 hr PO (adult: 100 mg q 6 hr)	Do not use in children <1 mo; avoid alcohol Tox: nausea, vomiting, rash
Furosemide (Lasix) Sol'n: 10 mg/ml Tab: 20, 40, 80 mg Amp: 10 mg/ml	1 mg/kg/dose q 6-12 hr IV initially (may repeat q 2 hr IV prn); 2 mg/kg/dose q 2-12 hr PO initially; may increase dose by 1 mg/kg increments (maximum: 6 mg/kg/dose PO, IM, IV)	Rapid acting; Table 16-3 Tox: hypokalemia, hyponatremia, alkalosis, prerenal azotemia, ototoxicity
Gentamicin (Garamycin) Vial: 10, 40 mg/ml	5.0-7.5 mg/kg/24 hr q 8 hr IM, IV (maximum: 300 mg/24 hr) (NB: 5 mg/kg/24 hr q 12 hr) (adult: 3-5 mg/kg/24 hr q 8 hr)	Therapeutic peak level: 6-12 µg/ml; caution in renal failure (adjust dose); slow IV infusion Tox: renal, VIII nerve
Glucagon Amp: 1 mg (1 unit)/ml	0.03-0.1 mg/kg/dose q 20 min SQ, IM, IV prn (NB: 0.1-0.2 mg/kg/dose q 4 hr prn) (adult: 0.5-1.0 mg/dose)	Hypoglycemia: not adequate as only glucose support, esp in NB; treatment of propranolol (beta-blocker) overdose
Glucose (see Dextrose)		
Griseofulvin Microsize (Grisactin, Grifulvin V) Susp: 125 mg/5 ml Tab/cap: 125, 250, 500 mg Ultramicrosize (Gris-PEG, Fulvicin P/G) Tab: 125, 250, 330 mg	Microsize: 10 mg/kg/24 hr q 24 hr PO (adult: 500-1,000 mg q 12-24 hr PO) Ultramicrosize: 5 mg/kg/24 hr q 24 hr PO (adult: 250-500 mg/24 hr q 12-24 hr PO)	Give with meals; either formulation is adequate; treatment period of 4-6 wk Tox: renal, hepatic, neutropenia, rash, headache
Heparin (Liquaemin, Panheprin) Vial: 100, 1,000, 5,000, 10,000, 20,000, 40,000 units/ml	Load: 50 units/kg IV bolus Maint: 10-25 units/kg/hr IV infusion **or** 100 units/kg/dose q 4 hr IV Adult: load (5,000 units) with maint (20,000-30,000 unit q 24 hr IV continuous infusion **or** 5,000-10,000 q 4 hr)	Titrate to maintain PTT at 2 times control; antidote: protamine Tox: bleeding, allergy rash, wheezing, anaphylaxis
Hydralazine (Apresoline) Tab: 10, 25, 50, 100 mg Amp: 20 mg/ml	Crisis: 0.1-0.2 mg/kg/dose (1.7-3.5 mg/kg/24 hr) q 4-6 hr IM, IV prn (adult: 10-40 mg/dose) Maint: 0.75-3 mg/kg/24 hr q 6-12 hr PO (adult: 10-75 mg/dose q 6 hr PO)	Vasodilator, prompt (10-30 min response if IV) decrease BP; Table 18-2 Tox: tachycardia, angina, SLE-like syndrome; reduce dose with renal failure

Drugs	Dosages	Comments
Hydrochlorothiazide (Esidrix, HydroDiuril) Tab: 25, 50, 100 mg	1-2 mg/kg/24 hr q 12 hr PO (NB: 2-3 mg/kg/24 hr PO) (adult 25-100 mg q 12-24 hr)	Table 16-3 Tox: hyponatremia, hypokalemia, alkalosis; reduce dose with renal failure
Hydrocortisone (Solu-Cortef) Susp: 10 mg/5 ml Tab: 5, 10, 20 mg Vial: 100, 250, 500, 1,000 mg	Maintenance: 0.5 mg/kg/24 hr q 8 hr PO Septic shock: 50 mg/kg/dose (maximum: 500 mg/dose) IV Asthma: 4-5 mg/kg/dose q 6 hr IV	Table 74-2
Hydroxyzine (Atarax, Vistaril) Syr/susp: 10, 25 mg/5 ml Tab (Atarax): 10, 25, 50 mg Cap (Vistaril): 25, 50, 100 mg Vial: (Vistaril): 25, 50 mg/ml	2 mg/kg/24 hr q 6 hr PO (adult: 200-400 mg/24 hr q 6 hr PO) 0.5-1 mg/kg/dose q 4-6 hr IM prn (adult: 25-100 mg/dose q 4-6 hr IM prn)	Antihistamine, potentiates meperidine, barbiturates Tox: sedation, anticholinergic (Chapter 55)
Ibuprofen (Motrin) Tab: 300, 400, 600, 800 mg	40 mg/kg/24 hr q 6-8 hr PO (adult: 1.2-2.4 g/24 hr)	Not approved in children <12 yr; available over-the-counter (Nuprin, Advil 200 mg Tab) (adult: 200-400 mg q 4-6 hr PO; maximum: 1.2 g/24 hr) Tox: GI irritant, keratopathy, retinopathy, rash
Immune serum globulin	Exposure to measles <1 yr of age (0.25 ml/kg IM) or immunocompromised (0.5 ml/kg IM); viral hepatitis type A contact within 14 days of exposure (0.02 ml/kg IM); and selected immunodeficiency disease. Hepatitis B immune globulin (HBIG) is used with significant exposure to HBsAG-positive blood within 24 hr and 1 mo later (0.06 ml/kg/dose IM) (p. 489)	
Indomethacin (Indocin) Cap. 25, 50 mg	1-3 mg/kg/24 hr q 6-8 hr PO (maximum: 100-200 mg/24 hr)	Not approved in children <14 yr; may be used to close PDA (with CHF) in neonate: 0.1-0.2 mg/kg/dose q 12 hr up to maximum 0.6 mg/kg IV Tox: nausea, vomiting, headache, corneal opacity
Insulin	Table 74-4	

Many oral drugs may be given 3-4 times per day with more flexibility than implied by the specific intervals noted. BR, Excreted in breast milk; NB, newborns under 7 days of age; Pen, penicillin; SR, sustained release; Tox, toxicity of drug.

Drugs	Dosages	Comments
Ipecac, syrup of	6-12 mo (10 ml/dose PO) 12 mo (15 ml/dose PO) Adult (30 ml/dose PO) Give initial dose and may repeat × 1	Do not use in children <6 mo; push fluids; contraindicated in caustic ingestions and patients who are comatose or having seizures; Chapter 54
Iron, elemental (Fe) (Fer-In-Sol, Feosol) Drop: 75 mg (15 mg Fe)/0.6 ml Syr: 90 mg (18 mg Fe)/5 ml Tab: 200 mg (40 mg Fe), 325 mg (65 mg Fe)	Therapeutic: 6 mg elemental Fe/kg/24 hr q 8 hr PO Prophylactic: 1-2 mg elemental Fe/kg/24 hr q 8-24 hr PO (maximum: 15 mg elemental Fe/24 hr)	Ferrous sulfate is 20% elemental iron (Fe) (Chapter 26) Tox: GI irritant (reduce by giving with food); overdose (Chapter 55)
Isoetharine (Bronkosol, Bronkometer) Sol'n: 1% (10 mg/ml) Aerosol	Nebulizer: 0.25-0.5 ml diluted in 2.5 ml saline q 4 hr prn Aerosol: 1-2 puffs q 2-4 hr prn	Administer by nebulizer with or without IPPB Tox: tachycardia, hypertension
Isoniazid (INH) Syr: 50 mg/5 ml Tab: 50, 100, 300 mg	10-20 mg/kg/24 hr q 12-24 hr PO (adult: 300 mg/24 hr)	Supplemental pyridoxine (10 mg/100 mg INH) needed in adolescents, adults Tox: peripheral neuropathy, hepatic, seizure, acidosis; BR
Isoproterenol (Isuprel) Amp: 200 µg/ml Neb: 1:100, 200 Aerosol	Shock: 0.05-0.5 µg/kg/min IV infusion; begin at 0.05 µg/kg/min and increase by 0.1 µg/kg/min increments (maximum: 1.5 µg/kg/min) Nebulizer: 0.5 ml diluted in 2.5 ml saline q 4 hr prn Aerosol: 1-2 puffs q 2-4 hr prn **Dilute** (for infusion in shock) 0.6 mg × weight (kg) in 100 ml D5W. Rate of infusion in 0.1 µg/kg/min = ml/hr (1 ml/hr delivers 0.1 µg/kg/min); or 200 µg (1 ml) in 200 ml D5W = 1 µg/ml	Tables 5-2 and 6-3
Kanamycin (Kantrex) Vial: 37.5, 250, 333 mg/ml	15 mg/kg/24 hr q 8 hr IM, IV (maximum: 1 g/24 hr) (NB: 15 mg/kg/24 hr q 12 hr)	Therapeutic peak level: 25-30 µg/ml; caution in renal failure (adjust dose); infusion IV slowly Tox: renal, hearing

Drugs	Dosages	Comments
Levothyroxine (Synthroid) Tab: 25, 50, 100, 200, 300 μg Vial: 500 μg	Infancy: 7-9 μg/kg/24 hr PO; thereafter 100 μg/m²/24 hr PO (child: 3-5 μg/kg/24 hr PO)	Monitor T4 and thyroid-stimu- lating hormone
Lidocaine (Xylocaine) Vial (IV): 10, 20 mg/ml Vial (anesthetic): 10 mg (1%), 20 mg, 40 mg/ml	Load 1 mg/kg dose q 5-10 min IV prn to maximum of 5 mg/ kg Maintenance: 20-50 μg/kg/min IV infusion Adult: load same; maintenance: 2-4 mg/min **Dilute** 150 mg × weight (kg) in 250 ml D5W. Rate of in- fusion in μg/min = 10 × ml/hr	Antidysrhythmic; therapeutic level: 1.5-5 μg/ml; may be given ET; Table 6-3 Tox: seizures, drowsiness eu- phoria, muscle twitching, dys- rhythmias
Magnesium hydroxide (see aluminum hydroxide) (Maalox)		
Magnesium sulfate Crystal: Epsom salt Vial: 10%, 12.5%, 25%, 50%	Catharsis: 250 mg/kg/dose PO (adult: 30 g/dose PO) Hypomagnesemia: 25-50 mg/ kg/dose q 4-6 hr × 3-4 doses IM or IV (adult: 1-4 g/ 24 hr Anticonvulsant: 1 g 10% sol'n IV or 25/50% sol'n IM)	Caution in renal failure; follow magnesium and calcium levels; Chapter 54 Tox: hypotension
Mannitol Vial: 20% (200 mg/ml) 25% (250 mg/ml)	Diuretic: 750 mg/kg/dose IV: do not repeat with persis- tent oliguria (adult: 300 mg/ kg/dose); Cerebral edema: 0.25-0.5 g/kg IV slow over 10-15 min q 3- 4 hr prn (maximum: 1 g/kg/ dose IV)	Maintain serum osmolality <320 mOsm/L; may get CNS re- bound, intracranial monitor indicated Tox: hypovolemia, volume over- load, hyperosomolality
Mebendazole (Vermox) Tab (chew), 100 mg	Pinworm: 100 mg PO, repeat in 1 wk Ascaris, hookworm: 100 mg q 12 hr PO for 3 days	Not studied in children <2 yr Tox: diarrhea

Many oral drugs may be given 3-4 times per day with more flexibility than implied by the specific intervals noted. BR, Excreted in breast milk; NB, newborns under 7 days of age; Pen, penicillin; SR, sustained release; Tox, toxicity of drug.

Drugs	Dosages	Comments
Meperidine (Demerol) Syr: 50 mg/5 mg Tab: 50, 100 mg Vial: 25, 50, 100 mg/ml	1-2 mg/kg dose q 3-4 hr PO, IM, IV prn (adult 50-150 mg/dose) (maximum: 100 mg/dose in children)	75 mg meperidine = 10 mg morphine DPT, sedative cocktail (ratio 4:1:1) Meperidine (Demerol) 1-2 mg/kg/dose (maximum: 50 mg/dose) Promethazine (Phenergan) 0.25-0.5 mg/kg/dose (maximum 12.5 mg/dose) Chlorpromazine (Thorazine) 0.25-0.5 mg/kg dose (maximum: 12.5 mg/dose) Also potentiated by hydroxyzine Tox: CNS, resp depression, seizure, overdose (Chapter 55); BR
Metaraminol (Aramine) Vial: 10 mg/ml	0.01 mg/kg/dose IV prn **or** 1-4 µg/kg/min IV infusion	Tox: tachycardia, dysrhythmia, local tissue slough
Methicillin (Staphcillin) Vial: 1, 4, 6 g	100-200 mg/kg/24 hr q 4-6 hr IM, IV (maximum: 12 g/24 hr) (NB: 50-75 mg/kg/24 hr q 8-12 hr)	Equivalent to nafcillin, oxacillin Tox: interstitial nephritis (hematuria), bone marrow suppression; see Penicillin G
Methsuximide (Celontin) 150,300 mg	Adult: 300 mg/24 hr q 24 hr PO × 1 wk; 300 mg/24 hr/wk increments q 3 wk as necessary (maximum: 1.2 g/24 hr)	Petit mal seizures Tox: CNS symptoms, behavioral change, caution in liver, renal disease
Methyldopa (Aldomet) Tab: 125, 250, 500 mg Vial: 50 mg/ml Susp: 250 mg/5 ml	Crisis: 2.5-5 mg/kg/dose q 6-8 hr IV (maximum: 20-40 mg/kg/24 hr or 500 mg/dose IV) Chronic: 10 mg/kg/24 hr q 6-12 hr PO (maximum: 40 mg/kg/24 hr or total dose 2 g/24 hr	Table 18-2 Tox: somnolence, hemolytic disease, ulcerogenic; reduce dose with renal failure
Methylene blue Vial: 1% (10 mg/ml)	1-2 mg/kg/dose IV q 4 hr prn	Use for methemoglobinemia; Table 54-4
Methylprednisolone (Solu-Medrol) Vial: 40, 125, 500, 1,000 mg	Septic shock: 30-50 mg/kg/dose IV Asthma: 1-2 mg/kg/dose q 6 hr IV	Table 74-2

Drugs	Dosages	Comments
Metolazone (Zaroxolyn, Diulo) 2.5, 5, 10 mg	Adult: 2.5-10 mg/24 hr PO	Little experience in children; useful when no response to other diuretics and glomerular filtration rate; Table 16-3 Tox: azotemia, ↓ K$^+$, hypotension, lethargy, coma
Metronidazole (Flagyl) Tab: 250 mg, 500 mg	*Haemophilus vaginalis*/vaginitis: 500 mg q 12 hr PO for 7-10 day *Trichomonas vaginalis:* 5 mg/kg/dose q 8 hr PO for 7 days (adult: 250 mg q 8 hr for 7 days) *Giardia lamblia:* 5 mg/kg/dose q 8 hr PO for 10 days (adult: 250 mg q 8 hr for 10 days) Amebiasis: 35-50 mg/kg/24 hr q 8 hr PO for 10 days (adult: 750 mg q 8 hr for 10 days)	IV form available for severe anaerobic infections Tox: nausea, diarrhea, neutropenia, urticaria, do not give to pregnant patient; BR
Miconazole (Monistat) Vag cream (2%) Supp: 200 mg (Monistat 3)	*Candida (Monilia)* vaginitis: 1 applicator-full before bed for 7-14 days; supp: 200 mg before bed x 3 days	Systemic form available
Morphine Vial: 8, 10, 15 mg/ml	0.1-0.2 mg/kg/dose (maximum: 15 mg/dose) q 2-4 hr IM, IV	Antidote, naloxone (Chapter 55) Tox: CNS, respiratory depression, hypotension; BR
Moxalactam (Moxam) Vial: 1, 2 g	150 mg/kg/24 hr q 6-8 hr IV, IM (maximum: 200 mg/kg/24 hr) (NB: 100 mg/24 hr q 12 hr IV) (gram-negative neonatal meningitis: load with 100 mg/kg) (adult: 2-6 g/24 hr; maximum: 12 g/24 hr)	Cephalosporin, excellent for *H. influenzae,* less active against gram-positives; reduce dose in renal failure; monitor PT Tox: eosinophilia, phlebitis, bleeding, hypersensitivity (cross-reacts with pen), diarrhea, renal, hepatic
Nafcillin (Unipen) Vial: 0.5, 1, 2 g	50-200 mg/kg/24 hr q 4-6 hr IM, IV (maximum: 12 g/24 hr) (NB: 40 mg/kg/24 hr q 12 hr)	Equivalent to methicillin, oxacillin; IM painful; oral form available Tox: allergy, see Pen; low renal toxicity

Many oral drugs may be given 3-4 times per day with more flexibility than implied by the specific intervals noted. BR, Excreted in breast milk; NB, newborns under 7 days of age; Pen, penicillin; SR, sustained release; Tox, toxicity of drug.

Drugs	Dosages	Comments
Naloxone (Narcan) Amp: (0.4, 1.0 mg/ml) 0.02 mg/ml (neonate)	0.1 ml/kg/dose (maximum: 0.8 mg) IV; if no response in 10 min and opiate suspected, give 2 mg IV	Narcotic antagonist; propoxyphene (Darvon) and pentazocine (Talwin) require very large doses to reverse; Chapter 55; may have role in septic shock
Naproxen (Naprosyn) Tab: 250, 375, 500 mg	Adult: 250 mg q 6-8 hr PO (maximum: 1,250 mg/24 hr) Dysmenorrhea: load 500 mg PO, then 250 mg q 6-8 hr PO	Nonsteroidal antiinflammatory Tox: GI irritant, vertigo, headache, platelet dysfunction; not approved for children
Nitrofurantoin (Furadantin, Macrodantin) Susp: 25 mg/5 ml Tab: 50, 100 mg Cap: 25, 50, 100 mg	5-7 mg/kg/24 hr q 6 hr PO; chronic: 2.5-5 mg/kg/24 hr (adult: 50-100 mg/dose q 6 hr PO; chronic: 50-100 mg before bed PO)	Do not use for renal disease, G6PD deficiency, child <1 mo, pregnancy Tox: hypersensitivity
Nitroprusside (Nipride) Vial: 50 mg	0.5-10 μg/kg/min (avg: 3 μg) IV infusion **Dilute** 6 mg × weight (kg) in 100 ml D5W. Rate of infusion in μg/kg/min = ml/hr or 50 mg (1 vial) in 100 ml of D5W = 500 μg/ml	Precise, rapid (1-2 min) BP control; requires constant monitoring; light sensitive; Table 18-2 Tox: hypotension, cyanide poisoning (monitor thiocyanate level)
Norepinephrine (Levophed) Vial: 1 mg/ml	0.1-1.0 μg/kg/min IV infusion **Dilute:** 0.6 mg × weight (kg) in 100 ml D5W. Rate of infusion in 0.1 μg/kg/min = ml/hr (1 ml/hr delivers 0.1 μg/kg/min); or 1 mg (1 ml) in 100 ml of D5W = 10 μg/ml	Table 5-2; titrate response
Nystatin (Mycostatin) Cream: 100,000 unit/g Susp: 100,000 unit/ml Tab (vag): 100,000 unit	Thrush: 1 ml in each side of the mouth q 4-6 hr PO Diaper rash (*Candida*): apply with diaper changes (q 2-6 hr) Vaginitis: 1 tab in vagina before bed for 10 days	Continue oral and topical therapy for 2-3 days after clearing

Drugs	Dosages	Comments
Oxacillin (Prostaphin) Sol'n: 250 mg/5 ml Cap: 250, 500 mg Vial: 0.5, 1, 2, 4 g	50-100 mg/kg/24 hr q 6 hr PO (adult: 500-1,000 mg q 6 hr PO); 50-200 mg/kg/24 hr q 4-6 hr IM, IV (maximum: 8 g/24 hr) (NB: 25-50 mg/kg/24 hr q 8-12 hr IM, IV)	Equivalent to methicillin, nafcillin; oral form optimally given on empty stomach Tox: see Penicillin G
Pancuronium (Pavulon) Vial: 1, 2 mg/ml	Load: 0.04-0.1 mg/kg/dose IV (intubation: 0.06-0.1 mg/kg/dose IV) (NB: 0.02 mg/kg/dose IV) Maint: 0.01-0.02 mg/kg/dose q 20-40 min IV prn (NB: adjust on basis of loading dose)	Peak effect in 2-3 min; duration 40-60 min; must be able to support respirations
Paraldehyde Sol'n: 1 g/ml Amp: 1 g/ml	Sedative: 0.15 ml (150 mg)/kg/dose PO, PR, IM Anticonvulsant: 0.3 ml (300 mg)/kg/dose q 4-6 hr PR prn (NB: 0.1-0.2 ml [100-200 mg]/kg/dose diluted in 0.9%NS q 4-6 hr PR prn; 0.15 ml/kg/dose q 4-6 hr IM, IV prn)	For PR, dissolve 1:1 in cottonseed, olive, or mineral oil; for IM, give deep; IV must be given slowly (5 min) after mixing 0.15 ml/kg/dose diluted 1:20 with saline in glass syringe and infused; may repeat IV dose in 20-40 min (avoid extravasation); do not give if hepatic or pulmonary disease is present (p. 134) Tox: IV (pulmonary edema, CHF), IM (sterile abscess), PR (proctitis), respiratory depression
Penicillin G (sodium or potassium salt) Susp: 125, 250 mg/5 ml Tab: 125, 250, 500 mg Vial: 1, 5, 20 million units	25-50 mg (40,000-80,000 units)/kg/24 hr q 6 hr PO (adult: 300,000-1.2 million units/24 hr PO); 50,000-250,000 units/kg/24 hr q 4 hr IM, IV (NB: 50,000-150,000 units/kg/24 hr q 8-12 hr IM, IV)	1 mg = 1600 units; salt content (1 million units contains 1.68 mEq Na$^+$ or K$^+$): PO erratically absorbed, give on empty stomach Tox: allergy (anaphylaxis, rash, urticaria), superinfection (*Candida*), hemolytic anemia, interstitial nephritis; adjust dose with renal failure; BR

Many oral drugs may be given 3-4 times per day with more flexibility than implied by the specific intervals noted. BR, Excreted in breast milk; NB, newborns under 7 days of age; Pen, penicillin; SR, sustained release; Tox, toxicity of drug.

Drugs	Dosages		Comments
Penicillin G benzathine and Penicillin G procaine (Bicillin C-R 900/300) 900,000 units benz and 300,000 units proc/2 ml	*Weight (lb)*	*Benzathine pen G (Bicillin L-A)*	*Benzathine/procaine pen G (Bicillin C-R (900/300)*
	<30	300,000 units	300,000:100,000
	31-60	600,000 units	600,000:200,000
	61-90	900,000 units	900,000:300,000
	>90	1,200,000 units	Not available

Penicillin V (Pen-Vee K, V-Cillin K)
Susp: 125, (200,000 units), 250 (400,000 units) mg/5 ml
Tab: 125, 250, 500 mg

25-50 mg (40,000-80,000 units)/ kg/24 hr q 6 hr PO (adult: 250-500 mg q 6 hr PO)

More resistant to destruction by gastric acid
Tox: see Penicillin G

Pentobarbital (Nembutal)
Elix: 20 mg/5 ml
Cap: 30, 50, 100 mg
Supp: 30, 60, 120, 200 mg
Vial: 50 mg/ml

Sedation: 6 mg/kg/24 hr q 8 hr PO, PR, IM, IV (adult: 30 mg q 6-8 hr)
Cerebral edema: load: 3-20 mg/kg slow IV; maint: 1-2 mg/kg/hr IV

Short-acting barbiturate; treatment of increased intracranial pressure must include monitor
Pentobarbital to maintain intracranial pressure <15 mm Hg and barbiturate level 25-40 μg/ml; support respirations, monitor BP
Tox: CNS excitement, respiratory depression, hypotension (Chapter 55)

Phenazopyridine (Pyridium)
Tab: 100, 200 mg

6-12 yr of age: 100 mg q 8 hr PO (adult: 200 mg q 8 hr PO)

Use until dysuria gone and diagnosis made; urine color orange/red; avoid with G6PD deficiency
Tox: hemolytic anemia, methemoglobinemia

Phenobarbital (Luminal)
Elix: 20 mg/5 ml
Tab: 8, 15, 30, 60, 90, 100 mg
Vial: 65, 130 mg/ml

Seizures: load: 10-15 mg/kg PO, IM (erratic absorption), IV (<25-50 mg/min); with status epilepticus and no response in 20-30 min, repeat 10 mg/kg IV (adult: 100 mg/ dose IV q 20 min prn × 3)
Maint: 3-5 mg/kg/24 hr q 12-24 hr PO (adult: 200-300 mg/24 hr PO)
Sedation: 2-3 mg/kg/dose PO, IM q 8 hr prn

May be used as first-line drug in status epilepticus (IM, IV) or after seizures controlled by diazepam (Valium); Chapters 21 and 81
Therapeutic level: 10-25 μg/ml
Tox: drowsiness, irritability, learning problems, CNS and respiratory depression with high doses (Chapter 55)
Reduce dose with renal failure; BR

Drugs	Dosages	Comments
Phentolamine (Regitine) Vial: 5 mg/ml	0.05-0.1 mg/kg/dose q 1-4 hr IV (adult: 2.5-5 mg/dose IV)	Specific for pheochromocytoma and MAO-induced hypertension; rapid onset; dose, esp PO, must be individualized; may be given as continuous infusion; Table 5-2 Tox: dysrhythmia, hypotension
Phenytoin (Dilantin, diphenylhydantoin) Susp: 30, 125 mg/5 ml Tab (chew): 50 mg Cap: 30, 100 mg Amp: 50 mg/ml	Seizures: load: 10-20 mg/kg PO, IV (<40 mg/min); maint: 5-10 mg/kg/24 hr q 12-24 hr PO (adult: 200-400 mg/24 hr PO) Dysrhythmia load: 5 mg/kg IV (<40 mg/min) (adult: 100 mg/dose q 5 min prn up to 1 g IV); maint: 6 mg/kg/24 hr q 12 hr PO (adult: 300 mg/24 hr PO)	Therapeutic level: 10-20 µg/ml: good for digoxin- and tricyclic antidepressant–induced dysrhythmias; Chapters 6, 21, and 81 Tox: nystagmus, ataxia, hypotension, gingival hyperplasia, SLE-like syndrome, hirsutism
Physostigmine (Antilirium) Vial: 1 mg/ml	Child: 0.5 mg IV (over 3 min) q 10 min prn (maximum: 2 mg) Adult: 1-2 mg IV (over 3 min) q 10 min prn (maximum: 4 mg in 30 min)	Anticholinesterase; use in anticholinergic overdose (Chapter 55 and Table 54-4)
Polystyrene sodium sulfonate (Kayexalate) Powder: 450 g	1 g/kg/dose q 6 hr PO or q 2-6 hr PR (adult: 15 g PO or 30-60 g PR q 6 hr)	1 level tsp = 3.5 g; 4.1 mEq Na^+/g: exchanges 1 mEq K^+ for 1 g resin, which delivers 1 mEq Na^+ for each 1 mEq K^+ removed; mix 30%-70% suspension in D10W, 1% methylcellulose, or 10% sorbitol Tox: electrolyte problems, constipation
Pralidoxime (Protopam, 2-PAM) Vial: 1 g	20-50 mg/kg/dose (maximum: 2 g/dose) IV slow (<50 mg/min) q 8 hr prn × 3	Cholinesterase reactivator; use after atropine in organophosphate overdose (Chapter 55); oral preparation for prophylaxis

Many oral drugs may be given 3-4 times per day with more flexibility than implied by the specific intervals noted. BR, Excreted in breast milk; NB, newborns under 7 days of age; Pen, penicillin; SR, sustained release; Tox, toxicity of drug.

Drugs	Dosages	Comments
Prednisone Tab: 5, 10, 20 mg Susp: 5 mg/5 ml	Maintenance: 0.1-0.15 mg/kg/24 hr q 12 hr PO Asthma: 1-2 mg/kg/24 hr q 6 hr PO	Table 74-2
Primidone (Mysoline) Susp: 250 mg/5 ml Tab: 50, 250 mg	10-25 mg/kg/24 hr q 6-8 hr PO; start at 125-250 mg, increase in 125-250 increments at 1-wk intervals (adult: initial 250 mg/24 hr PO; maintenance 750-1,500 mg/24 hr q 6 hr PO)	Therapeutic level: 7-15 μg/ml (or phenobarbital 10-25 μg/ml) Table 81-6 Tox: sedation, nausea, vomiting, diplopia: reduce dose with renal failure; see Phenobarbital
Probenecid (Benemid) Tab: 500 mg	Load: 25 mg/kg PO; maint: 40 mg/kg/24 hr q 6 hr PO (adult: 2 g/24 hr); 25 mg/kg (adult: 1 g) PO before ampicillin or penicillin treatment of *Neisseria gonorrhoeae*	Not recommended for children <2 yr Tox: GI irritant
Procainamide (Pronestyl) Tab/cap: 250, 375, 500 mg Vial: 100, 500 mg/ml	Load: 2-6 mg/kg/dose IV slow (<50 mg/min) (adult: 100 mg/dose IV slow q 10 min prn up to total load of 1 g IV) Maint: 20-80 μg/kg/min IV (adult: 1-3 mg/min IV) or 15-50 mg/kg/24 hr q 4-6 hr PO (adult: 250-500 mg/dose q 4-6 hr PO)	IV must be given slowly at concentration <100 mg/ml; do not use with heart block; Table 6-3 Tox: GI irritant, SLE-like syndrome dysrhythmias
Prochlorperazine (Compazine) Syr: 5 mg/5 ml Tab: 5, 10, 25 mg Supp: 2.5, 5, 25 mg Amp: 5 mg/ml	0.4 mg/kg/24 hr q 6-8 hr PO, PR (adult: 5-10 mg q 6-8 hr PO or 25 mg q 12 hr PR) 0.2 mg/kg/24 hr q 6-8 hr IM (adult: 5-20 mg/dose IM) (maximum: 40 mg/24 hr)	Only chidren >2 yr and >10 kg Tox: phenothiazine (extrapyramidal, anticholinergic) (Chapter 55)
Promethazine (Phenergan) Syr: 6.25, 25 mg/5 ml Tab: 12.5, 25, 50 mg Supp: 12.5, 25, 50 mg Amp: 25, 50 mg/ml	Nausea, vomiting: 0.25-0.5 mg/kg/dose q 4-6 hr PO, PR, IM prn (adult: 12.5-25 mg/dose) Sedation: 0.5-1 mg/kg/dose q 6 hr PO, PR, IM prn (adult: 25-50 mg/dose)	Often mixed with meperidine and chlorpromazine for DPT cocktail (see DPT cocktail—Meperidine) Tox: phenothiazine (sedation, extrapyramidal, anticholinergic) (Chapter 55)

Drugs	Dosages	Comments
Propranolol (Inderal) Tab: 10, 20, 40, 80 mg Vial: 1 mg/ml	Dysrhythmias: load: 0.01-0.1 mg/kg/dose (maximum: 1 mg/dose) IV over 10 min (adult: 1 mg/dose IV q 5 min up to total of 5 mg); maint: 0.5-1 mg/kg/24 hr q 6 hr PO (adult: 10-30 mg/dose q 6-8 hr PO) Hypertension: 0.5-1.0 mg/kg/24 hr q 6-12 hr PO (maximum: 320 mg/24 hr PO) Tetralogy spells: 0.1-0.2 mg/kg/dose IV repeated in 15 min prn Migraine prophylaxis: 10-60 mg q 8 hr PO Thyrotoxicosis: 10-20 mg q 6-8 hr PO	Beta-blocker; contraindicated in patient with asthma or CHF; Tables 6-3 and 18-2 Tox: dysrhythmias, hypoglycemia, hypotension, cardiac failure, bronchospasm, weakness; overdose treated with glucagon 0.1 mg/kg/dose IV
Propylthiouracil (PTU) Tab: 50 mg	Load: 5 mg/kg/24 hr q 6-8 hr PO (adult: 300 mg/24 hr); maint: $\frac{1}{3}$-$\frac{1}{2}$ of loading dose once patient is euthyroid (adult: 100-150 mg/24 hr)	Tox: blood dyscrasia, hepatic, dermatitis, urticaria, neuritis; BR
Protamine Amp: 10 mg/ml	1 mg IV for each 100 units of heparin given concurrently; 0.5 mg IV for each 100 units of heparin given in previous 30 min, and so on; maximum: 50 mg/dose	Heparin antidote Tox: hypotension, bradycardia, flushing
Pseudoephedrine (Sudafed) Syr: 30 mg/5 ml Tab: 30, 60 mg	4-6 mg/kg/24 hr q 4-6 hr PO (adult: 60 mg q 4-6 hr PO)	Tox: irritability; use with caution in hypertensive patient
Pyrantel (Antiminth) Susp: 250 mg/5 ml	11 mg (~0.2 ml)/kg/dose PO once (maximum: 1 g/dose); repeat in 1 wk	Do not use with preexisting liver disease, pregnancy Tox: nausea, vomiting, hepatic
Quinacrine (Atabrine) Tab: 100 mg	Giardiasis: 6 mg/kg/24 hr q 8 hr PO for 7 days (adult: 100 mg q 8 hr PO)	Tox: GI irritant, bone marrow depression; skin transiently turns yellow; caution in G6PD deficiency

---

Many oral drugs may be given 3-4 times per day with more flexibility than implied by the specific intervals noted. BR, Excreted in breast milk; NB, newborns under 7 days of age; Pen, penicillin; SR, sustained release; Tox, toxicity of drug.

Drugs	Dosages	Comments
Quinidine Tab: 100, 200, 300, 202 (SR), 300 (SR) mg Cap: 200, 300 mg	15-60 mg/kg/24 hr q 6 hr PO (adult: 300-400 mg q 6 hr PO)	Table 6-3 Tox: GI irritant dysrhythmias, hypotension, blood dyscrasia
Ranitidine (Zantac) Tab: 150 mg Vial: 25 mg/ml	2.5-3.8 mg/kg/24 hr q 12 hr PO (adult: 150 mg q 12 hr PO; 50 mg q 6-8 hr IV; maximum: 400 mg/24 hr IV)	Little experience in children; similar to cimetidine, less drug interactions
Reserpine (Serpasil) Elix. 0.25 mg/5 ml Tab: 0.1, 0.25, 0.5, 1 mg Vial: 2.5 mg/ml	0.02-0.04 mg/kg q 4-12 hr IM (adult: 0.25-4.0 mg/dose) 0.01-0.02 mg/kg/dose q 12 hr PO (adult: 0.1-0.25 mg/24 hr)	Usually used in combination with another drug; rarely used; Table 18-2 Tox: severe depression, bradycardia, ulcerogenic: BR
Rifampin (Rimactane, Rifadin) Cap: 300 mg	10-20 mg/kg/24 hr q 12-24 hr PO (maximum: 600 mg/24 hr) Meningococcal prophylaxis: 10 mg/kg q 12 hr PO for 2 days (adult: 600 mg q 12 hr) *H. influenzae* prophylaxis: 20 mg/kg q 24 hr for 4 days (adult: 600 mg q 24 hr × 4)	Tox: hepatic, GI irritant, hemolytic anemia; turns urine red; lower dose in children <1 mo
Secobarbital (Seconal) Elix: 22 mg/5 ml Cap: 30, 50, 100 mg Vial: 50 mg/ml	2-6 mg/kg/24 hr q 8 hr PO (adult: 60-120 mg/24 hr q 8-12 hr PO)	Short-acting barbiturate Tox: drowsiness, respiratory depression
Spectinomycin (Trobicin) Vial: 400 mg/ml	40 mg/kg/dose IM ×1 (adult: 2 g IM ×1)	*N. gonorrhoeae* treatment; not good for syphilus Tox: dizziness, vertigo
Spironolactone (Aldactone) Tab: 25, 50, 100 mg	1-3 mg/kg/24 hr q 6-12 hr PO (adult: 25-100 mg/24 hr	Useful adjunctive diuretic to maintain potassium; reduce dose with renal failure; Table 16-3
Succinylcholine (Anectine) Amp: 20 mg/ml Vial: 0.5, 1 g	1 mg/kg/dose IV (NB: 2 mg/kg/dose IV); maint: 0.3-0.6 mg/kg/dose q 5-10 min IV	Must be able to control airway; optimally premedicate with atropine
Sulfisoxazole (Gantrisin) Susp: 500 mg/5 ml Tab: 500 mg	Load: 75 mg/kg PO: maint: 120-150 mg/kg/24 hr q 6 hr PO (adult: 500-1,000 mg q 6 hr PO) (maximum: 4-6 g/24 hr)	Do not use in children <2 mo old: maintain good urine flow Tox: rash, Stevens-Johnson, neutropenia; reduce dose with renal failure; BR

Drugs	Dosages	Comments
Terbutaline (Brethine) Vial: 1 mg/ml	0.01 ml (0.01 mg)/kg/dose (maximum: 0.25 ml/dose) q 15-20 min SQ prn Aerosol: 0.03-0.05 mg (0.03-0.05 ml)/kg in 1-2.5 ml saline given q 4 hr (adult: 0.5 mg/dose)	Beta agonist for reactive airway disease; may have more prolonged effect than epinephrine Tox: sympathomimetic
Terfenadine (Seldane) Tab: 60 mg	Adult: 60 mg q 12 hr PO	No experience in children <12 yr; antihistamine without sedation
Tetracycline (Achromycin, Tetracyn) Syr: 125 mg/5 ml Tab/cap: 250, 500 mg Vial: 250, 500 mg (IM has lidocaine)	25-50 mg/kg/24 hr q 6 hr PO (adult: 250-500 mg q 6 hr PO) 15-25 mg/kg/24 hr q 8-12 hr IM (adult:200-300 mg/24 hr q 8-12 hr IM) 20-30 mg/kg/24 hr q 8-12 hr IV over 2 hr (adult: 250-500 mg/dose q 8-12 hr IV over 2 hr)	Do not use in children <9 yr Tox: GI irritant, hepatic, photosensitization, superinfection; BR
Theophylline (Table 84-1)	Load: 6 mg/kg PO; maint: 4-5 mg/kg/dose q 6 hr PO Load: 5 mg/kg IV slowly: maint: 0.6-0.9 mg/kg/hr IV	Therapeutic level: 10-20 μg/ml; Chapter 84 Tox: nausea, vomiting, irritability, seizures, dysrhythmias
Thioridazine (Mellaril) Susp: 25, 100 mg/5 ml Tab: 10, 15, 25, 50, 100 mg	0.5-1 mg/kg/24 hr q 8-12 hr PO (adult: 75-300 mg/24 hr q 8-12 hr PO) (maximum: 800 mg/24 hr)	Do not use in children <2 yr; titrate dose to response Tox: phenothiazine (Chapter 55)
Thiopental (Pentothal) Vial: 0.5, 1 g	Anesthesia: 2 mg/kg/dose IV (adult: 3-5 mg/kg/dose IV)	Respiratory support imperative; use 2.5% sol'n
Ticarcillin (Ticar) Vial: 1, 3, 6 g	200-300 mg/kg/24 hr q 4-6 hr IM, IV (maximum: 18-24 g/24 hr) (NB: 150-225 mg/kg/24 hr q 8-12 hr)	Similar to carbenicillin; adjust dose in renal failure; used in combination therapy

Many oral drugs may be given 3-4 times per day with more flexibility than implied by the specific intervals noted. BR, Excreted in breast milk; NB, newborns under 7 days of age; Pen, penicillin; SR, sustained release; Tox, toxicity of drug.

Drugs	Dosages	Comments
Tobramycin (Nebcin) Vial: 10, 40 mg/ml	3-7.5 mg/kg/24 hr q 8 hr IM, IV (maximum: 300 mg/24 hr) (NB: 4 mg/kg/24 hr q 12 hr)	Therapeutic peak level: 6-10 μg/ml: caution in renal failure (reduce dose); slow IV infusion Tox: renal, VIII nerve.
Trimethaphan (Arfonad) Vial: 50 mg/ml	50-150 μg/kg min IV infusion (adult: 0.5-1 mg/min)	Constant monitoring required; tachyphylaxis: Table 18-2 Tox: ganglionic blocker (paralysis of pupils, bladder, bowels)
Trimethoprim(TMP)-sulfamethoxazole(SMX) (Bactrim, Septra) Susp: 40 mg TMP/200 mg SMX/5 ml Tab: 80 mg TMP/400 mg SMX: 160 mg TMP/800 mg SMX Amp: 80 mg TMP/400 mg SMX/5 ml	6-12 mg TMP/30-60 mg SMX/kg/24 hr q 12 hr PO (adult: 80-160 mg TMP/400-800 mg SMX q 12 hr PO) *Pneumocystis:* 15-20 mg TMP/75-100 mg SMX/kg/24 hr q 6-8 hr PO, IV *Severe UTI, Shigella:* 8-10 mg TMP/40-50 mg SMX/kg/24 hr q 6-8 hr PO, IV	Do not use in children <2 mo; rare indications for IV route; reduce dose in renal failure Tox: bone marrow suppression, GI irritation; BR
Valproic acid or valproate (Depakene) Syr: 250 mg/5 ml Cap: 250 mg	15-60 mg/kg/24 hr q 8-24 hr PO	Therapeutic level: 50-100 μg/ml; Table 81-6; use in acute management of seizures is controversial Tox: sedation, vomiting, rash, headache, hepatotoxic; increases phenobarbital level (20%) and decreases phenytoin level (50%-100%)
Vancomycin (Vancocin) Vial: 500 mg	40 mg/kg/24 hr q 6 hr IV (<500 mg/30 min) (maximum: 2 g/24 hr) (NB: 30 mg/kg/24 hr q 12 hr)	Reduce dosage if renal impairment Tox: ototoxic, renal, rash, peripheral neuropathy
Verapamil (Isoptin, Calan) Amp: 2.5 mg/ml	0.1-0.2 mg/kg/dose IV over 2 min repeated in 10-30 min prn (adult: 5-10 mg/dose IV)	Table 6-3 Tox: bradycardia, hypotension
Vitamin K (Aquamephyton) Vial: 2, 10 mg/ml	NB, infant: 1-2 mg/dose IM, IV Child, adult: 5-10 mg/dose IM, IV	May give IV (<1 mg/min) but associated with hypotension and anaphylaxis
Warfarin (Coumadin) Tab: 2, 5, 7.5, 10 mg	Adult: 2-10 mg/24 hr q 24 hr PO after loading with 10-15 mg/24 hr PO for 2-3 days	Adjust dose to maintain PT at 2 times normal; antidote is vitamin K Tox: dermatitis

Appendix D-2: Simplified schedule for administration of pediatric resuscitation drugs

Drug (availability)	Single dose	Route	Dose (ml) administered by weight (kg)									
			5 kg	10 kg	15 kg	20 kg	25 kg	30 kg	35 kg	40 kg	45 kg	50 kg
EPINEPHRINE (1:10,000) (0.1 mg/ml)	0.01 mg/kg 0.1 ml/kg	IV,ET	0.5	1	1.5	2	2.5	3	3.5	4	4.5	5
SODIUM BICARBONATE (1 mEq/ml)	1 mEq/kg 1 ml/kg	IV	5	10	15	20	25	30	35	40	45	50
ATROPINE (0.1 mg/ml)	0.02 mg/kg 0.2 ml/kg	IV,ET	1	2	3	4	5	6	7	8	9	10
CALCIUM CHLORIDE 10% (100 mg/ml)	20 mg/kg 0.2 ml/kg	IV	1	2	3	4	5	5	5	5	5	5
LIDOCAINE (20 mg/ml)	1 mg/kg 0.05 ml/kg	IV,ET	0.25	0.5	1.75	1.0	1.25	1.5	1.75	2.0	2.25	5
FUROSEMIDE (Lasix) (10 mg/ml)	1 mg/kg 0.1 ml/kg	IV	0.5	1	1.5	2	2.5	3	3.5	4	4.5	5
DIAZEPAM (Valium) (5 mg/ml)	0.2 mg/kg 0.04 ml/kg	IV	0.2	0.4	0.6	0.8	1	1.2	1.4	1.6	1.8	2

Before using this schedule, it is essential to be certain that the concentration used is identical to that cited here. Clinical response and patient condition may modify this schedule (see Table 4-1).

Mixing dopamine, dobutamine, and nitroprusside for continuous infusion*

Wt. (kg) of child	Add this amount (mg)	to this volume (ml)	
2.0	12.5	104	
2.5		84	Often mixed double strength
3.0		69	(twice amount of milligrams
3.5	↓	59	in stated volume) to minimize
4.0	25	104	volume administered
4.5		92	
5.0		83	
5.5		75	
6.0		69	
6.5		64	
7.0		59	
7.5		55	
8.0	↓	52	
8.5	50	98	
9.0		92	
9.5		88	
10.0		83	
11.0		76	
12.0		69	
13.0		64	
14.0		59	
15.0		55	
16.0		52	
17.0		49	
18.0		46	
19.0		44	
20.0	↓	42	
22.0	100	76	
24.0		69	
26.0		64	
28.0		59	
30.0	↓	55	
35.0	200	95	
40.0		83	
45.0		74	Often mixed ¼ strength (¼
50.0		67	amount of milligrams in stat-
55.0		60	ed volume) to facilitate mix-
60.0		55	ing
65.0	↓	51	
70.0	400	96	
75.0		88	
80.0		84	
85.0		78	
90.0		74	
95.0		70	
100.0	↓	66	

Common doses (see Table 5-2). Dopamine: 5-20 μg/kg/min; dobutamine; 1-15 μg/kg/min; nitroprusside; 0.5-10 μg/kg/min.
*Single strength: number of ml/hr = number of μg/kg/min, e.g., for 2.5 kg child, mix 12.5 mg in 84 ml; if run at 2 ml/hr, administer 2 μg/kg/min to child.

Mixing isoproterenol, epinephrine, and norepinephrine for continuous infusion*

Wt. (kg) of child	Add this amount (mg)	to this volume (ml)	
2.0	1.25	104	Often mixed double strength (twice amount of mg in stated volume) to minimize volume administered
2.5		84	
3.0		69	
3.5		59	
4.0	2.5	104	
4.5		92	
5.0		83	
5.5		75	
6.0		69	
6.5		64	
7.0		59	
7.5		55	
8.0		52	
8.5	5.0	98	
9.0		92	
9.5		88	
10.0		83	
11.0		76	
12.0		69	
13.0		64	
14.0		59	
15.0		55	
16.0		52	
17.0		49	
18.0		46	
19.0		44	
20.0		42	
22.0	10.0	76	
24.0		69	
26.0		64	
28.0		59	
30.0		55	
35.0	20.0	95	
40.0		83	
45.0		74	
50.0		67	Often mixed ¼ strength (¼ amount of mg in stated volume) to facilitate mixing
55.0		60	
60.0		55	
65.0		51	
70.0	40	96	
75.0		88	
80.0		84	
85.0		78	
90.0		74	
95.0		70	
100.0		66	

Common doses (see Table 5-2). Isoproterenol: 0.1-1.5 µg/kg/min; epinephrine: 0.05-0.5 µg/kg/min; norepinephrine: 0.1-1 µg/kg/min.

*__Single strength:__ number of ml/hr = number of µg/kg/min, e.g., for 2.5 kg child, mix 1.25 mg in 84 ml and if run at 2 ml/hr, administer 0.2 µg/kg/min to child.

Appendix D-3: Pediatric specific equipment list

A. AIRWAY
1. Laryngoscope blades: 0, 1, 2 and 3 straight and curved; laryngoscope handle with extra bulbs
2. Endotracheal tubes; 2.5-5.5 mm uncuffed and 5.5-9.0 mm cuffed
3. Oropharyngeal airway: infant, small, medium, and large
4. Newborn and pediatric 100% bag-valve resuscitator with premature, newborn, infant, child, and adult masks
5. Yankauer suction handle with suction and catheters
6. Suction catheters: 6-14 Fr
7. Magill forceps: small and large
8. Oxygen tubing, masks, and cannulas
9. Chest tube tray with tubes sizes 10-42 Fr
10. Bulb syringe
11. Cricothyroidotomy tray with tracheostomy tubes 00-4

B. CARDIOVASCULAR
1. Cardiac monitor and defibrillator with 0-400 watt-sec range and pediatric and adult paddles. Cream or paste
2. Blood pressure cuffs: newborn, infant, child, and adult. Doppler amplifier
3. IV supplies
   a. Catheters and butterflies: 14-25 gauge
   b. Solutions of 250, 500, and 1000 ml containing D5W.9%NS, D5WLR, 0.9%NS, LR, D5W. 45%NS, D5W.2%NS
   c. Armboards
   d. Administration equipment including buretrol and infusion pump
   e. CVP catheters and monitoring equipment
4. Blood and IV solution warmer
5. Venous cutdown tray
6. Equipment for intraosseous infusion
7. Equipment for obtaining laboratory specimens
8. Consider thoracotomy tray

C. GENERAL
1. Nasogastric or feeding tubes: 5 and 8 Fr feeding tubes and 8-18 Fr NG tubes
2. Urinary catheters: 5 and 8 Fr feeding tubes and 8-12 Fr catheters
3. Pediatric scale
4. Miscellaneous sponges, tape, stopcocks, blood gas syringes, disinfecting solutions, diapers, formula, etc.
5. Spinal needle and tray
6. Overhead infant warmer (optional)
7. Oximeter (optional)

D. MEDICATIONS (see Pediatric emergency measures on front cover and Table 4-1)
1. Antibiotics: ampicillin, gentamicin, chloramphenicol, nafcillin, and cefotaxime (or equivalent)
2. Charcoal and $MgSO_4$

Appendix D-4: Antiparasitic drugs

AMEBIASIS (*Entamoeba histolytica*)
Asymptomatic carrier — Iodoquinol (previously diiodohydroxyquin) 40 mg/kg/24 hr q 8 hr PO (adult: 650 mg/dose) × 21 days; **or** diloxanide furoate (Furamide) (CDC) 20 mg/kg/24 hr q 8 hr PO (adult: 500 mg/dose) × 10 days

Mild to moderate colitis — Metronidazole (Flagyl) 35 mg/kg/24 hr q 8 hr PO (adult: 750 mg/dose) × 10 days; **plus** iodoquinol, as above

Severe colitis — Metronidazole, as above × 10 days; **plus** iodoquinol, as above

Extraintestinal — Metronidazole, as above × 10 days; **plus** iodoquinol, as above

ASCARIASIS (*Ascaris lumbricoides*) — Mebendazole (Vermox) 100 mg q 12 hr PO × 3 days (children >2 yr); **or** pyrantel pamoate (Antiminth) 11 mg/kg/dose, (Maximum: 1g) PO × 1 (one dose only)

BALANTIDIASIS (*Balantidium coli*) — Tetracycline 40 mg/kg/24 hr q 6 hr PO (children >8 yr only) (adult: 500 mg/dose) × 10 days; **or** iodoquinol 40 mg/kg/24 hr q 8 hr PO (adult: 650 mg/dose) × 21 days

CUTANEOUS LARVA MIGRANS or CREEPING ERUPTION (cutaneous hookworm) — Thiabendazole (Mintezol) 50 mg/kg/24 hr (maximum: 1.5 g/dose) q 12 hr PO × 3 days

CYSTICERCOSIS (*Taenia solium*) — Surgical excision most satisfactory; niclosamide (Niclocide, Cesticide) 11-34 kg: single dose 1 gm (2 tab) PO; >34 kg: single dose 1.5 g (3 tab) (adult: 2g or 4 tab PO)

DIENTAMOEBIASIS (*Dientamoeba fragilis*) — Iodoquinol 40 mg/kg/24 hr q 8 hr PO (adult: 650 mg/dose) × 21 days

FILARIASIS, ONCHOCERCIASIS (*Onchocerca volvulus*) — Diethylcarbamazine (Hetrazan) 1.5 mg/kg/24 hr q 8 hr PO (maximum: 25 mg/24 hr) × 3 days, then 3 mg/kg/24 hr q 8 hr PO (maximum: 50 mg/24 hr) × 3-4 days, then 4.5 mg/kg/24 hr q 8 hr PO (maximum: 100 mg/24 hr) 3-4 days, then 6 mg/kg/24 hr q 8 hr PO (maximum: 150 mg/24 hr) × 14-21 days

Other forms (LOA LOA, TROPICAL EOSINOPHILIA) (*Wuchereria bancrofti, Brugia malayi*) — Diethylcarbamazine (Hetrazan) 25-50 mg/24 hr q 24 hr PO (maximum: 50 mg/24 hr) × 1 day; then 75-150 mg/24 hr q 8 hr PO (maximum: 150 mg/24 hr) × 1 day; then 150-300 mg/24 hr q 8 hr PO (maximum: 300 mg/24 hr) × 1 day; then 6 mg/kg/24 hr q 8 hr PO × 17 days; surgical excision of subcutaneous nodules; allergic reactions may require steroids or antihistamines

FLUKES
Sheep liver (*Fasciola hepatica*)
Lung (*Paragonimus westermani*)
Chinese liver (*Clonorchis sinensis*) — Praziquantel (Biltricide) 25 mg/kg/dose PO × 3 doses (doses to be taken in 1 day)

GIARDIASIS (*Giardia lamblia*) — Furazolidone (Furoxone) 6-8 mg/kg/24 hr (adult: 100 mg/dose) q 6 hr PO × 7-10 days; **or** quinacrine (Atabrine) 6 mg/kg/24 hr (adult: 100 mg/dose) q 8 hr PO × 5-10 days; **or** metronidazole (Flagyl) 15 mg/kg/24 hr (adult: 250 mg/dose) q 8 hr PO × 5-10 days

HOOKWORM
Necator americanus
Ancylostoma duodenale — Mebendazole (Vermox) 100 mg q 12 hr PO (children >2 yr) × 3 days; **or** pyrantel pamoate (Antiminth) 11 mg/kg/dose (maximum: 1 g) PO × 1 dose

---

CDC: Available from the Centers for Disease Control Parasitic Drug Service, Atlanta; phone: (404) 329-3670. For emergencies on nights, weekends, and holidays: (404) 329-3644.

LEISHMANIASIS
Leishmania donovani (kala azar)
L. braziliensis (American mucocutaneous leishmaniasis)
L. mexicana, L. tropica

Stibogluconate sodium (Pentostam, Tricostam) (CDC) 10-20 mg/kg/24 hr (maximum: 600-800 mg/24 hr) q 24 hr IM, IV × 20 days; may need to repeat

MALARIA
Prophylaxis
For areas without chloroquine resistant *Plasmodium falciparum*

Chloroquine 5 mg base/kg (adult: 300 mg base) q wk PO, beginning 1 week before potential exposure and continuing for 6 weeks after last exposure; **plus** primaquine phosphate 0.3 mg base/kg (adult: 15 mg base) q 24 hr PO × 14 days after departure from endemic area

For areas with chloroquine-resistant *P. falciparum*

For **short term** (<3 wk) travel: chloroquine 5 mg base/kg (adult: 300 mg base) q week PO, beginning 1 wk before potential exposure and continuing for 6 wk after last exposure; **plus,** patient should be given single treatment dose of pyrimethamine-sulfadoxine (Fansidar)* and advised to take promptly if febrile illness develops, no medical care is available, and there is no known intolerance (2-11 mo: ⅛ tab/wk; 1-3 yr; ¼ tab/wk; 4-8 yr: ½ tab/wk; 9-14 yr: ¾ tab/wk; >14 yr (adult): 1 tab/wk PO) For **long-term** travel to high-risk area: chloroquine, as above; **plus** consider pyrimethamine-sulfadoxine, as above

Treatment
P. vivax, P. ovale

Chloroquine phosphate (Aralen, Nivaquine) 10 mg base/kg then 5 mg base/kg at 6 hr, 24 hr, and 48 hr after initial dose (adult: 600 mg base, then 300 mg base at 6 hr, 24 hr, and 48 hr **plus** primaquine 0.3 mg base/kg (adult: 15 mg base) q 24 hr PO × 14 days; parenteral chloroquine (CDC) is available for CNS disease

P. malariae

Chloroquine, as above

P. falciparum (non-chloroquine-resistant)

Chloroquine, as above

P. falciparum (chloroquine-resistant)

Quinine 25 mg/kg/24 hr (adult: 650 mg/dose) q 8 hr PO × 3 days; **plus** pyrimethamine 1 mg/kg/24 hr (adult: 25 mg/dose) q 12 hr PO × 3 days; **plus** sulfadiazine 120-150 mg/kg/24 hr (adult: 500 mg/dose) q 6 hr PO × 5 days; parenteral therapy (CDC) is administered for severe disease

PINWORMS (*Enterobius vermicularis*)

Mebendazole (Vermox) 100 mg PO once (children >2 yr) (repeat in 1 wk) **or** pyrantel (Antiminth) 11 mg/kg/dose (maximum: 1 g) PO once (repeat in 1 wk)

PNEUMOCYSTIS PNEUMONIA (*Pneumocystis carinii*)

Trimethoprim (TMP)-sulfamethoxazole (SMX) (Bactrim, Septra) 20 mg TMP, 100 mg SMX/kg/24 hr q 6-8 hr PO, IV × 10-14 days

SCHISTOSOMIASIS
Schistosoma haematobium
S. japonicum
S. mansoni

Praziquantel (Biltricide) 20 mg/kg/dose PO × 3 doses in 1 day

---

*Associated with serious adverse reactions, including erythema multiforme, Stevens-Johnson, toxic epidermal necrolysis and serum sickness. Discontinue if any mucocutaneous lesions develop. Presumptive treatment with pyrimethamine-sulfadoxine (Fansidar): 2-11 mo: ¼ tab; 1-3 yr: ½ tab; 4-8 yr: 1 tab; 9-14 yr: 2 tabs; >14 yr (adult): 3 tab as single dose PO.

Continued

Appendix D-4: Antiparasitic drugs—cont'd

TAPEWORMS
Taenia saginata
Taenia solium (see Cysticercosis)
Hymenolepis nana
Diphyllobothrium latum

Niclosamide (Niclocide, Cesticide) 11-34 kg: single dose 1g (2 tab) PO; >34 kg: single dose 1.5 g (3 tab) PO (adult: 2 g or 4 tab PO)
For *H. nana*, treat with 11-34 kg: single dose 1 g (2 tab) PO, then 0.5 g (1 tab)/24 hr PO × 6 days: >34 kg: single dose 1.5 g (3 tab) PO, then 1 g (2 tab)/24 hr PO × 6 days (adult: 2 g or 4 tab/24 hr PO × 7 days)

TOXOPLASMOSIS *(Toxoplasma gondii)*

Pyrimethamine (Daraprim) 2 mg/kg/24 hr (adult: 25 mg/24 hr) q 12 PO x 3 days, then 1 mg/kg/24 hr q 12 hr PO × 4 wk (supplement with folinic acid 5-10 mg/24 hr); **plus** trisulfapyrimidines or sulfadiazine 120-150 mg/kg/24 hr (adult: 4-6 g/24 hr) q 6 hr PO × 28 days

TRICHINOSIS *(Trichinella spiralis)*

Thiabendazole (Mintezol) 50 mg/kg/24 hr q 12 PO (maximum: 3 g/24 hr); **or** mebendazole (Vermox) 200-400 mg/dose (children >2 yr) q 8 hr PO × 5-10 days

TRYPANOSOMIASIS, CHAGAS' DISEASE
(Trypanosoma cruzi)

Nifurtimox (Bayer 2502) (CDC) 5 mg/kg/24 hr q 6 hr PO increasing by 2 mg/kg/24 hr q 2 wk until the maximum dose of 16 mg/kg/24 hr is reached and then continued for total course of 4 mo

VISCERAL LARVA MIGRANS *(Toxocara canis)*

Thiabendazole (Mintezol) 50 mg/kg/24 hr q 12 hr PO (maximum: 3 g/24 hr) × 5 days or longer

WHIPWORM *(Trichuris trichiura)*

Mebendazole (Vermox) 100 mg q 12 hr PO × 3 days

REFERENCE

Abramowicz, M., editor: Drugs for parasitic infections, Med. Let. Drug. Ther. **28**:9, 1986.

INDEX

A

A-aO$_2$ difference (gradient) in pulmonary contusion, 357
Abdomen
 in child abuse, 146t
 distention of
  in hepatitis, 488
  in intussusception, 499
  in pancreatitis, 491
 examination of, in multiple trauma management, 311-312
 inflammation in, chest pain in, 89t
 pain in
  in abortion, 518
  acute, 142-144
  in appendicitis, 494-495
  dysmenorrhea, 508-509
  in ectopic pregnancy, 519-520
  in Henoch-Schönlein purpura, 610
  initial assessment of, 4t
  in intussusception, 498
  in Meckel's diverticulum, 500
  in pancreatitis, 491
  in pelvic inflammatory disease, 511
  in psychophysiolgic illness, 578
  in volvulus, 502
 trauma to, 365-373
  blunt, 365
   management of, 369, 371-372
   mechanism of, 365
   peritoneal lavage in, 367, 370
  chest pain in, 89t
  diagnostic findings in, 366-368
  management of, 368-373
   blunt trauma in, 369-373
   general principles in, 368-369
  mechanism of injury in, 365-366
  penetrating, 365-366
   management of, 372-373
   mechanisms of, 365-366

Page numbers in *italics* indicate boxed material and illustrations.
Page numbers followed by *t* indicate tables.

Abdomen—cont'd
 trauma to—cont'd
  penetrating—cont'd
   peritoneal lavage in, 367, 370
  x-ray studies of; *see* X-ray(s), abdominal
Abdominal thrust for foreign body in airway, 601
Abdominal wall defects, postnatal, 68
Abducens (VI) nerve, palsy of, in coma, 93
ABE antitoxin, trivalent, for botulism, 537
Abortion, 518-519
 vaginal bleeding in, 221t
Abruptio placentae, 520-521
 vaginal bleeding in, 221t
Abscess(es)
 cellulitis differentiated from, 434
 cerebellar, ataxia and, 161t
 CNS, vomiting and, 223t
 dental, headache and, 194t
 headache and, 194t
 intracranial
  coma in, 94
  seizures in, 560t
 orbital, periorbital cellulitis differentiated from, 434t
 peritonsillar, 458-459
  dysphagia in, 176t
  respiratory distress in, 126t
 retropharyngeal, 462-463
  cough in, 168t
  cyanosis in, 111t
  dysphagia in, 176t
  respiratory distress in, 126t
 subperiosteal, periorbital cellulitis differentiated from, 434t
Absence seizures, 563t
Abuse, 145-151
 child, 145-149; *see also* Child abuse
 sexual, 150-151
A-C separation; *see* Acromioclavicular separation
Acclimatization in high-altitude sickness prevention, 250

Accutane; *see* Isotretinoin
Acetaminophen, 660
 for fever, 182-183
 for pharyngotonsillitis, 461
 poisoning from, 278-279
Acetazolamide, 660
 in high-altitude sickness prevention, 250
 for pseudotumor cerebri, 558
 for pulmonary edema in congestive heart failure, 105t
Acetylcysteine, 660
 for acetaminophen overdose, 274, 279
Achromycin; *see* Tetracycline
Acid(s)
 absorption of, prevention of, 266
 poisoning from, 282-284
Acid-base balance, 50-53
 abnormalities of, 54-55
Acidemias, organic, seizures in, 561t
Acidosis
 metabolic, 54
  in acute renal failure, management of, 619
  in poisoning, 277
  in near-drowning, 245
  in shock, management of, 31
  vomiting and, 225t
Acne, 430
Acquired immune deficiency syndrome (AIDS), hemophilia and, 526
Acromioclavicular separation, 393-394
ACTH; *see* Adrenocorticotropic hormone
Activated charcoal
 for phenobarbital overdose, 297
 for poisoning, 271-272
 for theophylline overdose, 302
Acute necrotizing gingivitis, 449-450
Acute renal failure; *see* Kidney(s), failure of, acute
Acute tubular necrosis, 376; *see also* Kidneys, failure of, acute
Acyclovir, 660

Face—cont'd
trauma to—cont'd
dislocations in, 327-330
fractures in, 327-330
management of, 325
in multiple trauma management,
312
soft tissue injuries in, management of, 325-327
Factors of blood
deficiencies of
bleeding disorders and, screening tests for, 164t
hemophilia and, 525-529; see
also Hemophilia
for disseminated intravascular coagulation, 523
replacement of, for hemophilia,
527-528
Factor VIII, 668
Factor IX, 668
Fahrenheit conversion, 655
Fainting, 137-139
Fallot tetralogy
cyanosis in, 112
syncope in, 138t
Familial hematuria, benign, 199t
Fansidar; see Pyrimethamine-sulfadoxine
Fasciola hepatica, drugs for, 688t
Fat pad sign, 397
Fear, diarrhea in, 173t
Febrile seizures, 560t, 564-568
Fecal impaction, diarrhea in, 173t;
see also Constipation
Fecal leukocytes in diarrhea, 482-483
Feeding techniques, vomiting and,
226t
Felon, 407
Female(s)
postpubescent, vulvovaginitis from,
515-516
prepubescent, vulvovaginitis and
vaginal discharge in, 514-
515
Femoral artery puncture, 626
Femoral epiphysis, capital, slipped,
limp and, 208t
Femur
distal, fracture of, 413
head of
avascular necrosis of, 410-411
epiphyseal separation of, 411
shaft of, fracture of, 411
Fenbutal for migraines, 557
Fentanyl, 668
for orthopedic injuries, 389
Feosol; see Iron, elemental
FEP; see Free erythrocyte protoporphyrin

Fer-In-Sol; see Iron, elemental
Ferririn, serum, 154, 155
Ferrous fumarate, 294
Ferrous gluconate, 294
Ferrous sulfate, 155
Fetal circulation, persistent
cyanosis in, 109t
postnatal, 65-66
Fever; see also Temperature
initial assessment of, 4t
in Kawasaki's syndrome, 539
in meningitis, 551
parent instruction sheet for, 640-
641
in poisoning, 269t
in children under 2 years of age,
178-183
etiology of, 178-179
management of, 179-183
parental education on, 179
FFP; see Fresh-frozen plasma
Fibrillation
atrial
acute, treatment of, 40t
characteristics of, 34-35t
ventricular
acute, treatment of, 40t
characteristics of, 34-35t
life support and, 12
Fibrinogen for disseminated intravascular coagulation, 523
Fibrinolytics for deep venous thrombosis, 429
Fibroids, vaginal bleeding in, 221t
Fibula, fracture of, 414
Fifth disease, maculopapular exanthems in, 219t
Filariasis onchocerciasis, drugs for,
688t
Finger
dislocation of, 403-404
mallet, 404
swollen, ring on, 407
Fingertip injuries, 405-406
Fiorinal for migraines, 557
Fishhook removal, 386
Fistula, tracheoesophageal, postnatal,
67
Fitz-Hugh-Curtis syndrome, 511
Flagyl; see Metronidazole
Flail chest, 354
Flexor digitorum profundus, evalua-
tion of, 401
Flexor digitorum sublimis, evaluation
of, 401
Flexor tendons, evaluation of, 401
Florinef; see Fludrocortisone for ad-
renal insufficiency
Fludrocortisone for adrenal insuffi-
ciency, 468t, 469

Fluid(s)
balance of, for acute renal failure,
618
body, electrolyte composition of,
55
and electrolytes, balance of, 43-55
abnormalities of, 53-55
body fluid composition in, 55
dehydration and, 44-51; see also
Dehydration
maintenance of, 52-53
intravenous; see Intravenous infusions
loss of, 52
pleural, analysis of, 637-638
from subdural space, analysis of,
636
Fluid therapy
for bacterial meningitis, 555
for burns, 239-240
for dehydration, 46-49
for diabetic ketoacidosis, 470-471
for heat cramps, 252
for heat stroke, 254
for pulmonary edema, 123
in congestive heart failure, 104
for sickle cell disease, 535
size and, in multiple trauma management, 313
for toxic shock syndrome, 548
Flukes, drugs for, 688t
Fluocinolone acetonide cream for
atopic dermatitis, 432
Fluorescein stains in eye trauma assessment, 332
Fluorescent (FA) antibody stain
pertussis and, 168t
rabies and, 544
Fluoroscopy for foreign body in airway, 600
Flutter, atrial
acute treatment of, 40t
characteristics of, 34-35t
Follow-up, parent instruction sheet
for, 641
Food poisoning, 482
diarrhea in, 172t
Foot (feet)
bones of, dislocations of, 417
dressing and splints of, for soft tissue injury management,
384, 386
soft tissue injuries of, suture repair
of, 385t
splinter in, limp and, 207t
Fordyce's granule, 337
Forehead, contusion of, 320
Foreign body(ies)
in airways, 599-601

Head—cont'd
  trauma to, 315-322
    ancillary data on, 318-319
    ataxia and, 161*t*
    complications of, 318
    diagnostic findings in, 315-319
    disposition of, 322
    initial assessment of, 3*t*, 4*t*
    management of, 319-320
    meningitis and, 554
    parent instruction sheet for, 643
    parental education on, 322
    prognostic factors in, 318
    specific clinical entities in, 320-322
    x-rays in, 318, 321, 322
Headache, 192-195
  ancillary data on, 193
  diagnostic findings in, 193, 194-195
  differential diagnosis of, 192*t*
  initial assessment of, 4*t*
  management of, 193
  migraine, 556-558
    vomiting and, 225*t*
  in psychophysiologic illness, 578
Heart
  disease of
    cyanotic congenital, postnatal, 65
    dysphagia in, 177*t*
    syncope in, 138*t*
  failure of, congestive, 98-107; *see also* Congestive heart failure (CHF)
Heart block, syncope in, 138*t*
Heart rate in poisoning, 269*t*
Heat cramps, 252, 253*t*
Heat exhaustion, 252-253
  ataxia and, 161*t*
Heat illness, vomiting and, 226*t*
Heat stroke, 253-255
  coma in, 94
Hegar's sign of pregnancy, 518
Heimlich maneuver for foreign body in airway, 601
Hemangioma
  hematuria in, 199*t*
  rectal bleeding in, 186-187*t*
Hematemesis, 184-191
  diagnostic considerations in, 186-189*t*
Hematest, 158*t*, 185
Hematologic disorders, 522-536
  disseminated intravascular coagulation as, 522-525; *see also* Disseminated intravascular coagulation
  hemophilia as, 525-526; *see also* Hemophilia
  idiopathic thrombocytopenic purpura as, 529-531

Hematologic disorders—cont'd
  postnatal, 68-70
  sickle cell disease, 531-536, *see also* Sickle cell disease
Hematologic findings in hemolytic-uremic syndrome and, 609
Hematoma
  epidural
    coma in, 94
    irritability in, 205*t*
    x-ray appearance of, 322
  in hemophilia, 526
  intramural, vomiting and, 224*t*
  rectal bleeding in, 186-187*t*
  subdural
    coma in, 94
    irritability in, 205*t*
    vomiting and, 224*t*
    x-ray appearance of, 322
Hematuria, 196-199
  benign familial, 199*t*
  in glomerulonephritis, 607
  in hemophilia, 526
Hemiplegia, 210-213
Hemiplegic migraines, 557
Hemoccult packets, 185
Hemodialysis for hypothermia, 258-259
Hemofil, 528*t*
Hemoglobin in hemocytic-uremic syndrome, 609
Hemoglobinemia, hereditary, cyanosis in, 111*t*
Hemoglobinopathy, hematuria in, 199*t*
Hemolytic-uremic syndrome, 608-610
Hemoperfusion for poisoning, 273
Hemophilia, 525-529
  ancillary data on, 526-527
  arthritis and, 159*t*
  complications of, 526
  diagnostic findings in, 525-527
  disposition of, 529
  gastrointestinal bleeding and, 188-189*t*
  limp and, 209*t*
  management of, 527-528
Hemoptysis, 167, 170
Hemorrhage; *see* Bleeding
Hemostasis, for soft tissue injury management, 384
Hemothorax, 358-359
Henderson-Hasselbalch equation, 52-53
Henoch-Schönlein purpura, 610-611
  arthritis and, 158*t*
  hematuria/proteinuria in, 198*t*
  rectal bleeding and, 188-189*t*
Heparin, 669

Heparin—cont'd
  bleeding disorders and, screening tests for, 164*t*
  for deep venous thrombosis, 429
  for disseminated intravascular coagulation, 523*t*, 525
Hepatic damage, hypoglycemia in, 201*t*
Hepatic enzyme deficiency, hypoglycemia in, 201*t*
Hepatitis
  arthritis from, limp and, 207*t*
  chest pain in, 89*t*
  in hemophilia, 526
  vital, 487-490
    A, 487*t*, 488, 489
    ancillary data on, 487*t*, 488
    B, 487*t*, 488, 489-490
      vaccine for, recommendations for, 659
    classification of, 487
    complications of, 488
    diagnostic findings in, 487-488
    differential diagnosis of, 488-489
    management of, 489-490
    non-A/non-B, 487*t*
    preventive measures for, 487*t*, 489-490
    vomiting and, 223*t*
Hepatitis B immunoglobulin (HBIG)
  for hepatitis B prophylaxis, 490
  indications for, 659
Hepatitis B surface antigen, 488, 489-490
Hereditary disorders, bleeding, screening tests for, 164*t*
Hernia(s), 504-505
  diaphragmatic
    cough in, 169*t*
    cyanosis in, 111*t*
  hiatal, chest pain in, 90*t*
  incarcerated
    irritability in, 205*t*
    limp and, 209*t*
Heroin overdose, 274*t*
Herpes conjunctivitis, 476, 477, 478*t*
Herpes simplex
  congenital, 72
  meningoencephalitis and, 550*t*
  type 2, vulvovaginitis from, 517
  vesicular exanthems in, 217*t*
Herpes zoster
  chest pain in, 89*t*
  vesicular exanthems in, 217*t*
Herpetic whitlow, 408
Hetrazan; *see* Diethylcarbamazine
Hiatal hernia, chest pain in, 90*t*
High altitude, headache and, 195*t*
High altitude cerebral edema, 251*t*
High altitude pulmonary edema, 251*t*

FREQUENTLY USED PEDIATRIC DRUGS

ANTIBIOTICS

Amoxicillin (Amoxil, Larotid)
Susp: 125, 250 mg/5 ml — 50 mg/kg/24 hr q 8 hr PO
Cap: 125, 250 mg — Dose: 15 mg/kg/dose tid
Adult: 250-500 mg/dose

Ampicillin (Omnipen, Polycillin)
Susp: 125, 250 mg/5 ml — 75 mg/kg/24 hr q 6 hr PO
Cap: 250, 500 mg — Dose: 20 mg/kg/dose qid
Adult: 250-500 mg/dose

Augmentin (amoxicillin/clavulanic acid)
Susp: 125 mg AMX/31.25 mg CLA/5 ml 250 mg AMX/62.5 mg CLA/5 ml — 30-50 mg AMX/kg/24 hr q 8 hr PO
Tab: 250, 500 mg AMX/125 mg CLA — Dose: 10-15 mg AMX/kg/dose tid
Adult: 250-500 mg AMX/dose
(NOTE: dosing by amoxicillin)

Cephalosporins: cephalexin (Keflex); cephradine (Velosef); cefaclor (Ceclor)
Susp: 125, 250 mg/5 ml — 40 mg/kg/24 hr q 6 hr PO
Cap: 250, 500 mg — Dose: 10 mg/kg/dose qid
Adult: 250-500 mg/dose

Dicloxacillin (Dynapen)
Susp: 62.5 mg/5 ml — 40 mg/kg/24 hr q 6 hr PO
Cap: 125, 250 mg — Dose: 10 mg/kg/dose qid
Adult: 250 mg/dose

Erythromycin (Pediamycin, EES, Erythrocin, E-Mycin)
Susp: 200, 400 mg/5 ml — 40 mg/kg/24 hr q 6 hr PO
Chew cap: 200 mg — Dose: 10 mg/kg/dose qid
Tab: 250, 400, 500 mg — Adult: 250-500 mg/dose

Erythromycin/sulfisoxazole (Pediazole)
Susp: 200 mg ERY/600 mg SXZ/5 ml — 40 mg ERY/120 mg SXZ/kg/24 hr q 6 hr PO
Dose: 10 mg ERY/30 mg SXZ/kg/dose qid

Penicillin V (Pen-Vee K, V-Cillin K)
Susp: 125 mg (200,000 units), 250 mg (400,000 units)/5 ml — 40 mg (65,000 units)/kg/24 hr q 6 hr PO
Tab: 125, 250 mg — Dose: 10 mg (15,000 units)/kg/dose qid
Adult: 250-500 mg/dose

Penicillin G benzathine/penicillin G procaine (C-R Bicillin 900/300 in 2 ml)

Weight (lb)	Benzathine pen G (Bicillin LA)	Benzathine/procaine pen G (Bicillin C-R 900/300)
<30	300,000 units	300,000 : 100,000 units
31-60	600,000 units	600,000 : 200,000 units
61-90	900,000 units	900,000 : 300,000 units
>90	1,200,000 units	Not available

Sulfisoxazole (Gantrisin)
Susp: 500 mg/5 ml — 120 mg/kg/24 hr q 6 hr PO
Tab: 500 mg — Dose: 30 mg/kg/dose qid
Adult: 500 mg/dose

Trimethoprim-sulfamethoxazol (Bactrim, Septra)
Susp: 40 mg TMP/200 mg SMX/5 ml — 10 mg TMP/50 mg SMX/kg/24 hr q 12 hr PO
Tab: 80 mg TMP/400 mg SMX, 160 mg TMP/800 mg SMX — Dose: 5 mg TMP/25 mg SMX/kg/dose bid
Adult: 80-160 mg TMP/400-800 mg SMX/dose

ANTIHISTAMINES

Diphenhydramine (Benadryl)
Susp: 12.5 mg/5 ml — 5 mg/kg/24 hr q 6 hr PO
Cap: 25, 50 mg — Dose: 1.5 mg/kg/dose qid
Adult: 25-50 mg/dose

Hydroxyzine (Atarax, Vistaril)
Syr/susp: 10, 25 mg/5 ml — 2 mg/kg/24 hr q 6 hr PO
Tab (Atarax): 10, 25, 50 mg — Dose: 0.5 mg/kg/dose qid
Cap (Vistaril): 25, 50, 100 mg — Adult: 25 mg/dose

ADRENERGIC AGENTS

Epinephrine (1 : 1,000) — 0.01 ml/kg/dose SQ q 20 min prn × 3 (maximum: 0.35 ml/dose)

Terbutaline — 0.01 ml/kg/dose SQ q 20 min prn × 3 (maximum: 0.25 ml/dose); nebulizer: 0.03-0.05 ml/kg (adult: 0.5 ml) in 1-2.5 ml saline q 4 hr

Isoetharine 1% (Bronkosol) — Nebulizer: 0.25-0.5 ml in 2-2.5 ml saline q 20 min prn

Metaproterenol 5% (Alupent) — Nebulizer: 0.1 (<2 yr)-0.3 (>7 yr) ml in 2-2.5 ml saline q 20 min prn

Racemic epinephrine 2.25% (Micronephrine)
Nebulizer: 0.25-0.50 ml in 2.5 ml saline q 2 hr prn

THEOPHYLLINE (see p. 584 and Table 84-1)

Age	Loading dose (mg/kg)	Maintenance dose (mg/kg/hr IV)
<12 mo	5-6	0.7
1-9 yr	5-6	0.9
10 yr and over	5-6	0.6

STEROIDS

Prednisone
Tab: 5, 10, 20 mg — 1-2 mg/kg/24 hr q 12-24 hr PO
Susp: 5 mg/5 ml — Dose: 0.5-1 mg/kg/dose bid
Adult: 40-80 mg/dose

Dexamethasone (Decadron)
Vial: 4, 24 mg/ml — 0.25-0.5 mg/kg/dose q 6 hr IM/IV